Revision
Total Hip
Arthroplasty

Revision Total Hip Arthroplasty

Editors

Marvin E. Steinberg, M.D.
Professor and Vice Chairman
Department of Orthopaedic Surgery
Hospital of the University of Pennsylvania
Philadelphia, Pennsylvania

Jonathan P. Garino, M.D.
Assistant Professor of Orthopaedic Surgery
Hospital of the University of Pennsylvania
Philadelphia, Pennsylvania

Illustrator

Theodore G. Huff & Associates
Ann Arbor, Michigan

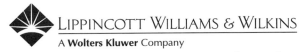
LIPPINCOTT WILLIAMS & WILKINS
A **Wolters Kluwer** Company
Philadelphia • Baltimore • New York • London
Buenos Aires • Hong Kong • Sydney • Tokyo

Acquisitions Editor: Kathey Alexander
Managing Editor: Susan Rhyner
Manufacturing Manager: Kevin Watt
Production Manager: Robert Pancotti
Production Editors: Christina Zingone and Frank Aversa
Cover Designer: QT Design
Indexer: Mary Kidd
Compositor: Tapsco, Inc.
Printer: Quebecor Kingsport

Printed in the United States of America

9 8 7 6 5 4 3 2 1

Library of Congress Cataloging-in-Publication Data

Revision total hip arthroplasty/[edited by] Marvin E. Steinberg, Jonathan P. Garino.
    p. cm.
    Includes bibliographical references and index.
    ISBN 0-7817-1424-9
    1. Total hip replacement—Reoperation. I. Steinberg, Marvin E.
II. Garino, Jonathan P.
    [DNLM: 1. Arthroplasty, Replacement, Hip—methods.
2. Reoperation—methods. 3. Prosthesis Failure. 4. Hip Prosthesis.
5. Postoperative Complications—prevention & control.   WE 860R4542   1999]
RD549.R443   1999
617.5′810592—dc21
DNLM/DLC
for Library of Congress   98-19477
                                                                                                      CIP

To my wife, Delores, our children, David, Jim, Susan, and Julie, and to my residents, fellows, and colleagues who provided the inspiration for this text.

M.E.S.

To my mentors, Marvin E. Steinberg and Paul A. Lotke, who have given me skills, judgment, and the opportunity to successfully address many of the problems covered in this text. Also to my wife, Jennifer, whose additional sacrifice and commitment to me have made my efforts in this work possible.

J.P.G.

Contents

Contributors

William L. Bargar, M.D.
Assistant Clinical Professor, Department of Orthopaedics, University of California, Davis School of Medicine; Attending Surgeon, Department of Surgery, Sutter General Hospital, 2801 L Street, Sacramento, California 95816

Robert L. Barrack, M.D.
Professor, Department of Orthopaedic Surgery, Tulane University Medical School; Director, Adult Reconstructive Surgery, Tulane University Medical Center, 1415 Tulane Avenue, New Orleans, Louisiana 70112

Daniel J. Berry, M.D.
Assistant Professor, Department of Orthopaedics, Mayo Medical School; Consultant in Orthopaedic Surgery, Mayo Clinic, 200 First Street, SW, Rochester, Minnesota 55905

Jonathan Black, Ph.D., F.B.S.E.
Professor Emeritus of Bioengineering, Clemson University; IMN Biomaterials, 409 Dorothy Drive, King of Prussia, Pennsylvania 19406-2004

J. Dennis Bobyn, Ph.D.
Associate Professor, Departments of Surgery and Biomedical Engineering, McGill University; Director of Orthopaedic Research, Division of Orthopaedic Surgery, Montreal General Hospital, 1650 Cedar Avenue, Montreal, Quebec, Canada H3G 1A4

Robert B. Bourne, M.D., F.R.C.S.(C)
Professor, Department of Orthopaedic Surgery, University of Western Ontario; Orthopaedic Surgeon, London Health Sciences Center, 339 Windermere Road, London, Ontario, Canada N6A 5A5

Pieter Buma, Ph.D.
Orthopaedic Research Laboratory , Catholic University Nijmegen; P.O. Box 9101, 6500 HB Nijmegen, The Netherlands

Miguel E. Cabanela, M.D., M.S.
Professor of Orthopaedics, Mayo Medical School; Consultant, Department of Orthopedics, Chairman, Division of Adult Reconstructive Surgery, Mayo Clinic, 200 First Street, S.W., Rochester, Minnesota 55905

John J. Callaghan, M.D.
Professor, Department of Orthopaedics, University of Iowa College of Medicine; University of Iowa Hospital and Clinic, 200 Hawkins Drive, Iowa City, Iowa 52242

Charles W. Cha, M.D.
Resident in Orthopaedic Surgery, University of Pittsburgh Medical Center; Resident in Orthopaedic Surgery, Lilliane Kaufmann Building, 3471 5th Avenue, #1010, Pittsburgh, Pennsylvania 15213

Russell G. Cohen, M.D.
Staff Orthopaedic Surgeon, Department of Orthopaedic Surgery, Tucson Medical Center, 2424 North Wyatt Drive, Suite 260, Tucson, Arizona 85712

Dennis K. Collis, M.D.
Associate Clinical Professor, Department of Orthopaedics, Oregon Health Sciences University, 3181 SW Sam Jackson Park Road, Portland, Oregon 97201

H. A. Crawford, M.B., ChB, F.R.A.C.S.
London Health Sciences Centre, University Campus, The University of Western Ontario, London, Ontario, Canada N6A 5A5

John M. Cuckler, M.D.
Professor and Director, Department of Orthopaedic Surgery, University of Alabama at Birmingham; Director, Division of Orthopaedic Surgery, University Hospital, 619 South 19th Street, Birmingham, Alabama 35233

Murray K. Dalinka, M.D.
Professor of Musculoskeletal Radiology, Department of Radiology, University of Pennsylvania; Chief of Musculoskeletal Radiology, Hospital of the University of Pennsylvania, 3400 Spruce Street/1 Silverstein, Philadelphia, Pennsylvania 19104

Lawrence D. Dorr, M.D.
Center for Arthritis and Joint Implant Surgery, University of Southern California, 1510 San Pablo Street, #634, Los Angeles, California 90033

Clive P. Duncan, M.D., F.R.C.S.(C)
Professor and Chairman, Department of Orthopaedics, University of British Columbia; Medical Director and Head, Department of Orthopaedics, Vancouver Hospital and Health Sciences Centre, 3rd floor, 910 West 10th Avenue, Vancouver, British Columbia, Canada V5Z 4E3

C. Anderson Engh, Jr., M.D.
Assistant Clinical Professor, University of Maryland School of Medicine, Baltimore, Maryland; Staff Orthopaedic Surgeon, INOVA Center for Joint Replacement at Mount Vernon Hospital, Arlington, Virginia; Anderson Orthopaedic Research Institute, P.O. Box 7088, 2501 Parker's Lane, Suite 200, Arlington, Virginia 22306

Charles A. Engh, Sr., M.D.
Associate Clinical Professor, University of Maryland School of Medicine, Baltimore, Maryland; Medical Director, INOVA Center for Joint Replacement, Alexandria, Virginia; Anderson Orthopaedic Research Institute, P.O. Box 7088, 2501 Parker's Lane, Suite 200, Arlington, Virginia 22306

John L. Esterhai, Jr., M.D.
Associate Professor, Department of Orthopaedic Surgery, Hospital of the University of Pennsylvania, 3400 Spruce Street/2 Silverstein, Philadelphia, Pennsylvania 19104

Robert H. Fitzgerald, Jr., M.D.
Chairman, Department of Orthopaedic Surgery, Hospital of the University of Pennsylvania, 3400 Spruce Street/2 Silverstein, Philadelphia, Pennsylvania 19104

Donald S. Garbuz, M.D., F.R.C.S.(C)
Clinical Instructor, Department of Orthopaedics, Faculty of Medicine, University of British Columbia; Associate Staff, Department of Orthopaedics, Vancouver Hospital and Health Sciences Centre, 910 West 10th Avenue, Third Floor, Vancouver, British Columbia, Canada V5Z 4E3

Jean W. M. Gardeniers, M.D., Ph.D.
Senior Staff Member, Department of Orthopaedics, University of Nijmegen; Orthopaedic Surgeon, Sint Radboud Hospital, Th. Craanenlaan 7/Postbus 9101, 6525 GH Nijmegen, The Netherlands

Jonathan P. Garino, M.D.
Assistant Professor, Department of Orthopaedic Surgery, University of Pennsylvania School of Medicine, 3400 Spruce Street, Philadelphia, Pennsylvania 19104

Graham A. Gie, F.R.C.S. Ed. (Orth)
Honorary Fellow, Department of Engineering Science, University of Exeter; Consultant Orthopaedic Surgeon, Princess Elizabeth Orthopaedic Centre, Barrack Road, Exeter, United Kingdom EX2 4LE

Andrew H. Glassman, M.D.
Director, Joint Replacement Program, Department of Orthopaedic Surgery, Pentagon City Hospital, 2455 Army Navy Drive, Arlington, Virginia 22206

Amy L. Graziani, Pharm.D.
Adjunct Assistant Professor of Pharmacy, Department of Medicine, Infectious Disease Section, University of Pennsylvania School of Medicine; Clinical Pharmacist Specialist, Anti-Infectives, Department of Pharmacy Services, University of Pennsylvania Medical Center, 3400 Spruce Street, Philadelphia, Pennsylvania 19104

Allan E. Gross, M.D., F.R.C.S.(C)
Professor of Surgery, University of Toronto; Head, Division of Orthopaedic Surgery, Mount Sinai Hospital, 600 University Avenue, Suite 476-A, Toronto, Ontario, Canada M5G 1X5

Stephen M. Herrington, B.S.M.E.
Director of Research Services, Joint Implant Surgeons, Inc., 720 East Broad Street, Columbus, Ohio 43215

Janet M. Hines, M.D.
Assistant Professor, Department of Medicine, University of Pennsylvania; Associate Director, Immunodeficiency Program, Department of Medicine, Hospital of the University of Pennsylvania, 3400 Spruce Street, Philadelphia, Pennsylvania 19104

William J. Hozack, M.D.
Associate Professor, Thomas Jefferson University, Attending Orthopaedic Surgeon, Pennsylvania Hospital and Thomas Jefferson University Hospital, Philadelphia, Pennsylvania; Rothman Institute, 800 Spruce Street, Philadelphia, Pennsylvania 19107

David S. Hungerford, M.D.
Professor, Department of Orthopaedic Surgery, Johns Hopkins University; Chief, Division of Arthritis Surgery, Good Samaritan Hospital, 5601 Loch Raven Boulevard, Suite G-1, Baltimore, Maryland 21239

Carol R. Hutchison, M.D., M.Ed.
Assistant Professor, Department of Surgery, University of Toronto; Director of Surgical Skills Center, Mount Sinai Hospital, 600 University Avenue, Suite 476-C, Toronto, Ontario, Canada M5G 1X5

Joshua J. Jacobs, M.D.
Professor, Department of Orthopaedic Surgery, Rush Medical College; Senior Attending Physician, Rush-Presbyterian-St. Luke's Medical Center, 1653 West Congress Parkway, Chicago, Illinois 60612

Norman A. Johanson, M.D.
*Associate Professor, Department of Orthopaedic Surgery, Temple University School
of Medicine, Temple University Hospital, Philadelphia, Pennsylvania; 115 Glenn
Road, Ardmore, Pennsylvania 19003*

Alan D. Kalvin, Ph.D.
*Research Staff Member, Thomas J. Watson Research Center, IBM Corporation,
30 Sawmill River Road, Hawthorne, New York 10532*

J. Bruce Kneeland, M.D.
*Associate Professor of Radiology, Department of Radiology, Hospital of the
University of Pennsylvania, 3400 Spruce Street/1 Silverstein, Philadelphia,
Pennsylvania 19104*

David G. Lewallen, M.D.
*Professor, Department of Orthopaedic Surgery, Mayo Medical School; Consultant in
Orthopaedic Surgery, Mayo Clinic/Mayo Foundation, 200 First Street, SW,
Rochester, Minnesota 55905*

Robin S. M. Ling, O.B.E., M.A., B.M.(Oxon), Hon. F.R.C.S.(Ed), F.R.C.S.
2 The Quadrant, Wonford Road, Exeter EX2 4LE, United Kingdom

Adolph V. Lombardi, Jr., M.D., F.A.C.S.
*Assistant Clinical Professor, Departments of Orthopaedic Surgery and Biomedical
Engineering, Ohio State University; Director of Medical Research, Department of
Orthopaedics, Ohio Orthopaedic Institute, Grant Medical Center, 111 South Grant
Avenue, Columbus, Ohio 43215*

Donald B. Longjohn, M.D.
*Assistant Professor, Department of Orthopaedic Surgery, Center for Arthritis and
Joint Implant Surgery, University of Southern California, 1510 San Pablo
Street #634, Los Angeles, California 90033*

Jess H. Lonner, M.D.
*Assistant Professor, Department of Orthopaedic Surgery, Adult Constructive
Surgery, University of Pennsylvania School of Medicine, 3400 Spruce Street/2
Silverstein, Philadelphia, Pennsylvania 19104*

Paul A. Lotke, M.D.
*Professor of Orthopaedic Surgery, Chief of Implant Service, Hospital of the
University of Pennsylvania, 3400 Spruce Street/2 Silverstein, Philadelphia,
Pennsylvania 19104*

Rob Roy MacGregor, M.D.
*Professor, Department of Medicine, University of Pennsylvania School of Medicine;
Director, AIDS Clinical Trials Unit, Hospital of the University of Pennsylvania, 3400
Spruce Street, Philadelphia, Pennsylvania 19104*

Thomas H. Mallory, M.D., F.A.C.S.
Clinical Assistant Professor, Division of Orthopaedic Surgery, Ohio State University Medical Center; Chairman, Grant Medical Center, 111 South Grant Avenue, Columbus, Ohio 43215

William J. Maloney, M.D.
Associate Professor, Department of Orthopaedic Surgery, Washington University School of Medicine; Chief of Service and Head of Joint Replacement, Barnes-Jewish Hospital, One Barnes-Jewish Plaza, Suite 11300, West Pavilion, St. Louis, Missouri 63110

Bassam A. Masri, M.D., F.R.C.S.(C)
Clinical Associate Professor, Department of Orthopaedics, University of British Columbia; Head, Division of Reconstructive Orthopaedics, Vancouver General Hospital and Health Sciences Center, Room 3114, 910 West 10th Avenue, Vancouver, British Columbia, Canada V5Z 4E3

Craig G. Mohler, M.D.
Clinical Instructor, Department of Orthopaedic Surgery, Oregon Health Sciences University; Orthopaedic Surgeon, Orthopaedic Healthcare NW, 1200 Hilyard Street, Suite 600, Eugene, Oregon 97401

Michael A. Mont, M.D.
5601 Loch Raven Boulevard, Baltimore, Maryland 21239

Amy S. Morgan, Pharm.D., B.C.P.S.
Assistant Professor of Pharmacy, Philadelphia College of Pharmacy, University of the Sciences in Philadelphia, 600 South 43rd Street, Philadelphia, Pennsylvania 19104-4495

Carl L. Nelson, M.D.
Professor and Chairman, Department of Orthopaedic Surgery, University of Arkansas for Medical Sciences; Staff Physician, University Hospital of Arkansas, 4301 West Markham Street, Slot 531, Little Rock, Arkansas 72205

Ohannes A. Nercessian, M.D.
Associate Clinical Professor, New York Orthopaedic Hospital, College of Physicians and Surgeons of Columbia University; Associate Attending Physician, Department of Orthopaedic Surgery, Columbia Presbyterian Medical Center, 161 Fort Washington Avenue, New York, New York 10032

Wayne G. Paprosky, M.D.
Associate Professor, Department of Orthopaedic Surgery, Rush University; Attending Staff, Rush-Presbyterian-St. Luke's Medical Center, 1653 West Congress Parkway, Chicago, Illinois 60612

Cecil H. Rorabeck, M.D., F.R.C.S.(C)
Professor and Chief, Department of Surgery, Division of Orthopaedic Surgery, University of Western Ontario; Consultant, London Health Sciences Center, University Campus, 339 Windermere Road North, London, Ontario, Canada N6A 5A5

Aaron G. Rosenberg, M.D.
Professor, Department of Orthopaedics, Rush Medical College; Attending Surgeon, Rush-Presbyterian-St. Luke's Medical Center, 1725 West Harrison Avenue, Suite 1063, Chicago, Illinois 60612

Harry E. Rubash, M.D.
Visiting Professor, Department of Orthopaedic Surgery, Harvard Medical School; Chief, Department of Orthopaedic Surgery, Massachusetts General Hospital, 55 Fruit Street, WHT 601, Boston, Massachusetts 02114

Eduardo A. Salvati, M.D.
Clinical Professor of Surgery, Department of Orthopaedics, Cornell University Medical College; Director, Hip and Knee Service, Hospital for Special Surgery, 535 East 70th Street, New York, New York 10021

Mari Schenk, M.D.
Department of Radiology, Hospital of the University of Pennsylvania, 3400 Spruce Street/1 Silverstein, Philadelphia, Pennsylvania 19104

B. Willem Schreurs, M.D., Ph.D.
Orthopaedic Surgeon, Department of Orthopaedics, Academic Hospital Nijmegen, P.O. Box 9101, 6500 HB Nijmegen, The Netherlands

Jeffrey E. Schryver, M.S.
Vice President, Implant Product Development, Smith & Nephew Inc., 1450 Brooks Road, Memphis, Tennessee 38116

Todd D. Sekundiak, M.D., F.R.C.S.(C)
Assistant Professor, Department of Orthopaedic Surgery, University of Manitoba; Surgeon, St. Boniface Hospital, 409 Tache Avenue, Room Z-3053, Winnipeg, Manitoba, Canada R2H 2A6

Arun S. Shanbhag, Ph.D.
Assistant Professor, Department of Orthopaedic Surgery, Massachusetts General Hospital, Harvard Medical School, GRJ 1126, 55 Fruit Street, Boston, Massachusetts 02114

Raj K. Sinha, M.D., Ph.D.
Assistant Professor, Department of Orthopaedic Surgery, University of Pittsburgh Medical Center, 3471 5th Avenue, Suite 1010, Pittsburgh, Pennsylvania 15213

Tom J. J. H. Slooff, M.D., Ph.D.
Professor in Orthopaedics, Department of Orthopaedic Surgery, University Hospital Sint Radboud, P.O. Box 9101, 6500 HB Nijmegen, The Netherlands

Paul N. Smith, B.M.B.S., F.R.A.C.S.
Division of Orthopaedic Surgery, University of Western Ontario, London Health Sciences Center, University Campus, 339 Windermere Road, P.O. Box 5339, Postal Station A, London, Ontario, Canada N6A 5A5

Marvin E. Steinberg, M.D.
Professor and Vice Chairman, Department of Orthopaedic Surgery, University of Pennsylvania, School of Medicine; Director, Joint Reconstruction Center, Hospital of the University of Pennsylvania, 3400 Spruce Street, Philadelphia, Pennsylvania 19104

Michael Tanzer, M.D., F.R.C.S.(C)
Associate Professor, Department of Surgery, McGill University; Assistant Chief, Division of Orthopaedic Surgery, Montreal General Hospital, 1650 Cedar Avenue, Room A2144, Montreal, Quebec, Canada H36 1A4

Leo A. Whiteside, M.D.
Director, Biomechanical Research Laboratory, Missouri Bone and Joint Center; Orthopaedic Surgeon, Barnes-Jewish West County Hospital, 12634 Olive Boulevard, St. Louis, Missouri 63141

Bill Williamson
Senior Imaging Systems Engineer, Integrated Surgical Systems, 1850 Research Park Drive, Davis, California 95616

Ye-Yeon Won, M.D.
Department of Orthopaedic Surgery, Ajou University, Suwon, South Korea

Preface

The modern era of total hip replacement arthroplasty spans more than three decades. During that time, it has been estimated that over 5,000,000 hips have been inserted worldwide. More than 200,000 total hip arthroplasties are now performed annually in the United States alone. This number will increase as our population continues to age.

Because most hips have been inserted in older individuals, most will live out their normal lifespan with their hips in place and functioning well. However, the best total hip replacement has a finite life expectancy and approximately 10% of all total hip replacements are revision procedures. As the life expectancy of senior citizens continues to increase, hips will need to function for longer periods of time. There is a growing number of patients in the community with hips that have been in place for over 20 years. With the success of these joints, there has also been a trend toward inserting these components in younger individuals. These factors ensure that the number of revisions required in the future will continue to increase.

During the 1970s and 1980s, orthopaedists focused on improving components and techniques for performing primary total hip replacement arthroplasty. Today these procedures are relatively commonplace and are well taught in virtually every training program in the United States and abroad. The past several years have seen a shift in interest toward the revision total hip replacement. Revisions embody the same principles, techniques, and components used in primary total hip replacement. However, with revisions one can encounter problems with the removal of failed components and cement, deficient bone stock, and reinsertion of new components. Therefore, planning is far more crucial than in straightforward primary total hip replacement. Knowledge of different and often extensile surgical exposures is essential. Familiarity with various reconstructive techniques is necessary, including a variety of grafting procedures, and the use of special instruments and components. The rate of intraoperative and postoperative complications is higher than in primary total hip replacement. The surgeon must be aware of these complications, how to prevent them, and how to treat them if they do occur. This text is designed to meet these various requirements.

Many excellent publications on surgery of the hip are currently available. Most of these devote only a relatively small portion to revision total hip arthroplasty. There is need for a text book that focuses on the failed total hip and how to revise it. When plans for this book were initiated, it was felt that it would be relatively brief. As we became more involved with the subject matter, it became obvious that the scope would have to be expanded considerably to cover this complicated subject adequately. The present volume therefore consists of 40 chapters. We are fortunate in having been able to recruit authors with national and international reputations who are experts in their respective fields. This text has been designed to serve as a working manual for the clinician faced with the often difficult task of evaluating and treating the patient with a failed total hip arthroplasty. It begins by giving us an insight into the causes and mechanisms of failure, goes on to discuss how to evaluate the patient with a failed hip, and concludes with a detailed description of the specific techniques and devices available for surgical revision. The result is a practical, concise, yet comprehensive text on revision total hip arthroplasty which will be of considerable value to both the general orthopaedist and the experienced hip surgeon.

The introductory chapter gives an overview of the etiology of failure of total hip arthroplasty. The first section on basic science covers many of the factors that lead to failure. It starts by reviewing the pathogenesis as well as the clinical picture of osteolysis and aseptic loosening, the most common mode of failure. It next discusses the effects of various acetabular and femoral designs on long-term survivorship. It concludes by reviewing the role played by different materials and surgical techniques. The second section deals with the evaluation of a painful total hip from both a clinical and a radiographic point of view. It ends with a pragmatic discussion of when to and when not to revise a painful total hip arthroplasty.

The third and most comprehensive section of the book contains 15 chapters giving considerable detail on specific techniques for revising the aseptic total hip. This section begins with a discussion of preoperative planning, surgical exposures, and removal of components and cement. It goes on to outline the selection of acetabular and femoral components, then gives an in-depth review of the various types of bone grafting procedures available to reconstruct deficient acetabula and femora, including structural grafts, cancellous grafts, and impaction grafting techniques. It then focuses on specific approaches to acetabular and femoral revision, using both cemented and uncemented components. The section concludes with a review of postoperative management and an analysis of the results of revision surgery.

The fourth section is concerned specifically with revising the infected total hip. It begins with an approach to diagnosis and evaluation, proceeds to a discussion of the infecting organisms and the appropriate antibiotics, and ends with a description of the surgical techniques designed specifically for treating the infected total hip and the results of treatment. The fifth section reviews intraoperative and postoperative complications, how to avoid them, and how to treat them if they occur. It includes a discussion of deep venous thrombosis, pulmonary embolism, dislocation, heterotopic ossification, femoral shaft fracture, and trochanteric nonunion and abductor compromise. The concluding section, entitled "Special Considerations," covers resection arthroplasty, arthroplasty of the arthrodesed hip, conversion of cup arthroplasty and femoral endoprostheses to total hip replacement, use of customized components and robotics, and methods for blood conservation and replacement.

It should be noted that this publication serves as a companion to *Revision Total Knee Arthroplasty,* edited by Paul A. Lotke and Jonathan P. Garino, and published by Lippincott Williams & Wilkins. As far as possible, these texts have followed a similar format. We thank our colleague, Dr. Paul Lotke, for his many suggestions regarding the content and organization of this publication. It also serves as a complement to *The Adult Hip,* edited by John J. Callaghan, Aaron G. Rosenberg, and Harry E. Rubash, also published by Lippincott–Raven. This excellent and comprehensive publication covers the broader topic of adult hip surgery, whereas the present publication focuses specifically on total hip revision.

We have enjoyed preparing this text and have learned a great deal in the process. We hope that it will be of assistance to our colleagues when faced with the often challenging problem of revision total hip arthroplasty.

We thank our authors and co-authors for preparing authoritative, well written, and timely manuscripts on their assigned topics. This appreciation extends to the many secretaries, research assistants, and photographers who have helped them. We are especially grateful to the team at Lippincott Williams & Wilkins, our publisher, who functioned so effectively to see this project through to its completion. They were all a delight to work with and made our editorial tasks easy. Special thanks go to Emilie M. Linkins and Susan Rhyner, developmental editors, and especially to Kathryn L. Alexander, vice-president and editor-in-chief, who initiated the idea for a text on this subject and who worked closely with us throughout. Our artist Theodore G. Huff and his associates did a superb job in interpreting the needs of our authors and in providing a large set of original drawings that are both aesthetically pleasing and technically effective in illustrating the material described in the text. We also thank Margaret M. Perry, Christine Coppertino, and Karen M. Hartman in our department for the many hours they have devoted to this book.

Marvin E. Steinberg, M.D.
Jonathan P. Garino, M.D.

Revision
Total Hip
Arthroplasty

Revision Total Hip Arthroplasty,
edited by Marvin E. Steinberg and Jonathan P. Garino,
Lippincott Williams & Wilkins, Philadelphia © 1999.

1

Etiology of Failure: An Overview

Jonathan P. Garino and Marvin E. Steinberg

The creation of this textbook on revision total hip arthroplasty implies that primary total hip replacements not only fail but also create numerous reconstructive problems for the surgeon performing the revision when they do. What is not implied is that constant improvements in primary total hip replacement from a materials, design, and technique standpoint are reducing the failure rate. These modifications, however, are becoming increasingly more reliant on information derived from analysis of failed components. Revision total hip arthroplasty has one main goal—restoration of function. However, through evaluation of failed implants, the surrounding tissue environment and devices recovered at autopsy, our understanding of the causes of failure is enhanced. This chapter is a brief overview of many of the reasons for failure.

MATERIAL FAILURE

Aseptic loosening is the leading cause of failure. It is cited as the reason for nearly 90% of revision total hip arthroplasties performed. Many factors influence the longevity of prosthetic implants. Perhaps the most important consideration in successful total joint replacement is the material from which the components are derived. Poorly designed components rarely fail within the first 2 to 3 years, but poor material choices have resulted in catastrophic failures, often within the first few years after implantation. The use of

J. P. Garino: Department of Orthopaedic Surgery, Hospital of the University of Pennsylvania, Philadelphia, Pennsylvania 19104

M. E. Steinberg: Department of Orthopaedic Surgery, University of Pennsylvania School of Medicine, Philadelphia, Pennsylvania 19104.

polytetrafluoroethylene (Teflon) in the original low-friction arthroplasty (5) and the use of titanium heads (2) in the early 1980's are two such examples. Although each material had its own set of favorable mechanical properties, neither demonstrated good wear characteristics. Each was, therefore, a poor choice for articulating surfaces. Stem fractures were common in the infancy of hip replacement, but with metallurgic improvements the strength of the newer alloys has made stem fracture a rarity. Because the diseased femoral head and corresponding acetabulum are not replaced with living bone and cartilage, the substitutes we have chosen represent a compromise. Living bone can respond to stress or lack thereof with hypertrophy or disuse osteoporosis. This ability to remodel and adapt is something that is lacking in inanimate replacement devices. However, it would seem, at least in the laboratory, that current hip replacements would be up to the challenge. Unfortunately, unlike the mechanical hip simulator, components are placed in a highly dynamic and ever-changing environment and are constantly at the mercy of the mechanical and metabolic stresses and adaptations taking place around them.

Clearly not all materials are suitable for prolonged service in such an environment. First of all, the material must be biologically inert. Compounds that are subject to considerable corrosion or biodegradation or that stimulate the immune system will not do well over time. With the prospect of facing forces in excess of three times the body weight on a continual basis, the chosen material must have great strength. Taking these primary factors into consideration, stainless steel was a logical initial selection. In spite of the relative strength of stainless steel over bone, femoral stem-component fractures were not uncommon in the early days of total hip replacement. The primary solution to this problem, was to use a material with greater fatigue strength. Enhanced fatigue strength was obtained with a combination of material change and manufacturing techniques. Specifically, use of a cobalt chromium alloy that was forged rather than cast enhanced the fatigue strength of the femoral stem. Forged titanium alloys have performed well with respect to resisting fatigue failure. Unfortunately, no aspect of the elements of a successful hip replacement are isolated in a vacuum. There is constant interplay with the dynamic environment in which they are placed. For example, reports of increased stem breakage with a "modern" component have surfaced (9). This increase in breakage is attributed to both debonding of cement with loss of proximal fixation and to the strength of the forged cobalt chromium stem. In this case, manufacturing techniques may have contributed to the failures: a laser etching on the surface of the stem produced a focal area of mechanical weakness through which the fractures occurred (Fig. 1).

Enhancing the strength of stems may result in increasing the stiffness of the component. Although definitely seen as an improvement, there is always a price to be paid. In this case, stiffer components usually result in increased stress shielding. At the current time, titanium and cobalt chromium, and to a lesser extent stainless steel, remain the most popular materials from which prosthetic components are manufactured. These materials are used both with and without cement with reasonable success, indicating that they all have the minimum requirements with respect to strength and stiffness. Their malleability allows for an infinite number of design possibilities and application of metallic and nonmetallic coatings. Although the initial metallurgic enhancements afforded by the use of superalloys and forging represented an improvement, no dramatic additional improvements in this regard have occurred in the last 10 to 15 years. Controversies still exist, primarily regarding the qualities of these metals with respect to the optimum material in cemented and uncemented situations (8). Research continues in regard to metal and composite components with the goal of developing a material that has sufficient strength and fatigue resistance while possessing a modulus of elasticity similar to that of bone. Techniques and technologies in genetic engineering may allow development biologic solutions that orthopedic surgeons can apply in situations formerly managed with hip replacement.

The original designs of hip replacement consisted of essentially two components, femoral and acetabular. Each of these components had the dual role of providing fixation, either through cement or bone ingrowth, and functioning as an effective articulating surface. From a materials standpoint, these two roles are very different, yet the early designs used a single material on either side of the joint to do both. The introduction of

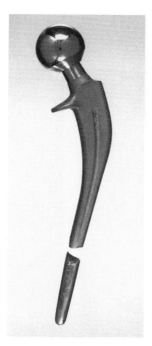

Figure 1. Fracture of a modern pre-coated prosthesis.

modularity resulted in uncoupling of these two separate functions and with it the potential for optimization of biomaterials for these two separate roles. In the early monoblock designs of both acetabular and femoral components, the failures were often blamed on cement and "cement disease," indicating that fixation was the problem to be conquered for long-term success. The uncoupling of the fixation and the articulation biomaterials led to improved understanding of the important qualities of each of the components within the system. The 1980's were the decade in which the perceived weak link of fixation, acrylic cement, was addressed. Although improvements were made in cementing techniques, it was concluded that cement was not the culprit it was once thought to be. Attention was focused on the polyethylene articular surface.

Although demonstrating reasonable wear properties and satisfactory 20-year long-term survivorship in certain series, polyethylene is now looked on as the long-term limiting factor in total hip replacement systems. Much attention has turned to polyethylene with the recognized importance of minimizing wear debris and particle formation. Attempts have been made to improve the durability of polyethylene, but this has often resulted in reduction in other properties of this material below the critical threshold, resulting in early failure. Carbon reinforcement of the polyethylene is such an example (7). Titanium, bone, and cement in particulate form can elicit inflammatory responses or become loose in the articulating area and accelerate wear of the polyethylene by a third-body wear mode. Polyethylene wear debris can be generated from multiple areas, including the back side of the cup, and the particles can generate an inflammatory reaction, resulting in extensive osteolysis even though components remain well fixed. Concerns have been raised regarding the importance of the technique of sterilization of polyethylene components. It is uniformly agreed that gamma sterilization in air can result in accelerated oxidation of the subsurface polyethylene caused by production of free radicals and degradation of the quality of the subsurface polyethylene over time. This appears to be a bigger problem with knee replacement than hip replacement because of the different wear modes in these joints. Gamma sterilization in a vacuum or in an inert environment, such as argon or nitrogen, and ethylene oxide sterilization are becoming the preferred methods of treatment to prevent this late oxidative phenomenon. With polyethylene wear representing a serious factor in hip replacement failure, alternative bearing materials, such as ceramic on ceramic

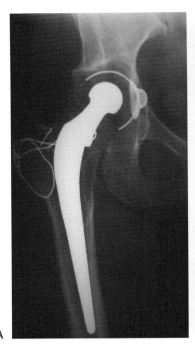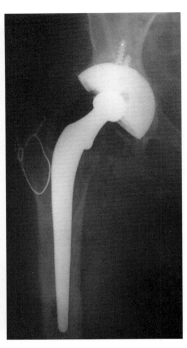

A   B

Figure 2. Material failure. **A:** Prerevision radiograph of a 60-year-old woman 22 years after total hip replacement with a standard Charnley prosthesis and radiolucent cement. Considerable wear has taken place, as has proximal migration of the component. **B:** Revision with slightly oversized, cementless, hemispheric cup.

and metal on metal, both with more than a 25-year history, are being reevaluated and reengineered for their potential as more durable articulations.

The materials from which prosthetic components are manufactured play an extremely important role in the long-term success of a prosthesis. Although there have been improvements in materials since the 1960's, some of the same materials used then remain in use today. Perhaps the most important advance with respect to biomaterials has been the recognition that fixation and articulation are two separate functions and require different biomaterials for optimum performance. This has given us invaluable insight into the material aspects of failure and the requirements for long-term success (Fig. 2).

FAILURES OF PROSTHETIC DESIGN

Perhaps the most difficult task in evaluating failures is drawing some conclusion or reference between prosthesis design and failure. The difficulty in this evaluation revolves around the fact that satisfactory long-term follow-up information exists only for a small number of designs. Even in those cases, rarely are the components available in their original form. A variety of modifications and many new devices have been introduced to address theoretic problems and hypothetical shortcomings. These changes have not always resulted in an improvement. Perceived or real niches in the evolving marketplace have driven design alteration. This has a negative effect on our ability appropriately to evaluate design factors in long-term survivor series, because the reported results are on a component no longer available. Our underappreciation of both design and material properties led to numerous device failures during the 1980's. In recent times there has been a great appreciation for the successful designs, and surgeons have migrated back to these types of components. This has resulted in a consolidation of prosthetic choices. Most of the leading manufacturers are now producing similar designs.

Although the optimum total hip design has not yet been developed, we have learned some lessons with regard to what designs do not work. Stems designed for cement should not be curved or have sharp edges. Porous coated stems should not rely on minimal proximal porous coating for fixation, and the porous coatings should be firmly fixed to the component. This demonstrates that design has an extremely important role in the long-term success of hip replacements. Components made of similar materials may have widely different failure rates on the basis of design features alone. The prosthetic designs also vary with the needs of the situation. Revision components usually have a variety of enhancements to compensate for bone and soft-tissue deficits. The plurality of designs of total hip replacements that have been developed and used over the course of the last two decades essentially have leveled the playing field with respect to the mode of fixation that seems to work best. There are ample examples of cemented designs and cementless designs that have not met expectations and have had high rates of early failure. On the other hand, there are examples of both cemented and cementless devices that have performed reasonably well over the long term. With so many examples of successes and failures in both categories, one must speak more in terms of the results of a specific device rather than the general category of cemented or cementless fixation.

With the failure of specific component designs, an explanation of the cause of early failure was often apparent. Frequently, design changes addressing one shortcoming would result in compromise of unrecognized, but often more important design features. Our understanding of the requirements of successful design has become increasingly more defined with each recognized design flaw. A number of devices on the market have reasonable track records in revision situations. There are also numerous new devices with features that in many ways attempt to mimic the qualities of the successful components. One must be particularly cautious in choosing a particular implant for revision purposes. Specific design features available in one prosthesis may enable the surgeon to enhance the potential for long-term fixation and function while addressing suboptimal anatomy and bone stock in that particular circumstance. Components with only proximal coating, for example, may be quite successful in the primary operation but fail at an unacceptably high rate in revisions because of lack of quality bone for ingrowth(1).

In essence, in the 1980's and early 1990's much fine tuning of the myriad design features of both cemented and cementless components occurred. The critical features for midterm success have been identified and are discussed in the ensuing chapters. Cementless cup designs of thin polyethylene or poorly supported polyethylene have a tendency to generate wear debris and occasionally to fracture. In many circumstances these cups were used with 32-mm femoral heads, further reducing the thickness of the polyethylene and increasing the opportunity for volumetric polyethylene wear (4). Screw-in acetabular cups, although once quite popular because of the excellent initial fixation they provided, loosened in a large percentage of instances at short- and midterm intervals. Use of femoral components with minimal proximal coating or poor attachment of the porous coating medium to the stem resulted in a number of failures. As the 1990's approached, emphasis for cementless fixation was placed on maximizing the proximal fit and the distal fill of the prosthesis. Techniques were devised for intraoperative manufacture of custom-designed femoral components without any type of roughened or coated surface. In spite of the theoretical advantage of a component with optimized fit and fill, these devices demonstrated high rates of early failure. These are just a few examples of the many design modifications that did not result in enhanced long-term fixation of components but rather hastened failure. In many instances an analysis of these failures enhanced our understanding and modified our thinking with respect to the design features that truly are important for excellent long-term results. The subtle enhancements and qualities that will likely lead to long-term success remain controversial. This is in part related to the interdependence of materials and technique (Fig. 3).

Revision total hip arthroplasty represents an even more difficult situation when planning an optimum reconstruction. Many of the components available for primary replacement with reasonable mid- or long term results may not fare as well in the revision situation because of problems with soft tissues and reduction in the quantity and quality of the bone stock available. Revision operations are opportunities to maximize the interdependence between the choice of prosthesis and the technical details with which it

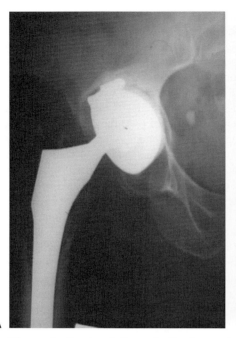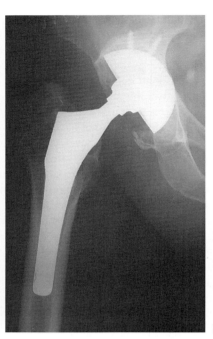

A   B

Figure 3. Design failure. **A:** Radiograph shows failed acetabular component with thin polyethylene liner. **B:** Revision to slightly oversized, cementless, hemispheric cup.

is implanted. That is, in the primary situation, slight lapses in component design or implantation technique may still provide a patient with long-term good quality results. This is a much less likely scenario in the revision situation, in which the slightest shortcomings in optimization of either prosthetic design or implantation technique can result in relatively early failure.

TECHNIQUE-RELATED FAILURES

Total hip arthroplasty is a surgical technique that has evolved over the past three decades. It was developed through careful scientific planning and meticulous surgical preparation. One can argue that technique represents the third limb in a triad that includes materials and design required for successful total hip replacement. Substantial improvements and long-term survivorship have been demonstrated with enhanced quality of cementation of prosthetic components. That is, second-generation femoral cementing techniques are better than their first-generation counterparts, and this is mostly a technique issue (6). Components that are inserted in varus or other forms of malposition are usually directly or indirectly related to inferior results (3). The creation of periprosthetic fractures or suboptimal implant fixation are all technique issues that more often than not have a negative effect on long-term results. Technique cannot be overemphasized. Trochanteric osteotomy was an exposure technique strongly advocated by Charnley. However, complications caused by this osteotomy were frequent. Nonunion, fibrous union, and even frank failure of the trochanteric reattachment were not uncommon. Charnley modified his technique for reattaching the trochanter on several occasions. Impaction grafting is a new technique in which crushed cancellous allograft is used for bone grafting during revision total hip replacement. The technique is very demanding, requiring special instrumentation and patience to pack the bone tightly and properly. The technique often requires careful placement of wire mesh to cover defects and rebuild the calcar. The use of reconstruction rings often demands ample exposure and firm attachment of the device to the ischium and the ilium. Use of whole acetabular transplants is technically demanding in terms of recreating a relatively normally positioned socket while obtaining appropriate fixation to host bone. If a technically poor job is performed, particularly with regard to structural grafting, relatively early failure of the device can be expected.

Surgeons have the responsibility to continue to update their skills through a variety of educational programs. In revision operations, technique reaches its peak of importance. It is carefully and thoroughly intertwined with intraoperative judgment as to what must be done to optimize the result. The unpredictability of revisions usually involves selection of well-thought-out compromises based on bone and soft tissue loss, the prosthetics components, specific techniques, and the resources available to the surgeon. In Section III of this textbook, the myriad of reconstructive techniques and the situations in which they are best used are fully discussed. The fact that this represents the largest section in the text emphasizes the importance of sound intraoperative judgment based on an extensive fund of knowledge. An expression that can be applied is "The eye sees what the mind knows." One must carefully examine the situation and be looking to use specific techniques if they meet the needs of the reconstruction. The only way this can be done is to have all the techniques for a particular situation immediately available. Section III aids the reader in both "seeing" and "knowing" (Figs. 4 and 5).

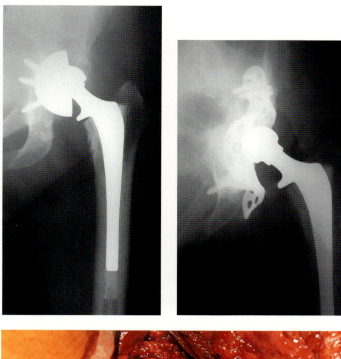

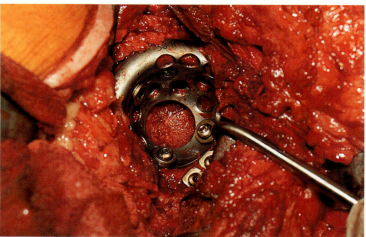

Figure 4. A: Cup malposition with transverse acetabular fracture. **B:** Intraoperative view of antiprotrusio cage placement. **C:** Postoperative radiograph shows reconstruction. The cage supports the cemented acetabular component and acts as a plate with a screw attachment to both sides of the pelvis.

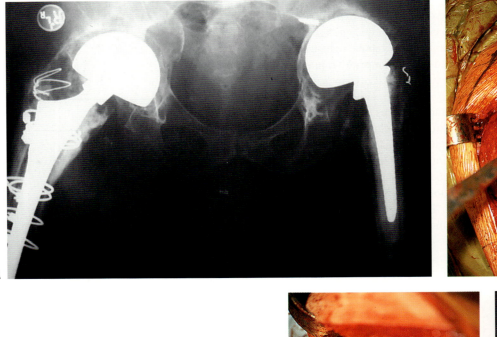
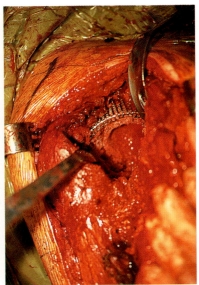
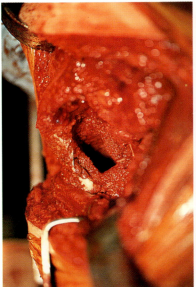
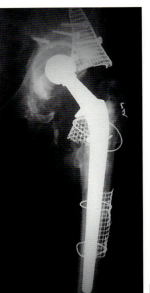

Figure 5. A: Poor judgment exercised when surgeon chose to perform third revision on the left side with a bipolar component. **B:** Intraoperative view of impaction grafting of acetabular side. Mesh augmentation of the posterosuperior margin of the acetabulum is present. **C:** Intraoperative view of neocortex made by impaction grafting technique on the femoral side. **D:** Postoperative radiograph.

BIOLOGIC FAILURES

Why do some patients with obvious wear on follow-up radiographs demonstrate no marked osteolysis and other patients with no demonstrable signs of wear have tremendous osteolysis? Clearly there are biologic aspects of failure that have to be addressed. Is there such a thing as hypersensitivity to polyethylene? What about hypersensitivity to metals, such as chromium or titanium? These are questions that remain unanswered and more than likely remain underappreciated. What causes the osteolysis in these patients? Can osteoclasts be modified or regulated with a variety of pharmaceuticals? Some of these areas are being investigated. Studies looking specifically at a reduction of osteoclast response to particulate debris in the presence of disphosphonates are showing some degree of promise. Further data are necessary to develop a better understanding of how particulate debris stimulates osteoclast formation or activity, resulting in aseptic loosening and why this response is variable from patient to patient. Biologic failure means more than aseptic loosening. Transplant recipients and other patients who have immunocompromise are also candidates for joint replacements. These patients are at increased risk for infection. The wounds of patients with collagen vascular diseases heal wounds slowly and with reduced quality. These patients are highly susceptible to wound difficulties and infection. Perhaps the most helpful approach in many of these cases is preoperative identification of the patient groups at risk and subsequent modification of techniques, procedures, and protocols to enhance the outcome of joint replacement among these patients.

One can argue that arthritis in itself is a biologic failure. The technologic advancements of the future that could bring about a durable prosthesis may show that the optimal reconstruction would be re-creation of a normal joint. Tissue engineering is an exploding area within medicine. The techniques developed in this arena may eventually be applied to restoration of normal and healthy joints.

Biologic failure can occur when bony ingrowth into a cementless but coated component does not take place, although stable fibrous ingrowth often may yield a satisfactory initial outcome. The use of steroids can retard the potential for biologic fixation.

NONSURGICAL FAILURES: MINIMIZING THE COMPLICATIONS

Perhaps there is no more frustrating circumstance to an orthopedic surgeon who has just performed a successful joint replacement, than finding that a serious postoperative complication has developed. Unfortunately from the surgeon's standpoint most of these complications are usually related to a failure to execute proper intraoperative or postoperative "technique." On the other hand, when complications arise from presumably preventable circumstances, there is some reassurance in being able to identify the mechanism leading to the complication and take preventive measures. Although simplistic in its concept, the factors leading to complications and even more so the preventive measures necessary can be difficult to isolate. Nonetheless, perhaps more so than any other aspect of hip replacement surgery, complications have been reduced to only a fraction of what was encountered during the infancy of this reconstructive procedure. Infection was a chief concern of John Charnley when he first developed hip replacement and encountered nearly a 10% infection rate. Charnley's extensive efforts to understand the causes of infection in this procedure and the subsequent steps taken to prevent this catastrophic circumstance from arising with such frequency resulted in many improvements and alterations in technique.

The changes were incremental. First was the perioperative use of antibiotics. This may be the most important adjunct to preventing infection in hip replacement next to sterile technique itself. Charnley also recognized that although a wound is sterile, the environment, specifically the air flow around a wound may not be sterile. He therefore instituted laminar flow with highly filtered air, which enters and leaves the room in a single direction and does not allow recirculation. Full-body exhaust suits were added next. Studies in which agar plates were placed around surgical sites without the presence of total-body exhaust suits demonstrated that surgeons, their assistants, and other persons near the wound "shed" a certain amount of bacterial particles per minutes into the surrounding environment. Through careful thought and a systematic approach, this problem, which once was nearly overwhelming, has been reduced to a near fraction of what it once was.

During the past decade of primary and revisional surgery, much attention has been paid to intra- and perioperative details that tend to reduce complications. Such details include prophylaxis of deep venous thrombosis, dislocation precautions, perioperative use of antibiotics, and rehabilitation protocols. There are many other important perioperative complications that throughout the last few decades surgeons have sought to minimize. Deep venous thrombosis has generated a great deal of interesting controversy. Rarely does a meeting focused on joint replacement take place without at least one discussion of prophylaxis of deep venous thrombosis. A variety of mechanical and chemoprophylactic regimens have been attempted and evaluated over the years, each with a varying degree of success.

Patient education has come a long way. Having a patient thoroughly understand some of the do's and the don'ts following hip replacement and preoperative delineation of the expectations following joint replacement have been identified as important factors. The patient remains a true partner in successful joint replacement. This is no more important than in the case of dislocations. Dislocations after primary total hip replacement take in most instances in the first 3 months after the operation. Most of these patients do not go on to experience chronic dislocation. The dislocation more than likely occurs because the patient does not follow instructions, not because component malposition occurs. If the latter were the case, one would expect chronic dislocation to be more frequent.

Additional emphasis has been placed on these aspects of total hip surgery because managed care has increased the pressure on surgeons and hospitals to maximize both quality and efficiency. Section V is devoted to the prevention and management of complications with special emphasis on the needs of the patients undergoing revision.

SUMMARY

This chapter emphasizes the fact that total hip replacement can fail for any number of reasons. Perhaps better stated, long-term success is multifactorial and dependent on optimization of a number of important factors. Suboptimal conditions in any of the important arenas will jeopardize long-term success and, in most circumstances, bring about a premature failure. Appreciation of what seems to work and perhaps more important knowledge of what does not work is essential in maximizing the long-term success of both primary and revision hip replacements. The routine performance of hip replacement, the availability of quality components, and streamlining of instrumentation have enhanced total hip replacement surgery tremendously. This sanitation of the procedure can deemphasize the importance of meticulous technique and can result in complacency. In addition to providing state-of-the-art information on revision total hip arthroplasty, this text should serve as a strong reminder that the surgeon makes these complex reconstructions possible. Perhaps more so than in any other type of operation performed in the field of orthopedics are experience, judgment, and technique so critical for maximizing the opportunity for long-term success. The information contained in the ensuing chapters provides the reader with some enhancement of all of those qualities.

REFERENCES

1. Berry DJ, Harmsen WS, Ilstrup D, Lewallen DG, Cabanela ME. Survivorship of uncemented proximally porous coated femoral components. *Clin Orthop* 1995;319:168–177.
2. Charnley J, Kamanger A, Longfield MD. The optimum size of prosthetic heads in relation to wear of plastic sockets in total replacement of the hip. *Med Biol Eng* 1969;7:31–39.
3. Eftekhar NS. Results in primary total hip arthroplasty. In: *Total hip arthroplasty.* St. Louis: Mosby–Year Book, 1993:1343–1414.
4. Hernandez JR, Keating EM, Faris PM, Meding JB, Ritter MA. Polyethylene wear in uncemented acetabular components. *J Bone Joint Surg Br* 1994;76:263–266.
5. Malchau H, Herberts P, Ahnfelt L. Prognosis of total hip replacement in Sweden: follow-up of 92,675 operations performed between 1978 to 1990. *Orthop Scand* 1993;64:497–506.
6. Mulroy WF, Estok DM, Harris WH. Total hip arthroplasty with use of so called second generation cementing techniques. *J Bone Joint Surg Am* 1995;77:1845–1852.
7. Pryor GA, Villar RN, Coleman N. Tissue reaction and loosening of carbon reinforced polyethylene arthroplasties. *J Bone Joint Surg Br* 1992;74:156–157.
8. Sotereanos DG, Engh CA, Glassman AH, Macalino GE, Engh CA Jr. Cementless femoral components should be made from cobalt chrome. *Clin Orthop* 1995;313:146–153.
9. Woolson ST, Milbauer JP, Bobyn JD, Yu ES, Maloney WJ. Fatigue fracture of a forged colbalt-chromium-moylbdenum femoral component inserted with cement: a report of 10 cases. *J Bone Joint Surg Am* 1997;79:1842–1848.

SECTION I

Basic Science

Revision Total Hip Arthroplasty,
edited by Marvin E. Steinberg and Jonathan P. Garino,
Lippincott Williams & Wilkins, Philadelphia © 1999.

2

Osteolysis and Aseptic Loosening: Pathogenesis

William J. Maloney

Osteolysis and aseptic loosening are the most common and important long-term complications following total hip arthroplasty. With time, the likelihood of these problems increases, limiting the longevity of the reconstruction (28). Charnley first identified the osteolytic process associated with cemented total hip replacement but attributed it to infection. Harris et al. (11) later identified localized bone resorption in the femur around loose cemented stems. Histologic analysis of the material in the lytic lesions showed predominantly macrophages associated with birefringent material that could not be further identified at that time. Jasty et al. (15) described a similar process around well-fixed cemented stems. The periprosthetic bone resorption that occurred with aseptic loosening of cemented femoral components was referred to as *cement disease*. We now know that is a misnomer.

The phenomenon then referred to as cement disease was in part one of the driving forces behind the development and subsequent popularity of cementless technologies. Unfortunately, eliminating cement did not eliminate the problem of osteolysis. Brown and Ring (3) were among the first to identify the problem with implants inserted without cement. They reported on osteolytic changes in the proximal part of the femurs of patients who had extensively porous coated, cobalt chromium femoral components. Maloney et al. (23) reported on 16 patients with osteolysis predominantly in the diaphysis of the femur; the patients had radiographically stable titanium alloy and chromium cobalt components. A more recent report demonstrated osteolysis of the pelvis in association with stable cementless acetabular components (24).

The term *focal osteolysis* has become commonly used to describe periprosthetic bone

---

W. J. Maloney: Department of Orthopaedic Surgery, Washington University Medical School, and Orthopaedic Surgery Service, Barnes-Jewish Hospital, St. Louis, Missouri 63110.

resorption around cementless implants. Although aseptic loosening and osteolysis have been historically considered separate processes, from a biologic standpoint, they are essentially identical. The biologic process of aseptic loosening as it relates to the linear pattern of osteolysis that develops at the interface between implant and bone, whether it be metal or cement, is identical to that of the expansile, focal type of osteolysis that has classically been associated with cementless implants. The differences lie in the radiographic pattern of bone resorption that is determined not by the underlying biologic features but by issues related to access of joint fluid and wear debris in the implant–bone interface and surrounding bone.

The process of periprosthetic bone resorption, whether it be linear or expansile in its radiographic appearance, is related to three main factors. The first is generation of particulate debris. The second relates to access of particle-laden joint fluid to the implant–bone interface or periprosthetic bone. Finally, the biologic reaction to the implant debris results in macrophage and osteoclast activation and bone resorption. This chapter focuses on the pathophysiologic aspects of aseptic loosening and osteolysis and concentrates on these three areas.

GENERATION OF PARTICULATE DEBRIS

Particulate wear debris has emerged as a serious problem in the long-term survival of total hip replacements. Particles can be generated not only by wear but also by fretting and fragmentation. The most common source of wear particles in total hip arthroplasty is the articulation between femoral head and acetabular liner. On the basis of volume of polyethylene wear and average particle size, McKellop et al. (30) estimated that as many as 500,000 particles of polyethylene less than 1 μm in diameter can be generated with each gait cycle. Several factors that are under the surgeon's control are important as they relate to polyethylene wear. The first is head size. Most laboratory and clinical studies have suggested that volumetric wear of polyethylene is proportional to the size of the femoral head. The larger the femoral head, the greater is the sliding distance between metal and polyethylene. This results in higher volumetric wear. For this reason, 32-mm heads have been abandoned by many surgeons in preference for 28- or 26-mm heads and in some cases 22-mm heads. It is advisable to avoid thin polyethylene liners when at all possible. In general it is preferable to have at least 6 to 8 mm of polyethylene. Although finite-element studies suggest that in a constrained environment such as the hip, polyethylene thickness is not a factor, it is clear from clinical experience that very thin polyethylene liners have not performed well. Congruity and stability between liner and shell may be another important variable that relates to wear. Implant design has evolved to address these issues. Both factors are important in minimizing motion between the polyethylene and metal shell, which can lead to wear on the backside of polyethylene liners.

Other factors that influence polyethylene wear include oxidation of the material and counterface abrasions. Oxidative degradation over time of polyethylene implants that have been sterilized with gamma radiation in air is a topic of growing concern. Radiation produces free radicals, which are chemically reactive sites. These free radicals can react with oxygen to form ketone, ester, and carboxylic acid groups, which prevent recombination and decrease the molecular weight of the material, its tensile strength, and its fracture toughness. This has led the biomaterials industry to sterilize polyethylene by using radiation in the absence of oxygen or by using alternative methods of sterilization, such as ethylene oxide.

Counterface abrasions are potentially another important factor in accelerated polyethylene wear. Fisher et al. (6) reported that whereas 5 years of oxidation led to a threefold increase in polyethylene wear, roughening the surface of the counterface to the degree one might see in a damaged femoral head led to a tenfold increase in wear rate. It is important for the surgeon to handle the femoral head carefully during implantation to avoid scratching.

Although the articulation is the most important source of particles, other potential particle generators must be considered. Modular connections have been shown to be a source of particulate debris (Fig. 1). Urban et al. (41) demonstrated that corrosion products from modular head–neck junctions can migrate to the periprosthetic tissues and to the polyethylene bearing surface. The corrosion products identified as chromium orthophosphate hydrate-rich material appears to develop as a result of crevice corrosion. At histologic examination they appear to be biologically active; they have been shown to be present within histiocytes and surrounded by foreign-body giant cells. Because they are hard particles, these corrosion products have the potential to play a role in three-body wear at the articulation. Any modular connection can generate particles and therefore the benefits of using modularity on a widespread basis must be weighed against this potential long-term problem.

Braided wires or cables that are commonly used around the hip joint for reattachment of trochanteric osteotomies or wiring of femoral allografts have shown to be a source of particulate debris. In general, these particles are relatively large and are therefore biologically probably not tremendously important. However, they have been shown to migrate into the articulation between femoral head and acetabular liner and therefore are an important source of three-body wear. Other sources of wear particles include the cement–metal interface, fragmentation of bone cement, the bone–cement interface, and the metal–bone interface in cementless applications.

Several authors have reported on the size and morphologic features of wear particles. Maloney et al. (26) reported on 35 membranes obtained during revision hip replacements of failed cementless components (Fig. 2). The tissue from the implant–bone interface was harvested and digested with papain. The particles were isolated and characterized by means of both light and scanning electron microscopic examination and by x-ray microanalysis and automated particle analysis. The mean size of the polyethylene particles was 0.5 μm. The metal particles were similar in size at 0.7 μm. Ninety percent of all particles isolated were less than 0.95 μm. To quantitate the number of particles per gram of tissue, hip capsules from primary total hip arthroplasties were digested by means of a similar method. The number of "biologic particles" was compared with the number of particles obtained from revision membrane. A mean of 1.7 billion particles per gram of tissue were obtained from the revision membranes compared with only 143 million particles per gram of tissue for the control samples. On average, the total number of particles associated with bipolar acetabular components was twice that associated with the fixed acetabular components. There also was a trend toward a larger mean size of polyethylene particles associated with the bipolar cups.

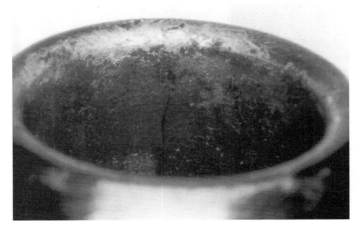

Figure 1. Corrosion at a modular head-neck junction. Corrosion on the modular head is a source of particulate wear debris.

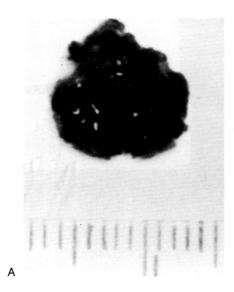

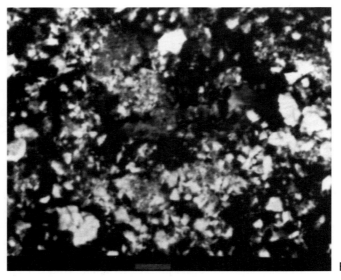

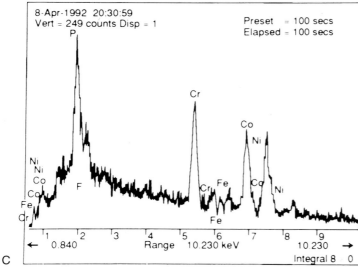

Figure 2. A: Interface membrane from a failed cobalt chrome total hip arthroplasty approximately 1 cm in diameter. **B:** Scanning electron micrograph of the particles obtained from the membrane in **A** after enzymatic digestion with papain. **C:** X-ray microanalysis of retrieved particles demonstrates a pattern consistent with cobalt chrome alloy.

ACCESS TO THE IMPLANT–BONE INTERFACE AND PERIPROSTHETIC BONE

The prevalence and location of osteolytic lesions after cemented or cementless total hip arthroplasty depend not only on generation of particles but also on access of the particles to the implant–bone interface and periprosthetic bone. Schmalzried et al. (35) call this area the *effective joint space*. The effective joint space is defined by all periprosthetic regions accessible to joint fluid and wear debris. With activities of daily living, the fluid present in the hip joint is subject to high pressures. The fluid is dispersed along the path of least resistance. With the fluid, particles present in joint fluid primarily from the articulation are transported to the periprosthetic tissues. The path of least resistance is determined by the type of fixation, implant design, and bone remodeling around the implant (34,45). Examples are given later to illustrate this point.

CEMENTED VERSUS CEMENTLESS SOCKETS

Autopsy studies after cemented acetabular replacement have demonstrated that the subchondral bone plate reforms. This is a relative barrier for joint fluid and particles to

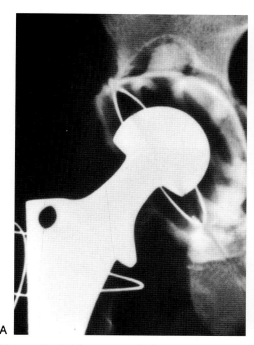
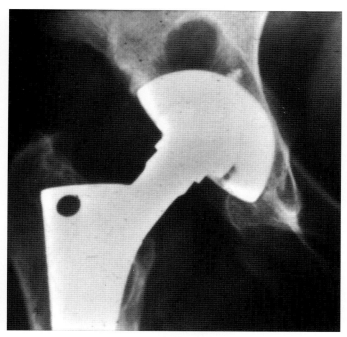

Figure 3. A: Linear osteolytic pattern around a loose cemented acetabular component. **B:** Focal expansile osteolytic pattern around a well-fixed cementless acetabular component.

gain access to trabecular bone in the ilium. Schmalzried et al. (36) demonstrated that the soft-tissue membrane that forms, which is essentially an extension of the joint pseudo-capsule, migrates along the interface between cement and subchondral bone and resorbs bone as it progresses toward the dome of the acetabulum. This results in the linear pattern of osteolysis seen radiographically around cemented sockets (Fig. 3A). As the interface is disrupted and disruption progresses to the dome of the acetabulum, loss of fixation results. Cemented acetabular components tend to migrate into this radiolucency. Although cystic or expansile osteolytic lesions are uncommon with cemented sockets, extensive bone loss still results.

In contrast, autopsy and animal studies have shown that after cementless acetabular replacement, one tends to see dense areas of ingrowth into the porous coating. This pattern of ingrowth tends to be patchy. As a result, with a bone-ingrown socket, the path of least resistance is through noningrown areas (gaps or fibrous tissue) around the periphery of the socket and through screw holes into the trabecular bone of the ilium, ischium, and pubis. This results in a more focal, expansile type of osteolysis (Fig. 3B). The consequence of this pattern of osteolysis is progressive bone loss. Unlike the situation with a cemented socket, loosening does not result until there is extensive bone loss, and loosening is usually acute and catastrophic. The patient often has no symptoms until this event occurs.

CIRCUMFERENTIAL VERSUS PATCH POROUS COATED STEMS

Another example of the consequences of the effective joint space is seen in a comparison of the patterns of osteolysis with circumferentially porous coated and patch porous coated cementless femoral components. In patch porous coated implants, the path of least resistance is often along the smooth portion of the stem into the diaphysis of the femur (Fig. 4). As a result, these types of stems are prone to diaphyseal osteolysis. Bobyn et al. (2) demonstrated this in an animal study in which partially porous coated rods were implanted into the distal femur of a rabbit.

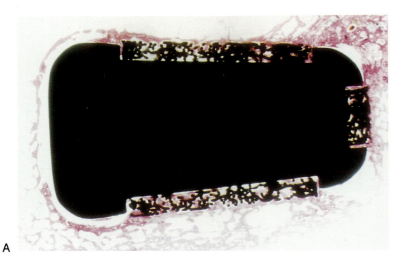

A

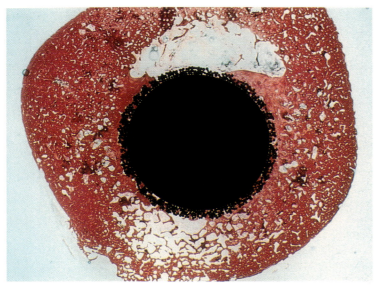

B

Figure 4. A: Bone remodeling pattern around a patch porous coated implant. Dense bone ingrowth into the titanium fiber mesh pads is present, as is a periprosthetic cavity around the smooth portion of the stem, which represents a potential access channel to the diaphysis. **B:** Bony remodeling pattern around a circumferentially porous coated stem. There is dense circumferential ingrowth. This is a relative barrier for ingress of joint fluid and polyethylene wear debris. (*4A*–Photo courtesy of Joshua Jacobs, MD. *4B*–Photo courtesy of Charles Engh, MD.)

Polyethylene particles were then injected into the joint. Histologic analysis demonstrated that the areas of bone ingrown were relative barriers to the ingress of joint fluid and polyethylene debris. In contrast, around the smooth portion of the implant, a periprosthetic cavity formed uniformly. The tissue in that cavity contained abundant polyethylene particles. Similar findings have been found at autopsy studies of patched porous coated implants used to treat humans (42). Two implant designs were compared in clinical studies: the Harris-Galante femoral component and the Multilock stem (Zimmer, Warsaw, Ind.) (29). The Harris-Galante femoral component is a titanium stem that has a fiber mesh patch porous coating on the anterior, posterior, and medial surfaces. The Multilock stem is a second-generation titanium alloy cementless stem that has circumferential porous coating. A matched-pairs study was performed by Maloney et al. that demonstrated that there was a 50% incidence of diaphyseal osteolysis in the Harris-Galante group compared with no diaphyseal osteolysis in the Multilock group after similar follow-up periods (Fig. 5). The findings are similar with the APR-I anatomic porous replacement (Intermedics, Austin, Tex.) stem which has patched porous coating, and with the initial S-ROM stem (Joint Medical Products, Stamford, Conn.), which had a seam that allowed access of joint fluid into the diaphyseal region of the femur. These studies pointed out the importance of implant design in the prevalence and location of osteolysis (1,4,5,7–10).

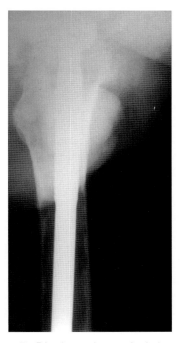

Figure 5. Diaphyseal osteolysis in association with a stable, proximal, patch
porous coated, cementless femoral
component. Extensive endosteal resorption is present in the diaphysis of
this femur.

THE BIOLOGIC PROCESS OF OSTEOLYSIS

When one is referring to aseptic loosening or osteolysis, the cause of bone loss appears
to be the same from the standpoint of the histopathologic features. This process has been
delineated through a variety of studies, including analysis of autopsy specimens, analysis
of material taken at revision operations, animal studies, and cell culture studies
(1,4,5,7–10,12–15,17–22,25,26,31,32,34,37–39,43,44). In general, the process of
periprosthetic bone resorption has been attributed to a biologic reaction to particulate wear
debris (25). Autopsy studies have been helpful in allowing us to understand the effects of
wear particles on periprosthetic tissues by demonstrating what that interface looks like in
the absence of particulate debris. They provide a unique opportunity to examine tissues
after a period of time with an implant *in vivo* and allow correlation of the mechanical
stability of the implant with the findings at the implant–bone interface.

Extensive studies have been done analyzing the cement–bone interface on both the
acetabular and femoral sides and the implant–bone interface with cementless hip
arthroplasties. These studies have shown repeatedly that the interface between bone and
implant in stable reconstruction, whether cemented or cementless, bulk biomaterials,
including bone cement, titanium and titanium alloys, and chrome cobalt alloys, are well
tolerated from a biologic standpoint. There appears to be no adverse reaction related to
toxicity of bone cement or ion release from metallic implants at least locally at the
interface between implant and bone.

These studies also have demonstrated that particulate wear debris is uniformly present
in an area of periprosthetic bone resorption. For example, analysis of cemented sockets
routinely demonstrates a soft-tissue membrane at the cement–bone interface. It dissects
the interface between implant and bone and resorbs bone beginning at the periphery of the
cemented socket and progressing toward the dome, eventually effecting implant stability.
Histologic analysis of this membrane reveals that it consists mainly of macrophages.

There is evidence of large amounts of submicron-sized polyethylene. Immunohistochemical staining has confirmed that the predominant cell in this soft-tissue membrane is a macrophage. *In situ* hybridization techniques have demonstrated that macrophages release interleukin-1β, a potent bone-resorbing cytokine. The histologic features of the pseudocapsule were first described by Willert (43). He found granulation tissue in the joint capsule and reported that the tissue appeared to be capable of inducing bone resorption. He further postulated that this phenomenon could result in loosening of the implant. Because of the limitations of light microscopic examination at the time of his report, Willert concluded that the wear particles, predominantly polyethylene, were relatively large compared with the metallic debris. Subsequent studies showed that the polyethylene wear particles are predominantly submicron-sized. Goldring et al. (9) described a synovium-like membrane at the cement–bone interface of patients with loose femoral components. This soft-tissue membrane was studied in tissue culture, and the investigators reported that the tissue had the capacity to produce both prostaglandin-E$_2$ and collagenase. They postulated that release of these substances, which were known to play a role in bone resorption, might explain the progressive lysis at the bone–implant interface.

These and other studies demonstrated that the histologic features of the soft-tissue membrane that forms between implant and bone are those of foreign-body granuloma (Fig. 6A). The granuloma appears to form in response to biomaterials that are incapable of being degraded or removed. The principle cell type in this granuloma is the macrophage

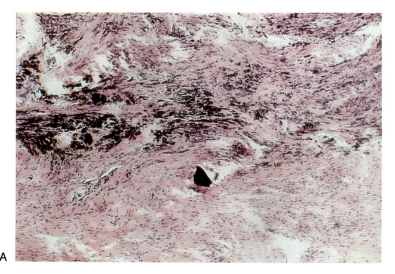

A

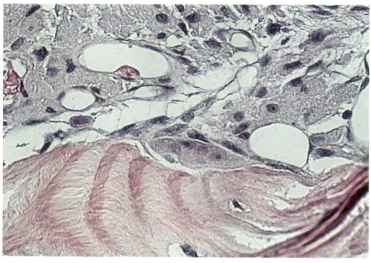

B

Figure 6. A: Interface membrane retrieved from a failed titanium cementless femoral component. Abundant titanium wear debris is *black* on this photomicrograph. **B:** Biopsy specimen from an osteolytic lesion. The membrane with osteoclastic giant cell is present at the membrane–bone interface.

(19). However, there often are relatively large numbers of fibroblasts and giant cells. Lymphocytes generally are not a prominent histologic feature, although they have been reported in small percentages. In addition, examination of the bone at the implant–bone interface has demonstrated what appear to be activated osteoclasts with resorption pits (Fig. 6B).

Santavirta et al. (33) examined tissue obtained from patients at revision total hip arthroplasty performed because of aggressive osteolytic lesions. They compared that tissue with tissue from patients who underwent revision joint replacement because of aseptic loosening without severe osteolysis. They found that with osteolysis, granulomatous lesions tended to lack activated fibroblasts. The investigators postulated that there was uncoupling of the macrophage-mediated clearance of particles in the fibroblast-mediated synthesis of extracellular matrix in the osteolytic lesions. They concluded that there may be two distinct histopathologic entities. However, these findings might also be explained on the basis of a continuum of the biologic response to particulate wear debris. It is possible that the normal response involving clearance and repair breakdown at high particle loads. The process subsequently cannot be walled off and focal osteolysis results.

Animal studies have been used to investigate the biologic responses to orthopedic implant materials. Cohen (5) was one of the first to investigate the foreign-body reaction to implant particles. He injected particulate metals subcutaneously into hamsters and rats and found they elicited an inflammatory reaction. Gelb et al. (7) used an air-pouch model to examine the effect of particle size, morphologic features, and surface area on the inflammatory response in rats. They demonstrated that small particles of bone cement caused more inflammation than large particles for a given mass. Irregularly shaped particles produced a greater response than spherical particles. There was also a difference in terms of production of bone-resorbing factors, larger particles producing a higher level of prostaglandin-E_2, and the presence of smaller particles resulting in higher levels of tumor necrosis factor. The investigators postulated that surface area may play a role in the type of response the particle induces.

Jasty et al. (16) used an animal model to examine the potential role of the immune system in response to wear particles. They implanted particles in mice with varying immunologic capacities. The mice included immunocompetent mice and mice deficient in T cells, T and B cells, and natural killer cells. They demonstrated that all mice, regardless of immunodeficiency, had a foreign-body response consisting of macrophages and giant cells when exposed to subcutaneous injection of polymethylmethacrylate powder. The investigators concluded that the immune system did not appear to play an important role in the cellular reaction to wear debris.

Cell culture studies have been used extensively to examine the reaction of cells to specific biomaterials. Although these studies do not mimic the dynamic situation that occurs in vivo, they allow quantitation of the effect of particles on cellular metabolism. These studies have predominantly examined the reaction of two cell types, macrophages and fibroblasts, to a variety of particulate biomaterials to determine the effect of these materials on cell viability and their effect on production and secretion of a variety of bone-resorbing factors.

Because the macrophage is the predominant cell type in periprosthetic granuloma, most cell culture studies have focused on these cells. Shanbhag et al. (39) reported on the ability of titanium alloy, commercially pure titanium, polyethylene produced in the laboratory, and polyethylene retrieved from membranes obtained at revision operations to stimulate macrophages to release bone-resorbing agents. In their study, titanium alloy particles were the most inflammatory on the basis of release of interleukin-1β, interleukin-6, and prostaglandin E_2. Similarly, Maloney et al. (22) challenged human macrophages with titanium alloy particles from interfacial membranes retrieved at revision surgery. The metabolic response of the macrophages included increased release of prostaglandin E_2, interleukin-1β, interleukin 6 and tumor necrosis factor α. Analysis of the macrophage response to particles of different sizes, concentrations, and compositions demonstrated that a variety of particulate biomaterials, including commercially pure titanium, bone cement, and polystyrene, stimulate the release of inflammatory cytokines such as interleukin-1 and prostaglandin-E_2 in a dose- and time-dependent manner (40). Titanium particles in the size range of 1 to 3 μm stimulated maximal bone-resorbing activity at concentrations that corresponded to the maximal release of interleukin-1. Anti-interleukin antibodies partially suppressed the bone-resorbing activity but did not completely suppress it. In addition, indomethacin also suppressed the bone-resorbing activity of the macrophage-conditioned medium, but the suppression was not complete. These data demonstrate that particulate biomaterials activate macrophages *in vitro* in a manner analogous to that observed around failed arthroplasties.

Most studies concerning cellular reactivity to wear debris have focused on the macrophage. The fibroblast is believed to be primarily responsible for synthesis and deposition of type I collagen, which provides structural integrity to the tissue. However, in addition to collagen synthesis, fibroblasts are capable of producing cytokines and enzymes that may influence tissue remodeling. Manlapaz et al. (29) studied the effect of titanium alloy particles obtained from revision membranes on human fibroblasts in culture. They demonstrated that these particles were potent stimulators of interleukin-6. Yao et al. (44) explored the response of fibroblasts to titanium particles and demonstrated that they responded with significantly increased expression of collagenase and stromelysin. In addition, the conditioned medium from the fibroblast cultures significantly decreased messenger ribonucleic acid (mRNA) levels of procollagen in osteoblast cells. These data suggest that the reaction of fibroblasts to particulate biomaterials may play a role in periprosthetic bone resorption.

The final common pathway in the osteolytic process is bone resorption. Although the osteoclast is the primary cell that resorbs bone, some data suggest that activated macrophages are capable of low-grade bone resorption. Murray and Rushton (31) studied this phenomenon by adding latex, which is considered to be inert, and zymosan, which is inflammatory, to cells in culture. They also studied the effect of polymethylmethacrylate and polyethylene particles. They then took the conditioned medium from these cultures and added it to neonatal mouse calvaria into which had been injected radioactive calcium. The investigators were able to measure the radioactive calcium release as an indicator of bone resorption. All the particles appeared to activate macrophages, and the presence of the resulting medium led to bone resorption when compared with the situation among controls. Zymosan as expected was the most stimulatory and latex the least. Both polymethylmethacrylate and polyethylene had an intermediate effect. Quinn et al. (32) examined the potential of macrophages to resorb bone by looking at macrophage cultures alone or in coculture with fibroblasts or osteoblasts. When these cells were stimulated with methyl methacrylate particles and slices of cortical bone were added to the cultures, low-grade bone resorption was seen at 7 days and increased by 14 days. Similarly, Athanasou et al. (1) demonstrated that small resorption pits formed when macrophages and macrophage polycaryons from the pseudocapsule of failed revision joint replacements were cultured on slices of cortical bone. Despite the evidence that macrophages may be capable of low-grade bone resorption, osteoclast activation is likely to be the main process by which aggressive bone resorption occurs, on the basis of the unique capability of osteoclasts to resorb bone.

SUMMARY

Osteolysis and aseptic loosening are believed by most orthopedic surgeons to be the most common and important long-term complications associated with total hip arthroplasty whether the operation is performed with or without bone cement. This process appears to be fueled by the biologic reaction to particulate wear debris and is likely to depend on several factors. These include the type, amount, and rate of wear debris production; access of this debris to the implant–bone interface and periprosthetic bone; and the biologic reaction to the wear debris, which may vary from one person to the next. Factors related to implant design and polyethylene manufacturing and sterilization may influence not only the generation of wear debris but also access of the debris to the implant–bone interface.

Future efforts to minimize this problem target several areas of research. First, one would like to minimize production of wear debris. Because most wear debris comes from the articulation, there is renewed interest in alternative bearing surfaces, such as metal-on-metal and ceramic-on-ceramic articulations. Work is ongoing to improve the wear characteristics of polyethylene. Despite technologic advances, it is unlikely that wear debris will be completely eliminated. It is important that we continue to study the underlying mechanisms of periprosthetic osteolysis. Further understanding of this process may make it possible to modulate or prevent this reaction pharmacologically.

REFERENCES

1. Athanasou NA, Quinn J, Bulstrode CJ. Resorption of bone by inflammatory cells derived from the joint capsule of hip arthroplasties. *J Bone Joint Surg Br* 1992;74:57–62.
2. Bobyn JD, Jacobs JJ, Tanzer M, et al. The susceptibility of smooth implant surfaces to peri-implant fibrosis and migration of polyethylene wear debris. *Clin Orthop* 1995;311:21–39.
3. Brown IW, Ring PA. Osteolytic changes in the upper femoral shaft following porous-coated hip replacement. *J Bone Joint Surg Br* 1985;67:218–221.
4. Chiba J, Rubash HE, Kim KJ, Iwaki Y. The characterization of cytokines in interface tissue obtained from failed cementless total hip arthroplasty with and without femoral osteolysis. *Clin Orthop* 1994;300:304–312.
5. Cohen J. Assay of foreign-body reaction. *J Bone Joint Surg Am* 1959;41:152–166.
6. Fisher J, Hailey JL, Chan KL, et al. The effect of aging following irradiation on the wear rate of UHMWPE. Transactions of the 41st Annual Meeting of the Orthopaedic Research Society, Orlando, FL, February 13–16, 1995. Vol. 1, p. 120.
7. Gelb H, Schumacher HR, Cuckler J, Baker DG. *In vivo* inflammatory responses to polymethylmethacrylate particulate debris: effect of size, morphology, and surface area. *J Orthop Res* 1994;12:83–92.
8. Glant T, Jacobs JJ, Molnar G, Shanbhag AS, Valyon M, Galante JO. Bone resorption activity of particulate stimulated macrophages. *J Bone Miner Res* 1993;8:1071–1079.
9. Goldring SR, Schiller AL, Roelke N, Rourke CM, O'Neil DA, Harris WH. The synovial-like membrane at the bone cement interface in loose total hip replacements and its proposed role in bone lysis. *J Bone Joint Surg Am* 1983;65:575–584.
10. Goodman SB, Fornasier VL, Kei J. The effects of bulk versus particulate polymethylmethacrylate on bone. *Clin Orthop* 1988;232:255–262.
11. Harris WH, Schiller AL, Scholler JM, Freiberg RA, Scott R. Extensive localized bone resorption in the femur following total hip replacement. *J Bone Joint Surg Am* 1976;58:612–618.
12. Haynes DR, Rogers SD, Hay S, Pearcy MJ, Howie DW. The differences in toxicity and release of bone resorbing mediators induced by titanium and cobalt chromium alloy wear particles. *J Bone Joint Surg Am* 1993;75:825–834.
13. Horowitz SM, Gautsch TL, Frondoza CG, Riley L. Macrophage exposure to polymethylmethacrylate leads to mediator release in injury. *J Orthop Res* 1991;9:406–413.
14. Jasty M, Bragdon C, Jiranek W, Chandler H, Maloney WJ, Harris WH. Etiology of osteolysis around porous coated cementless total hip arthroplasties. *Clin Orthop* 1994;308:111–126.
15. Jasty M, Floyd WE III, Schiller AL, Goldring SR, Harris WH. A localized osteolysis in stable, non-septic total hip replacement. *J Bone Joint Surg Am* 1986;68:912–919.
16. Jasty M, Jiranek W, Harris WH. Acrylic fragmentation in total hip replacements and its biological consequences. *Clin Orthop* 1992;285:116–128.
17. Jiranek WA, Machado M, Jasty MJ, et al. Production of cytokines around loose cemented acetabular components: analysis with immunohistochemical techniques and *in situ* hybridization. *J Bone Joint Surg Am* 1993;75:863–879.
18. Kim KJ, Chiba J, Rubash HE. *In vivo* and *in vitro* analysis of membranes from hip prostheses inserted without cement. *J Bone Joint Surg Am* 1994;76:172–180.
19. Kim KJ, Rubash HE, Wilson S, D'Antonio JA, McClain EJ. Histological and biochemical comparison of the interface tissues in cementless and cemented hip prostheses. *Clin Orthop* 1993;287:142–152.
20. Lee SH, Brennan FR, Jacobs JJ, Urban RM, Ragasa DR, Glant TT. Human monocyte/macrophage response to cobalt-chromium corrosion products and titanium particles in patients with total joint replacements. *J Orthop Res* 1997;15:40–49.
21. Maloney WJ, James RE, Smith RL. Human macrophage response to retrieved titanium alloy particles *in vivo*. *Clin Orthop* 1996;322:268–278.
22. Maloney WJ, Jasty MJ, Harris WH, Galante JO, Callaghan JJ. Endosteal erosion in association with stable uncemented femoral components. *J Bone Joint Surg Am* 1990;72:1025–1034.
23. Maloney WJ, Peters P, Engh CE, Chandler H. Severe osteolysis of the pelvis in association with acetabular replacement without cement. *J Bone Joint Surg Am* 1993;75:1627–1635.
24. Maloney WJ, Smith RL. Periprosthetic osteolysis in total hip arthroplasty: the role of particulate wear debris. *J Bone Joint Surg Am* 1995;77:1448–1461.
25. Maloney WJ, Smith RL, Castro F, Schurman DJ. Fibroblast response to metallic debris in vitro enzyme induction cell proliferation and toxicity. *J Bone Joint Surg Am* 1993;75:835–844.
26. Maloney WJ, Smith RL, Schmalzried TP, Chiba J, Huene D, Rubash, H. Isolation and characterization of wear particles generated in patients who have had failure of a hip arthroplasty without cement. *J Bone Joint Surg Am* 1995;77:1301–1310.
27. Maloney WJ, Woolson ST. Increasing incidence of osteolysis in association with uncemented Harris-Galante total hip arthroplasty. *J Arthroplasty* 1996;11:130–134.

28. Maloney WJ, Woolson ST, Conlon T, Rubash HE. Influence of stem design on the location and prevalence of femoral osteolysis: support for the gasket theory. Presented at the 64th Annual Meeting of the American Academy of Orthopaedic Surgeons; 1997 Feb 13–17; San Francisco.
29. Manlapaz M, Maloney WJ, Smith RL. In vitro activation of human fibroblast by retrieved titanium alloy wear debris. *J Orthop Res* 1996;17:465–472.
30. McKellop HA, Campbell P, Park SH, et al. The origin of submicron polyethylene wear debris in total hip arthroplasty. *Clin Orthop* 1995;311:3–20.
31. Murray DW, Rushton N. Macrophages stimulate bone resorption when they phagocytose particles. *J Bone Joint Surg Br* 1990;72:988–992.
32. Quinn J, Joyner C, Triffitt JT, Athanasou NA. Polymethylmethacrylate-Induced Inflammatory Macrophages resorb bone. *J Bone Joint Surg Br* 1992;74:652–658.
33. Santavirta S, Konttinen YT, Bergroth V, Eskola A, Tallroth K, Lindholm TS. Agressive granulomatous lesions associated with hip arthroplasty. immunopathological studies. *J Bone Joint Surg Am* 1990;72:252–258.
34. Schmalzried TP, Guttman D, Greculam HC. The relationship between design, position and articular wear of acetabular components inserted without cement and the development of pelvic osteolysis. *J Bone Joint Surg Am* 1994;76:677–688.
35. Schmalzried TP, Jasty M, Harris WH. Periprosthetic bone loss in total hip arthroplasty: polyethylene wear debris and the concept the effected joint space. *J Bone Joint Surg Am* 1992;74:849–863.
36. Schmalzried TP, Kwong LM, Jasty MJ, et al. The mechanism of loosening of cemented acetabular components in total hip arthroplasty: analysis retrieved at autopsy. *Clin Orthop* 1992;274:60–78.
37. Schmalzried TP, Maloney WJ, Kwong LM, Jasty M, Harris WH. Autopsy studies of the cement–bone interface of well-fixed cemented total hip replacements. *J Arthroplasty* 1993;8:179–188.
38. Shanbhag AS, Jacobs JJ, Black J, et al. Cellular media secreted by interfacial membranes obtained at revision total hip arthroplasty. *J Arthroplasty* 1995;10:498–506.
39. Shanbhag AS, Jacobs JJ, Black J, Galante JO, Glant TT. Human monocyte response to particulate biomaterials generated in vivo and in vitro. *J Orthop Res* 1995;13:792–801.
40. Shanbhag AS, Jacobs JJ, Black J, Galante JO, Glant TT. Macrophages/particle interaction: effect size, composition and surface area. *J Biomed Mater Res* 1994;28:81–90.
41. Urban RM, Jacobs JJ, Gilbert JL, Galante JO. Migration of corrosion products from modular hip prostheses. *J Bone Joint Surg Am* 1994;76:1345–1359.
42. Urban RM, Jacobs JJ, Sumner D, Peters CL, Voss FR, Galante JO. The bone implant interface of femoral stems with non-circumferential porous coating. *J Bone Joint Surg Am* 1996;76:1068–1081.
43. Willert HG. Reactions of the articular capsule to wear products of artificial joint prostheses. *J Biomed Mater Res* 1977;11:157–164.
44. Yao J, Glant TT, Lark MW, et al. The potential role of fibroblasts in periprosthetic osteolysis: fibroblast response to titanium particles. *J Bone Miner Res* 1995;10:1417–1427.
45. Zicat B, Engh CE, Gokcen E. Patterns of osteolysis around total hip components inserted with and without cement. *J Bone Joint Surg Am* 1996;77:432–439.

Revision Total Hip Arthroplasty,
edited by Marvin E. Steinberg and Jonathan P. Garino,
Lippincott Williams & Wilkins, Philadelphia © 1999.

3

Osteolysis and Aseptic Loosening: Clinical Picture

Charles W. Cha, Raj K. Sinha,
Arun S. Shanbhag,
and Harry E. Rubash

Total hip arthroplasty has evolved since its inception in 1959 by Sir John Charnley. The original concept, using polytetrafluoroethylene as a low-friction bearing surface, had unsatisfactory results because of poor wear resistance (5). In the ensuing decade, Charnley introduced polyethylene as a bearing surface and polymethylmethacrylate as a fixative for the components. The low coefficient of friction and superior wear characteristics of polyethylene improved the longevity of the implants, and established total hip arthroplasty as a treatment option for end stage arthritis of the hip.

In the 1970's, femoral component loosening in the absence of infection emerged as a cause of implant failure. The endosteal bone resorption that preceded loosening of these early cemented implants presented radiographically as linear periprosthetic radiolucencies (17). With time, the bone loss tended to progress evenly and diffusely around the entire prosthesis (45). The underlying pathologic process was referred to as *aseptic loosening* and was initially considered an adverse biologic reaction to the acrylic cement. Two separate approaches developed in an effort to solve the problem of aseptic loosening. Surgeons improved cementing techniques to increase the strength of the cement. Long-term results showed that the new cementing methods effectively reduced the incidence of mechanical failure (18,21,33,34). A second approach was to eliminate the use of acrylic cement and rely on biologic fixation for component stability. In association with these first-generation cementless implants, a new clinical entity emerged that was

---

C. W. Cha, R. K. Sinha, A. S. Shanbhag, and H. E. Rubash: Department of Orthopaedic Surgery, University of Pittsburgh, Pittsburgh, Pennsylvania 15213.

distinctly different from the aseptic loosening that was occurring in cemented implants. Focal radiolucencies at the implant–bone interface had a propensity to occur early and expand rapidly and became known as *osteolysis*. In general these lesions affected femoral stems and did not compromise implant stability unless bone loss was considerable. The ensuing failure would then necessitate a revision operation.

Though aseptic loosening and osteolysis tend to be differentiated radiographically, these two patterns of interfacial bone loss share a common etiologic mechanism. Particulate debris generated by the articulating prosthetic components is phagocytosed by macrophages in the periprosthetic environment (31). In response, the stimulated macrophages release a variety of inflammatory mediators into the surrounding tissues, which then stimulate osteoclastic resorption of periprosthetic bone (6,16,24). The specific pattern of interfacial bone loss seen radiographically appears to depend on the distribution and local concentration of wear particles at the interface. The joint fluid acts as the vehicle responsible for deposition of debris to the interface (42). An even distribution of wear debris at the interface is believed to lead to the linear bone resorption that is generally associated with aseptic loosening of cemented components. In contrast, localized concentrations of wear debris at the interface may produce the focal and expansile osteolysis associated with cementless implants (22), although this situation also may occur with cemented stems (2).

Given the etiologic features in common with bone loss, regardless of the radiographic pattern, it seems appropriate to use a singular term to describe the pathologic condition. This chapter uses the term *osteolysis* to represent the process of wear debris–mediated interfacial bone resorption. To differentiate between the two radiographic patterns, *focal osteolysis* refers to the focal and expansile lesions commonly seen with cementless implants, and *linear osteolysis* refers to the linear pattern of periprosthetic bone loss that was previously termed *aseptic loosening*.

RADIOGRAPHIC FEATURES OF OSTEOLYSIS

Patients with radiographic evidence of osteolysis often have no clinical asymptoms and may continue to have none despite substantial bone loss (28). Clinical symptoms may not occur until progressive bone loss has compromised implant stability. An unstable implant is prone to mechanical failure and may precipitate fracture of the surrounding periprosthetic bone. Early intervention may be necessary to prevent these catastrophic failures (Fig. 1) and the associated complications. The importance of close patient follow-up examinations with serial radiographs cannot be understated.

The radiographic patterns of osteolysis, whether linear or focal, are variable and depend on the distribution of wear debris at the periprosthetic interface. The mode of fixation and location of the implant determine which periprosthetic regions are accessible to the particle-rich joint fluid. The ensuing patterns of wear-debris accumulation at the interface ultimately define the radiographic appearance of the resultant lesions. It is important, therefore, to separately consider femoral and acetabular patterns of osteolysis for both cemented and uncemented implants. To facilitate radiographic description, the standardized radiographic zones for the femur as defined by Gruen et al. (17), modified by Johnston et al. (22), and for the acetabulum delineated by DeLee et al. (8) are used.

Cemented Implants

Radiographic analysis of cemented cups shows that linear osteolysis tends to begin peripherally, especially at the superior edge (zone 1). Analysis of 63 cemented cups demonstrated radiolucencies in 92% of instances, 85% occurring in zone 1 (51). A review of 680 instances of cemented total hip arthroplasty revealed radiolucent lines in zone 1 in 47% of instances as early as 6 months postoperatively, compared with 7% in zone 2 and 10% in zone 3 (14). Though these peripheral demarcations are prevalent, they are not clinically significant. When operative findings were directly compared with radiographic appearance, only 7% of cups with radiolucencies restricted to the outer third were loose (20).

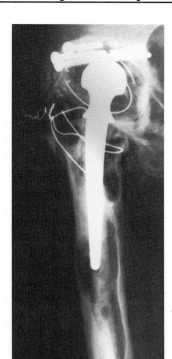

Figure 1. Lateral radiograph of a right cemented total hip arthroplasty. Catastrophic failure of the implant has occurred because of substantial focal and linear periprosthetic bone loss. Periprosthetic fracture is imminent.

In due course, osteolysis may progress medially until the entire cement–bone interface is disrupted (43). Radiographically this appears as a complete linear radiolucency in all three zones (Fig. 2), which strongly correlates with clinical loosening (20,51). Zicat et al. (51) found that 75% of patients who needed revision of a cemented cup had a continuous radiolucent line around the cup. Direct operative comparisons revealed that complete radiographic demarcation of a cup at least 1 mm thick correlated with clinical loosening 94% of the time (20). It appears that the extent of linear osteolysis along the interface best correlates with loss of implant stability.

Biologic and mechanical events at the cement–bone interface of cemented sockets dictate the radiographic presentation. Because the path of least resistance for wear particles is at the cement–bone interface, the resultant bone resorption is expected to begin at the peripheral margin of the cup that is in direct contact with the particle-laden synovial fluid (43). Reconstitution of subchondral bone at the cement–bone interface partially blocks the access of particles to the underlying trabeculae. Particles are thereby dispersed evenly at the interface, which results in a uniform pattern of circumferential bone resorption that is manifested radiographically as a linear osteolysis (43,51).

Analogous to the resorptive process for cemented cups, whether linear or focal osteolytic lesions develop around cemented femoral implants depends primarily on the pattern of access and distribution of particulate debris in the periprosthetic environment. With early cemented femoral implants, linear osteolysis frequently formed along the entire prosthesis (17). Improved cementing techniques decreased the incidence of linear osteolysis to 3% at 11 years (33), and the lesions formed predominantly in the proximal femur (Fig. 3). These changes may be attributed to several factors. The relatively small femoral surface exposed to the joint fluid limits the amount of debris introduced. In addition, the improved cement mantle diminishes access of particulate debris and reduces production of cement particles because of stem

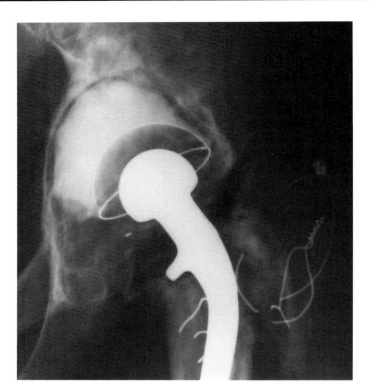

Figure 2. Anteroposterior radiograph of a left cemented total hip arthroplasty. A linear radiolucent line has developed along the entire bone–cement interface of the acetabular component. Broken wires can accelerate polyethylene wear if they migrate into the articulation and act as third bodies.

debonding and cement fracture. The net result is that less debris collects at the interface and the incidence and progression of osteolysis are reduced.

Though documented to occur proximally (33), focal osteolysis around cemented femurs is primarily seen distally, adjacent to the stem tip. Several mechanisms have been proposed to account for this radiographic finding. High intraarticular pressures generated during the gait cycle may force particles into the cement–implant interface and along the implant to the distal regions (2). The resultant debonding of the cement and implant predominantly appears radiographically as a radiolucent line between the stem and cement in zone 1. Gruen et al. (17) found this debonding among 10% of their patients. In a 10-year follow-up review of 54 total hip arthroplasty procedures, 17 of 54 implants exhibited debonding in zone 1 (39). Particles within the cement–implant interface may exit to the endosteal bone through defects in the distal cement mantle and stimulate the biologic response that leads to focal bone resorption (2). Review of 29 loose Iowa implants documented a consistent progression of radiographic findings that culminated in the development of focal osteolysis in a manner consistent with this mechanism. Radiographs initially displayed superolateral debonding. This was followed by development of a progressive cement–implant radiolucency. Twenty of 29 loose hips formed osteolytic lesions, and the most were distal (32).

Other investigators proposed that the wear particles access the bone–cement interface directly. An experimental joint capsule was fabricated over femurs containing a cemented total hip implant. Colored pigment was injected into the capsule, and its distribution at the interfaces was monitored after cyclic pressurization of the joint fluid. The pigment localized predominantly to the bone–cement interface (38).

Acrylic cement rather than the intraarticular wear debris has been postulated as a cause of focal bone loss. Radiographic analysis by Maloney et al. (29) identified focal osteolytic lesions in zones 2 and 5. Sixty percent of the lesions were associated with either a defect of the cement mantle or an area of thin cement. Further histologic analysis of tissue retrieved from the lesions

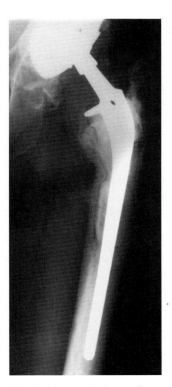

Figure 3. Anteroposterior radiograph of a left cemented total hip arthroplasty. Even distribution of wear debris along the bone–cement interface has led to formation of a linear radiolucent line around the proximal cement mantle.

did not show any evidence of polyethylene debris. However, particulate polymethyl methacrylate was present at histologic examination. The authors suggested that poor operative technique led to the development of areas within the cement mantle that were mechanically predisposed to fragmentation. High local concentrations of particulate cement were generated and believed to have stimulated the biologic cascade that resulted in focal osteolysis.

Uncemented Implants

With cementless cups, whether a linear or focal pattern of bone loss occurs depends on the amount and location of bony ingrowth into the component. This is a function of implant design and operative technique. Many of the original acetabular components were hemispheric with a porous metal backing. These were initially placed into the acetabulum by means of line-to-line or exact-fit techniques (the outer diameter of the cup matches the diameter of the final acetabular reamer). Because of lack of interference with the adjacent bone with this technique, many of these cups relied on screw fixation for initial postoperative stability. Though screw placement facilitates good bone contact where the cup is secured, there is a propensity for peripheral gap formation. In a radiographic analysis of 83 Harris-Galante porous coated (HGP; Zimmer, Warsaw, Ind.) cups, Schmalzried et al. (41) found peripheral gaps on immediately postoperative radiographs in 50% of instances. The lack of bone apposition and bone ingrowth at the cup margins may make this region unstable and allow for micromotion, which results in sclerosis of the adjacent bone and fibrous membrane formation at the interface. Consequently the peripheral gap that forms allows particulate debris in the intraarticular fluid to gain access to the bone–implant interface. Particulate induced bone resorption then proceeds in a process similar to the mechanism described earlier for cemented cups. The peripheral gaps expand and migrate medially in a circumferential manner (43) that presents radiographically as linear osteolysis. On subsequent follow-up evaluation of the 83 cups, Schmalzried et al. (41) found that the peripheral gaps were associated with a 39% incidence of progressive linear osteolysis compared with a 14% incidence of linear osteolysis when peripheral gaps were not present. In the series, only one focal osteolytic lesion and no continuous linear radiolucencies were found. In another analysis of 136 HGP cups after an average follow-up period of 7 years, discontinuous radiolucent lines were observed in 34 hips, mostly in peripheral zones 1 and 3. Only two hips displayed focal osteolysis (25) (Fig. 4).

In contrast to the HGP cup, the anatomic medullary locking (AML; DuPuy, Warsaw, Ind.) and the porous coated anatomic (PCA; Howmedica, Rutherford, N.J.) cups are press fit into the acetabulum by seating a larger-diameter cup into an underreamed socket. These components rely on peripheral bone contact for initial stability and bone ingrowth for ultimate stability. The areas of peripheral bony ingrowth serve as barriers to the ingress of particulate debris. However, well-ingrown areas occupy only a small percentage of the implant surface. The remaining noningrown areas rest in direct contact with trabecular bone, because bony reconstitution and sclerosis do not occur in the absence of motion (11,28). The path of least resistance for particles is gaps between areas of ingrowth or an alternative portal of entry, such as screw holes or polar holes, that provide access to the soft cancellous bone of the pelvis (43). This particle migration stimulates local bone resorption that expands focally into the surrounding pelvis. The radiographic manifestation of this process is a focal, expansile, ballooning radiolucency (28,40).

Radiographic reviews of the AML cup indicate a 20% incidence of acetabular osteolysis, predominantly in zone 3 at intermediate follow-up times (9,51). Although the PCA cup seems to have a lower rate of pelvic lysis, varying from 4% to 9% at intermediate follow-up times (23,37,50), the incidence of osteolysis with this component may increase considerably with time. Owen et al. (37) found that the osteolysis rate was 8% less than

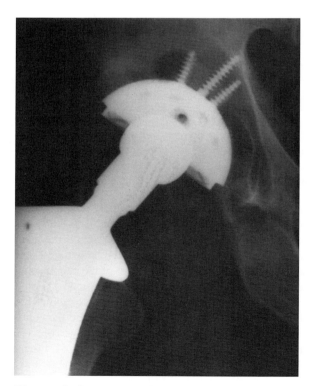

Figure 4. Anteroposterior radiograph of a right uncemented total hip arthroplasty. A focal osteolytic lesion has formed adjacent to the hemispheric acetabular component in the vicinity of a screw (zone 2).

5 years after implantation compared with 36% more than 5 years after implantation. The clinical significance of these lesions and their propensity for progression will be clarified as long-term results become available.

The threaded acetabular designs are associated with high rates of osteolysis (13). The lesions are seen radiographically as early as 3 years postoperatively and tend to expand rapidly (13). Unlike osteolysis with other designs, these lesions have a dramatic clinical effect; the prevalence of painful loosening ranges from 20% to 31% at 5 years (13).

Because the radiographic appearance of osteolysis in uncemented cups is a function of bone ingrowth, it would be advantageous to be able to assess radiographically the adequacy of acetabular bone ingrowth and pelvic bone loss. However, histologic correlations with follow-up radiographs indicates that use of conventional radiographic views leads to overestimation of bone apposition and underestimation of gap areas (11). It has also been shown that radiographs underestimate the size of osteolytic lesions (28). The addition of Judet views in the radiographic assessment of uncemented cups may improve the ability to detect lucencies (34). In a radiographic analysis of HGP cups, the use of judet views increased the detection of interface gaps by 46% (41). Whether these additional views can improve estimations of bone apposition is not yet clear.

With cementless stems, prosthetic design features markedly affect the radiographic picture. The HGP implant is a straight titanium alloy stem with proximally placed titanium fiber-metal mesh pads on the anterior, posterior, and medial surfaces. The HGP and other patch porous coated designs such as the anatomic porous replacement (APR-l; Intermedics, Austin Tex.) have smooth seams between the areas of porous coating proximally, which form low resistance pathways for access of debris to the distal portions of the interface (3). The particles adjacent to the smooth diaphyseal portion of the stem stimulate a scalloped pattern of endosteal bone loss (Fig. 5). The incidence of focal, endosteal osteolysis associated with HGP implants ranges from 8% to 52% and increases with the

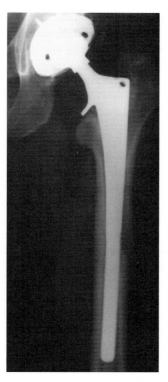

Figure 5. Anteroposterior radiograph of a left uncemented total hip arthroplasty. Focal osteolysis is adjacent to the femoral implant in the middiaphyseal region (zone 2).

duration of implantation. These studies uniformly report the lesions to be located in the diaphysis, predominantly Gruen zones 3, 4, and 5 (15,29,30,46). Osteolysis developed around the APR-l implant in 40% of instances. Like the HGP implant, the lesions occurred in the middle to distal femoral regions (47).

Unlike patch porous coated implants, circumferentially porous coated designs (AML and PCA) lack smooth proximal seams between the porous pads. The particles do not have an easy passage into the femoral diaphysis; therefore to enter the interface the debris must migrate into gaps between bone ingrown areas. Local accumulation of debris is generally restricted to the proximal femur, and the characteristic radiographic appearance consists of focal cystic lesions localized to the greater and lesser trochanters. Two large studies of the AML prosthesis found the incidence of osteolysis to be about 20%. All of the lesions were situated in either zone 1 or zone 7 (9,51). Reviews of use of PCA implants showed a similar incidence of femoral osteolysis as with AML implants. However, the lesions were not restricted to the proximal femur; both midstem and distal lesions have been documented to occur with this design (19,23,50). The debris presumably gained access to the diaphysis in these instances through noningrown areas along the porous surface. Extended duration of implantation or a greater particulate burden from the large 32-mm femoral heads often used with the PCA implant may have contributed to the bone loss.

If bone ingrowth does not occur around the entire porous coating of a cementless femoral implant, the prosthesis may still be stabilized with fibrous tissue at the interface (10). Initial micromotion at the interface stimulates reconstitution of the endosteal bone, which manifests radiographically as reactive lines adjacent to the implant. Linear osteolysis can occur that is similar to that seen with cemented femoral implants.

LOOSENING: CLINICAL PRESENTATION

When a patient has a painful hip after total hip arthroplasty, the main concern is that progressive osteolysis has loosened the implant. Other possible causes include sepsis, periprosthetic fracture, tendinitis, referred spinal pain, heterotopic ossification, subluxation, dislocation, and trochanteric nonunion after osteotomy (12). A detailed and thorough history and physical examination are essential to narrow the differential diagnoses. It is especially important to eliminate sepsis.

Key points in the medical history and physical examination can help make the distinction. Patient age and activity level are important. Younger and more active patients have a higher rate of aseptic loosening. Location of the pain can help identify the pain source. Thigh pain suggests a femoral disorder, and groin and buttock pain often point to the acetabular component. During the evaluation, the timing of pain onset, duration, presence of a painless interval, pain quality, aggravating features, concurrent medical illness or procedures, previous infection, and associated systemic symptoms all must be recorded. Patients with no clinical symptoms and an aseptically loose hip usually have weight-bearing or activity-related pain that is relieved by rest. They experience symptoms many years after the initial total hip replacement and have an associated pain-free interval before the onset of symptoms. At physical examination, a limp or Trendelenburg gait may be seen. The limb may be shortened and held in external rotation, and there may be pain with passive rotation of the affected extremity.

Patients with septic loosening report night or rest pain that is constant and not associated with activity. The onset of pain is usually earlier than with aseptic loosening, and sepsis should be suspected if the pain has persisted since implantation (12). The physical findings are similar to those for aseptic loosening, and a thorough inspection for possible sources of infection should be undertaken. A draining wound, delayed postoperative fever, history of infection, and systemic illness such as rheumatoid arthritis support an infections causation (12).

These are generalized clinical scenarios that do not apply to all cases. A patient may have overlapping findings common for both aseptic and septic loosening, making diagnosis difficult. For example, patients with aseptic loosening of implants may have night pain and may seek treatment as early as 12 months postoperatively. Pain suggestive of loosening can be misleading because stable uncemented femoral implants can cause thigh pain in as many as 18% of instances (19,23). Extensive osteolysis can be asymptomatic, and loose, uncemented implants secured with fibrous tissue can be painless. It becomes clear that the diagnosis of loosening whether septic or aseptic is difficult to make solely on the basis of medical history.

Laboratory studies can complement the medical history by helping to differentiate septic and aseptic loosening. White blood cell count, erythrocyte sedimentation rate (ESR), and C-reactive protein (CRP) values are commonly obtained to identify the infected hip prosthesis (12). The white blood cell count can be helpful if elevated, though many patients with septic arthroplasties have with a normal level. ESR and CRP are acute-phase reactants that become elevated in certain inflammatory states, such as infection. An ESR greater than 30 mm/h and a CRP greater than 20 mg/L with a consistent clinical presentation suggest an infected implant (1).

LOOSENING: CLINICAL INCIDENCE

Outcomes associated with the various techniques and implant designs serve as a basis of comparison to promote further improvement. However, outcome reviews are difficult to summarize because the defined clinical end point varies between studies. Some reports define clinical failures strictly as cases of loosening confirmed during revision operations. Others use one of the many radiographic criteria of loosening to mark the clinical end point. To avoid confusion, this summary defines the radiographic criteria that identify a loose implant and reports the clinical incidence of prosthetic loosening as a combination of surgically revised cases and cases that are definitely loose radiographically.

Cemented Implants

Harris et al. (18) defined three categories to assess the stability of cemented femoral components. The implant is considered *definitely loose* if plain radiographs display evidence of subsidence, radiolucency at the stem–cement interface, a crack in the cement mantle, or stem fracture. Stems are *probably loose* if a complete radiolucent zone surrounds the entire cement mantle. *Possibly loose* stems demonstrate a radiolucent zone over 50% to 100% of the cement–bone interface.

There are more than three decades of experience with total hip arthroplasty. Long-term follow-up studies with the initial patients treated with first-generation cementing techniques (hand mixing and finger packing of the cement) have surpassed the 20-year mark. Reports with follow-up periods of at least 10 years indicate that loosening of first-generation cemented femoral components occurs in 7% to 30% of instances (39,45). Improvements in cementing technique, so-called second-generation technique, such as use of medullary plug, lavage of the intramedullary canal, and retrograde delivery of cement with a cement gun, have dramatically improved the durability of cemented femoral implants. The outcome at an intermediate follow-up time was excellent with a rate of loosening that was less than 3% up to 10 years (33). Though this rate has increased to 7% at 15 years, the overall impact of these technical innovations is significant (34). Third-generation cementing techniques, which include centralization of the stem, porosity reduction, and surface modification, are being used. Short to intermediate-term results are consistent with those of second-generation techniques (15,32). The long-term effect of these modern improvements has yet to be revealed.

At radiographic evaluation of the acetabulum, a cemented cup is considered definitely loose if the component has migrated or the cement mantle has cracked. *Impending loosening* refers to cups with a continuous radiolucent zone around the cement mantle that is at least 2 mm thick (36). Studies indicate that radiographic assessment of cemented femoral component loosening is more accurate than that of cemented acetabular loosening (36). O'Neill et al. (36) analyzed plain radiographs of 61 patients undergoing revision operations and correctly predicted loosening of 89% of the femoral components, whereas they correctly identified loosening of only 37% of the cemented cups preoperatively.

Carlsson et al. (4) found that only 31% of cemented cups that on radiographs showed a continuous radiolucency greater than 2 mm actually were loose. They also found that 35% of sockets showing radiographic evidence of migration were stable at operation.

In contrast to these findings, Hodgkinson et al. (20) were able to correlate operative findings with radiographic signs of loosening. All cups that had migrated on surveillance radiographs were loose surgically. Cups with radiographic demarcation around the entire interface were loose 94% of the time. If radiolucencies were restricted to two zones, then 71% of cups were loose, and if restricted to one zone, only 7% were loose.

The inconsistencies associated with radiographic detection of socket loosening may relate to difficulty in differentiating radiographic signs. Socket migration is more difficult to discern radiographically than stem migration (36). Clinically insignificant linear radiolucencies are commonly seen around cemented sockets. Exact reproduction of pelvic position on conventional radiographic views is difficult, and conventional views do not adequately represent the entire periprosthetic acetabular interface. Clearly, plain radiographic assessment of implanted cups is of limited accuracy.

Supplementing plain radiography with an arthrographic evaluation may improve detection of aseptically loose cups. Specific arthrographic criteria to diagnose loosening generally include penetration of contrast medium into the cement–implant interface or extended penetration of contrast medium between the cement and surrounding bone (36). For cemented cups, contrast medium in at least two adjacent zones allowed prediction of 90% to 100% of loose implants. These results represent considerable improvement over the documented accuracy of plain radiography. In instances of suspected socket loosening without radiographic evidence of migration, arthrograms may play a useful diagnostic role. Though arthrographic predictions of femoral loosening were impressive, they did not offer appreciable diagnostic advantage over plain radiographic assessment.

The early results with cement-fixed polyethylene cups were encouraging. However, with first-generation techniques, the incidence of cup loosening increased dramatically after 10 years, approaching 30% in some studies. Unlike cementing of femurs, newer cementing techniques did not improve the clinical outcome with cemented cups. Mulroy and Harris (34), using second-generation cement, found that 44% of cups were loose 14 years postoperatively. With cemented cups, the exposed surface in continuity with the effective joint space is relatively large compared with the volume of the associated cement–bone interface. The generous amount of debris that can gain access through the peripheral margins can affect implant cup stability in the long term and may account for the high rates of cemented-cup loosening. The persistence of late acetabular loosening despite modern techniques led investigators to cite acetabular loosening as one of the main problems in modern total hip arthroplasty.

Cementless Implants

Radiographic criteria to identify loose cementless components are not well established, partly because of the wide variety of cementless implant designs. Regarding porous coated femoral components, Engh et al. (10) identified certain radiographic signs that were indicative of successful bone ingrowth and others that indicated femoral component instability. Absence of reactive lines adjacent to the porous surface and endosteal "spot welds" correlated strongly with successful bone ingrowth. Additional signs that suggested successful bone ingrowth included proximal stress shielding and cortical density at the stem tip. Femoral loosening was definitely evident if progressive implant migration was seen radiographically. Divergent reactive lines, calcar hypertrophy, pedestal formation, shedding of the porous coating, and progressive radiolucencies adjacent to the porous coating also suggested an unstable femoral implant.

Intermediate-term data indicate that the clinical performance of cementless prostheses depends on implant design features and anatomic location. Though some of the early cementless stems have outperformed early-generation cemented stems, whether they will compare favorably with the stems implanted with second- and third-generation cementing techniques will be clarified as long-term data become available. The Bias (Zimmer) and

Identifit femoral components (Thackery, Leeds, England) experienced high rates of loosening, on the order of 35% and 28%, respectively (26,35). With the HGP prosthesis, diaphyseal osteolysis led to loosening in 9% to 32% of cases 44 to 74 months after implantation (15,30,49). Though porous coated stems, such as the AML and PCA implants, had high rates of focal osteolysis in the proximal zones, these lesions generally did not jeopardize implant fixation. At 5 to 7 years, loosening rates for the PCA implant varied between 2% and 7% (23,37,50). In their analyses, both Owen et al. (37) and Kim et al. (23) found that all loosened stems were undersized and did not adequately fill the intramedullary canal. Kim et al. (23) found that all stable stems were adequately sized. It appears that strict preoperative planning and confirmation of intramedullary fill with two radiographic views may dramatically improve clinical results with the PCA stem. In a large review of use of the AML stem, after average 11-year follow-up period, the rate of loosening was only 1.5%. This compares favorably with the success of second-generation cemented stems (9).

Regardless of loosening rates, the incidence of thigh pain with some cementless stem designs, even when stable, has compromised the clinical results. Thigh pain is associated with 14% to 26% of implanted cementless prostheses (19,23). Described as a dull ache after extended weight bearing, this pain, which occurs less frequently with cemented stems, may be attributed to irritation of the endosteum by a mobile stem tip.

To address the problems of osteolysis and thigh pain, second-generation cementless components have emerged. Modifications, including proximal implant wedging, distal implant fluting, and surface hardening, have been implemented to improve the clinical results with cementless implants. Early follow-up evaluation of a series of 130 second-generation implants reveal a high level of implant stability and no femoral or pelvic osteolysis. Only one patient had intermittent thigh pain (7). If this early clinical success persists in the long term, both cemented and cementless fixation will be viable methods of femoral component implantation.

As with cemented cups, radiographic determination of loosening for cementless cups is difficult, because osteolysis is found frequently and pelvic orientation often is inconsistent between radiographs. Migration is the hallmark of a loose cementless socket. Associated radiographic signs include implant fracture, screw breakage, shedding of the porous surface, and progressive periprosthetic radiolucencies (48).

The performance of cementless sockets relies heavily on component design. Threaded cups, which are screwed into the acetabulum, initially were very stable. However, considerable periprosthetic bone resorption around these cups resulted in high rates (40%) of failure (13). Hemispheric cup designs rely on either peripheral bony interference due to underreaming or transimplant screw fixation for stability. Taken collectively, these implants have outperformed cemented acetabula at intermediate follow-up evaluations. With regard to the AML cup, only a small percentage need revision despite the frequent occurrence of periprosthetic osteolysis. In one large study, 6 of 146 cups were revised because of aseptic loosening at 7 years, whereas 20% of patients had osteolytic lesions on radiographs (9). Analysis of the PCA cup reveals that osteolysis and loosening occur at similar rates, 5% to 7% on average (23,37,50). The clinical and radiographic performance of the HGP cup has been excellent at intermediate follow-up evaluations; associated osteolysis and loosening are almost nonexistent (30,40,44,49). A multicenter retrospective review of more than 1,000 HGP cups found osteolysis in 2.3% of instances and implant migration of only three cups (27). However, the propensity for late loosening of cemented sockets dictated that long-term follow-up data on the HGP cups be available before definite conclusions are drawn.

CONCLUSION

Though the clinical presentation of osteolysis varies, the pathogenesis of the disease can be consolidated into a single mechanism. Basic scientific studies have demonstrated that osteolysis is a wear debris-mediated phenomenon. The ultimate pattern of bone resorption that occurs in response to wear debris depends on the quantity and distribution of wear particles at the bone–cement or bone–implant interface, which is a function of anatomic location, implant design, and mode of fixation. Large, localized collections of wear debris, which can accumulate adjacent to cement cracks or cementless implants, stimulate formation of rapidly expansile and focal osteolysis. Even dispersal of particles at the interface of cemented or fibrous stable cementless implants leads to a more slowly progressive pattern of linear osteolysis.

Loosening of components due to progression of interfacial bone loss was a concern with early total hip arthroplasty. At present, because of technological improvements over the past three decades, the problem of component loosening has decreased. Time has shown that hemispheric, metal-backed acetabular components implanted without cement and femoral components placed with contemporary cement techniques have low rates of loosening at long-term follow-up evaluation. Modern cementless femoral designs may prove to be equally as effective as long-term data become available. Though the incidence of loosening has diminished considerably, osteolysis remains a concern and is the chief problem facing modern total hip arthroplasty.

To solve the problem of osteolysis, future efforts must be directed at decreasing the production of particulate debris and modifying the biologic response to it. Improvements in the manufacture, sterilization, and storage of polyethylene or the development of alternative bearing materials such as ceramics or metal-on-metal articulations may effectively reduce formation of particulate wear debris. Efforts to modulate the host response to the debris by pharmacologic or immunologic means may inhibit bone resorption. Until such technology becomes available, orthopedic surgeons must become familiar with the peculiarities of the many implant designs so that osteolysis can be detected early, followed closely, and managed in a timely manner.

REFERENCES

1. Aalto K, Osterman K, Peltola H, Rasanen J. Changes in erythrocyte sedimentation rate and C-reactive protein after total hip arthroplasty. *Clin Orthop* 1984;184:118–120.
2. Anthony PP, Gie GA, Howie CR, Ling RSM. Localised endosteal bone lysis in relation to the femoral components of cemented total hip arthroplasties. *J Bone Joint Surg* 1990;72:971–979.
3. Bobyn JD, Jacobs JJ, Tanzer M, Urban et al. The susceptibility of smooth implant surfaces to periimplant fibrosis and migration of polyethylene wear debris. *Clin Orthop* 1995;311:21–39.
4. Carlsson AS, Gentz C. Radiographic versus clinical loosening of the acetabular component in noninfected total hip arthroplasty. *Clin Orthop* 1984;185:145–150.
5. Charnley J. Arthroplasty of the hip. *Lancet* 1961;1:1129–1132.
6. Chiba J, Rubash HE, Kim KJ, Iwaki Y. The characterization of cytokines in the interface tissue obtained from failed cementless total hip arthroplasty with and without femoral osteolysis. *Clin Orthop* 1994;300: 304–312.
7. Conlan TK, Fenwick J, Rubash HE, Bobyn JD, Mehta S, Trakru S. The Multilock uncemented femoral prosthesis: a clinical and radiographic review with minimum two-year follow-up. Presented at the 64th Annual Meeting of the American Academy of Orthopaedic Surgons; 1997 Feb 13–17; San Francisco.
8. Delee JG, Charnley J. Radiological demarcation of cemented sockets in total hip arthroplasty. *J Clin Invest* 1979;64:1386–1392.
9. Engh CA, Hooten JPJ, Zettl-Schaffer KF, et al. Porous-coated total hip replacement. *Clin Orthop* 1994; 298:89–96.
10. Engh CA, Massin P, Suthers KE. Reoentgenographic assessment of the biologic fixation of porous-surfaced femoral components. *Clin Orthop* 1990;257:107–128.
11. Engh CA, Zettl-Schaffer KF, Kukita Y, Sweet D, Jasty M, Bragdon C. Histological and radiographic assessment of well functioning porous-coated acetabular components. *J Bone Joint Surg Am* 1993;75:814–824.
12. Evans BG, Cuckler JM. Evaluation of the painful total hip arthroplasty. *Orthop Clin North Am* 1992;23:303–311.
13. Fox GM, McBeath AA, Heiner JP. Hip replacement with a threaded acetabular cup. *J Bone Joint Surg Am* 1994;76:195–201.
14. Garcia-Cimbrelo E, Munuera L. Early and late loosening of the acetabular cup after low-friction arthroplasty. *J Bone Joint Surg* 1992;74:1119–1129.
15. Goetz DD, Smith EJ, Harris WH. The prevalence of femoral osteolysis associated with components inserted with or without cement in total hip replacements. *J Bone Joint Surg Am* 1994;76:1121–1129.
16. Goldring SR, Schiller A, Roelke M, Rourke, CM, O'Neill DA, Harris WH. The synovial-like membrane at the bone-cement interface in loose total hip replacements and its proposed role in bone lysis. *J Bone Joint Surg Am* 1983;65:575–584.
17. Gruen TA, McNeice GM, Amstutz HC. "Modes of failure" of cemented stem-type femoral components. *Clin Orthop* 1979;141:17–27.
18. Harris WH, McCarthy JC, O'Neill DA. Femoral component loosening using contemporary techniques of femoral cement fixation. *J Bone Joint Surg Am*1982;64:1063–1067.

19. Heekin RD, Callaghan JJ, Hopkinson WJ, Savory CG, Xenos JS. The porous-coated anatomic total hip prosthesis, inserted without cement. *J Bone Joint Surg Am* 1993;75:77–91.
20. Hodgkinson JP, Shelley P, Wroblewski BM. The correlation between the roentgenographic appearance and operative findings at the bone-cement junction of the socket in Charnley low friction arthroplasties. *Clin Orthop* 1988;228:105–109.
21. Hozack WJ, Rothman RH, Booth REJ, Balderston RA. Cemented versus cementless total hip arthroplasty. *Clin Orthop* 1993;289:161–165.
22. Johnston RC, Fitzgerald RHJ, Harris WH, Poss, R, Muller ME, Sledge, CB. Clinical and radiographic evaluation of total hip replacement: a standard system of terminology for reporting results. *J Bone Joint Surg Am* 1990;72:161–168.
23. Kim Y, Kim VEM. Uncemented porous-coated anatomic total hip replacement. *J Bone Joint Surg Br* 1993;75:6–14.
24. Kim KJ, Rubash HE, Wilson SE, D'Antonio JA, McClain EJ. A histological and biochemical comparison of the interface tissues in cementless and cemented hip prosthesis. *Clin Orthop* 1993;286:142–152.
25. Latimer HA, Lachiewicz PF. Porous-coated acetabular component with screw fixation. *J Bone Joint Surg Am* 1996;78:975–981.
26. Lombardi AV, Mallory TH, Eberle RW, Mitchell MB, Lefkowitz MS, Williams JR. Failure of intraoperatively customized non-porous femoral components inserted without cement in total hip arthroplasty. *J Bone Joint Surg Am* 1995;77:1836–1844.
27. Maloney WJ, Anderson MJ, Jacobs JJ, et al. Polyethylene wear and pelvic osteolysis in association with the Harris-Gallante socket in primary total hip replacement. Presented at the 63rd Annual Meeting of the American Academy of Orthopaedic Surgeons; Feb. 22–26, 1996; Atlanta.
28. Maloney WJ, Engh CA, Chandler H. Severe osteolysis of the pelvis in association with acetabular replacement without cement. *J Bone Joint Surg Am* 1993;75:1627–1635.
29. Maloney WJ, Woolson ST. Increasing incidence of femoral osteolysis in association with the uncemented Harris-Galante total hip arthroplasty. *J Arthroplasty* 1996;11:130–134.
30. Martell JM, Pierson RH, Jacobs JJ, Rosenberg AG, Maley M, Galante JO. Primary total hip reconstruction with a titanium fiber–coated prosthesis inserted without cement. *J Bone Joint Surg AM* 1993;75:554–571.
31. Mirra JM, Marder RA, Amstutz HC. The pathology of failed total joint arthroplasty. *Clin Orthop* 1982;170:175–183.
32. Mohler CG, Kull LR, Martell JM, Rosenberg AG, Galante, JO. Total hip replacement with insertion of an acetabular component without cement and a femoral component with cement. *J Bone Joint Surg Am* 1995;77:86–96.
33. Mulroy RD, Jr, Harris WH. The effect of improved cementing techniques on component loosening in total hip replacement. *J Bone Joint Surg Br* 1990;72:757–760.
34. Mulroy WF, Estok DM, Harris WH. Total hip arthroplasty with use of so-called second-generation cementing techniques. *J Bone Joint Surg Am* 1995;77:1845–1852.
35. Nashed RS, Becker DA, Gustilo RB. Are cementless acetabular components the cause of excess wear and osteolysis in total hip arthroplasty? *Clin Orthop* 1995;317:19–28.
36. O'Neill DA, Harris WH. Failed total hip replacement: assessment by plain radiographs, arthrograms, and aspiration of the hip joint. *J Bone Joint Surg Am* 1986;66:540–546.
37. Owen TD, Moran CG, Smith SR, Pinder IM. Results of uncemented porous-coated anatomic total hip replacement. *J Bone Joint Surg Br* 1994;76:258–262.
38. Roberts EB, Noble PC, Carlyle TA, Tullous HS. Pathways for periprosthetic transport of particulate debris in cemented total hip arthroplasties. [abstract]. Presented at the 43rd Annual Meeting of the Orthopaedic Research Society; 1997;Feb 9–13; San Francisco.
39. Salvati EA, Wilson PD, Jr, Jolley MN, Vakili F, Aglietti P, Brown GC. A ten-year follow-up study of our first one hundred consecutive Charnley total hip replacements. *J Bone Joint Surg Am* 1981;63:753–767.
40. Schmalzried TP, Guttman D, Grecula M, Amstutz HC. The relationship between the design, position and articular wear of acetabular components inserted without cement and the development of pelvic osteolysis. *J Bone Joint Surg Am* 1994;76:677–688.
41. Schmalzried TP, Harris WH. The Harris-Galante porous-coated acetabular component with screw fixation. *J Bone Joint Surg Am* 1992;74:1130–1139.
42. Schmalzried TP, Jasty MJ, Harris WH. Periprosthetic bone loss in total hip arthroplasty. *J Bone Joint Surg Am* 1992;74:849–863.
43. Schmalzried TP, Kwong LM, Jasty MJ, et al. The mechanism of loosening of cemented acetabular components in total hip arthroplasty. *Clin Orthop* 1992;274:60–78.
44. Schmalzried TP, Wessinger SJ, Hill GE, Harris WH. The Harris-Galante porous acetabular component press-fit without screw fixation. *J Arthroplasty* 1994;9:235–242.
45. Stauffer RN. Ten-year follow-up study of total hip replacement. *J Bone Joint Surg Am* 1982;64:983–990.
46. Tanzer M, Maloney WJ, Jasty MJ, Harris WH. The progression of femoral cortical osteolysis in association with total hip arthroplasty without cement. *J Bone Joint Surg Am* 1992;74:404–410.
47. Wan Z, Dorr LD. Natural history of femoral focal osteolysis with proximal ingrowth smooth stem implants. *J Arthroplasty* 1996;11:718–725.
48. Whirlow J, Rubash HE. Aseptic loosening in total hip arthroplasty. In: Callaghan JJ, Denis DA, Paprosky WG, Rosenberg AG, eds. Orthopaedic knowledge update: hip and knee reconstruction. Rosemont, IL: American Academy of Orthopaedic Surgeons, 1995:147–156.
49. Woolson ST, Maloney WJ. Cementless total hip arthroplasty using a porous-coated prosthesis for bone ingrowth fixation. *J Arthroplasty* 1992;7:381–388.
50. Xenos JS, Hopkinson WJ, Callaghan JJ, Heekin RD, Savory CG. Osteolysis around an uncemented cobalt chrome total hip arthroplasty. *Clin Othop* 1994;317:29–36.
51. Zicat B, Engh CA, Gokcen E. Patterns of osteolysis around total hip components inserted with and without cement. *J Bone Joint Surg Am* 1995;77:432–439.

Revision Total Hip Arthroplasty,
edited by Marvin E. Steinberg and Jonathan P. Garino,
Lippincott Williams & Wilkins, Philadelphia © 1998.

4

Effect of Acetabular Design on Long-term Survivorship

Jeffrey E. Schryver

It is now apparent that the longevity of total hip replacement is influenced to a great extent by the performance of the acetabular construct. Long-term studies of cemented hips have shown that although femoral loosening may be reduced with modern techniques, acetabular component loosening has been relatively insensitive to these improvements. Mulroy and Harris (27) reported a 42% rate of acetabular loosening compared with a 3% rate of femoral stem loosening after a minimum follow-up period of 10 years. The increasing incidence of osteolysis attributable to polyethylene debris, particularly evident in cementless designs, further implicates the acetabular cup as a leading contributor to modern total hip failure (12,36). Acetabular component design also is influential in short-term outcomes, because dislocation, a function of the maximum range-of-motion (ROM) of the implant, component position, and joint tension, remains the most common postoperative complication in total hip arthroplasty (18).

Current design practices for acetabular components must focus on two performance criteria: mechanical integrity of the joint construct and reduction of wear debris. Achieving mechanical stability requires a sufficiently stable ROM without dislocation, absence of liner disassociation, and absence of liner micromotion. Current design proposals for wear debris reduction include lowering polyethylene contact stress, minimizing abrasive surfaces in contact with polyethylene in both the primary articulating and the secondary backside wear interfaces, reducing motion between nonarticulating surfaces, avoiding deleterious material property changes from sterilization, and enhancing material properties through polyethylene fabrication methods and changes in material chemistry.

J. E. Schryver: Department of Implant Product Development, Smith & Nephew Orthopaedics, Memphis, Tennessee 38816.

Acetabular cups can be divided into three interfaces of interest for considering design features and device performance. The primary articulation interface between the femoral ball and polyethylene liner influences ROM and is the main site for production of polyethylene wear debris. The secondary articular interface, or so-called backside surface, has been associated with increased production of polyethylene wear debris. In two-piece devices this debris is formed through abrasion at the internal interface of metal-backed cups against their polyethylene liners. These devices may be subject to accelerated damage from increased liner stress in areas of unsupported polyethylene and sharp contact surfaces in the shell interior. The third acetabular interface lies between the prosthesis and bone. In both cemented and cementless designs, loss of fixation and aseptic loosening at this interface constitute the chief cause of acetabular revision.

DESIGN ISSUES

Polyethylene Thickness, Conformity, and Contact Stress

Of the many design criteria that affect function and longevity after total hip arthroplasty, none has been highlighted more than a desire for increased polyethylene thickness for the purpose of reducing contact stress. The root of this understanding comes from Bartel et al., (1) who described the effect of nonconformity between metal and polyethylene surfaces in hip and knee total joints. Load transfer from the rigid metal-bearing surface to the deformable polyethylene can result in high local stress in the polyethylene. The magnitude of this stress for a given load depends on the conformity, or difference of curvature, between the metal and polyethylene surfaces. The failure of knee tibial bearings through delamination and subsurface cracking can be attributed to high contact stress induced by the large difference of curvature between knee femoral components and their tibial inserts. This stress is central to the observed failure modes of cylinder-on-flat knee designs and is influenced by the degree of nonconformity and the thickness, stiffness, and fatigue strength of the polyethylene.

In acetabular cups the same criteria for contact stress apply. However, the amount of nonconformity in a hip is substantially lower than that in the articular surface of a knee because of the congruous matching of the femoral ball and liner. International cup design standards (International Standards Organization 7206-2) specify a manufactured gap between a hip ball and liner of 0.05 to 0.15 mm to prevent initial seizure. This greatly contrasts to the 2 to 3 mm radial difference between metal and plastic in knee components in the medial lateral direction and more than 30 mm of radial curvature differential in the anterior-posterior direction during flexion. Thus the typical hip articulation has 30 to 300 times less gap (nonconformity) than the average knee. The analysis by Bartel et al. (1) showed that highly conforming surfaces produce low contact stress and that contact stress in fully conforming surfaces is independent of thickness. This implies that conformity, as opposed to thickness, is the primary concern in reducing contact stress in polyethylene bearings. This is difficult to achieve in the articulating bearing surfaces of a knee but quite easy to achieve in ball-and-socket hip bearings. However, although primary articular contact stress is low in hips, the same concerns about high contact stress and increased wear due to nonconformity and point loading apply to both sides of the liner. This brings specific attention to the need for conformity between the exterior surface of the liner and the interior surface of the shell.

Rosner et al. (34) measured conformity in contemporary metal-backed acetabular components. Gaps between the liner and shell of less than 0.2 mm were labeled as conforming, and estimates of the total unsupported liner were made with this gap criterion. The percentage of unsupported polyethylene ranged from 10.3% to as high as 96.9% in this study of 20 different cup designs. It is likely that many of these gaps will be reduced during the load cycle; a process that may lead to wear through repetitive motion. In addition, contemporary metal-backed cups have a variety of screw holes, sharp edges, and relatively abrasive surfaces, which could produce marked contact stress and potential damage on the polyethylene liner at this backside interface.

The potential for vascular damage from screw fixation (19), the desire to place screws preferentially in the superior quadrant of the acetabulum, and the concern for multiple areas of unsupported polyethylene have prompted the development of clustered screw-hole cups. Most often these designs have between two and six holes for bone screws placed in one quadrant of the shell. Placement of screws in the superior area of the acetabulum results in fixation in line with the load vector of the hip and thus in typically strong, dense bone. However, a result is that most gait loading is transmitted through the polyethylene to the shell in an area where the screw-hole relief provides diminished support of the liner. The design of the hole itself and the potential for overlapping with adjacent holes can result in sharp edges and high-stress, low-area contact points. Figure 1 shows a contemporary cup design with overlapping screw holes. Close placement of the holes results in sharp points and low areas of contact directly in line with the greatest loads between the polyethylene and shell. Lieberman et al. (21) observed extrusion of the liner into screw holes in the weight-bearing region in every modular acetabular cup tested *in vitro*. In each design with a sharp edge at screw holes, this extrusion resulted in a shearing of the polyethylene surface, described as *punch-out*. In cups with generously rounded edges around the screw holes the punch-out was absent, indicating that local shear stresses caused by sharp edges can be eliminated through design. Also observed were areas of gouging where sharp edges of locking mechanisms attached to the liner. These findings paralleled retrieval data showing backside wear of liners abraded by the metal shell (4,35).

Avoiding high local stress and polyethylene damage at the backside interface is probably critical to long-term acetabular cup performance. It is achievable through proper design and manufacturing practices. Conformity at the liner-shell interface must be considered a high design priority to reduce debris production. Features or edges that would tear a surgical glove may be a warning sign of impending polyethylene damage and increased wear. Nonconformity can and should be minimized through exact size matching between the liner and shell and by eliminating points and sharp edges that would damage the liner.

Abrasive Backside Wear

The secondary articular surface, or backside of the polyethylene liner has been shown to be a source of debris generation (26). Even cemented cups are not immune to abrasive wear at this interface. Wroblewski et al. (39) found that 19 of 59 cemented high-density polyethylene sockets removed at revision operations showed wear on the outside of the polyethylene socket. Since the advent of metal backing, a wide variety of investigations have focused on the effects of this newly studied interface.

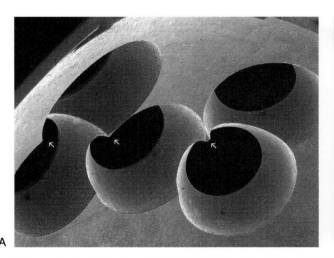
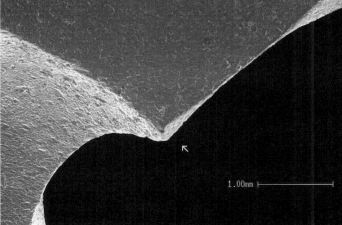

A   B

Figure 1. Acetabular shell interior showing areas of high contact stress and minimal support in the load-bearing liner support region. **A:** Low-power view. **B:** Magnified view.

Dowson et al. (5) showed that the wear rate of polyethylene against a metal surface is proportional to average roughness of that surface (Ra). Thus a surface ten times rougher than a femoral head would produce ten times greater wear debris for a given area of contact and sliding distance. It is also clear that the presence of metal edges above the support surface results in a remarkable increase in polyethylene wear rate (6). The inside surfaces of acetabular cups have average surface roughness that range up to two orders of magnitude greater than that of femoral heads. In addition, the machined surface finishes commonly found at this interface provide an abundance of imperfections and raised edges. Finally, the surface area of the convex side of the liner may approach five times that of the articular surface. Considering these relations, the amount of micromotion between the liner and shell during gait, the inside shell roughness, and the large available polyethylene surface area may have a marked effect on debris generation at the backside surface. The retrieved liner shown in Fig. 2 shows abrasive wear of the backside of the polyethylene liner. The circular raised areas are the original surface of the liner that have not been worn by the metal shell. The rough, depressed areas between the screw hole signatures show substantial abrasive wear on the liner by the shell interior.

Acetabular cups are generally manufactured from cast cobalt chrome or wrought titanium alloy. A variety of different production methods and finishing steps are commonly used in cup manufacturing, and each results in different roughness and final surface topographies. The abrasive potential of these surfaces against polyethylene is related to their roughness and is magnified by the presence of sharp edges or peaks. Investment casting, used for manufacturing cobalt chrome cups, typically leaves a randomly rough surface. An example of the three-dimensional texture of the inside of a cast cobalt chrome cup surface is shown in Fig. 3A. The vertical height of the box illustrates maximum and minimum bounds for the surface roughness peaks and measures 23 μm in this example. Machining of cups is required for holding closer tolerances and details that cannot be cast into the parts. The lathe-turning process used to machine titanium implants to final dimension typically results in concentric rings of fine grooves and ridges as seen in Fig. 3B (total vertical height 5 μm). Matte finishing through glass bead blasting after machining can leave a randomly textured surface, as shown in the titanium cup in Fig. 3C (total height 6 μm). In comparison with the cup surface textures shown, a femoral head would be a flat, featureless plane. These typical textures of interior surfaces of acetabular cups illustrate the variety of topographic features that may present additional sources of polyethylene wear. The contribution of these sources of debris relative to that of primary articulation is unclear and merits further study. The clinical observation of wear at these interfaces and the increasing incidence of debris-related osteolysis suggest that design-related improvements to reduce secondary wear may be advantageous.

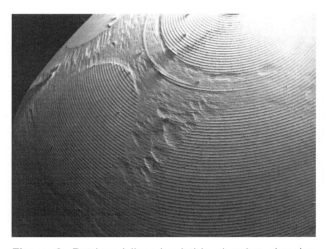

Figure 2. Retrieved liner backside showing abrasion from shell.

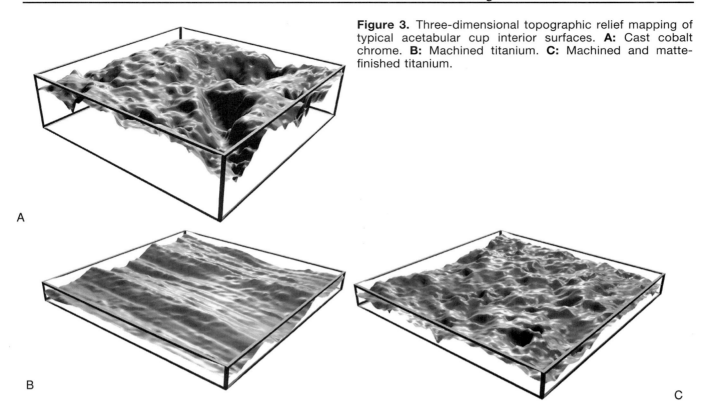

Figure 3. Three-dimensional topographic relief mapping of typical acetabular cup interior surfaces. **A:** Cast cobalt chrome. **B:** Machined titanium. **C:** Machined and matte-finished titanium.

Liner Micromotion

In examining long cycle performance of cups in torsion, Chen et al. (3) found marked differences in the stability of polyethylene liner locking-mechanism designs. In five cup types these rotational motions ranged from undetectable to as high as 0.96 degrees of rotation per cycle and produced abrasion of the polyethylene surface. In axial loading without torsion, Lieberman et al. (21) found burnishing and abrasion of the convex side of the liners of five different designs ranging from 2% to 23% of their backside surface area. These authors (3,21) concluded that smooth interior acetabular shell surfaces, the absence of sharp edges and points at the shell–liner interface, and stable locking mechanisms are recommended to minimize backside production of polyethylene debris. Williams et al. (37) combined torsion and axial loading to examine the micromotion and backside wear of six commonly used cup designs. The results showed liner micromotion values and abrasive wear scores that differed by two orders of magnitude between the designs. The purpose of the cup locking mechanism is to allow intraoperative orientation, assembly, and removal of the liner with sufficient locking integrity to eliminate in-service disassociation and micromotion. The clinical incidence of liner disassociation, a concern in early designs, is now seldom reported. However, in sufficient magnitude cyclic motion at the liner–shell interface can constitute noncatastrophic failure. It is now the primary concern in liner locking-mechanism design. Therefore the consideration of long-term stability of liner locking mechanisms with minimized micromotion is essential.

Range of Motion and Dislocation

Dislocation is the most common postoperative complication of total hip arthroplasty. The reported incidence generally ranges from 3% to 5% (18). There is general agreement in the literature that surgical experience decreases risk for dislocation. Hedlundh et al. (16) illustrated a learning curve for inexperienced surgeons that leveled off at a 3% dislocation rate after 30 operations and correlated with the number of operations per year for experienced surgeons.

Surgical approach has been reported to affect dislocation rates (25). The posteriolateral approach in the lateral position is more likely to lead to dislocation than anterior and transtrochanteric approaches in the supine position. A hip that undergoes multiple operations is at greater risk for dislocation. Some surgeons have seen 75% to 80% of dislocations occurring in revision operations (7,10). Many surgical factors influence dislocation rates, but there is general agreement that cup position is a primary concern (12,26,27).

Cup Position Requirements for Reconstruction

Dislocation due to incorrect orientation is usually caused by placing the cup too vertically or too anteverted (18). Dislocation may be initiated by impingement between the femoral neck and cup producing lever out or by tissue impingement. Placement of the prosthetic acetabulum in 30 to 50 degrees of abduction and 20 to 40 degrees of flexion has been recommended as safe for anatomic range of motion ROM (25). McCollum and Gray (25) found that the orientation of the pelvis in the lateral surgical position can flex by as much as 35 degrees from the standing position. Common landmarks used in positioning the cup can vary by as much as 40 degrees. The variability of cup orientation carries important design requirements in that the prosthetic ROM without impingement must be greater than the physiologic ROM to allow for positioning uncertainties during the operation.

Design and Prosthetic Range of Motion

Two primary factors control ROM with respect to the external prosthetic acetabular axis: head-to-neck diameter ratio and orientation of the articular surface. The maximum angular excursion for a femoral head is limited by the intersection of the ball spherical diameter with the prosthesis neck. In cup–liner articulation both the geometric features of the liner and the thickness of the femoral neck at point of contact control ROM. Liner designs that place the head center of rotation below the liner surface reduce the maximum ROM as the neck abuts the raised flange. In liners it is not uncommon to find head centers below the face by 2 to 5 mm. This depression usually is chamfered internally to the bore and can cause increased risk for dislocation by reducing ROM. The original Charnley prosthesis with a head diameter of 22.2 mm and neck diameter of 12.5 mm would have a calculated maximum theoretic ROM of 111 degrees. Any liner material that stood above the bore equator, such as a flange or a deep bore, would reduce this possible range. A 2 mm thick face flange or deep bore in the Charnley cup design would reduce the calculated ROM by 20 degrees. This is consistent with a report of 90 degrees ROM for the Charnley prosthesis (3).

Although the theoretic increase in ROM for a larger head diameter with a given neck diameter is not at question, clinical results have not always confirmed the stability of large heads (15). It is important to note, however, that in this series the neck diameter for the 32 mm head (Lubinus) was larger than the neck of the 22 mm head (Charnley) and that the head-neck ratios, thus the ROM, in the two stems was equivalent. Hedlundh et al. (15) also found that the increase in risk for recurrent dislocation of the hip was twice as high with a 22 mm head than with a 32 mm head. Garellick et al. (11) reported a significantly lower rate of dislocation for a 32 mm hip with an increased ROM than for a 22-mm Charnley head in a randomized study of 410 hips with a mean follow-up period of 7 years.

The discussion of head size is germane to acetabular design for two reasons. For a given system the choice of head size influences polyethylene thickness, and it affects the range of motion. The current understanding of the thickness of polyethylene as it relates to contact stress and wear is strong motivation to reduce head size in a given acetabular component. Choosing a smaller head size for the given femoral prosthesis increases polyethylene thickness but decreases the ROM of the component. Given this possible trade-off in decreased stability for decreased wear, it is important to establish designs for the femoral stem, neck, and head and for the acetabular liner that allow full ROM without impingement. The goal of reduced wear may not be fully realized if a smaller but skirted head abuts and wears the liner rim during physiologic ROM. Similarly, recurrent dislocation negates the benefit of reduced wear.

Neutral, Extended-Lip, and Offset Liners

Until the past decade the general design of the liner face has been axis-symmetric and neutral with respect to the cup rim. These so-called zero-degree liners allow the greatest ROM, but the cone of possible motion is limited to the orientation of the acetabulum or position of the metal shell. Nordin and Frankel (29) found that the position of the normal acetabulum was 60 degrees abduction and 40 degrees anteversion. Equatorial containment of a hemispheric prosthesis in the normal acetabulum therefore may result in more abduction and anteversion than is typically recommended (25). Flanged, cemented, all-polyethylene cups such as the Charnley PIJ design (2) allow containment and pressurization of the cement with increased flexibility in angular orientation of the bearing surface. Many second-generation cemented metal-backed cups introduced an offset liner that rotated the axis of the bearing hemisphere and allowed shell containment in the acetabulum along with adjustment of the orientation of the bearing axis. This approach is now a common option in current cemented and cementless cup designs.

The proposed advantage of the offset liner is primarily to increase stability in a particular orientation. This is done by repositioning the hemisphere of head–liner contact, hence reorienting the limits of instability and head dislocation relative to that of a neutral or zero-degree liner. Figure 4A shows one type of offset design that maintains the center of rotation of the ball within the socket. The inner hemisphere is rotated, in this example 20 degrees, resulting in a semicircle of raised polyethylene. However, this design approach reduces the total ROM cone. The neck contacts the raised equator earlier during total ROM excursion, as shown by the dark, striped cone compared with the gray, transparent ROM cone for the same head–neck configuration in a zero-degree liner. Advantages to this approach over other designs are maintaining concentric placement of the head in the acetabulum, minimizing unsupported polyethylene, and providing greater effective rotation of the articulation hemisphere. Figure 4B illustrates a second offset alternative, which rotates the polyethylene-bearing hemisphere about the liner outside edge. The advantage is that the total ROM cone is not reduced relative to the neutral liner but is reoriented relative to the acetabular rim. This, however, causes lateralization of the head center, which tends to increase the joint reaction force with possible implications in wear. Other trade-offs include increased unsupported polyethylene and a limitation of the degree of maximum tilt. In the edge-rotated design, the practical limit is 10 degrees of tilt, because the extended rim rises twice as much as in the center-rotated design (see Fig. 4A).

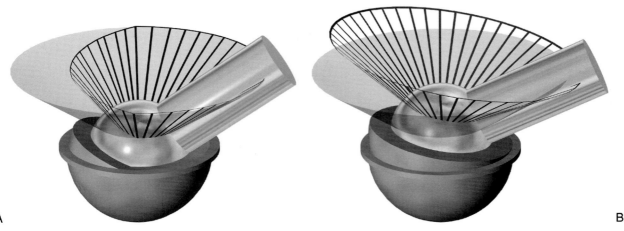

A   B

Figure 4. Range of motion (ROM) comparison for 20-degree center rotation (**A**) and 10-degree edge rotation (**B**). ROM cones for offset liners are shown by *dark line* and boundaries with neutral liner comparisons in *gray*.

Reorientation of the articulation hemisphere is an attempt to optimize the balance between increasing the stability by proper coverage of the femoral ball and increasing the dislocation due to lever out. Charnley used this type of design approach in the long-posterior-wall design and found marked reduction in the frequency of posterior dislocations (2). However, excessive anteversion of the liner rim such as is possible by anteversion of the shell with posterior placement of an extended rim can cause impingement and increase the chance of dislocation. This is especially apparent during external rotation in extension. Figure 5 illustrates an inferior view of a hemipelvis with various positions of a femoral neck during ROM limits. The cup is aligned with the acetabular rim (55 degrees of abduction and 15 degrees of anteversion in this example). Position 1 corresponds to the natural femoral neck axis in a standing condition (0 degrees flexion, 0 degrees abduction, 0 degrees rotation). Position 2 flexes the hip to 105 degrees. At this point increased adduction and internal rotation would tend to cause dislocation in the posterior inferior direction. Rotation of the articular surface to increase coverage in this area can be accomplished with a combination of anteversion and possibly an extended lip liner. However, doing so excessively may increase the chance of anterior dislocation when the hip is in position 6 (0 degrees flexion, 45 degrees external rotation). Position 3 occurs at 40 degrees abduction at 0 degrees flexion, position 4 is at 20 degrees adduction, and position 5 is at 45 degrees internal rotation (all at 0 degrees flexion). Charnley cautioned that anteversion of the long-posterior-wall cup could cause excessive protrusion of the posterior wall and impingement in extension with anterior dislocation (2).

The relative merits of current approaches to modifying the articular orientation relative to the acetabular rim are design specific and must be considered in conjunction with the femoral stem and head. It is generally agreed that offset liners are not a substitute for correct cup placement but that in some cases the joint stability of a securely fixed acetabular component may be finitely improved by orientation of an asymmetric liner.

Liner Design and Joint Tension: The Lateralized Liner

Charnley (2) believed that correct joint tension and proper cup position, achieved in his hands through a supine position transtrochanteric approach with trochanteric advance-

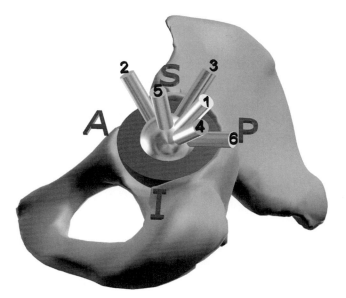

Figure 5. Neck positions from common anatomic range of motion tests. **1:** Neutral standing (0 flexion, 0 abduction, 0 rotation). **2:** 105 degrees flexion. **3:** 40 degrees abduction (0 flexion). **4:** 20 degrees adduction (0 flexion). **5:** 45 degrees internal rotation (0 flexion). **6:** 45 degrees external rotation (0 flexion).

ment, were central to reducing dislocation. In one series of 4,076 patients, this soft tissue balancing in conjunction with a long posterior wall liner allowed Charnley to reduce the frequency of dislocations to 0.4% (9). Using computed tomographic measurements, Pierchon (31) found no difference between the alignment of prosthetic components in a group of 38 dislocated hips compared with a control group of 14 hips that underwent uneventful arthroplasty. Soft-tissue laxity was thought to be the most likely contributor to instability in this series. It is possible that correct device position is necessary but not always sufficient to avoid dislocation.

Some acetabular devices now offer a liner with a center of rotation lateralized by 4 mm or more in addition to concentric centers of rotation as an option to adjust joint tension. This approach can serve a dual purpose for reducing dislocation in that it may be possible to restore sufficient joint tension without the need to use skirted heads. This would increase the total ROM by reducing the effective neck diameter (head to neck ratio) while increasing stability through joint tension. Lateralization of the head center, however, reduces the abductor moment arm and increases joint reaction forces. Thus the use of lateralized liners may be best considered in restoring the natural acetabular center of rotation in conjunction with proper prosthetic stem offset.

PROSTHESIS TYPES

The Cemented Acetabulum

Cemented cup designs today retain most of the features found in first-generation components produced three decades ago. All-polyethylene cemented cups are commonly found in both neutral and hooded or offset designs. Design practices for cement fixation to the polyethylene typically include shallow grooves to enhance interface shear resistance. They should not protrude deeply into the cup, a good depth is typically 1 mm to 1.5 mm, so as to avoid loss of liner structural strength and bearing surface thickness (32). Pressurization of the acetabular cement has been shown to correlate with reduced risk for revision (23). The presence of an equatorial flange may assist in pressurization on component insertion. Centralization of the cup to avoid thinning of the cement mantle and bone contact against the liner is essential. Spacing pods on the back of cemented cups are typically machined into the unitary liner or may be polymethyl methacrylate pods mechanically attached to the cup. The mantle spacer design should provide a smooth extension in the exterior cup surface to avoid sharp discontinuities in the cement mantle and to allow placement in the bone bed without catching on predrilled cement fixation holes.

The survivorship of cemented acetabular components past the first decade of implantation has raised concerns by some authors. Mulroy and Harris (27) defined a 42% incidence of radiographic loosening and a 4.8% acetabular revision rate in 105 cemented acetabular cups at a minimum of 10 years. Kavanaugh et al. (17) reported probable acetabular loosening in 12% of instances (n = 24) at 10 years. Garellick et al. (11) reported four cups definitely loose and two revised in 410 hips with an acetabular survivorship of 97.4% at 11 years.

Metal-Backed Cemented Cups

Concerns with the difficulties of cemented polyethylene cups prompted introduction of a metal shell backing by Harris (13) in 1971. The design included a cobalt chrome shell, a thick polyethylene liner (13 mm for a 50 mm shell) achieved through eccentric placement of the articular surface within the cup, a 26 mm diameter femoral head for increased ROM over the Charnley cup, and the ability to replace the liner during revision operations without disrupting the cement–bone interface. Interestingly, the hypothesis of a reduction in cement mantle stress as a result of metal backing was not highlighted in the initial design rationale for metal backing. A follow-up study involving 48 patients showed a survivorship probability of 87.4% at 10 years.

A review of the literature showed no support for the long-term efficacy of metal-backed cemented cups. The necessity of securely locking the metal and polyethylene together is clear. The Swedish National Registry (24) shows survivorship of one cemented cobalt chrome hip design with a metal-backed cup at 87.9% (n = 1,362) compared with the same stem with an all polyethylene cup at 99.2% (n = 939) at 9 years. The manufacturer's data indicated that when this design of metal-backed cup failed it was most often through fracture of the liner locking mechanism as a result of stem-neck impingement that resulted in disassociation of the liner.

Although metal-backed cups were widely believed to reduce stress in the cement mantle, the reasons for their generalized early failure remain unclear. Nashed et al. (28) reported a 31% incidence of osteolysis with a titanium metal-backed cemented cup after 7.8 years of follow-up study compared with no (0%) osteolysis using the same stem and head with a cemented all-polyethylene cup at 9.4 years. Although many authors have implicated the reduction of polyethylene thickness in metal-backed cups as contributing to increased wear, in this series the penetration rates were similar (0.13 mm/year metal backed, 0.10 mm/year all polyethylene). The loss of polyethylene liner thickness from the use of a metal shell in this design was small (1.5 mm). One notable difference in these cemented metal-backed components from their polyethylene counterparts is the addition of a second wear interface between the liner and shell. Figure 6 shows a commonly implanted, cemented metal-backed cup in a disassembled state. This design, like many metal-backed cemented cups, was factory assembled because there was no need for intraoperative assembly. The interior roughness of the metal shell is two orders of magnitude greater than that found in primary articulating surfaces. This rough texture in combination with micromotion at the liner–shell interface could be expected to generate additional polyethylene debris. The relations between these design features and their possible effect on production of wear debris merit further investigation. They may be important in the proper design of metal-backed acetabular components.

Uncemented Cup Design

Long-term fixation of noncemented cups is achieved either through mechanical means as in the case of threaded cups or through biologic fixation with roughened surfaces,

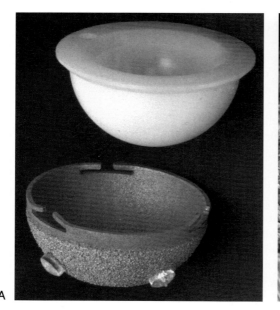
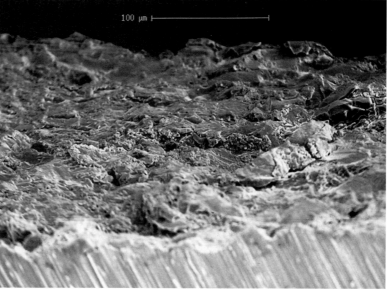

A   B

Figure 6. A: Two-piece, metal-backed cemented cup disassembled to show interior surface. **B:** Low-incidence, magnified view of inside shell surface. Near field (*light striped*) and far field (*dark*) are front and back edges of surface sample.

porous beads, wire mesh, or calcium hydroxyapatite (HA) coatings. Uncoated threaded cups have generally performed less well than other forms of acetabular fixation. The early failure rate by means of aseptic loosening in some designs was 21% at 3.9 years (8) and 21% at 6 years (14). In contrast, the Norwegian Registry has shown results for some designs of HA-coated threaded cups equivalent to those of porous coated devices (14). Threaded cups have essentially been abandoned in North America.

Cementless Fixation

The initial use of cementless cups involved a hemispheric or low-profile hemispheric cup placed in a spherically reamed acetabulum of equal size. Concerns for insufficient stability of this technique prompted use of bone screw–augmented designs for initial fixation sufficient to allow bone ingrowth. The disadvantages of use of screws include metal debris from motion between the screw head and shell, unintentional vascular penetration, and access of polyethylene debris to the bone bed through the screw hole. Screws apply a tensile load to the shell that is counteracted and unloaded by the compressive forces of gait. Subsidence of the shell or nonrecoverable compression of the acetabular bone results in loss of contact between the screw head and the shell. The impression of screw heads into the polyethylene is a common observation in revised liners (4) and suggests that the screw primarily counteracts transverse forces and acts as a toggle point. *In vitro* stability testing indicates that a non–press-fit cup with screw fixation is less stable than a press-fit cup without screws and that the addition of screws to a press-fit construct does not necessarily increase initial stability (20,38). Alternative approaches to adjunctive fixation include spikes or pegs to provide transverse interface stability. One design using three fixed axial spikes has shown less stability at the illiac interface but additional stability at the pubis and ischium over screw-augmented hemispheric press-fit fixation (30). The use of fixed spikes requires exact positioning in the acetabulum during component seating because off-center placement results in spike fixation without coincident surface contact between the shell hemisphere and the acetabular bone. The use of modular pegs or spikes placed after full seating of the acetabular component has the surgical advantage of allowing adjustment of shell orientation and concentric contact of the shell and bone before placement of the dowel. However, the long-term clinical benefit of the modular spike design is unknown.

The use of cup fixation without adjunct bone screws is increasing. This desire has produced a variety of cup designs to enhance the initial press-fit fixation. These include an interference fit with oversized hemispheric cups, stepped nonhemispheric cups with an increased peripheral equatorial diameter, and ellipsoid cups. Press fitting of oversized hemispheric components is now a common practice for initial fixation. The advantage is avoiding the drawbacks of screw fixation. The disadvantages include loss of medial dome contact and possible acetabular rim fracture (22). The amount of press fit required for stability varies with bone quality, the design of the hemispheric shell, the size of the shell, and the perceived size of the prepared acetabulum. Low-profile shells typically remove a 4 mm band of material from the shell equator and thereby reduce the shell height. Thus the radius of curvature of the shell is the stated cup size, but the final diameter of the shell rim is less than an equivalent full hemisphere. Because most friction fixation of an oversized shell occurs at the rim, these low-profile cups require a greater labeled size effectively to engage the acetabular rim. Likewise, the guidelines of oversizing for a low-profile shell can be excessive if applied to a full hemispheric design and possibly increase the chance of rim fracture. It is also likely that the dimension of press-fit suitable for a 48 mm cup is different from that required for a 70 mm cup (33). Finally, the surgical technique of reaming, the hardness and homogeneity of the acetabulum, and the sharpness and size of the reamer all influence the final diameter of the prepared bed. Use of hemispheric dome-sizing gauges for accurate measurement of the reamed acetabulum is recommended for determining true size to assess the proper amount of press fit.

CONCLUSION

To improve survivorship and performance, contemporary design tenets are directed toward reducing articular wear, eliminating debris at nonarticular interfaces, maintaining long-term prosthesis-to-bone fixation, and restoring a full range of function without dislocation. The greatest concern for long-term failure of total hip arthroplasty is osteolysis caused by the presence of polyethylene and metallic wear debris produced at the acetabular cup. The design-based sources of debris and current proposals for debris reduction are a primary consideration in the choice of acetabular components. It is now clear that the introduction of metal backing and its associated requirements of new manufacturing methods, locking mechanisms, internal conformity, and adjunctive fixation for cementless application have brought substantial lessons in design. We find that the worthy goal remains of trying to better the longevity of acetabular arthroplasty over the original Charnley-designed polyethylene cemented cup.

REFERENCES

1. Bartel DL, Burstein AH, Toda MD, Edwards DL. The effect of conformity and plastic thickness on contact stresses in metal-backed plastic implants. *J Biomech Eng* 1985;107:193–199.
2. Charnley J. *Low friction arthroplasty of the hip: theory and practice.* Berlin: Springer-Verlag, 1979.
3. Chen PC, Mead EH, Pinto JG, Colwell CW. Polyethylene wear debris in modular acetabular prosthesis. *Clin Orthop* 1995;317:44–56.
4. Collier JP, Mayor MB, Jensen RE, et al. Mechanisms of failure of modular prosthesis. *Clin Orthop* 1992;285:129–139.
5. Dowson D, Diab MMEH, Gillis BJ, Atkinson JR. Influence of counterface topography on the wear of ultra high molecular weight polyethylene under wet or dry conditions. In: Lee, LH, ed. *Polymer wear and its control.* American Chemical Society Symposium Series No. 287. Washington DC: American Chemical Society, 1985.
6. Dowson D, Taheri S, Wallbridge NC. The role of counterface imperfections in the wear of polyethylene. *Wear* 1987;119:277–293.
7. Eftekhar NS. Dislocation and instability complicating low friction arthroplasty of the hip joint. *Clin Orthop* 1976; 121:120–125.
8. Engh C, Griffin W, Marx C. Cementless acetabular components. *J Bone Joint Surg Br* 1990;72:53–59.
9. Etienne A, Cupic Z, Charnley J. Postoperative dislocation after Charnley low-friction arthroplasty. *Clin Orthop* 1978;132:19–23.
10. Evanski PM, Waugh TR, Orofino CF. Total hip replacement with the Charnley prosthesis. *Clin Orthop* 1972;95:69.
11. Garellick G, Malchau H, Herberts P. Charnley versus Spectron. Presented at the 47th Congress of the Scandinavian Orthopaedic Association; 1994; Reykavik, Iceland.
12. Harris WH. The problem is osteolysis. *Clin Orthop* 1995;311:46–53.
13. Harris WH. A new total hip implant. *Clin Orthop* 1971;81:105–113.
14. Havelin LI, Vollset SE, Endesaeter LB. Revision for aseptic loosening of uncemented cups in 4,352 primary total hip prostheses. *Acta Orthop Scand* 1995;66:494–500.
15. Hedlundh U, Ahnfelt L, Hybbinette CH, Wallinder L, Weckstrom J, Fredin H. Dislocations and the femoral head size in primary total hip arthroplasty. *Clin Orthop* 1996;333:226–233.
16. Hedlundh U, Ahnfelt L, Hybbinette CH, Weckstrom J, Fredin H. Surgical experience related to dislocations after total hip arthroplasty. *J Bone Joint Surg Br* 1996;78:206–209.
17. Kavanaugh BF, Dewitz MA, Ilstrup DM, Stauffer RN, Coventry MB. Charnley total hip arthroplasty with cement. *J Bone Joint Surg Am* 1989;71:1496–1503.
18. Khan MAA, Brakenbury PH, Reynolds ISR. Dislocation following total hip replacement. *J Bone Joint Surg Br* 1981;63:214–218.
19. Kirkpatrick JS, Callaghan JJ, Vandemark RM, Goldner RD. The relationship of intrapelvic vasculature to the acetabulum: implications in screw-fixation acetabular components. *Clin Orthop* 1990;258:183–190.
20. Kwong LM, O'Connor DO, Sedlacek RC, Krushell RJ, Maloney WJ, Harris WH. A quantitative in vitro assessment of fit and screw fixation on the stability of a cementless hemispherical acetabular component. *J Arthroplasty* 1994;9:163–170.
21. Lieberman JR, Kay RM, Hamlet WP, Park SH, Kabo JM. Wear of the polyethylene liner-metallic shell interface in modular acetabular components. *J Arthroplasty* 1996;11:602–608.
22. MacKenzie JR, Callaghan JJ, Pedersen DR, Brown TD. Areas of contact and extent of gaps with implantation of oversized acetabular components in total hip arthroplasty. *Clin Orthop* 1994;298:127–136.
23. Malchau H. On the importance of stepwise introduction of new hip implant technology [thesis]. Goteborg: Goetborg University, 1995.
24. Malchau H, Herberts P. Prognosis of total hip replacement. Scientific exhibit at the 63rd Annual Meeting of the American Academy of Orthopaedic Surgeons; 1996;Feb 22–26; Atlanta.
25. McCollum DE, Gray WJ. Dislocation after total hip arthroplasty. *Clin Orthop* 1990;261:159–170.
26. McKellop HA, Campbell P, Park SH, et al. The origin of submicron wear debris in total hip arthroplasty. *Clin Orthop* 1995;311:3–20.
27. Mulroy RD, Harris WH. The effect of improved cementing techniques of component loosening in total hip replacement. *J Bone Joint Surg Br* 1990;72:757–760.

28. Nashed RS, Becker DA, Gustilo RB. Are cementless acetabular components the cause of excess wear in total hip arthroplasty? *Clin Orthop* 1995;317:19–28.
29. Nordin M, Frankel BH. *Basic biomechanics of the musculoskeletal system,* 2nd ed. Philadelphia: Lea & Febiger, 1989.
30. Perona PG, Lawrence J, Paprowsky WG, Pathwardhan AG, Sartori M. Acetabular micromotion as a measure of initial implant stability in primary hip arthroplasty. *J Arthroplasty* 1992;7:537–547.
31. Pierchon F, Pasquier G, Cotton A, Fontaine C, Clarisse J, Duquennoy A. Causes of dislocation of total hip arthroplasty. *J Bone Joint Surg Br* 1994;76:45–48.
32. Oh I, Sander TW, Treharne RW. Total hip acetabular cup flange design and its effect on cement fixation. *Clin Orthop* 1985;189:308–312.
33. Ries MD, Harbaugh M, Shea J, Lambert L. Effect of cementless acetabular cup geometry on strain distribution and press-fit stability. *J Arthroplasty* 1997;12:207–212.
34. Rosner BI, Postak PD, Greenwald, AS. Cup/liner conformity of modular acetabular designs. Scientific exhibition at the 62nd Annual Meeting of the American Academy of Orthopaedic Surgeons, 1995; Feb.
35. Salvati EA, Lieberman JR, Huk OL, Evans BG. Complications of femoral and acetabular modularity. *Clin Orthop* 1995;319:85–93.
36. Willert HG, Bertram H, Buchorn GH. Osteolysis in alloarthroplasty of the hip. *Clin Orthop* 1990;258:95–107.
37. Williams VG, Whiteside LA, White SE, McCarthy DS. Fixation of ultrahigh-molecular-weight polyethylene liners to metal-backed acetabular cups. *J Arthroplasty* 1997;12:25–31.
38. Won CH, Hearn TC, Tile M. Micromotion of cementless hemispherical acetabular components. *J Bone Joint Surg Br* 1995;76:484–489.
39. Wroblewski BM, Lynch M, Atkinson JR, Dowson D, Isaac GH. External wear of the polyethylene socket in cemented total hip arthroplasty. *J Bone Joint Surg Br* 1987;69:61–63.

Revision Total Hip Arthroplasty,
edited by Marvin E. Steinberg and Jonathan P. Garino,
Lippincott Williams & Wilkins, Philadelphia © 1998.

5

Effect of Femoral Design on Long-term Survivorship

J. Dennis Bobyn, Michael Tanzer, and
Andrew H. Glassman

After more than three decades of experience with total hip arthroplasty, the science and surgical principles guiding revision surgery for aseptic loosening have become increasingly clear and refined. Aseptic loosening accounts for more than 80% of all revision hip operations. Different philosophies exist for the treatment of loose femoral prostheses. These are dictated partially by the extent of associated host bone damage and partially by the surgeon's preference for either cemented or uncemented fixation. The fact that no single approach is suitable or superior for all revision operations attests to the complexity of the problem and the need for further research and development in this field. This chapter reviews the most current thinking in revision hip surgery with specific focus on femoral implant design and its influence on clinical results. For each fixation philosophy, informative, representative, and recent literature publications are included for a balanced perspective.

Revision hip arthroplasty is commonly associated with varying degrees of bone loss. The factors contributing to femoral bone loss include osteolysis caused by the presence of particulate debris (polyethylene, cement, metal), stress shielding, mechanical erosion of bone from loose and migrating stems, osteopenia from the aging process, and infection. Because of the special circumstances surrounding revision surgery for infection, it is not included in the data review or discussion of implant design. The challenge of achieving

J. D. Bobyn: Departments of Surgery and Biomedical Engineering, McGill University and Montreal General Hospital, Montreal, Quebec, Canada H3G 1A4.

M. Tanzer: Department of Surgery, McGill University and Montreal General Hospital, Montreal, Quebec, Canada H3G 1A4.

A. H. Glassman: Anderson Orthopaedic Research Institute, Arlington, Virginia 22206.

enduring fixation becomes increasingly difficult with increasing bone stock damage. Because fixation philosophy and the clinical results can depend on the extent of host bone damage by the loosening process, it is helpful to define some common terms for the various deficiencies.

According to the classification of the American Academy of Orthopaedic Surgeons (AAOS) Committee on the Hip, femoral abnormalities can be described as segmental (uncontained lesion or loss of bone in the supporting femoral cortical shell), cavitary or ectatic (contained lesion representing an excavation or expansion of cancellous or cortical bone), combined (cavitary and segmental), malaligned (rotational or angular), stenotic (relative or absolute narrowing of the femoral canal), or discontinuous (absence of bony integrity that occurs with femoral fractures) (7). In addition to these six types of femoral abnormality, the classification system includes a definition of levels of involvement. Level 1 is defined as bone proximal to the inferior aspect of the lesser trochanter. Level 2 includes the region from the inferior aspect of the lesser trochanter to 10 cm distal. Level 3 involves all bone distal to level 2. Most defects associated with failed femoral implants are incorporated within levels 1 or 2. Level 3 deficiencies are the most extreme and typically result from either femoral fractures or loosening of long-stem prostheses. Descriptions of femoral deficiencies have been added by Peters et al. (35). For example, a stage I femur has cancellous cavitary defects limited to level 1 or 2. A stage II femur has either cortical or ectatic cavitary defects limited to level 1, cancellous cavitary defects in level 2, or segmental defects of less than 1 cm in level 1. A stage III femur has cortical or ectatic cavitary defects in level 1, 2, or 3 or segmental defects of less than 1 cm in levels 2 or 3 or both. A stage IV femur has cortical or ectatic cavitary defects in levels 1, 2, and 3; segmental defects of at least 1 cm in levels 1, 2, or 3; or a fracture of the femur. Most reports in the literature use a modification of this system or a different system altogether. Within reasonable limits of interpretation herein, information from the various reports is standardized to this terminology when possible.

Any review or discussion of revision hip surgery is complicated by the broad range of osseous abnormalities, reason for revision, method of treatment, and method of reporting results. Cases in which multiple revisions have been performed are particularly difficult to analyze or compare on an equal basis. Most multiple revisions are for aseptic loosening and hence are associated with increasing loss of bone stock. The second most common indication for multiple revision is recurrent dislocation, associated with loss of the abductor mechanism because of deficient soft tissues, limb shortening, and component malposition. In certain cases, trochanteric detachment and subsequent loss of abductor function further complicates subsequent reconstruction. Recurrent instability often leads to loosening of the acetabular cup because of the high forces exerted on the implant during dislocation. All these factors make it impossible to isolate the influence of implant design on the clinical outcome. For the most part, this review considers only the literature in which a single revision for aseptic femoral loosening was performed. The most critical measure of success after revision arthroplasty is whether implant fixation is established and maintained. Hence, emphasis is placed on reporting rates of revision, radiographic loosening, and survivorship with revision and loosening as end points. With minor exceptions, the rates of radiographic loosening include both definite and probable (radiolucencies surrounding 50% to 100% of the cement–bone interface) loosening. Because resection arthroplasty for infection cannot usually be attributed to implant design, the revision and loosening data do not include failures for infection. Discussion of clinical scores, limp, pain, and details of radiographic features such as radiopaque lines is not included.

REVISION WITH CEMENT

The longest clinical history of revision hip arthroplasty involves the use of bone cement for stem fixation. Traditionally this involved cementing the prosthesis into the femur without associated bone graft. More recently techniques have evolved to reconstruct more severely damaged femurs by means of impaction grafting before cementing the femoral prosthesis. The results of these techniques are discussed separately.

First–Generation Cementing Technique

There are many reports on the results of cemented revision hip arthroplasty, but because of improvements in cementing techniques over the years, only the more recent publications are strictly relevant to current clinical practice. The published results of cemented revision using so-called first-generation cementing (without bone plug or pressurization) demonstrated unacceptably high re-revision rates at relatively short-term follow-up times (Table 1). Loosening rates as high as 44% and re-revision rates as high as 7.5% have been reported with average follow-up periods from only 2.1 to 4.5 years. In 1985, Pellicci et al. (34) reported a 17% femoral component loosening rate and a 12% re-revision rate in an 8.1 year average follow-up study of 99 cases. In many of these earlier reports, the implants possessed design features such as sharp corners and narrow medial borders that are now known to increase stress in adjacent cement and therefore increase the likelihood of cement fracture and subsequent stem loosening.

In a recent report of femoral revision using first-generation cementing, Stromberg and Herberts (42) described 51 femoral revisions at a 10-year average follow-up period (range, 8 to 13 years). Prerevision femoral bone deficiencies were primarily cavitary defects confined to levels 1 (73%) and 2 (25%). Almost all implants were cobalt chrome Lubinus (Link, Hamburg, Germany) and stainless steel Charnley designs (Thackray, Leeds, U.K.). There was a very high mechanical failure rate (revised plus radiographically loose) of 59% with a re-revision rate of 41%. Although an increase in the severity of bone deficiency was found at the last follow-up examination compared with prerevision radiographs, the influence of the bone deficiency on the results was not described.

Garcia-Cimbrelo et al. (12) reviewed 155 consecutive cemented stem revisions with Charnley implants and first-generation cementing technique after an average follow-up period of 11.5 years (range, 0.1 to 20 years). Most of the cases consisted of cavitary lesions confined to levels 1 (69%) and 2 (23%). No bone graft was used for any of the reconstructions. The probability of stem revision was 12% at 10 years and 16% at 16 years. The probability of radiographic stem loosening was 17% at 10 years and 22% at 16 years. Radiographic stem loosening was more frequent with the more severe prerevision bone deficiencies, although not statistically different.

Combined First- and Second-Generation Cementing Technique

Second-generation cementing includes operations in which a distal cement plug was used in conjunction with a gun for cement delivery and pressurization. In several published reports, both first- and second-generation cement techniques were used (Table 2). Mohler and Collis (28) reported on 96 cemented stem revisions after a mean follow-up

Table 1. *Data related to representative studies of first-generation cementing techniques*

Investigators	No. of cases	Patient age (yr; mean and range)	Follow-up period (yr; mean and range)	Implant, alloy	Survivorship[a] (revision)	Survivorship[b] (revision or loosening)	Revision rate[c]	Mechanical loosening rate[d]
Pellicci et al. (34)	99	64 (29–89)	8.1 (5–12.5)	NA	NA	NA	12%	29%
Stromberg and Herrberts (42)	51	47 (31–55)	10 (8–13)	Lubinus, Co Cr Charnley, SS	NA	NA	41%	59%
Garcia Cimbrelo et al. (12)	155	59 (22–82)	11.5 (0.1–20)	Charnley, SS	88% @ 10 yr 84% @ 16 yr	71% @ 10 yr 62% @ 16 yr	NA	NA

[a] Revision for aseptic loosening as end point.
[b] Revision or radiographic loosening (definite or probable) as end points.
[c] Revision for aseptic loosening.
[d] Includes revision and radiographic loosening (definite or probable).
NA, not available; SS, stainless steel.

Table 2. *Data related to representative studies of combined first- and second-generation cementing techniques*

Investigators	No. of cases	Patient age (yr; mean and range)	Follow-up period (yr; mean and range)	Implant, alloy	Survivorship[a] (revision)	Survivorship[b] (revision or loosening)	Revision rate[c]	Mechanical loosening rate[d]
Mohler and Collis (28)	96	65 (28–84)	5.5 (1–7)	Iowa, Co Cr TR-28, Co Cr	NA	80% @ 9–10 yr	7%	13%
Raut et al. (37)	399	65 (26–92)	7.5 (3–19)	Charnley, SS	94% @ 10 yr	92% @ 10 yr	5%	7.8%
Raut et al. (38)	39	55 (26–81)	7.3 (2–19)	Charnley, SS	NA	NA	NA	5.1%
Iorio et al. (15)	107	63 (NA)	7.7 (2–20)	Charnley, SS	NA	99% @ 5 yr 77% @ 10 yr	3.8%	16%
Marti et al. (25)	60	71 (26–86)	8.9 (5–14)	Weber, Co Cr	NA	NA	5%	32%

[a-d] See Table 1.
NA, not available; SS, stainless steel.

period of 5.5 years (range, 1 to 17 years). Second-generation cement technique was used in 86% of cases. Although a variety of stem designs were used, the Iowa (67%) and TR-28 (23%) stems composed the vast majority. Preoperatively, bone defects were absent or mild in 75 cases (78%). Cavitary cortical defects of 1 to 3 cm were present in 13 cases (14%), and cavitary defects extending more than 3 cm or segmental defects occurred in 8 cases (8%). Survivorship analysis revealed that 80% of the femoral components remained *in situ* 9 to 10 years after the operation. Thirteen components (13%) were mechanically loose, including 7 (7%) that were re-revised for aseptic loosening. Ten stems longer than 200 mm were used; in this subgroup there were three cases of loosening (30%). The overall good results were attributed to the high proportion of cases with no or minimal bone stock damage and the relatively elderly profile of the patient population (mean age, 65 years).

Reports from the Wrightington Hospital for Joint Disease on the use of stainless steel Charnley stems and mostly second-generation cementing yielded results superior to those obtained with first-generation cementing technique alone. Raut et al. (37) reviewed 283 revisions for aseptic loosening and 116 revisions for stem fracture with a mean follow-up period of 7.5 years (range, 3 to 19 years). The prerevision bone stock was normal or minimally damaged in 49% of cases, moderately damaged in 42%, and severely damaged in 9%. Associated femur fracture was present in 7.3% of cases. Four or more Gruen zones had cavitary or ectatic lesions in 28.3% of the cases. At last follow-up evaluation 7.8% (31) of the stems were radiographically loose. Of these, a total of 20 (5%) required re-revision for mechanical stem failure: 14 (3.5%) for aseptic loosening and 6 (1.5%) for stem fracture. Survivorship was 94% at 10 years with stem revision as the end point and 91% at 10 years with radiographic loosening as the end point. No correlation was found between fixation results and the state of prerevision femoral bone stock.

Raut et al. (38) also reviewed a subset of cemented femoral revisions among 39 patients with rheumatoid arthritis at an average follow-up time of 7.3 years (range, 2 to 19 years). This represented a relatively low-demand patient series; 60% of the patients were in Charnley class C. Although the frequency of acetabular failure was high, only 5.1% of patients (2) showed radiographic stem loosening at last follow-up examination.

Survivorship of 107 cemented revisions with an average follow-up period of 7.7 years (range, 2 to 20 years) was described by Iorio et al. (15). All patients were treated with stainless steel Charnley stems (Thackray), and second-generation cementing technique was used in 73% of the operations. Bone grafting was used in 9% of the operations, and long-stemmed prostheses were used to bypass segmental defects in 11% of the operations. At last follow-up examination, the radiographic loosening rate was 16% and the stem revision rate was 3.8%. Survivorship with radiographic loosening as an end point was 99% at 5 years and 77% at 10 years.

Marti et al. (25) reviewed the 8.9-year average results (range, 5 to 14 years) of 60 cemented revisions with the Weber prosthesis, a curved cobalt chromium stem with a modular trunnion-bearing cobalt chromium head. Two thirds of the operations were performed with first-generation cementing technique. The study emphasized that only three femoral components (5%) had been revised for mechanical loosening. However, 16 additional stems were unstable, for an overall mechanical loosening rate of 32%. This study did not provide any details about the extent of bone damage for the different revision procedures.

Second-Generation Cementing Technique

Izquierdo and Northmore-Ball (16) reviewed 139 cases of cemented femoral revision in a patient series with an average follow-up period of 6.5 years (range, 2 to 11 years) (Table 3). The series was different from most in that one third of the patients had undergone a previous revision and one third had an established deep infection. In almost all operations Charnley components were used. Cement was contained and pressurized in all instances, and antibiotics were added for the patients with infections. No details of the extent of bone damage were provided other than that 23% of the patients had segmental defects that were occluded before cementing. The radiologic survival rate was 90.5% at 10 years. Excluding recurrent infection (4 patients), the re-revision rate was 2.2% and the radiographic stem loosening rate was 4.4% at an average of 6.5 years.

Weber et al. (44) described the results of 48 cemented revisions for aseptic loosening with a precoated Iowa component (Zimmer, Warsaw, Ind.) after an average follow-up time of 6.2 years (range, 5 to 8 years). An osseous femoral defect greater than 2 cm was present in 40% of patients; the other 60% had defects smaller than 2 cm. Of the defects greater than 2 cm, 36% were segmental and 64% were cavitary. Most of the defects (88%) were confined to levels 1 and 2. At final follow-up examination, four patients had radiographic evidence of loosening (8.3%), one of whom (2.1%) had undergone revision arthroplasty. The probability of survival of the femoral component, with revision or radiographic evidence of definite or probable loosening as the end point, was 96% at 5 years and 81% at 8 years. A long-stemmed prosthesis (at least 200 mm) had been used in one third of the operations to bypass cortical defects; these operations were associated with a significantly increased femoral loosening rate. The presence of a 2-cm or larger osseous defect did not correlate significantly with a higher rate of loosening.

Table 3. *Data related to representative studies of second-generation cementing technique*

Investigators	No. of cases	Patient age (yr; mean and range)	Follow-up period (yr; mean and range)	Implant, alloy	Survivorship[a] (revision)	Survivorship[b] (revision or loosening)	Revision rate[c]	Mechanical loosening rate[d]
Izquierdo and Northmore-Ball (16)	139	67 (19–82)	6.5 (2–11)	Charnley, SS	NA	90.5% @ 10 yr	2.2%	4.4%
Weber et al. (44)	48	66 (39–84)	6.2 (5–8)	Iowa, Co Cr	NA	96% @ 5 yr 81% @ 8 yr	2.1%	8.3%
Estok and Harris (11)	38	57 (NA)	11.7 (9.8–14.3)	HD-2, Co Cr Calcar, Co Cr	90% @ 10 yr	86% @ 10 yr[e]	10.5%	21%[e]
Mulroy and Harris (31)	35	57 (NA)	15.1 (14.2–17.5)	HD-2, Co Cr Calcar, Co Cr	NA	0	20%	26%[e]
Katz et al. (18)	50	64 (23–89)	11.9 (10–16)	Charnley, SS Iowa, Co Cr	NA	0	9.5%	26%
Ballard et al. (1)	27	84 (80–90)	5 (1–7)	Iowa, Co Cr	100%	100%	0%	0%
Stromberg and Herberts (43)	57	47 (29–55)	7 (4–18)	NA	95% @ 6 yr 85% @ 8 yr	0	7%	21%
Pierson and Harris (36)	29	49 (NA)	8.5 (5.2–11)	HD-2, Co Cr Calcar, Co Cr	NA	0	6.9%	14%

[a-d] See Table 1.
[e] Does not include instances of probable loosening.
NA, not available; SS, stainless steel.

The results of a small series of cemented femoral revisions for aseptic loosening were described by Estok and Harris (11) and Mulroy and Harris (31) at two long follow-up intervals. At 11.7 years (range, 9.8 to 14.3 years) 38 hips were reviewed (11). A cobalt chrome HD-2 stem (Howmedica, Rutherford, N.J.) was used in 61% of the operations and a cobalt chrome calcar replacement stem (Howmedica) in 39%. No stems longer than 180 mm were used, and none of the implants was precoated. Prerevision bone damage was judged mild in 34%, moderate in 47%, and severe in 19% of instances. Radiographic evidence of definite loosening (not including probable loosening) was present in 8 cases (21%), 4 of which (10.5%) necessitated re-revision. No correlation could be drawn between osseous damage and the fixation results. A 15.1-year average follow-up study (range, 14.2 to 17.5 years) for this patient series described the results for the 35 surviving hips (31). The overall loosening rate, including revisions and those radiographically loose (not including probable loosening), was 26% (9 hips) with a re-revision rate of 20% (7 hips).

Katz et al. (18) reported on the results of improved cementing technique in a group of 50 revised hip replacements with an 11.9-year mean follow-up period (range, 10 to 16 years). Charnley and Iowa stem designs were used in about an equal number of operations. Prerevision bone deficiencies were not severe for the most part. Forty-nine (98%) of the patients had stage I or II loss. At last follow-up examination, the rate of aseptic revision was 9.5%, and the rate of radiologic loosening was 26%.

The effect of advanced age on the longevity of cemented revision was reported by Ballard et al. (1) in a study of 27 operations on patients at least 80 years of age. The average age at the time of revision was 84 years (range, 80 to 90 years), and the average follow-up period was 5 years (range, 1 to 7 years). Twelve patients (44%) had Charnley class C involvement. An Iowa femoral component was used in all revisions. There were no re-revisions, and no instances of radiographic loosening at the last follow-up examination, reflecting the lower activity level of the patient group.

Stromberg and Herberts (43) reviewed the results of cemented revision among patients younger than 55 years recorded in 25 hospitals of the Swedish Total Hip Registry. Fifty-seven hips were followed for an average of 7 years (range, 4 to 10 years). The average age at revision was 47 years (range, 29 to 55 years). Only 10% of the patients were in Charnley class C. The probabilities of stem survivorship with revision as the end point were 95% at 6 years and 85% at 8 years. Four stems were revised for aseptic loosening and 8 others were radiographically loose for a combined mechanical failure rate of 21%. No details of stem design other than length were provided. Because of the multicenter nature of the review it is likely that several different designs were used. Although only general statements were made about the extent of bone deficiencies at the time of revision, a statistically significant correlation was reported to exist between the severity of bone defects and aseptic loosening.

Pierson and Harris (36) reviewed the results of cemented revision among 29 patients with moderate or extensive femoral osteolysis caused by a loosened cemented component. The mean follow-up period was 8.5 years (range, 5.2 to 11 years). All but three of the patients were treated with HD-2 or calcar replacement stem designs (Howmedica). At last follow-up examination only 2 replacements (6.9%) had been rerevised for aseptic loosening, and 86% of the stems were well fixed. Only 2 patients (6.9%) had a recurrence of osteolysis.

Summary: Cementing Without Bone Graft

It is impossible to compare the various reports on cemented femoral revisions on an equal basis because of differences in patient series, follow-up periods, and methods of reporting. Certain general conclusions can be drawn, however. The implant should be manufactured of either forged cobalt chromium alloy or stainless steel. Both these materials have a twofold higher modulus of elasticity compared with titanium alloy. Finite-element studies have shown that higher stem stiffness helps reduce the stresses in the cement mantle and may influence longevity of fixation. Both materials are harder than titanium alloy and therefore more abrasion resistant. This has been shown to be important in reducing the extent of metallosis in cases of loosening and stem motion against the cement mantle. A few reports of stem fractures occurred in series with both cobalt chromium and stainless steel stems. In North America there is almost universal use of cobalt chromium alloy, but forged stainless steel has comparable fatigue strength. Judging from the various reports in the literature, the fracture rate of femoral stems in revision surgery exceeds that encountered in primary hip replacement.

For many years there has been general agreement on the need for rounded edges and a broad enough medial aspect to reduce cement stresses below the fracture limit. There is less agreement on the need for proximal macrotexturing or precoating with bone cement to enhance the stem–cement bond. Although precise descriptions of the stems used in the various reported series usually were not provided, most did not have macrotexturing features, and only in a couple of reports did some of the stems have precoating. Although precoating has been shown in the laboratory to enhance the strength of the stem–cement bond, it has not been associated with better clinical results in primary total hip arthroplasty than obtained with nonprecoated devices. It is therefore unlikely that precoating represents an important design feature for cemented revision implants.

Use of long-stemmed implants (longer than 200 mm) tends to be associated with poorer results, probably not because of an inherent weakness in the design so much as that longer stems are used when there are segmental defects and more extensive overall osseous deficiencies. Retpen and Jenson (39) reported that there is a substantially higher risk for failure if the long stem does not bridge the femoral defect by more than one width of the cortical shaft. It does not appear that a stem collar is an essential design feature. Similar revision and loosening at a minimum follow-up period of 10 years have been reported with use of stems with and without collars (11,18).

Good cement technique has been shown in several studies to improve the quality and longevity of fixation (41). Pressurization of cement into a plugged canal improves mechanical interlock with host bone. Several authors emphasize the importance of complete removal of the soft-tissue membrane and, if present, the neocortex to expose as much of the underlying cancellous bone as possible for good cement interdigitation. As in primary operations, a uniform cement mantle of at least 2 mm is important to reduce cement stresses, as is extension of cement beyond the stem tip by at least 1 to 2 cm. Several studies refer to worse results with decreasing quality of the cement mantle, emphasizing the need to avoid an incomplete mantle (39). Varus positioning of the stem has been associated with a higher rate of loose stems, although not all studies agree with this finding (39). Although it is generally believed that cement porosity decreases longevity of the construct, data from Raut et al. (37) suggest that good results can be obtained when mantle voids are prevalent. There are no substantial data on the results of cemented revision operations in which third-generation cement technique was used (second-generation with centralization and porosity reduction of cement).

As would be expected, implant survivorship decreases with increasing follow-up time. Reports with an average follow-up period of less than 9 or 10 years must be viewed cautiously. Reports with small patient numbers are less helpful. The results are generally worse among younger, more active patients (39). Some studies make brief reference to less favorable results with increasing severity of prerevision bone stock damage. Cavitary defects confined to level 1 are rarely associated with loosening as long as 10 years after the operation. Snorrasen and Karrholm (41) used roentgen stereophotogrammetric techniques to show increased stem instability with increasing bone deficiency. It is not possible to make definitive statements about the expected result with the more severe extent of osseous damage. With second-generation cementing techniques, the revision rate after an average of 7 to 10 years ranged from 5% to 7%, excluding the report by Ballard et al. (1), in which there were no revisions among a small group of sedentary and very old patients. Stem survivorship with revision or radiographic loosening as the end point ranged from 82% to 93% 8 to 11 years after the operation (Fig. 1). These results are not as good as with cemented primary total hip arthroplasty but are clearly improved over reports published in the 1980's. Some studies included only definite radiographic loosening in survivorship data, but most included both definite and probable loosening.

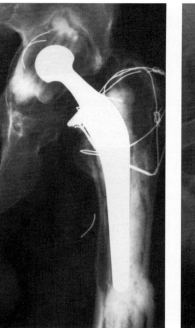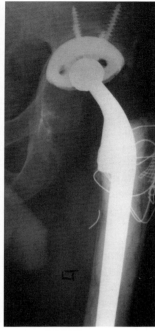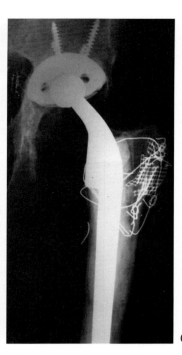

A,B   C

Figure 1. **A:** Prerevision radiograph shows a loose cemented stem with stage III bone loss. **B:** Radiograph obtained immediately after revision shows use of a long, cobalt chrome calcar, cemented prosthesis to bypass segmental defects. The cement mantle is thick, and cement–bone radiolucencies are apparent. **C:** Nine-year postrevision radiograph shows a stable component with no deterioration of the cement–bone interfaces. (Courtesy of W. H. Harris, MD.)

The latter, more conservative definition is preferable, because most stems with probable loosening culminate in a revision with a sufficient follow-up period. One last issue concerns the fact that the best results were obtained in centers for hip surgery in which the revisions were performed by a one experienced surgeon. The multicenter reports from the Swedish Hip Registry emphasize that these results probably cannot be expected from the orthopedic community at large (43).

CEMENTING WITH BONE GRAFT

An alternative technique to conventional cemented revision total hip arthroplasty is impaction grafting, a technique in which morselized cancellous bone graft is packed into the canal before stem cementing (13,23) (Table 4). Gie et al. (13) and Ling et al. (23) advocate use of a polished, collarless, double-tapered stem with a distal hollow centralizer that allows the implant to subside within the cement mantle. When loaded, the double-tapered wedge design results in predominantly radial compression of the surrounding cement and reduces shear at the implant–cement and bone–cement interfaces. This radial compression further impacts and loads the bone graft in the revised femur. Like any taper, as the stem subsides and engages the cement mantle, it becomes progressively more stable.

Despite the increasing popularity of and interest in this technique, there are only a few published reports on the results of impaction grafting for femoral revision. In the most recent report by Gie et al. (13), records of 50 patients who had undergone femoral revision with impaction grafting and implantation of the stainless steel Exeter stem (Howmedica) were reviewed. Three hips had bone loss with radiolucent lines confined to the upper half of the cement mantle with clinical signs of loosening; 34 had bone loss with generalized radiolucent lines and endosteal erosion of the upper femur leading to widening of the medullary canal; and 13 had bone loss with widening of the medullary canal by expansion of the upper femur. There were no cases of segmental bone loss in this study. Although

Table 4. *Data related to studies of cementing with impaction grafting*

Investigators	No. of cases	Patient age (yr; mean and range)	Follow-up period (yr; mean and range)	Implant, alloy	Survivorship[a] (revision)	Survivorship[b] (revision or loosening)	Revision rate[c]	Mechanical loosening rate[d]
Gie et al. (13)	50	68 (46–85)	NA (3.8–6.6)	Exeter, SS	NA	NA	0%	NA
Elting et al. (10)	56	65 (35–88)	2.6 (2–5.2)	CPT, Co Cr	NA	NA	0%	NA
Elting (9)	147	66 (33–89)	5.5 (2–8)	Exeter, SS CPT, Co Cr	NA	NA	1.4%	5.4%

[a–d] See Table 1.
NA, Not available; SS, stainless steel.

several hips required reoperation, primarily for femoral fractures, none required re-revision for aseptic loosening. Radiographic evaluation of the bone graft revealed cortical healing and trabecular remodelling in 32% of the cases, trabecular remodelling in 27%, cortical healing and trabecular incorporation in 16%, trabecular incorporation in 9%, cortical healing in 9%, bone resorption in 4% and no change in the graft in 2%. In all cases of bone resorption, the graft had been inadequately constrained. Subsidence of the stem in the cement mantle occurred in all cases. The subsidence was less than 1 mm in 18% of the hips, 1 to 2 mm in 32%, 3 to 4 mm in 32%, 5 to 7 mm in 11%, and 8 to 10 mm in 7%. Subsidence of the entire cement mantle within the femoral canal occurred in 20% of cases. The subsidence was less than 1 mm in 4.5% of the hips, 1 to 2 mm in 11.4%, 3 to 4 mm in 2%, and 5 to 7 mm in 2%. Despite the marked subsidence in many cases, the authors concluded that impaction grafting shows considerable promise and that in the short term clinical and radiographic results do not deteriorate.

Similar encouraging results were reported by Elting et al. (10) in a review of the treatment of 56 patients 31 months (range, 24 to 64 months) after femoral revision by means of the impaction grafting technique and use of a cobalt chrome CPT prosthesis (Zimmer). According to the AAOS classification, the bony defects were cavitary in 43% of cases, segmental in 13%, and combined in 31%. Two hips needed rerevision for sepsis, but there were no revisions for aseptic loosening. Three hips needed reoperation for postoperative femur fractures, and 2 needed revision for recurrent dislocation. At radiographic examination the bone grafts appeared to show cortical repair and trabecular incorporation in 63% of the cases, cortical repair and trabecular remodelling in 20%, trabecular incorporation in 9%, trabecular remodelling in 4%, and cortical repair in 2%. Two percent of the cases showed no change in appearance of the graft material. Forty-eight percent of the stems demonstrated subsidence in the cement mantle, which averaged 2.8 mm (range, 1 to 8 mm). Nonprogressive subsidence of the cement mantle within the allograft reconstruction occurred in 7% of cases and averaged 1.7 mm (range, 1 to 3 mm). Based on these results, the conclusion was that impaction grafting provides a reliable method for femoral revision, reconstruction, and reconstitution.

Elting (9) also reported on 147 patients who underwent impaction grafting after follow-up examinations averaging 5.5 years (range, 2 to 8 years). Only two revisions (1.4%) were needed for aseptic loosening with symptomatic subsidence of stem and cement mantle, both by patients taking intermittent high-dose steroids and each at 6 years. The combined revision and radiographic loosening rate was 5.4%. Subsidence of the stem within the mantle occurred frequently within the first 2 years (48%) but was less than 2 mm. Subsidence of the entire construct was observed in 5% of cases, but it was also less than 2 mm. The graft was judged to be radiographically incorporated in 96% of cases.

Summary: Cementing with Bone Graft

The reported experience with impaction grafting using a cemented, polished, collarless, double-tapered femoral stem is limited and of short follow-up duration. Nonetheless the early results have been encouraging. Radiographic and histologic evidence of at least partial bone remodelling of the impacted cancellous allograft has been reported. Histologic studies have shown that the grafted bone becomes organized into three zones (23,32). On the surface there is regenerated cortex with fatty marrow and a few islands of dead bone. The intermediate zone demonstrates direct contact between osteoid and bone cement with some areas of foreign-body giant cells or soft tissue. In some cases trabecular condensation in the intermediate zone produces a neocortex similar to that seen at histologic examination around stable, cemented femoral components. The deep layer contains necrotic bone embedded in the cement mantle. This bone remodelling is believed to be caused by the initial stability provided by the densely packed bone graft, the cement bond between the implant and the graft, and the compressive loads transmitted to the graft by the double-wedged-shaped, polished femoral component as it subsides into a stable position.

The combination of stem design, hollow distal centralizer, and bone cement creep are believed to act in concert to allow subsidence at the implant–cement interface. However, excessive subsidence or failure of the cement mantle to creep sufficiently can result in cement fractures (because of excessive radial tension within the mantle), which place the underlying bone at risk for osteolysis and the implant at risk for failure. Subsidence of the stem in the cement mantle as much as 8 to 10 mm has been reported, yet none of the stems were judged to be radiographically loose.

Although impaction grafting is promising for revising femurs with primarily proximal cavitary defects, the outcome of this technique for femurs with large segmental defects or

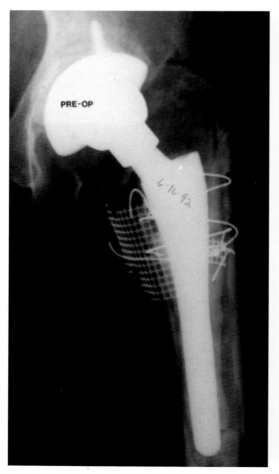
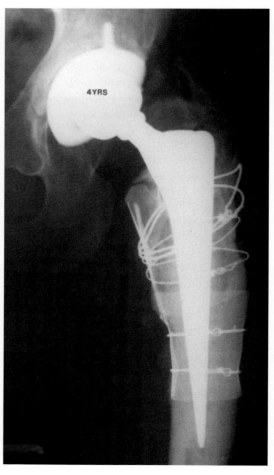

A   B

Figure 2. A: Prerevision radiograph shows loose cemented stem with stage III bone loss. **B:** Four-year postrevision radiograph shows tapered stainless steel Exeter stem with impaction grafting. Although the interfaces are difficult to visualize because of the mesh used to contain segmental defects, the implant appears stable, and there is clear restitution of bone stock. (Courtesy of J. J. Elting, MD.)

with osteolysis distal to a conventional-length stem is unknown. Furthermore, the high incidence of absence or deficiency of cement mantles with the Exeter impaction allografting system raises some concerns about the long-term survivorship of this implant (8,26).

The advantage of impaction grafting is that it can provide immediate implant stability and restore proximal femoral stock in the case of future revision (Fig. 2). However, the procedure can be technically demanding, it requires a large quantity of allograft bone, cement mantle deficiencies can occur with some of the present instrumentation, and the long-term outcome of the procedure remains unknown. Some centers are evaluating the technique with stems other than the double-taper polished design, but there are no longer-term results.

FIXATION WITHOUT BONE CEMENT

Diametrically opposed to the rationale of using cement for revision is the concept of biologic fixation by means of direct insertion of implants into host bone. As in primary operations, this concept relies on achieving sufficient initial implant stability to allow osseointegration of the implant into the surrounding host bone. This is a stringent requirement. Results of experimental studies with animals have suggested that bone ingrowth can occur only if motion at the bone–implant interface is less than about 40 μm. Beyond this limit there is increased tendency for less rigid fibrous tissue fixation (17). The two main approaches to solving the problems of revision surgery for aseptic loosening involve the use of implants with proximal porous coating, in which the metaphyseal portion of the implant can enhance secondary stability by ingrowth, or with extensive porous coating, in which most or all of the stem length is available for tissue ingrowth. The principal arguments for proximally porous coated devices in revision surgery include ease of removal and minimization of stress shielding and bone resorption. The main argument for using extensively coated stems is that the diaphysis is the most reliable and reproducible region for primary and secondary fixation, because metaphyseal bone stock is often compromised in revision operations. Alternative uncemented approaches include use of hydroxyapatite (HA)–coated stems and grit-blasted stems designed for secondary stabilization by bone ingrowth or osseointegration.

Implants with Proximal Porous Coating

Malkani et al. (24) reviewed 69 noncemented revisions with long-stemmed, curved prostheses at a mean follow-up time of 3 years (range, 2 to 5 years) (Table 5). The implant was made of cobalt chrome and was proximally coated with sintered beads (Omnifit; Osteonics, Allendale, N.J.). Level 1 cavitary bone loss was present in 15% of cases, level 2 cortical or cancellous cavitary bone loss was present in 76% of cases, and segmental bone loss occurred in the remaining 9%. Bone grafts were used extensively in the series, most of which were cancellous autograft and allograft. Subsidence of 5 mm or more was noted in 57% of cases. At last follow-up examination, six stems (9%) had been revised, five for aseptic loosening and one because of deep infection. With component revision as the end point, survivorship was 82% at 5 years. In the entire group, 34 patients (46%) incurred an intraoperative femoral fracture, which often resulted in a poor clinical result. If revision or moderate to severe pain was used as the definition of failure, the predicted survivorship among the patients with an intraoperative fracture was only 58%. Progressive radiolucent lines were common and were seen in Gruen zones 1 and 7 among half the patients.

Ninety-one operations in which a modular titanium proximally porous coated stem was used (S-ROM; Joint Medical Products, Stamford, Conn.) were reviewed by Cameron (5) with a follow-up period of 3.5 years (range, 2 to 6 years). A primary stem was used in 29 cases and a longer revision stem was used in 62. Revision stems were reserved for the more severe stage II and stage III reconstructions. None of the replacements with primary stems needed re-revision and none had an unstable radiographic appearance. Eight of the

Table 5. *Data related to studies of proximally porous coated stems*

Investigators	No. of cases	Patient age (yr; mean and range)	Follow-up period (yr; mean and range)	Implant, alloy	Survivorship[a] (revision)	Survivorship[b] (revision or loosening)	Revision rate[c]	Mechanical loosening rate[d]
Malkani et al. (24)	69	62 (NA)	3 (2–5)	Omnifit, Co Cr	82%	58%	9%	NA
Cameron (5)	91	57 (26–84)	3.5 (2–6)	S-ROM, Ti	100%	NA	0%	2.2%
Smith et al. (40)	66	65 (31–84)	3.4 (2–5)	S-ROM, Ti	100% @ 5 yr	88% @ 5 yr	0%	7.6%
Chandler et al. (6)	52	60 (NA)	3 (2–5.5)	S-ROM, Ti	NA	NA	4%	10%
Meding et al. (27)	32	64 (22–80)	3.6 (2–6)	PCA, Co Cr BiMetric, Ti	100%	NA	0%	18%
Mulliken et al. (30)	52	59 (36–79)	4.6 (4–6)	Mallory-Head, Ti	NA	NA	10%	23%
Buoncristiani et al. (4)	66	56 (29–83)	4.7 (3–7)	APR, Ti	NA	NA	4.5%	NA
Berry et al. (2)	375	60 (27–89)	4.2 (0–9)	Bias, HGP, Ti Omnifit, PCA, Co Cr	58% @ 8 yr	20% @ 8 yr	16%	NA
Woolson and Delaney (45)	28	55 (NA)	5.5 (4–8)	HGP, Ti	NA	NA	20%	52%
Peters et al. (35)	49	60 (52–82)	5.5 (3.8–7.3)	Bias, Ti	96% @ 6 yr	37% @ 6 yr	NA	NA
Hungerford (14)	91	55 (26–81)	6.5 (3–10)	PCA, Co Cr	NA	NA	10%	NA

[a–d] See Table 1.
APR, anatomic porous replacement; HGP, Harris-Galante porous coated; NA, not available; PCA, porous coated anatomic.

62 revision stems were revised, but none because of aseptic loosening. An unstable interface with divergent radiopaque lines was present in two cases (3.2%).

Use of the S-ROM stem was reviewed by Smith et al. (40) in a series of 66 hips with an average follow-up period of 3.4 years (range, 2 to 5 years). Among all reconstructions, 5 had segmental defects only, 16 had cavitary defects only, and 44 had combined defects. Most of the patients needed bone grafting to fill gaps or defects (79%), and some needed structural bone grafting for additional implant stability (7%). As in the series reviewed by Cameron, there was a relatively high rate of intraoperative femoral fractures (27%). There were no revisions for aseptic loosening. Five hips (7.6%) were judged to be radiographically loose. The 5-year survivorship including aseptic failure and radiographic loosening was 88%.

Chandler et al. (6) studied the results of 52 complex revision operations in which the S-ROM femoral component was used. The follow-up period averaged 3 years (range, 2 to 5.5 years). The patients generally had severe bone loss, leg length inequality, and instability. Twenty-two patients (42%) needed structural femoral allografts, and 8 patients (15%) had undergone previous resection arthroplasties for sepsis. The average number of previous hip operations was three. Mechanical loosening occurred in five hips (10%), two of which were undersized and re-revised (4%). Although many complications related to reconstruction were described, none was specifically associated with the stem design.

Meding et al. (27) studied 32 revision operations with long-stemmed (200 to 250 mm) uncemented implants after a mean follow-up period of 3.6 years (range, 2 to 6 years). The porous coated anatomic (PCA) stem (Howmedica) was used in 23 procedures and the BiMetric stem (Biomet, Warsaw, Ind.) in 9. Prerevision bone loss was primarily cavitary with stage I and II reconstructions. Five patients (16%) with PCA implants showed radiographic evidence of bead shedding. Six patients (18%) showed evidence of subsidence, progressive radiopaque lines, or instability.

Table 6. *Data related to studies of extensively porous coated stems*

Investigators	No. of cases	Patient age (yr; mean and range)	Follow-up period (yr; mean and range)	Implant, alloy	Survivorship[a] (revision)	Survivorship[b] (revision or loosening)	Revision rate[c]	Mechanical loosening rate[d]
Moreland and Bernstein (29)	175	62 (23–89)	5 (2–10)	AML, Co Cr Solution, Co Cr	NA	NA	2.5%	2.9%
Lawrence et al. (21,22)	174	57 (21–89)	7.4 (5–11)	AML, Co Cr	91% @ 10 yr	NA	3.4%	4.6%
Paprosky and Krishnamurthy (33)	297	60 (24–86)	8.3 (5–14)	AML, Co Cr	NA	NA	1.6%	2.4%

[a–d] See Table 1.
AML, anatomic medullary locking; NA, not available.

Mulliken et al. (30) reviewed 52 revision total hip arthroplasties with a 4.6-year average follow-up period (range, 4 to 6 years). A titanium alloy, long-revision stem with proximal plasma spray porous coating was used in all operations (Mallory-Head; Biomet). Preoperatively the femurs were classified with stage I bone loss in 16 cases (31%), stage II and III loss in 35 cases (67%), and stage IV loss in 1 case (2%). At last follow-up examination, 5 stems (10%) had been revised, and 7 others were unstable, for a radiographic loosening rate of 23%. Eleven of the 12 stem failures were in femurs with moderate or severe prerevision bone loss. Twenty (38%) femoral fractures occurred during stem insertion.

Buoncristiani et al. (4) reviewed the results of total hip arthroplasty using the anatomic porous replacement (APR) revision stem (Intermedics, Austin, Tex.), an anatomic (curved) titanium alloy design with proximal regions of inlaid cancellous structured porous coating. Sixty-six cases were reviewed after an average follow-up period of 4.7 years (range, 3 to 7 years). Thirty-one stems (47%) were plasma sprayed on the proximal porous areas with HA coating. Small cavitary lesions confined to level 1 were present before the revision operation in 26 cases (39.4%). Cavitary and segmental lesions extending to level 2 were present in 26 cases (39.4%). Damage in the remaining cases extended to level 3, with cavitary lesions in 3 cases (4.5%) and fractures or segmental lesions in 11 cases (16.7%). At the last follow-up examination, three stems (4.5%) needed revision because of instability. Radiographic evidence of bone ingrowth (spot welding) in Gruen zone 7 was observed in 53 cases (80%). This occurred more frequently among the group of stems with HA coating. This study differed from most in that a high proportion (48%) of reconstructions were augmented by demineralized strut cortical allografts.

Three hundred seventy-five revisions with six different proximally porous coated femoral components were reviewed by Berry et al. (2) on the basis of data from the Mayo Clinic Total Joint Registry. The titanium alloy implants included 51 standard-length Harris-Galante porous (HGP) and 94 long Bias stems (Zimmer), both designs with proximal, noncircumferential, fiber metal porous coating. The other implants were made of cobalt chrome alloy and included 72 Omnifit, 52 Omnifit long-stemmed, 49 PCA, and 57 PCA long-stemmed implants. The mean follow-up period was 4.2 years (range, 0 to 9 years). Prerevision bone deficiencies were present in level 1 in 29% of cases, level 2 in 58%, and level 3 in 10%; 3% of the patients had a periprosthetic fracture. At last follow-up examination, 16% of the patients needed component removal because of aseptic loosening. At 8 years, survivorship free of revision for aseptic failure was 58%, whereas survivorship free of revision or aseptic loosening was only 20%. More severe preoperative bone loss correlated statistically with poorer survivorship free of aseptic loosening and subsidence of more than 5 mm.

Woolson and Delaney (45) reviewed the results of 25 revisions with HGP prostheses (Zimmer) at a mean follow-up period of 5.5 years (range, 4 to 8 years). The preoperative femoral bone stock was classified as stage I in 17 hips (68%), stage II or III in 7 hips (28%), and stage IV in 1 hip (4%). Five patients (20%) underwent re-revision because of aseptic loosening. Subsidence of the femoral component of 5 mm or more occurred in 12 of the 25 hips (48%). Only 8 (32%) of the 25 patients had radiologic signs of bone ingrowth fixation of the stem. Radiographic evidence of instability was found in 13 cases (52%).

Peters et al. (35) reviewed the results of 49 revision hip arthroplasties at a mean follow-up period of 5.5 years (range, 3.8 to 7.3 years). All operations involved the use of a curved, long-stemmed titanium alloy implant (Bias; Zimmer) with proximal noncircumferential porous coating of commercially pure fiber metal. Prerevision bone damage was classified as stage I in 8 cases (16%), stage II in 20 cases (41%), and stage III in 21 cases (43%). Only two hips (4%) needed revision because of aseptic loosening. With revision as the end point, survivorship at 6 years was 96%. The main clinical problem with this series was component subsidence. At least 2 mm of subsidence occurred within the first year among 28 hips (57%). Subsidence of at least 2 mm occurred beyond the first postoperative year among 22 hips (45%). Radiolucent lines around these components were frequent. With revision or progressive subsidence (definite loosening) as the end points, survivorship at 6 years was only 37%. Stability of the femoral component was statistically worse in stage III compared with stage I reconstructions.

Hungerford (14) reviewed 91 hip replacements with the proximally coated cobalt chrome PCA prosthesis (Howmedica) at an average follow-up period of 6.5 years (range, 3 to 10 years). A revision rate of 10% was reported at last follow-up examination. None of the 9 patients with stage I bone loss underwent revision, whereas 14% of the 44 patients with stage III and IV loss underwent revision. Revision was attributed to undersizing and implant instability caused by intraoperative femoral fractures. Of the surviving hips, no details were provided regarding subsidence or the radiographic appearance of the bone–implant interfaces.

Summary: Proximal Porous Coating

The reported results with proximally porous coated implants do not extend beyond an average of 6.5 years of follow-up study and thus are not as reliable as the data on cemented revisions for providing an indication of long-term expectations. Although some of the short-term studies report no revisions and no loosening, others describe very poor results and relatively high revision rates. The study by Berry et al. (2) was particularly illuminating because it described results in a large series with six different stem designs made of both titanium and cobalt chrome alloy with and without collars. The results were extremely poor, much worse than reported for most series of cemented implants with longer follow-up periods.

There are fundamental deficiencies in the rationale for using proximally porous coated stems in revision surgery. First, the damaged, weakened bone often present in the proximal femur provides a suboptimal environment for initial stability and secondary stability by means of biologic fixation. The use of allogenic bone graft in the proximal femur to augment fixation and improve bone–implant contact generally does not result in bone ingrowth. Second, the distal portion of most proximally porous coated stems is typically smooth and cylindrical, sometimes with shallow flutes. The geometric features are generally designed for endosteal contact and press fit in the isthmus region. This does not provide the magnitude of initial torsional stability that can be obtained by means of actively engaging splines or cutting flutes into endosteal cortical bone (19). Long, straight stems, by virtue of additional area for endosteal contact, are helpful in bridging segmental defects or femoral fractures but have limited use in shorter or bowed femurs. Long, curved stems are better suited anatomically but it is not possible to insert a long anatomic stem into a bony envelope made by means of precision machining. Hence the fit often depends on several discrete regions of point or line contact. An inherent problem with uncemented long stems is that distal to the isthmus the intramedullary canal widens, reducing the potential extent or reliability of bone–implant contact. In all reports, the use of long stems, straight or curved, was associated with a high proportion of femoral fractures and associated complications. Of all the proximally coated devices, the titanium alloy S-ROM stem is the most versatile and appears to have the most promise for success in certain revision settings (Fig. 3). The modular proximal segment allows reproducible fit with instruments that machine the metaphysis, and the distal segment has cutting flutes that can engage with endosteal bone for increased stability. A distal slot or clothespin feature may be helpful in reducing risk for femoral fracture. Its effect on reducing stress shielding has not been quantified, although several studies have documented that titanium stems, by virtue of decreased stiffness, result in less periprosthetic bone resorption than those made of cobalt chrome alloy. With the exception of instances in which bone-stock damage is minimal, the same reproducibility of results cannot generally be expected with proximally coated stems as with cemented devices.

Extensively Porous Coated Stems

The rationale for using extensively porous coated stems is that the diaphysis is the most reliable segment of the femur for achieving primary stability and subsequent bone ingrowth. Because of frictional and mechanical resistance, torsional implant stability is increased if the stem is porous coated and press fit at the isthmus (19). Histologic studies have demonstrated that the extent of bone ingrowth and the fixation provided by ingrowth are maximized with close apposition to cortical bone.

Moreland and Bernstein (29) reviewed the results of 175 revision arthroplasties with extensively porous coated cobalt chrome stem designs (AML, Solution; Depuy, Warsaw, Ind.) (Table 6). The average follow-up period was 5 years (range, 2 to 10 years). Preoperatively the femoral bone-stock deficiency was classified as minimal in 25% of cases, moderate in 55%, and severe in 20%. At last follow-up examination, aseptic loosening was found in 5 cases (2.9%), in 4 of which (2.3%) the arthroplasty had been revised. The porous interfaces were classified as probable bone ingrowth in 83% of cases and stable fibrous interface in 15.5% of cases. Patients with mild prerevision bone-stock

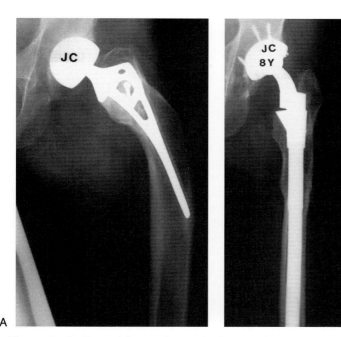

A   B

Figure 3. A: Prerevision radiograph shows a loose uncemented Moore stem with associated angular femoral deformity. **B:** Radiograph 8 years after revision shows use of a modular titanium S-ROM stem to bypass an osteotomy for correction of the deformity. The prosthesis is stable, and adaptive bone remodeling has occurred. (Courtesy of H. U. Cameron, MD.)

loss had a significantly higher rate of bone ingrowth than patients with moderate and severe loss. Bone resorption from stress shielding was judged severe in 7.6% of the cases of bone ingrowth.

Lawrence et al. (21,22) reviewed the results of 174 revision arthroplasties with a mean follow-up period of 7.4 years (range, 5 to 11 years). The prostheses were made of cobalt chrome alloy and most were the anatomic medullary locking design (AML; Depuy). All implants were either extensively (80%) or fully porous coated with multiple layers of sintered beads. Prerevision bone-stock damage was present in level 1 and mild in 43 cases (25%), in level 1 but extensive in 92 cases (53%), and in levels 2 and 3 in 39 cases (22%). At last follow-up examination, six stems had been revised because of aseptic loosening (3.4%) and two others were radiographically unstable for a total mechanical loosening rate of 4.6%. Including two revisions for stem fracture and two resection arthroplasties for infection, survivorship at 9 years was 91%. The more severely deficient femurs with damage in levels 2 and 3 were associated with a significantly higher failure rate. Among the stable implants, 89% were judged to have bone ingrowth and 11% to have stable fibrous interfaces. Similar data were reported by Lawrence et al. (22) for a subset of 83 patients with extensively porous coated cobalt chrome stems who participated in follow-up study for an average of 9 years (range, 5 to 13 years). This study added that there was a significant correlation between undersized stems and a higher rate of mechanical loosening.

Paprosky and Krishnamurthy (33) reported the results for a series of 297 patients who participated in follow-up study for a mean of 8.3 years (range, 5 to 14 years). All operations involved use of an extensively coated cobalt chrome AML prosthesis (Depuy). In one third of the cases prerevision bone-stock damage extended into levels 2 and 3. In 163 cases (55%) it was determined that the metaphysis was unable to support the implant proximally and distal diaphyseal stability was necessary. At last follow-up examination, 5 hips (1.6%) had been revised for aseptic loosening and 2 others had definite radiographic instability for a total mechanical failure rate of 2.4%. Bone ingrowth was evident in 82% of the cases and stable fibrous fixation in 15.6%. Overall, 84% of the femurs showed some improvement in bone stock from preoperative radiographs. Stress shielding of the femur was moderate in 13% and severe in 6% of cases but was not symptomatic or otherwise related to outcome.

Summary: Extensively Porous Coated Stems

The long-term results with extensively porous coated revision stems are derived almost exclusively from the cobalt chrome AML and Solution designs (DePuy). Because of strength issues related to metallurgic changes during the heat treatments used to bond porous coatings, cobalt chrome alloys are preferred for designs with extensive coating. Given that the diaphysis is generally the primary source of implant stability, the presence of a collar on the implant is probably not always necessary. It is clear from the different reports that the technique of diaphyseal fixation yields good, reliable, long-term survivorship. The revision and loosening rates are generally superior to those achieved with proximally porous coated implants and as good or better than the best reports of use of cement for fixation. As with all stem designs, survivorship of extensively porous coated stems decreases with increasing extent of prerevision bone-stock damage. The excellent reported results are not a reflection of an unusually high proportion of revision procedures with mild bone deficiencies. Compared with cemented series there does not appear to be a bias toward more operations with less severe damage in the reports on extensively porous coated stems.

The fibrous interface around porous implants is very different from that in cemented arthroplasty. If a cemented stem is primarily surrounded by a radiolucent seam, indicative of fibrous tissue at the interface, it is generally classified as probably or definitely loose and included in revision and loosening statistics. However, in the case of porous coated devices, a fibrous interface is most often considered stable because the ability of fibrous tissue to become mechanically attached to the implant surface provides supportive implant fixation. In reports on extensively porous coated stems, the proportion of patients with stable fibrous interfaces ranged between 11% and 15%. This represents a three- to four-fold higher proportion than is typically reported with the use of such devices in primary operations. This further illustrates the fact that revision operations represent a more challenging environment for obtaining implant stability. Although stable fibrous interfaces maintain their radiographic appearance beyond a decade after primary operations, one crucial question is whether the fibrous interfaces will continue to function in a stable manner with increasing follow-up times after revision arthroplasty. Given the general tendency for poorer bony implant support in revision operations, there may be increased mechanical demands on the fibrous interfaces, and some may deteriorate with time.

Criticism about the concept of diaphyseal fixation centers on difficulties in implant removal and the potential for exaggerated bone resorption from stress shielding. Although extremely challenging, techniques have been developed for the removal of well-fixed, extensively porous coated devices. The issue of stress shielding has long been debated, and there is unanimous agreement that minimizing stress-related bone resorption is ideal. At the same time, the primary goal of revision surgery is to establish and maintain fixation, and this goal can conflict with the desire to conserve bone stock. With current technology there is little choice but to use cobalt chrome alloy for extensively porous coated designs. The twofold higher modulus of cobalt chrome compared with titanium alloy renders such designs stiffer and therefore prone to more extensive stress shielding. The proportion of cases in which severe stress shielding develops is less that 10% in revision surgery and, as with primary arthroplasty, no complications directly related to bone loss from stress shielding have been reported after a decade or more of follow-up study (3). Furthermore, there is evidence that healing of bone defects occurs with extensively porous coated

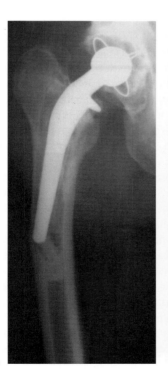
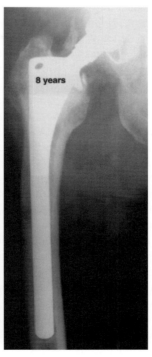

A   B

Figure 4. A: Prerevision radiograph shows loose cemented stem with varus angulation and stage II cavitary bone loss. **B:** Radiograph 8 years after revision shows use of a fully porous coated cobalt chrome alloy straight stem. The stem is stable, and periimplant bone resorption from stress shielding is relatively minor. (Courtesy of A. H. Glassman, MD.)

devices, even with larger, stiffer sizes (Fig. 4). Titanium alloy devices with extensive textured coatings have been developed for use in revision (Biomet, Osteonics). More innovative still is composite stem technology. One such example is a design consisting of a cobalt chrome inner core, a full length outer wrap of titanium porous fiber metal, and a flexible middle layer of low-modulus thermoplastic (polyaryletherketone) sandwiched between the two (Epoch; Zimmer). This design allows modulation of implant stiffness over the full stem length by varying the proportions of core and middle materials. It is too early to predict whether these developments with lower stiffness devices will be successful in reducing the extent of periimplant stress shielding while providing comparable fixation.

CONCLUSIONS

Revision total hip arthroplasty will always present greater challenges than primary hip arthroplasty, and the expectations for enduring implant fixation should generally be less. Despite the wide differences between various patient series and methods of reporting, some general conclusions can be drawn from review of the literature. Survivorship decreases with increasing follow-up time, hence 10 to 11 year average follow-up data are more informative and reliable than 5 to 6 year average follow-up data. With cemented implants for instance, the best survivorship rates with revision or radiographic loosening as end points are 95% to 99% at 5 years and 91% at 10 years. Similarly, the lowest revision rates with cemented implants range from about 2% at an average of 6 years to 10% at an average of 11 years of follow-up study. Many of the reports are based on relatively small patient series, which often precludes statistical analysis of factors possibly related to aseptic loosening. As with short follow-up periods, data based on only two or three dozen cases should generally be interpreted with a certain degree of caution.

The revision rates and survivorship data with proximally porous coated implants are generally worse than for other fixation modalities. Reports with proximally porous coated implants have typically involved smaller patient series. These series do not extend beyond a mean of 5 to 6 years of follow-up study and thus cannot be compared with long-term data on cemented or extensively porous coated stem designs. Excellent short-term fixation has been reported in femurs with mild bone-stock deficiencies, particularly with the modular S-ROM design. Hips with less severe metaphyseal bone damage generally do well with any implant design or fixation modality in the short term. With proximally coated revision stems that have smooth distal segments and hence less ability for mechanical purchase with diaphyseal bone, the results are decidedly unreliable or poor, especially with increasing degrees of bone defects.

Although cement fixation on the femoral side has historically been viewed as the standard for revision total hip arthroplasty, an objective review of the literature reveals inconsistent survivorship data, excluding results among very old, sedentary patients with low mechanical demands. Revision rates range from 2% to 7% after 6 to 7 years and from 5% to 10.5% after 8 to 12 years of follow-up study. Only some of this variability can be accounted for by differences among studies in patient age, activity level, and degree of bone-stock deficiencies. Perhaps more revealing are the combined rates of revision and radiographic loosening. These range from 4.4% to 21% at 6 to 7 years and 14% to 26% at 8 to 12 years. These statistics are important to consider because they include patients with probable or definite signs of radiographic loosening, a high proportion of which have been shown eventually to require revision for aseptic loosening. Cemented revision is most reliably indicated for more elderly, less active patients with larger intramedullary canals in which uncemented stems would tend to be stiffer and cause more stress shielding.

Although revision with cement and impaction grafting is of high interest and potential, it is difficult to gauge the prognosis for enduring fixation because the reports are few and the follow-up period is relatively short. Although low revision and radiographic loosening rates are reported, the concomitant high rates of subsidence are worrisome. Interpretation of the radiographic appearance of the cement–implant, cement–bone, and bone–bone interfaces is subjective and requires refinement and additional correlation with clinical and fixation results. Reporting from additional centers with a larger number of cases and longer follow-up periods is required to evaluate efficacy and consistency. A report by Masterson et al. (26) attests to the sensitivity of the operative technique and implant design for obtaining good short-term results. Of all fixation and design concepts, impaction grafting is in the earliest stages of research and development. Despite these reservations, it must be emphasized that there is corroboration from several centers that the technique is capable of restoring bone stock in deficient femurs. Although conventional cemented revision has been shown to be effective for preventing further endosteal cavitation, it does not provide the same potential for bone healing and restoration. Regardless of long-term survivorship, this attribute alone is of sufficient value to justify further trials and include impaction grafting as an option for a revision operation.

On balance, the survivorship data with extensively porous coated revision prostheses are the most consistent and encouraging of all. The reports from three centers are reliable because they are based on very large patient series. The rates of revision and radiographic loosening range from 2.4% to 4.6%. These rates do not appear to be biased because of more favorable patient demographics or extent of prerevision bone-stock deficiencies. These are distinctly superior statistics than obtained with cemented implant designs. Although the average follow-up period with extensively porous coated designs is somewhat shorter, even if all the cases with radiographic signs of instability were included as revisions in the next 2 to 3 years, the 10 to 11 year aseptic revision rate would tend to be lower than with cement at comparable follow-up periods. The caveat to this result is that the hips designated as having stable fibrous interfaces remain as such. Although there will always remain the concern about additional loss of bone with the larger and stiffer extensively porous coated prostheses because of stress shielding, it is noteworthy that periprosthetic bone healing and restoration are commonly observed after uncemented revision arthroplasty. This important advantage is shared with the impaction grafting technique.

The future holds several areas for improvement in prosthetic design and technique of revision hip arthroplasty. Development of less rigid extensively porous coated devices has been mentioned. The role of calcium phosphate implant coatings, with and without porous surfaces, will be elucidated for their potential in enhancing osteogenesis at bone–implant interfaces. The Wagner approach to revision with long, conical, fluted, stems with grit-blasted surfaces is gaining increasing acceptance and is approaching 5 years of follow-up study (20). By respecting the mechanics and biologic features of the reconstruction, the process of bone destruction associated with loosening can be arrested and even reversed. Increased awareness of this idea coupled with advances in surgical techniques, instrumentation, and implant materials should culminate in improved survivorship over the second decade of follow-up study of femoral revision operations.

REFERENCES

1. Ballard WT, Callaghan JJ, Johnston RC. Revision of total hip arthroplasty in octogenarians. *J Bone Joint Surg Am* 1995;774:585–589.
2. Berry DJ, Harmsen WS, Ilstrup D, Lewallen DG, Cabanela ME. Survivorship of uncemented proximally porous-coated femoral components. *Clin Orthop* 1995;319:168–177.
3. Bugbee WD, Culpepper WJ, Engh CA, Engh CA. Long-term clinical consequences of stress-shielding after total hip arthroplasty without cement. *J Bone Joint Surg Am* 1997;79:1007–1012.
4. Buoncristiani AM, Dorr LD, Johnson C, Wan Z. Cementless revision of total hip arthroplasty using the anatomic porous replacement revision prosthesis. *J Arthroplasty* 1997;12:403–415.
5. Cameron H. The 2 to 6 year results with a proximally modular non-cemented hip stem. *Clin Ortho* 1994;298:47–53.
6. Chandler HP, Ayres DK, Tan RC, Anderson I, Varma AK. Revision total hip replacement using the S-ROM femoral component. *Clin Orthop* 1995;319:130–140.
7. D'Antonio J, McCarthy JC, Bargar WL, et al. Classification of femoral abnormalities in total hip arthroplasty. *Clin Orthop* 1993;296:133–139.
8. Eldridge JDJ, Smith EJ, Hubble MJ, Whitehouse SL, Learmonth ID. Massive early subsidence following femoral impaction grafting. *J Arthroplasty* 1997;12:535–540.
9. Elting JJ., Raimondo RA, Smallman TV, Hubbell JC. Impaction grafting for femoral revision: five year results. *Trans Am Acad Orthop Surg* 1998; abstract,185.
10. Elting JJ, Mikhail WEM, Zicat BA, Hubbell JC, Lane LE, House B. Preliminary report of impaction grafting for exchange femoral arthroplasty. *Clin Orthop* 1995;319:159–167.

11. Estok DN, Harris WH. Long-term results of cemented femoral revision surgery using second generation techniques: average 11.7 years follow-up. *Clin Orthop* 1994;299:190–202.
12. Garcia-Cimbrelo E, Munuera L, Diez-Vazquez V. Long-term results of aseptic cemented Charnley revisions. *J Arthroplasty* 1995;10:121–131.
13. Gie GA, Linder L, Ling RSM, Simon JP, Slooff TJJH, Timperley AJ. Femoral reconstruction cement with graft. In: Galante JO, Rosenberg AG, Callaghan JJ, eds. *Total hip revision surgery*. New York: Raven Press, 1995:367–373.
14. Hungerford DS. Femoral stem revision using a proximally porous-coated prosthesis. In: Galante JO, Rosenberg AG, Callaghan JJ, eds. *Total hip revision surgery*. New York: Raven Press, 1995:375–385.
15. Iorio R, Eftekhar NS, Kobayashi S, Grelsamer RP. Cemented revision of failed total hip arthroplasty: survivorship analysis. *Clin Orthop* 1995;316:121–130.
16. Izquierdo RJ, Northmore-Ball MD. Long-term results of revision hip arthroplasty. *J Bone Joint Surg Br* 1994;76:34–39.
17. Jasty M, Bragdon C, Burke D, O'Connor D, Lowenstein J, Harris W. In vivo skeletal responses to porous-surfaced implants subjected to small induced motions. *J Bone Joint Surg Am* 1997;79:707–714.
18. Katz RP, Callaghan JJ, Sullivan PM, Johnston RC. Long-term results of revision total hip arthroplasty with improved cementing technique. *J Bone Joint Surg Br* 1997;79:322–326.
19. Kendrick JB, Noble PC, Tullos HS. Distal stem design and the torsional stability of cementless femoral stems. *J Arthroplasty* 1995;10:463–469.
20. Kolstad K, Adalberth G, Hallmin H, Milbrink J, Sahlstedt B. The Wagner revision stem for severe osteolysis. *Acta Orthop Scand* 1996;67:541–544.
21. Lawrence JM, Engh CA, Macalino GE. Revision total hip arthroplasty long-term results without cement. *Orthop Clin North Am* 1993;24:635–655.
22. Lawrence JM, Engh CA, Macalino GE, Lauro GR. Outcome of revision hip arthroplasty done without cement. *J Bone Joint Surg Am* 1994;76:965–973.
23. Ling RSM, Timperley AJ, Linder L. Histology of cancellous impaction grafting in the femur. *J Bone Joint Surg Br* 1993;75:693–696.
24. Malkani AL, Lewallen DG, Cabanela ME, Wallrichs SL. Femoral component revision using an uncemented, proximally coated, long-stem prosthesis. *J Arthroplasty* 1996;11:411–418.
25. Marti RK, Schuller HM, Besselaar PP, Haasnoot ELV. Results of revision hip arthroplasty with cement: a 5–14 year follow-up study. *J Bone Joint Surg Am* 1990;72:346–354.
26. Masterson EL, Masri BA, Duncan CP. The cement mantle in the Exeter impaction allografting technique. A cause for concern. *J Arthroplasty* 1997;12:759–764.
27. Meding JB, Ritter MA, Keating EM, Faris PM. Clinical and radiographic evaluation of long-stem femoral components following revision total hip arthroplasty. *J Arthroplasty* 1994;9:399–408.
28. Mohler CG, Collis DK. Femoral reconstruction: cement. In: Galante JO, Rosenberg AG, Callaghan JJ, eds. *Total hip revision surgery*. New York: Raven Press, 1995:359–365.
29. Moreland JR, Bernstein ML. Femoral revision hip arthroplasty with uncemented, porous-coated stems. *Clin Orthop* 1995;319:141–150.
30. Mulliken BD, Rorabeck CH, Bourne RB. Uncemented revision total hip arthroplasty. *Clin Orthop* 1996;325:156–162.
31. Mulroy WF, Harris WH. Revision total hip arthroplasty with use of so-called second-generation cementing techniques for aseptic loosening of the femoral component. *J Bone Joint Surg Am* 1996;78:325–330.
32. Nelissen RGHH, Bauer TW, Weidenhielm LR, LeGolvan DP, Mikhail WEM. Revision hip arthroplasty with the use of cement and impaction grafting: histological analysis of four cases. *J Bone Joint Surg Am* 1991;77:412–422.
33. Paprosky WG, Krishnamurthy A. Five to 14-year follow up on cementless femoral revisions. *Orthopaedics* 1996;19:765–768.
34. Pellicci PN, Wilson PD, Sledge CB, et al. Long-term results of revision total hip arthroplasty: a follow-up report. *J Bone Joint Surg Am* 1985;67:513–516.
35. Peters CL, Rivero DP, Kull LR, Jacobs JJ, Rosenberg AG, Galante JO. Revision total hip arthroplasty without cement: subsidence of proximally porous-coated femoral components. *J Bone Joint Surg Am* 1995;77:1217–1226.
36. Pierson JL, Harris WH. Cemented revision for femoral osteolysis in cemented arthroplasties. *J Bone Joint Surg Br* 1994;76:40–44.
37. Raut VV, Siney PD, Wroblewski BM. Outcome of revision for mechanical stem failure using the cemented Charnley's stem. *J Arthroplasty* 1996;11:405–410.
38. Raut VV, Siney PD, Wroblewski BM. Cemented revision Charnley low-friction arthroplasty in patients with rheumatoid arthritis. *J Bone Joint Surg Br* 1994;76:909–911.
39. Retpen JB, Jensen JJ. Risk factors for recurrent aseptic loosening of the femoral component after cemented revision. *J Arthroplasty* 1993;8:471–478.
40. Smith JA, Dunn HK, Manaster BJ. Cementless femoral revision arthroplasty: 2- to 5-year results with a modular titanium alloy stem. *J Arthroplasty* 1997;12:194–201.
41. Snorrasen F, Karrholm J. Early loosening of revision hip arthroplasty. *J Arthroplasty* 1990;5:217–229.
42. Stromberg CN, Herberts P. Cemented revision total hip arthroplasties in patients younger than 55 years old. *J Arthroplasty* 1996;11:489–499.
43. Stromberg CN, Herberts P. A multicenter 10-year study of cemented revision total hip arthroplasty in patients younger than 55 years old. *J Arthroplasty* 1994;9:595–601.
44. Weber KL, Callaghan JJ, Goetz D, Johnston RC. Revision of a failed cemented total hip prosthesis with insertion of an acetabular component without cement and a femoral component with cement. *J Bone Joint Surg Am* 1996;78:982–994.
45. Woolson ST, Delaney TJ. Failure of a proximally porous-coated femoral prosthesis in revision total hip arthroplasty. *J Arthroplasty* 1995;10 (Suppl):S22–S28.

Revision Total Hip Arthroplasty,
edited by Marvin E. Steinberg and Jonathan P. Garino,
Lippincott Williams & Wilkins, Philadelphia © 1999.

6

Effect of Material on Long-term Survivorship

Jonathan Black and Joshua J. Jacobs

Total replacement arthroplasty of the hip is one of the great biomedical success stories of the twentieth century. Hundreds of thousands of patients worldwide have been restored to full, painless mobility after, in some cases, decades of increasing pain, disability, and limitation of vocational and recreational activity. A small number of relatively standard approaches to design and fabrication of implants for total hip replacement (THR) arthroplasty have been developed, and long-term clinical follow-up data, in some cases collected for more than 20 years, are now available.

THR arthroplasty in the late 1990's is such a successful procedure that it is extremely difficult to generalize about the origins of the so-called failures encountered in clinical practice. Failure of THR arthroplasty (better termed, generally, maloutcome) that leads to the need for surgical revision is usually attributed to one or more of four sources: the design and manufacture of the device components, the surgeon's skill level, the patient's disease, and the use of the implant by the patient after the operation. This chapter addresses those aspects of the materials of fabrication of THR components and their interactions with the patient, which particularly in the longer term may contribute to the need for partial or total revision.

This consideration is a part of the larger subject termed *biological performance* of the manufactured materials used and can be further subdivided into a consideration of material response (degradation of materials by service requirements and environmental exposure) and host response (local, systemic, and remote site response to materials and their degradation products) (6).

J. J. Jacobs: Department of Orthopaedic Surgery, Rush-Presbyterian-St. Luke's Medical Center, Chicago, Illinois 60612.

J. Black: IMN Biomaterials, King of Prussia, Pennsylvania 19406.

BACKGROUND AND UNDERLYING ISSUES

Before discussion of the specific roles played by materials in long-term degradation of THR arthroplasty, several issues should be considered. In the first place, it must be emphasized just how rarely failures of outcome that necessitate revision occur. A 1994 U.S. consensus conference concluded the following: "Revision rates for cemented femoral components . . . have been reported to be less than 5 percent at 10 year follow up; revision rates for uncemented acetabular components are approximately 2 percent at 5-year follow up. To be deemed efficacious, new design features should be shown to have a mechanical failure rate equal to or less than these figures" (2). Are cumulative femoral revision rates of 5% 10 years after implantation (about 0.5%/year) and cumulative acetabular revision rates of 2% 5 years after implantation (about 0.4%/year) attributable to mechanical (design and manufacture) factors large or small?

The rate of revision (initial as well as second, third, and so forth) of THR arthroplasty in the United States, expressed as a percentage of installed total, appeared to reach a peak in 1991 and apparently declined monotonically since then to a 1995 value of about 1.6% of all implants *in situ* (4). That is, for every 1,000 THRs in use in patients at the beginning of 1995, approximately 16 underwent revision during that year. It is interesting to reflect that this is probably lower than the death rate among patients with clinically functional THRs during that year. It is further interesting to note that as long ago as 1988, it was estimated that 92.2% of all artificial joints (hips and knees) were never replaced during the patient's lifetime (43).

This remarkably low overall *incidence* of revision is obscured, for the average clinician, by a much higher *prevalence* in current practice. The rate of revision of THRs in the United States, expressed as a percentage of new primary THR arthroplasty procedures only, probably reached a peak in 1992 and appears to have remained constant or possibly declined modestly since then, to a current rate of about 20% (4). That is, for each five new THRs implanted in 1995, one revision of a previously implanted THR was necessary. Clinicians in teaching and secondary or tertiary centers experience a much greater local prevalence of revision, because of referral of complex cases.

It must be emphasized that such data are based on past practice. It is not currently possible to predict the long-term clinical outcome of the use of new component designs, even in instances in which relatively modest changes in materials and component shape are made. Discussing causes of long-term revision of THR arthroplasty in 1998 is to discuss the consequences of technologic choices and clinical practice in the mid 1980's and, in some cases, much earlier. One of the overwhelming difficulties in such discussions is that despite widespread evidence of clinical success of some THR designs and material combinations, commercial practice often removes device designs, and in some cases materials, from the marketplace before reliable long-term results become available.

Nevertheless, examination of data from the Swedish THR arthroplasty registry (36), as well as other sources, clearly suggests that by more than 7 to 10 years after implantation the survivorship curves for even quite successful devices turn downward, implying an increased annual rate of failure. This supports the assertion that the results of THR arthroplasty deteriorate with time and that it is useful to inquire what role biological performance of materials may play in such a decline. However, this conclusion must only be accepted with caution, because patient numbers in any series decrease with time, resulting in monotonically increasing uncertainty, reflected by wider error intervals (46).

Second, we must define what is meant by *long term*. In reporting evaluations of biomaterials, writers usually distinguish between intraoperative, acute, and chronic use of materials as implants. The term *chronic* is usually taken to mean implantation for periods of 30 days or longer. This is clearly not enough to define long-term effects in human THR arthroplasty, because the implant recipient is rarely even back to full daily activities within the first postoperative month. Older studies of surgical procedures on the hip tend to define long-term or late events as those occuring more than 6 months postoperatively. However, it is clear that bony remodeling, particularly around "osseointegrated" uncemented (adhered or ingrown) components may continue for 2 to 3 years, and semiobjective

TABLE 1. *Biomaterials used in contemporary total hip replacement arthroplasty components*

ASTM designation[a]	Material[b]
F-67	Unalloyed (CP) titanium
F-75	Cast cobalt-chromium-molybdenum alloy (Co28.5Cr6Mo)[c]
F-90	Wrought cobalt-chromium-tungsten-nickel alloy (Co20Cr10Ni15W)
F-136	Wrought titanium alloy (Ti6A14V ELI)
F-451	Polymethyl methacrylate cement [PMMA]
F-562	Wrought cobalt-nickel-chromium-molybdenum alloy (Co35Ni20Cr10Mo; MP35N)
F-563	Wrought cobalt-nickel-chromium-molybdenum-tungsten-iron alloy (Co20Ni20Cr3.5Mo3.5W5Fe; Syncoben)
F-603	Dense aluminum oxide [Alumina]
F-648	Ultrahigh-molecular-weight polyethylene [UHMWPE]
F-1185	Calcium hydroxyapatite ($Ca_{10}(PO_4)_6(OH)_2$; [HA])
F-1295	Wrought titanium-aluminum-niobium alloy (Ti6A17Nb)
F-1314	Wrought nitrogen containing stainless steel (Fe22Cr12.5Ni5Mn2.5Mo0.4N; Ortron 90)
F-1472	Wrought titanium alloy (Ti6A14V)
F-1537	Wrought cobalt-chromium-molybdenum alloy (Co28Cr6Mo)
—	Dense zirconium oxide [Zirconia]

Square brackets indicate commonly used abbreviations or names.

[a] ASTM specifications for biomaterials have the form F NNNN-MM, where (19)MM is the year last revised. This suffix is omitted here for simplicity.

[b] Not title of standard; please see ref. 2 for full title and latest revision date.

[c] Numbers preceding chemical symbol indicate nominal weight percentage of element.

ASTM, American Society for Testing and Materials; CP, commercially pure; ELI, extra low interstitial (high-purity) grade;—No ASTM standard currently exists but one is expected to be adopted in the near future.

evaluation scores, such as the Harris Hip Score, continue to improve as long as 3 years postoperatively in most prospective clinical series. For the sake of this chapter, the threshold between the postoperative and long-term or chronic eras in patient experience is regarded as occuring sometime between 2 and 3 years postoperatively. The focus is on materials-related outcomes, which can be expected to occur at the end of or after this postoperative interval.

Third, it is necessary to define the materials used in the fabrication of THR components and their fixation systems and in what combinations these materials are used in common designs.[1] Trial and error, in both laboratory and clinical settings, has restricted the selection of biomaterials used in contemporary designs of THR devices to little more than a dozen, including ten metallic alloys, two polymers, and three ceramics (Table 1). Table 2 shows that of the possible 90 applications (15 materials × 6 elements), less than half have been found to be successful in the long term (Designated by a check mark in Table 2). Figure 1 shows, with horizontal or inclined link lines, the materials choices and combinations believed to be in use today or that are currently considered technologically feasible.

Femoral Component Materials

Fixation on the femoral side is now divided between polymethyl methacrylate (PMMA) cemented components and uncemented ones with or without surface features, such as grooves or porosity, and with or without calcium hydroxyapatite (CaHAP) coatings. Choices of the metal for fabrication of the stem (structural element) also are varied. There appears to be however, a preference for titanium-base alloys for uncemented designs and

[1] This discussion of materials selection and combinations in use, with the accompanying two tables and figure, is adapted from Black J. Biomaterials overview. In: Callaghan JJ, Rosenberg AG, Rubash HE, eds. *The Adult Hip.* New York: Lippincott–Raven, 1998:87–96.

TABLE 2. *Application of biomaterials to contemporary total hip replacement arthroplasty components*

Material		Acetabular Component			Femoral Component		
ASTM designation	Common name	Articulation	Structural	Fixation	Articulation	Structural	Fixation
Metals							
F-67	CP Ti	✓	✓[a]				✓[a]
F-75	Cast CoCr	✓	✓	✓	✓	✓	✓
F-90	Wrt CoCr	✓	✓	✓	✓	✓	✓
F-136	Ti6A14VELI	✓	✓			✓	✓
F-562	MP35N	✓				✓	
F-563	—						
F-1295	Ti6A17Nb	✓				✓	
F-1314	High N SS				✓[b]	✓[b]	
F-1472	Wrt Ti6A14V		✓			✓	
F-1537	Wrt CoCrMo	✓[c]	✓		✓	✓	
Polymers							
F-451	PMMA			✓			✓
F-648	UHMWPE	✓	✓				
Ceramics							
F-603	Alumina	✓[c]	✓[b]		✓[d]	✓[e]	
F-1185	Hydroxyapatite			✓			✓
(ZrO$_2$)	Zirconia				✓[f]	✓[e]	

Check marks indicate successful application of this material.
[a] Applied to different metal alloy substrate, such as F-136, F-1472.
[b] Not in use in United States, in use elsewhere.
[c] Only used in articulation with itself; not in use in United States, in use elsewhere.
[d] Only used in articulation with UHMWPE in United States, used with itself elsewhere.
[e] As modular component on metal alloy stem, such as F-90.
[f] Only used in articulation with UHMWPE.
CP, commercially pure; PMMA, polymethyl methacrylate cement; UHMWPE, ultrahigh-molecular-weight polyethylene; Wrt, wrought.

cobalt-base (stainless steel outside the United States) for cemented designs. The use of cast cobalt chromium (CoCr)[2], and stainless steel femoral heads (articulation elements) is now mostly restricted to older monobloc (or unibloc) designs with or without cement. Newer modular designs, in which the stem is separate from the head and joined to it by a conical trunnion (on the stem) friction fitted into a mating bore (in the head), provide the option of use of wrought CoCr or cobalt chromium molybdenum (CoCrMo) alloys as well as alumina and zirconia ceramics for the femoral head. Ceramic articulation elements, although popular in European and worldwide markets, still constitute only 5% to 7% of U.S. usage. Zirconia in particular is articulated only with ultrahigh-molecular-weight polyethylene (UHMWPE) on the acetabular side (worldwide) and alumina-alumina and CoCrMo-CoCrMo articulation pairs, while undergoing clinical evaluation, are not currently approved for routine clinical use in the United States.

In the United States, the most popular choices of materials for the femoral component are titanium-base or cobalt-base alloy structural elements combined with wrought modular CoCr or CoCrMo articulation elements and a variety of fixation elements, PMMA cement probably modestly dominating.

Acetabular Component Materials

Fixation on the acetabular side was from the early 1960's until recently dominated by PMMA cementation. Within the last decade, the use of uncemented designs, involving threaded, structured, or porous surfaces and in many cases including CaHAP coatings, has been growing rapidly. This growth is related to increasing evidence of progressive

---

[2] See Table 2 for typical grades (ASTM designations).

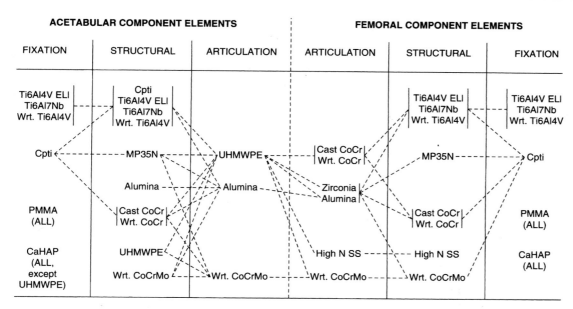

Figure 1. Material combinations used in total hip replacement arthroplasty. (From Callaghan JJ, Rosenberg AG, and Rubash HE. The adult hip. New York: Lippincott-Raven, 1998.)

loosening of PMMA cemented all-UHMWPE designs implanted with older, less sophisticated techniques than in use today in the more than 10-year postoperative period. The choice for the articulation (and structural) element of acetabular components is still primarily UHMWPE, combined in many cases with a thin titanium, titanium-base, or cobalt-base alloy structural or fixation shell. The compound structure allows use of a variety of uncemented fixation technologies, because UHMWPE performs poorly in direct contact with bone and has not as yet been successfully coated with CaHAP or other adhesion materials. UHMWPE is still the standard for the articulation surface, but there is increasing interest worldwide in use of alumina and wrought CoCrMo articulated on the femoral side, each mating respectively with itself on the acetabular side.

In the United States the most popular choices of materials for the acetabular component are titanium, titanium-base alloy, or cobalt-base alloy structural elements combined with UHMWPE articulation inserts and a variety of fixation elements; uncemented technologies, in many cases involving CaHAP, probably dominate. There is anecdotal evidence, however, that all-UHMWPE, PMMA cemented components are experiencing renewed clinical popularity.

RATIONALE FOR CHOICES OF MATERIALS

Metals

The choice of metals for structural elements of both femoral and acetabular components is among three alloy systems: stainless steel, cobalt-base, and titanium-base alloys. Stainless steel was used first and was supplanted by cobalt-base (cast CrCo and wrought CrCoMo) alloys, because of considerations of higher strength and lower corrosion rates. Stainless steel, primarily of more modern types, such as F-1314, remain in use, primarily outside the United States, where materials cost is a dominant factor. Interest in the use of titanium-base alloys sprang primarily from the lower modulus (intrinsic stiffness) of these materials combined with still lower corrosion rates than for cobalt-base alloys, less concern about biologic properties of corrosion products, and excellent fatigue resistance. This trend is being continued with the experimental introduction of so-called β alloys in contrast to Ti6A14V (F-136; F-1472), which is an α-β alloy. These alloys, such as Ti13Nb13Zr (developed by Smith and Nephew, Memphis) and Ti5Mo5Zr2Fe (developed by Howmedica, Rutherford, N.J.), have elastic moduli considerably lower than those of Ti6A14V. In addition to these alloys, commercially pure (*CP*) titanium is used, primarily on titanium-base alloy components, to take advantage of direct osseointegration of this elemental material with bone to provide uncemented fixation, and occasionally by itself as a combined structural and fixation element.

All these alloys are highly corrosion resistant, in engineering terms. However, their use in THR arthroplasty produces chronic elevations in serum and in some cases urine content of various metals by two- to fivefold over normal levels (28). In the case of incipient loosening or aggravated wear, related to fretting at interfaces, for example, or the use of metal-on-metal articulations, levels may rise even higher (29). However, no clinical associations have been made as yet between these findings and any adverse biologic effect.

Polymers

The only polymer used in THR arthroplasty for nonarticulation purposes is PMMA. With small variations affecting primarily handling characteristics and setting rates, this material continues to dominate cemented fixation applications, because no superior alternative has been found. The intrinsic physical properties of PMMA cements are known to depend to some degree on mixing techniques and are known to deteriorate with time in the body. However, there is no persuasive proof of accelerated late failure (loosening, cement fragmentation) related to these effects.

Ceramics

The only ceramic used in THR arthroplasty for nonarticulation purposes is CaHAP. It is now widely used as an adjunctive material in uncemented fixation on smooth, contoured, or porous metallic substrates and appears to enhance bone ingrowth. CaHAP is applied most generally in a largely crystalline film of about 50-μm thickness with the intention that the material remain *in situ* during the life of the device. Although clinical studies have now extended beyond 7 years and the material has been in used for 10 years (19), there is no persuasive proof of late failure (loosening) related to its use or deterioration. There is now some evidence of fragmentation and dissolution with time; fragments have been found within articulating interfaces, but no pattern of accelerated failure has been associated with such occasional findings.

RATIONALE FOR CHOICES OF INTERFACIAL COMBINATIONS

General Comments

Many of the problems associated with materials used in THR arthroplasty components come not from the intrinsic bulk or surface properties of the materials themselves but from interactions across interfaces, either between components of dissimilar materials or between components and surrounding tissues. Figure 2 shows the interfaces present after THR arthroplasty. On the left are interfaces associated with PMMA cemented conventional or uniblock components. On the right are those associated with uncemented modular components. Many hip reconstructions entail a hybrid approach; thus a typical patient may have a combination of interfaces rather than the array shown on one or the other side of Fig. 2. Some device designs have higher degrees of modularity than shown, including head inserts, proximal femoral sleeves, and distal canal-centering elements. Table 3 summarizes the interfaces shown here and lists the degradative phenomena known to be associated with each interface.

The question to be addressed is whether the degradative phenomena are seen from the beginning of the implantation period or develop or accelerate in the long-term period. The

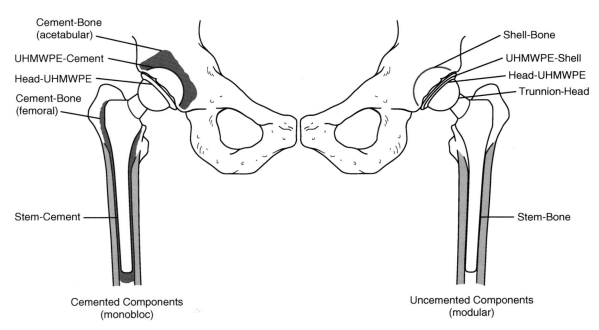

Figure 2. Interfaces in total hip replacement arthroplasty.

general rule is that all effects are present *de novo*. However, symptoms and biologic consequences may depend on accumulation of either damage to the interface or accumulation of degradation products. There are no persuasive data that show interfacial degradation phenomena *in vivo* once initiated accelerate with implantation duration.

Articulating Interfaces

The issue of osteolysis associated with the production of debris, primarily at articulating interfaces (5) is viewed as sufficiently important that it must be treated at length.[3] The standard or classic wear pair, as reflected in the Charnley and similar THR device designs, consists of a metal femoral head articulating with a UHMWPE articular surface. This wear pair (with stainless steel used initially rather than the current cast CoCr or wrought CoCrMo alloy) has been in use since 1961 and is associated with the well-known excellent performance of the conventional PMMA cemented THR arthroplasty. However, there are shortcomings to this technology. There is considerable wear of the UHMWPE, perhaps 75 to 150 μm/year (11) depending in part on the diameter of the femoral head (32) but apparently largely independent of other patient factors including period of implantation (58). Other shortcomings are a poorer outcome among younger patients (27) and a well-known incidence of osteolysis (24). However, it is the standard against which all alternative technologic choices must be compared.

Great concern has focused on how fabrication and sterilization of UHMWPE may affect its clinical performance (34,52). The basis for comparison must be the behavior of components machined from hot-pressed block, sterilized (and partially cross linked) with γ irradiation and stored in air before use. This combination was used for more than 95% of all acetabular components implanted before 1990. Results of laboratory studies suggest that other sterilization modes, which either reduce or eliminate the ionizing effects of γ irradiation and its cross-linking effects or modify the exposure to oxygen during sterilization and subsequent storage, appear to reduce *in vitro* wear in certain modes of testing but may actually increase wear rates in more complex simulator testing. Claims of superior behavior have been based on clinical follow-up findings without controls for the

---

[3] The subject of osteolysis is treated at length in Chapters 2 and 3.

TABLE 3. *Degradative phenomena*

Location	Mechanism	Long term effect?
Bulk		
Metal	Fatigue	Damage accumulation; fracture
Ceramic	Fatigue	Damage accumulation?
Polymer	Fatigue	Damage accumulation; fracture
	Oxidation	Reduced resistance to wear?
Surface		
Metal	Uniform corrosion	Constant or decreasing rate
	Localized corrosion	Constant or decreasing rate; increasing secondary to mechanical damage
	Fretting	Constant; increasing secondary to loss of fixation
Ceramic	Dissolution	Constant or decreasing rate
Polymer	Oxidation	No; early effects dominate
	Fretting	Constant; increasing secondary to loss of fixation or oxidation
Interface		
Cement-bone	Microfracture	Possible decrease in PMMA properties
	Osteolysis	Secondary to wear debris accumulation
UHMWPE-cement	Wear	Secondary to progressive loosening
	Microfracture	Possible decrease in PMMA properties
UHMWPE-shell (acetabular)	Wear	None; design related
Metal-bone	Osteolysis	Secondary to wear debris accumulation; Immune response? Chemical neoplasia?
Metal-cement	Debonding	Secondary to fatigue?
	Wear	Secondary to loosening
Head-UHMWPE	Uniform wear	None; wear rates constant or decreasing
	Third body wear	Secondary to hard debris accumulation
	Fatigue	Possible; data inconclusive

Possible mechanism. Clinical evidence scant or lacking; PMMA, polymethyl methacrylate cement; UHMWPE, ultrahigh-molecular-weight polyethylene.

use of extruded or individually (closed-die) molded acetabular components. The use of such alternative fabrication and sterilization routes in any great amount is of relatively recent initiation. These materials-processing changes are statistically confounded with device design changes, so no sound judgment can be made concerning whether they will prove to be superior or inferior to the historical practices in the long term. Care should be exercised in the application of these alternative technologies, because of the overall excellent long-term behavior of the prior art. It should be noted that certain attempts to improve UHMWPE, for example by means of inclusion of carbon fibers, have actually resulted in an inferior and unacceptable material.

The most common alternative to this combination is to replace the metal head with a ceramic head, fabricated from either aluminum oxide (alumina; Al_2O_3) or zirconium oxide (zirconia; ZrO_2) (14). The ceramic-UHMWPE wear pair has a long clinical history, alumina femoral heads being used since at least 1976 (55). There is also a clearly reduced rate of UHMWPE wear, perhaps as much as a 50% reduction after the first several years of use, from that expected with a conventional metal head (67). Despite this apparently superior technology, there are technical problems. The ceramic head is significantly more expensive than a metallic head, there is a small but real risk of head fracture, and osteolysis is still encountered (57). A broad reading of the available published results of series involving such components leads to the following suppositional conclusions:

1. Ceramic component fracture is relatively rare and appears to occur within a range of 1/1000 and 1/50,000 patient years. It depends in part on the type of ceramic and the precision of matching the junction between the head and the femoral component.

2. Many, but not all, such failures can be associated with events of trauma.

3. Component failure seems to be more common in the early experience of individual surgeons and individual hospitals. That is, as sequential reports of a clinical trial appear, reflecting increased trial duration and group size, the component failure rate decreases, despite the increase in clinical exposure. Furthermore, single-time-point reports of larger, longer term series appear to reflect lower failure rates than those for smaller, shorter series.

Ceramic heads generally have proved to be more expensive than the metallic heads they replace. This is an issue in the increasingly cost-conscious U.S. medical environment. Furthermore, as is the case with other alternative wear pairs, there is as yet no evidence of clinical benefit (as measured with annual or cumulative revision rate) from the use of this alternative.

An older alternative is to replace the UHMWPE articular surface with a metallic surface to produce a hard-hard or metal-on-metal wear pair. This approach actually predates Charnley's innovations with clinical systems in use, designed by Müller (44), Ring (51), and McKee and Watson-Farrar (37) as early as 1948. In 1988, Weber (64) "rediscovered" this approach and introduced a new generation of metal-metal THR components. The older systems clearly produced very much smaller amounts of wear debris than the conventional UHMWPE-metal systems with linear wear on the order of 2.5 to 5 μm per component per year (38). Early experience with the newer designs suggests similar wear rates (54). However, the metallic wear particles released appear to be extremely small (perhaps 0.02 to 0.4 μm primarily) with correspondingly very high specific surface area (15,61). The nature of the cobalt-base super alloys used in these systems raises concerns about local tissue necrosis and possibly elevated risk for some neoplastic transformation processes (8,20,21,60). The older systems show no clinical advantage, and there have been no definitive reports of the outcomes of the post-1988 designs.

Another alternative approach has been to replace both head and cup with alumina ceramic to form a ceramic-on-ceramic hard-hard wear pair. This approach was first introduced by Boutin (9) in 1972 and popularized by Mittelmeier (41) and Nizard et al. (47) and Sedel (55). Until the recent introduction of improved ceramic materials, this technology had been in use since 1977 (14). These bearings show even lower wear rates than metal-on-metal, perhaps as low as 0.5 to 2.5 μm per component per year (63). However, the breakage and cost issues associated with use of isolated ceramic heads are multiplied by the use of two components per joint replacement.

There are as yet, no data available from long-term, prospective comparisons of these alternative technologies. Materials effects on outcome cannot yet be separated from those of device design, surgical technique, and patient selection (42,45).

LONG-TERM HOST RESPONSE TO BIOMATERIALS

After implantation of THR components, patients accommodate to foreign materials in a variety of ways. Initial phases include acute inflammation, possible perioperative infection, and specific (type IV) hypersensitivity as well as the hoped-for remodeling and bony ongrowth or ingrowth that leads to osseointegration. These all represent normal aspects of healing after a massive injury, such as THR arthroplasty represents, modified by the presence of a long-term implant (6). However, our concern is with the consequences of the presence of the implanted components and their degradation products after initial tissue resolution has occurred. There are four phenomena, other than osteolysis, through which materials may contribute to long-term failure of the procedure.

Late Infection

Late infection associated with the presence of THR components is a deep infection. Improvements in perioperative antisepsis during the last decade have reduced the overall incidence of infection in THR arthroplasty to less than 1.0% but have resulted in a relative increase in late infections. These late infections have three recognized causes: hematogenous spread from another site of infection, such as the urogenital tract; reactivation of infection, for example after revision of a previously infected hip; and direct infection due to local trauma or regional communicating infections (53). *Staphylococcus aureus* and *Staphylococcus epidermidis* organisms, well known for their roles in primary infection, are also seen in late infection, as are *Escherichia coli* organisms and a variety of other organisms that can be spread hematogenously.

The microbiologic features of implant-site infection are still poorly understood (16). In general, implant surfaces provide protected culture substrates for bacteria, reducing the critical inoculum needed to sustain an infection, rendering some otherwise benign organisms more virulent, and providing protection from antibiotic treatment. Establishment of bacterial growth on an implant surface depends in part on what has been termed "the race for the surface" (22)—a competition between bacterial colonization of the implant surface and overgrowth of normal and encapsulating (relatively avascular) tissue. The virulence effect of implant surfaces is related to the ability of several microorganisms, especially *S aureus,* to elaborate a protective slimy film, the glycocalyx. A secondary effect may be related to the presence of iron-containing corrosion products in infected sites of steel implants. Infection is usually accompanied by an acidic pH shift (26), which generally increases corrosion. At the same time, such corrosion makes iron more available to iron-dependent bacteria. It is possible to show in animal models that sites with iron-containing implants, such as stainless steel, are easier to infect than ones containing iron-free implants, such as pure titanium (3). A secondary effect may be suppression of local immune resistance mechanisms, rendering the implant-tissue interface to a degree "immunoincompetent" (22).

The long-term materials-associated concerns about infection must therefore center on two issues. First, as time progresses, patients have a greater probability of being exposed to infections in other anatomic sites that might produce hematogenous seeding. Second, continued materials degradation will produce a local environment surrounding the implanted device that is more welcoming to infection while affording increased, newly formed surface area (wear debris) for colonization.

Immune Response

The role that a specific immune response to implants may play in loosening and failure is controversial and unresolved (17,40,48,50). Mechanisms for sensitization to nonbiologic materials are discussed elsewhere (6). The primary response seems to be a type-IV, cell-mediated delayed sensitivity to inorganic moieties that form a complex with native proteins or to self-proteins denatured by means of contact with high-energy surfaces. Humoral responses also are possible, because of detection of circulating antibodies to metal-containing haptens in patients after implantation of cobalt-base alloy THR components (66). Chromium, cobalt, nickel (65), and various components released from PMMA cements (23), have been established as potential sensitizers. Sensitization by relatively inert titanium alloy wear debris also has been reported (33).

Apart from incidental case reports and a body of suggestive studies, there is as yet no firm link between such sensitivity and painful, with or without associated loosening, THR arthroplasty. However, if such links become established, the long-term materials-associated concerns about immune response must center on two issues. First, as time progresses, unsensitized patients have a greater probability of being exposed to a potentially sensitizing episode. Second, continued materials degradation will produce moieties capable of haptenic binding as well as increased, newly formed surface area (wear debris) as sites for protein denaturation.

Neoplastic Transformation

One of the most troubling long-term concerns associated with THR arthroplasty has been the possibility of neoplastic transformation. More than two decades ago, one of us

(J. B.), was disturbed by an apparent paradox: Although potentially carcinogenic elements, such as nickel and chromium, were routinely used in the fabrication implants, such as THR components for long-term use by humans, there were few, if any, reliable reports of tumors associated with such implants. Because foreign-body carcinogenesis, common among lower animals, is essentially unrecognized in humans, the concern focused primarily on production of corrosion products and the ability of such products to initiate and promote neoplastic transformation (7,8). There has been extensive study of this issue in both laboratories and clinics. The following general conclusions can be stated.

More than two dozen chronic metallic implant–associated tumors, most THR arthroplasty sites, have been reported (28). Most of the tumors are reported to be malignant fibrous hysticytoma, and although many have occurred as late as 10 years after implantation, most are still considered to be secondary (metastatic) latent tumors, because the latency period for chemical carcinogenesis is frequently as long as 20 years or more (8).

Epidemiologic studies suggest no overall elevation of cancer risk associated with THR arthroplasty (49) for periods of up to 25 years after implantation. However, patients who received older metal-on-metal devices, especially the McKee-Farrar, appear to be at up to threefold elevated risk for leukemia or lymphoma (21,60).

A 1996 study of patients undergoing THR revision detected possible preneoplastic changes in bone marrow adjacent to 2 of 21 implants. No changes were seen in either distant marrow specimens or in 30 control specimens from patients undergoing primary arthroplasty (12). One implant had been *in situ* for 18 years and the other for 20 with two intervening revisions.

Apart from incidental case reports and a body of suggestive studies, no firm link has been established between THR arthroplasty and increased risk for neoplasia. If such links become established, the long-term materials-associated concerns about carcinogenesis must center on three issues. First, the primary risk identified so far appears to be modest elevations in the incidence of leukemia and lymphoma, apparently in the presence of high metal release devices. Second, as time progresses, patients are exposed to increasing body burdens of corrosion products and associated debris, especially in the presence of loose components. Third, the longer-term risk, if it exists, for true primary tumors of solid tissues produced or promoted by chemical stimuli may still become apparent as patient populations 20 years or more after implantation continue to expand.

Regional and Distant Distribution of Corrosion Products and Wear Debris

Studies of release of degradation products from implants have until recently focused on the implant site itself and have neglected systemic and remote site effects (6). Because this chapter is specifically concerned with maloutcome of THR arthroplasty, some of these more recent considerations are discussed only in passing. That is, although there are concerns about the consequences of systemic and remote dissemination of degradation debris (6,28), these appear to have little or no direct bearing on the actual function of the reconstructed joint.

In summary, the following may be stated:

1. Corrosion, both through uniform attack and fretting and crevice mechanisms, especially on bearing surfaces and at modular interfaces, releases corrosion products for all alloy systems. These products can be detected in elevated concentrations in serum, urine, and tissues, especially in reticuloendothelial cell–rich sites, such as lymph nodes, liver, and spleen (28).
2. Wear and precipitation of corrosion products (30,59) produce metallic, polymeric, and ceramic debris that can be found in regional lymph nodes (13,30,59), remote lymph nodes (13,56), bone marrow, liver, and spleen (13).
3. The most prevalent response to the presence of particle materials in remote sites is the same as that within the joint capsule itself—histiocytosis with accompanying foreign-body giant cells and occasional evidence of immunologic activation of macrophages and lymphocytes (13,25,59).

Such systemic and remote site accumulations of degradation products and the biologic response to these products are just becoming recognized as being perhaps the rule rather than the exception in THR arthroplasty. However, correlative studies of the long-term consequences of these phenomena largely remain to be performed. In the long term, we may come to appreciate the consequences of such widespread "internal pollution," but this field of investigation is still in its infancy. More detailed discussions of host response to implanted materials and their degradation products in an orthopedic context are found in references 6,18,30,31,35, and 62.

DETECTION OF MATERIAL-RELATED CLINICAL PROBLEMS

Diagnosis of the role of materials in maloutcome of THR arthroplasty procedures is still highly controversial. There are three main tools available to the clinician: a) radiography or other imaging of the THR construct *in situ*; b) examination of clinical symptoms; and c) after revision, histologic examination of removed tissues coupled with engineering examination of retrieved components. Limited studies of nonrevised constructs obtained at autopsy have shed light on the issue. Table 4 summarizes the materials-related findings, possible mechanisms of production, and implications of these findings, as seen through the use of each of these three primary clinical tools (6). Infection and engineering examination of retrieved devices are two topics that are deliberately omitted. The presence of foreign bodies, such as THR components, is associated with elevated early and late risk for infection relative to undisturbed tissues. However, extensive studies have failed to document any routine human clinical predisposition to elevated risk related to use of any specific one of the current materials used in fabrication of THRs and fixation systems. Excellent information may be found elsewhere (10,39). The systematic study of components retrieved during revision operations, now termed *device retrieval and analysis,* remains a research field and has not yet emerged as a real-time diagnostic aid, except in individual instances in which imaging or clinical symptoms provide *a priori* reasons to be interested in specific hardware. General findings from device retrieval and analysis studies have been mentioned throughout this chapter; more information on such studies may be found in references 1 and 34.

SUMMARY

There can be no question that choice of materials and to some degree processing of the particular materials into specific components play a role in the success or failure of THR arthroplasty. The issue addressed here is the role such factors play in long-term failure of the procedure. With a number of exceptions and unanswered questions, we now understand the behavior of implant materials enough to support the following argument: All implant materials degrade. All degradation products of implant materials appear to be more biologically active than their undegraded (bulk) precursors. The occurrence of adverse effects in the long term appears to depend on a balance between the production and accumulation rates of degradation products on one hand and the tolerance of individual patients on the other hand.

The last point is perhaps the most important message. THR arthroplasty is intended to be a definitive procedure; that is, the normal (diseased) hip is replaced with a construct containing foreign (nonbiologic) materials. Throughout the life of the patient, the implanted materials and their degradation products will interact with the patient locally, systemically, and in some cases at remote sites. Evaluation of outcomes of THR arthroplasty has traditionally focused on the mechanical function of the replaced joint, its radiographic appearance, and overall pain reduction. More complex questions of improvement of patient function and overall patient satisfaction now are being asked. Still to be explored are the more global issues of long-term effects on a patient's physiologic processes. Only when we fully understand the biologic performance of implanted materials can we provide definitive answers about the role of materials in determining the long-term outcome of THR arthroplasty.

TABLE 4. *Materials-related findings in total hip replacement arthroplasty*

Finding	Mechanism	Implication
Imaging		
PMMA fragments (early)	Operative debris	Third-body wear
		Single-cycle fracture
PMMA fragments (late)	Fatigue	Third-body wear
		Cup loosening
PMMA mantle fracture (early)	Inadequate bony support; single-cycle fracture	Stem subsidence
PMMA mantle fracture (late)	Inadequate bony support; fatigue	Stem subsidence
Broken cerclage wire	Fatigue	(early) Trochanteric dislodgement, nonunion; Wire migration; third body wear (late) Wire migration; third body wear
Stem deformation	Plastic deformation	Change in bony support
		Inadequate stem size or yield point
		Impending failure
Stem, cup or cup screw fracture	Fatigue	Manufacturing defect
		Chronic mechanical overload
		(early) Inadequate bony support
		(late) Change in bony support
Eccentric cup-head centers	Plastic deformation	UHMWPE creep
	Wear	Uniform wear
		Spalling; delamination?
Loose metallic debris	Wear	Third-body wear
		Fretting (loose component)
	Fatigue ± corrosion	Inadequate processing of porous coating
		Mismatching ± misassembly of modular components
Focal lytic lesion[a]	Particle phagocytosis	Excessive wear debris
	Immune response?	Metal sensitivity?
		(both) Progressive failure?
Progressive dissecting lesion[a]	Osteoclasis	Excessive wear debris
		Metal sensitivity?
		Neoplasm?
Clinical		
Hip pain[a]	Immune response	Metal sensitivity?
	Venous blockade	Excessive wear
Dislocation (late)	Pericapsular laxity	Excessive fretting, corrosion (modular junction)
	Fibrosis or necrosis	
Ectopic calcification	Wear debris nucleation?	Excessive wear
Dermatitis	Delayed hypersensitivity?	Metal sensitivity?
Eczema	Delayed hypersensitivity?	Metal sensitivity?
Bronchospasm	Delayed hypersensitivity?	Metal sensitivity?
Depressed leukocyte migration	Delayed hypersensitivity	Metal sensitivity?
Elevated (more than fivefold) urine Cr or Ti	Renal clearance	Excessive corrosion with or without fretting
Histologic		
Fibrous capsule	Local host response	Normal response
Histiocytosis with multinuclear cells	Chronic inflammation	Manufacturing defect
		Inappropriate material
		Excessive wear
Necrotic capsule, fascia	Local host response	Excessive wear with or without corrosion
		Metal sensitivity?
Lymphocytic infiltration with plasma cells	Delayed hypersensitivity?	Metal sensitivity?
		Polymer sensitivity?
Elevated cytokines, esp. interleukin-1, prostaglandin E_2	Chronic inflammation	Inappropriate material; Excessive wear
Fibrosarcoma	Neoplastic transformation	Chemical neoplasia?
Lymphoma	Neoplastic transformation	Chemical neoplasia?
Rhabdomyosarcoma	Neoplastic transformation	Chemical neoplasia?
Malignant fibrous histiocytoma	Neoplastic transformation	Chemical neoplasia?
Osteosarcoma	Neoplastic transformation	Chemical neoplasia?

[a] In absence of infection or loosening.

?, possible mechanism or implication; PMMA, polymethyl methacrylate cement; UHMWPE, ultrahigh-molecular-weight polyethylene.

Adapted from ref. 6, with permission.

ACKNOWLEDGMENT

The preparation of this chapter was supported by NIH grant AR 39310.

REFERENCES

1. Alexander H, Anderson JA, Duncan E. Implant retrieval symposium. *Trans Soc Biomater* 1992;15:1–104.
2. Anonymous. American Society for Testing and Materials: *1997 Annual Book of Standards, Vol. 13.01: Medical Devices; Emergency Medical Services*, West Conshohocken.
3. Arens S, Schlegel U, Printzen G, Ziegler WJ, Perren SM, Hansis M. Influence of materials for fixation implants on local infection. *J Bone Joint Surg Br*. 1996;78:647–651.
4. Black J. Prospects for alternate bearing surfaces in total hip replacement arthroplasty. In: Puhl W, ed. *Proceedings of 2. CERASIV: symposiums am 8 März 1997 in Stuttgart*. Stuttgart: Fredinand Enke Verlag, 1997:1–10.
5. Black J. Metal on metal bearings: a practical alternative to metal on polyethylene bearings? *Clin Orthop* 1996;329S:S244–S255.
6. Black J. *Biological performance of materials: fundamentals of biocompatibility. 2nd. ed.* New York: Marcel Dekker, 1992.
7. Black J. Does corrosion matter? *J Bone Joint Surg Br* 1988;70:517–520.
8. Black J. Metallic ion release and its relationship to oncogenesis. In: Fitzgerald RH Jr, ed. *The Hip*. St. Louis: Mosby, 1986:199–213.
9. Boutin P. Les prothèses totales de la hanche en alumine: l'ancrage direct sans ciment dans 50 cas. *Rev Chir Orthop* 1974;60:233–245.
10. Brause BD. Infected orthopedic prostheses. In: Bisno AL, Waldvogel FA, eds. *Infections associated with indwelling medical devices*. Washington: American Society for Microbiology, 1989:111–128.
11. Callaghan JJ, Pedersen DR, Olejniczak JP, Goetz DD, Johnston RC. Radiographic measurement of wear in 5 cohorts of patients observed for 5 to 22 years. *Clin Orthop* 1995;317:14–18.
12. Case CP, Langkmer VG, Howell RT, et al. Preliminary observations on possible premalignant changes in bone marrow adjacent to worn total hip arthroplasty implants. *Clin Orthop* 1996;329S:S269–S279.
13. Case CP, Langkmer VG, James C, et al. Widespread dissemination of metal debris from implants. *J Bone Joint Surg Br* 1994;76:701–712.
14. Christel P. Ceramics for joint replacement. In: Morrey BF, ed. *Biological, material, and mechanical considerations of joint replacement*. New York: Raven Press, 1993;303–314.
15. Doorn P, Campbell B, Benya P, et al. The application of transmission electron microscopy to the characterization of metal wear particles from metal on metal total hip replacements [Abstract]. *Trans Orthop Res Soc* 1997;22:70.
16. Dougherty SH. Microbiology of infection in prosthetic devices. In: Wadstrom T, Eliasson I, Holder I, Ljungh A, eds. *Pathogenesis of wound and biomaterial-associated infections,* London: Springer-Verlag, 1990:375–390.
17. Dujardin F, Février V, Lecorvaisier C, Poly P. Dermatoses d'intolérance aux implantes métalliques en chirurgie orthopédique. *Rev Chir Orthop Reparatrice Appar Mot* 1995;81:473–484.
18. Friedman RJ, Black J, Galante JO, Jacobs JJ, Skinner HB. Current concepts in orthopaedic biomaterials and implant fixation. *J Bone Joint Surg Am* 1993;75:1086–1110.
19. Geesink RGT, Hoefnagels NHM. Six-year results of hydroxyapatite-coated total hip replacement. *J Bone Joint Surg Br* 1995;77:534–547.
20. Gillespie WJ, Frampton CMA, Henderson RJ, Ryan PM. The incidence of cancer following total hip replacement. *J Bone Joint Surg Br* 1988;70:539–542.
21. Gillespie WJ, Henry DA, O'Connell DL, et al. Development of hematopoietic cancers after implantation of total joint replacement. *Clin Orthop* 1996;329S:S290–S296.
22. Gristina AG. Implant failure and the immuno-incompetent fibro-inflammatory zone. *Clin Orthop* 1994;298:106–118.
23. Haddad FS, Cobb AG, Bentley G, Levell NJ, Dowd PM. Hypersensitivity in aseptic loosening of total hip replacements: the role of constituents of bone cement. *J Bone Joint Surg Br* 1996;78:546–549.
24. Harris WH. The problem is osteolysis. *Clin Orthop* 1995;311:46–53.
25. Hicks DG, Judkins AR, Sickel JZ, Rosier RN, Puzas JE, O'Keefe RJ. Granular histiocytosis of pelvic lymph nodes following total hip arthroplasty. *J Bone Joint Surg Am* 1996;78:482–496.
26. Hierholzer S, Hierholzer G, Sauer KH, Paterson RS. Increased corrosion of stainless steel implants in infected plated fractures. *Arch Orthop Trauma Surg* 1984;102:198–200.
27. Hozack WJK, Rothman RH, Booth RE Jr, et al. Survivorship analysis of 1,041 Charnley total hip arthroplasties. *J Arthroplasty* 1990;5:41–47.
28. Jacobs JJ, Gilbert JL, Urban RM. Corrosion of metallic implants. In: Stauffer RN, ed. *Advances in operative orthopedics. Vol. 2.* St. Louis: Mosby; 1994;279–320.
29. Jacobs JJ, Skipor AK, Doorn PF, et al. Cobalt and chromium concentrations in patients with metal on metal total hip replacements. *Clin Orthop* 1996;329S:S256–S263.
30. Jacobs JJ, Urban RM, Gilbert JL et al. Local and distant products from modularity. *Clin Orthop* 1995;319:94–105.
31. Jacobs JJ, Urban RM, Wall J, Black J, Reid JD, Veneman L. Unusual foreign-body reaction to a failed total knee replacement: simulation of a sarcoma clinically and a sarcoid histologically—a case report. *J Bone Joint Surg Am* 1995;77:444–451.
32. Jasty M, Goetz DD, Bragdon CR et al. Wear of polyethylene acetabular components in total hip arthroplasty. *J Bone Joint Surg Am* 1997;79:349–358.
33. Lalor PA, Revell PA. T-lymphocytes and titanium aluminium vanadium (TiAlV) alloy: evidence for immunological events associated with debris deposition. *Clin Mater* 1993;12:57–62.

34. Li S, Chang JD, Barrena EG, Furman BD, Wright TM, Salvati E. Nonconsolidated polyethylene particles and oxidation in Charnley acetabular cups. *Clin Orthop* 1995;319:54–63.
35. Löhrs U, Bos I. The pathology of artificial joints. In: Berry CL, ed. *The pathology of devices*. Berlin: Springer-Verlag, 1994:1–52.
36. Malchau H, Herberts P, Ahnfelt L. Prognosis of total hip replacement in Sweden: follow-up of 92,675 operations performed 1978–1990. *Acta Orthop Scand* 1993;64:497–506.
37. McKee GK, Watson-Farrar J. Replacement of arthritic hips by the McKee-Farrar prosthesis. *J Bone Joint Surg Br* 1968;48:245–259.
38. McKellop H, Park SH, R Chiesa R, et al. *In vivo* wear of 3 types of metal on metal hip prostheses during 2 decades of use. *Clin Orthop* 1996;329S:S128–S140.
39. Merritt K, Panigutti MA, Kray MJ, Brown SA. Incidence of infection and analysis of contributing factors in revision joint arthroplasty over a two year period. *J Appl Biomater* 1994;5:103–108.
40. Merritt K, Rodrigo JJ. Immune response to synthetic materials: sensitization of patients receiving orthopaedic implants. *Clin Orthop* 1996;326:71–79.
41. Mittelmeier H. Report on the first decennium of clinical experience with a cementless ceramic total hip replacement. *Acta Orthop Belg* 1985;51:367–376.
42. Morris, R. Evidence-based choice of hip prostheses [editorial] *J Bone Joint Surg Br* 1996;78:691–693.
43. Moss AJ, Hamburger S, Moore RM, Jeng LL, Howie JL. Use of selected medical device implants in the United States, 1988. *Advanced data from vital and health statistics of the national center for health statistics.* Vol. 191. Hyattsville, MD: National Center for Health Statistics, 1991:1–24.
44. Müller ME. The benefits of metal-on-metal total hip replacements. *Clin Orthop* 1995;311:54–59.
45. Murray DW, Carr AC, Bulstrode CJ. Which primary total hip replacement? *J Bone Joint Surg Br* 1995;77:520–527.
46. Murray DW, Carr AC, Bulstrode CJ. Survival analysis of joint replacements. *J Bone Joint Surg Br* 1993;75:697–704.
47. Nizard RS, Sedel L, Christel P, Meunier A, Soudry M, Witvoet J. Ten-year survivorship of cemented ceramic-ceramic total hip prosthesis. *Clin Orthop* 1992;282:53–63.
48. Nordström D, Sanatavirta S, Gristina A, Konttinen YT. Immune-inflammatory response in the totally replaced hip: a review of biocompatibility aspects. *Eur J Med* 1993;2:296–300.
49. Nyrén O, McLaughlin JK, Gridley G, et al. Cancer risk after hip replacement with metal implants: a population-based cohort study in Sweden. *J Natl Cancer Inst* 1995;87:28–33.
50. Remes A, Williams, DF. Immune response in biocompatibility. *Biomaterials* 1992;13:731–743.
51. Ring PA. Complete replacement arthroplasty of the hip by the Ring prosthesis. *J Bone Joint Surg Br* 1968;50:720–731.
52. Satula LC, Collier JP, Saum KA, et al. Impact of gamma sterilization on clinical performance of polyethylene in the hip. *Clin Orthop* 1995;319:28–40.
53. Schmalzreid TP, Amstutz HC, AMK, Dorey FJ. Etiology of deep sepsis in total hip arthroplasty: the significance of hematogenous and late infections. *Clin Orthop* 1992;280:200–207.
54. Schmidt M, Weber H, Schön R. Cobalt chromium molybdenum metal combination for modular hip prostheses. *Clin Orthop* 1996;329S:S35–47.
55. Sedel L. L'alumine en chirurgie orthopédique. *Cah Enseignement SOFCOT* 1986;25:61–69.
56. Shea KG, Bloebaum RD, Avent JM, Birk GT, Samuelson KM. Analysis of lymph nodes for polyethylene particles in patients who have had a primary joint replacement. *J Bone Joint Surg Am* 1996;78:497–504.
57. Shih CH, Wu CC, Lee ZL, Yang WE. Localized femoral osteolysis in cementless ceramic total hip arthroplasty. *Orthop Rev* 1994;23:325–328.
58. Sychertz CJ, Moon KH, Hasimoto Y, Terefenko KM, Engh CA Jr, Bauer TW. Wear of polyethylene cups in total hip arthroplasty: a study of specimens retrieved post mortem. *J Bone Joint Surg Am* 1996;78:1193–1200.
59. Urban RM, Jacobs JJ, Gilbert JL, Galante JO. Migration of corrosion products from modular hip prostheses: particle microanalysis and histopathological findings. *J Bone Joint Surg Am* 1994;76:1345–1359.
60. Visuri Y, Koskenvuo M. Cancer risk after McKee-Farrar total hip replacement. *Orthopedics* 1991;14:137–142.
61. Wait ME, Walker PS, Blunn GW. Tissue reaction to CoCr wear debris from metal on metal total hip replacements [Abstract]. *Trans Eur Orthop Res Soc* 1995;5:160.
62. Wadstrom T, Eliasson I, Holder I, Ljungh A, eds. *Pathogenesis of wound and biomaterial-associated infections*. London: Springer-Verlag, 1990.
63. Walter IA. On the material and the tribology of alumina-alumina couplings for hip joint prostheses. *Clin Orthop* 1992;282:31–46.
64. Weber BG. The reactivation of the metal-metal pairing for the total hip prosthesis. In: Morscher E, ed. *Endoprosthetics*. Berlin: Springer-Verlag, 1995:50–59.
65. Yang J, Merritt K. Production of monoclonal antibodies to study corrosion products of CoCr biomaterials. *J Biomed Mater Res* 1996;31:71–80.
66. Yang J, Merritt K. Detection of antibodies against corrosion products in patients after Co-Cr total joint replacements. *J Biomed Mater Res* 1994;28:1249–1258.
67. Zichner L, Lindenfeld T. *In vivo* wear of ceramic-polyethylene and metal-polyethylene wear pairs [German] *Orthopade* 1997;26:129–134.

Revision Total Hip Arthroplasty,
edited by Marvin E. Steinberg and Jonathan P. Garino,
Lippincott Williams & Wilkins, Philadelphia © 1999.

7

Effect of Surgical Technique on Long-term Survivorship

Thomas H. Mallory,
Adolph V. Lombardi, Jr., and
Stephen M. Herrington

The long-term success of revision total hip replacement is based on three key factors. The first factor is appropriate management of host- or patient-related factors. Although a young, healthy patient is able to tolerate a joint replacement procedure, revision total hip replacement is usually more common in the geriatric population. Consequently a more radical procedure is imposed on a patient in less than optimum condition. Second, long-term survival after revision total hip replacement is affected by the surgical method used. For example, the surgical approach adequate for a primary total hip replacement may have to be modified to achieve the more extensile exposure required for the revision procedure. However, a more extensile surgical approach is associated with an increased incidence of postoperative dislocation. Furthermore, revision total hip replacement carries with it increased surgical risk, which can adversely affect the outcome. For example, a straightforward revision total hip replacement procedure can become quite complex when implant removal is attempted without adequate experience, instrumentation, or exposure.

    T. H. Mallory: Joint Implant Surgeons, Inc.; Division of Orthopaedic Surgery, The Ohio State University; Section of Joint Implant Surgery, The Ohio Orthopaedic Institute, Grant Medical Center, Columbus, Ohio 43215.
    A. V. Lombardi, Jr.: Joint Implant Surgeons, Inc.; Division of Orthopaedic Surgery, The Ohio State University; Department of Biomedical Engineering, The Ohio State University; Section of Orthopedics, The Ohio Orthopaedic Institute, Grant Medical Center, Columbus, Ohio 43215.
    S. M. Herrington: Research Services, Joint Implant Surgeons, Inc., Columbus, Ohio 43215.

Bone loss frequently adds a challenge unique to revision total hip replacement. The surgeon must have extensive knowledge of bone grafting techniques and have access to an inventory of bone graft material. Third, selection of a prosthesis must be based on knowledge and experience. The surgeon must be knowledgeable about the various design features of cementless components, jumbo acetabular components, reinforcement rings or cages for acetabular reconstruction, cement or cementless modes of fixation, and other prosthetic design features.

With these key factors identified, a straightforward and logical approach to revision total hip replacement is possible but not always easily defined. We use the following algorithmic approach to standardize management of revision total hip arthroplasty: (a) preoperative planning, (b) surgical approach, (c) implant removal techniques, (d) proper assessment of bony and soft-tissue deficiencies, (e) reconstruction, and (f) postoperative care. Proper execution of these steps will guide the surgeon in performing a revision total hip replacement that will most likely have successful long-term results.

PREOPERATIVE PLANNING

Preoperative planning is a critical part of the operative procedure and is often overlooked. The value of preoperative radiographs cannot be overemphasized. For example, if the femoral component is being revised because of aseptic loosening and associated osteolysis, stem length should be adjusted to extend adequately beyond the osteolytic lesion. By carefully evaluating preoperative radiographs, the surgeon can establish the appropriate inventory of prostheses necessary for successful completion of the procedure. Furthermore, assessment of preoperative radiographs allows the surgeon to identify any structural weakness in the existing bone–prosthesis composite and assists in avoiding perforation or subsequent fracture. Understanding the pathologic process that leads to failure of a prosthetic device is another important aspect of preoperative planning. For example, if osteolysis is caused by titanium polyethylene bearing surfaces, the osteolytic lesion is typically larger than actually shown by a radiograph. In this situation, extensive bone grafting can be required. Therefore understanding failure modes preoperatively influences the overall strategy of revision total hip replacement.

Familiarity with the existing implant system is an important factor to be considered in preoperative planning. Cemented devices have special considerations. For example, a femoral stem with an I-beam configuration and a channel on the anterior and posterior aspects can be particularly difficult to remove. Recognizing that a cemented precoated device is to be revised can be beneficial. It alerts the surgeon that the cement–implant interface may be difficult to debond. The surface finish of the existing device also affects ease of removal. A prosthesis with a grit-blasted or textured surface is more difficult to remove than a stem with a smooth surface. When revising cementless devices, it is important to know the extent and location of the porous coating, a factor that can play a role in determining surgical technique.

When dealing with cemented acetabular components, an all-polyethylene versus a metal-backed component can change revision strategy. Surface coatings, grit blasting, or undercut geometric features enhance cement fixation but can make removal difficult. Various design features of cementless acetabular devices can complicate their removal. Acetabular components with adjunct screw fixation may have to be removed with special instruments and a threaded component has to be removed with a special extraction device.

Thorough preoperative planning can determine the need for additional laboratory and radiographic evaluation. For example, extrusion of cement beyond the medial wall of the acetabulum necessitates an arthrogram to detect any possible arterial involvement. If periosteal elevation is seen on a preoperative radiograph, the surgeon should be alerted to the possibility of infection. Therefore, preoperative laboratory evaluation, radionuclide scans, and possible aspiration might be needed to rule out infection. Alerting a pathologist that intraoperative frozen section analysis is anticipated can be helpful. When large bone deficits are involved, computed tomographic scans can facilitate and enhance the surgeon's understanding of the size and orientation of the deficits.

Because infection rates are higher in revision total hip replacement than in primary total hip arthroplasty, prevention of infection is an important consideration. This preventive process begins preoperatively and extends throughout the operative procedure. Prophylaxis of perioperative infection may require various combinations of antibiotics and the expertise of an infectious disease consultant. If cement fixation is anticipated, addition of antibiotics to the cement should be considered. The use of clean-air operating rooms and personal isolator suits has been reported to reduce exposure to infection. The operating room team must be efficient to reduce surgical time and the exposure of the patient to infection.

SURGICAL APPROACH

The most commonly used approaches in total hip replacement revision operations are the transtrochanteric, posterolateral, and anterolateral. Experience with each of these approaches has been well documented in the literature. Although the effects of these approaches on long-term clinical survival of the prosthetic composite are not completely clear, surgical approach does affect dislocation rates, trochanteric nonunion rates, and other indicators of clinical success.

Transtrochanteric Approach

Three variations of the transtrochanteric approach exist: classic Charnley, trochanteric slide, and extended trochanteric osteotomy (see Chapter 12).

Classic Charnley Trochanteric Approach

The classic Charnley trochanteric approach was popularized by virtue of its use in primary total hip arthroplasty and therefore was easily applied to revision total hip arthroplasty. This approach allows excellent visualization of the lateral shaft of the femur, enhancing implant and cement removal. However, the classic Charnley approach is associated with a high incidence of trochanteric nonunion. Reattachment of the atrophied trochanteric fragment often requires adjunct fixation with cables, hooks, or bolts. These devices can break, migrate, or generate particulate debris and produce extensive granuloma (44).

Trochanteric Slide

The trochanteric slide is accomplished by means of anteromedial inclination of an osteotomy to provide a more stable interface for reattachment. The trochanteric slide has the advantage of maintaining muscle continuity. The disadvantage of this technique is decreased visualization of the acetabulum. Adjunct fixation of the trochanter is required with this approach. Glassman et al. (17) reported a 10% incidence of nonunion when this technique was used in revision hip arthroplasty.

Extended Trochanteric Osteotomy

With a 6 to 12 cm distal extension to the trochanteric fragment, a large lateral window is developed that enhances both prosthesis and cement removal. Trochanteric fixation is enhanced because the extended fragment increases the surface area available for fixation. Because extended trochanteric osteotomy requires extensive bone resection, proximal femoral bone stock can be compromised. As a result, proximal prosthetic support with a tapered device can force the trochanter fragment laterally, increasing the likelihood of nonunion. When an extended trochanteric osteotomy is used, the patient's postoperative physical therapy and rehabilitation course should be modified to protect the healing trochanteric fragment.

Posterolateral Surgical Approach

The posterolateral surgical approach is used commonly in revision total hip arthroplasty. The technique is used widely for endoprosthetic replacement in the treatment of subcapital fractures. The posterolateral approach also is quite popular for primary total hip replacement. This approach has the advantage of maintaining the integrity of the abductor mechanism. Although femoral exposure is adequate, acetabular exposure can be limited. This approach is associated with an increased incidence of dislocation. Another concern with this surgical exposure is its proximity to the sciatic nerve, which predisposes the patient to risk for nerve injury.

Anterolateral Surgical Approach

The anterolateral surgical approach has the advantage of improved visualization of the acetabulum and femur without the attendant trochanteric complications and proximity to the sciatic nerve. This approach is associated with a low incidence of dislocation. However, the abductor muscle is divided or split and therefore abductor dysfunction can occur postoperatively. There also can be an increased incidence of heterotopic ossification (3). However, we prefer the anterolateral approach for revision total hip replacement because it affords an extensile exposure with minimal risk of prosthetic dislocation. It also avoids the problem of trochanteric nonunion. In our experience abductor muscle dysfunction has not been a problem (12).

IMPLANT REMOVAL TECHNIQUES

Implant removal can have a serious effect on the outcome of revision total hip arthroplasty. A full assortment of instruments and a working knowledge of various techniques are necessary to perform this part of the procedure effectively. The goal of implant removal is expedient removal of the prosthetic device with minimal bone loss and soft-tissue damage.

Removal of the Femoral Component

Extraction of the femoral component requires adequate exposure of the implant and implant interface. For example, the prosthetic interface around the trochanteric fossa should be cleared of all debris and bone overgrowth before removal of the femoral component is attempted. Removal of a femoral component is facilitated by use of a universal femoral extraction device. Use of the extraction device is critical in removal of a femoral component with a modular head. If the femoral component cannot be removed easily, the interface should be further interrupted to free the femoral component. Development of an anterolateral femoral episiotomy relieves, or loosens, the grip of the femur, further freeing the implant. If the femoral component continues to remain well fixed, one can convert the episiotomy to an extended trochanteric osteotomy (50) or make a window on the anterolateral shaft of the femur. Removal of the cemented femoral component progresses from development of an anterolateral episiotomy to an anterior window (Fig. 1). Similarly, for removal of a cementless device, conversion of the episiotomy to an extended trochanteric osteotomy expedites component removal. A cementless device occasionally can be so well-fixed distally that transfemoral resection may be necessary (16).

Once the cemented femoral component is extracted, the cement must be carefully removed. Appreciation of the three zones of the femur—proximal, intramedullary, and distal—provides for a standardized approach to cement removal. In the proximal region, cement removal can be accomplished under direction visualization with hand tools or a high-speed burr. Special techniques are needed for cement removal in the intramedullary zone of the femur. If hand tools are used, one must be careful not to perforate or fracture the femur. Anterior femoral windows facilitate cement removal and lessen the incidence

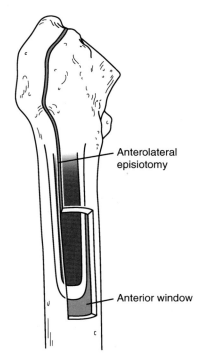

Figure 1. Femoral component removal is facilitated with the use of an anterior window.

of fracture. Controlled perforation is a recommended technique (6,47). A series of 8 mm holes are made along the anterior shaft of the femur at intervals twice the diameter of the bone (Fig. 2A). A high-speed reamer is advanced down the intramedullary canal under direct visualization through the apertures. An alternative method is advocated by Turner and Scheller (48), who recommend the use of fluoroscopy with use of high-speed drills or burrs. However, increased exposure to radiation is a concern to the patient and the surgical team when fluoroscopy is used to assist in cement removal. Cement removal in the distal zone of the femur can be expedited with the use of ultrasonic tools (26). The feedback of the ultrasonic tool differentiates bone and cement, making it easier to separate and define the interface (Fig. 2B). Ultrasonic instrumentation can be effective in a nonvisualized portion of the femur.

Acetabular Component Removal

Removing a failed acetabular component can be difficult because of exposure constraints and access to the acetabulum. The initial step in acetabular component removal is circumferential exposure of the rim of the acetabulum. The cement–component interface can be interrupted with curved osteotomes. With initial separation of the component from the cement, there is less chance of causing acetabular fracture or diminishing acetabular bone stock. Each step in removal of an acetabular component should be tempered by awareness of its potential for fracture or development of serious bone deficits. Levering an instrument against the bony acetabulum should be avoided because of the increased possibility of acetabular fracture. This becomes a critical issue when working in the posterosuperior portion of the acetabulum, because this important structure is critical for reconstruction. Cement that has extruded beyond the medial wall of the acetabulum should not be removed because of the likelihood of damage to vascular, neurologic, or urologic structures. Cement should be removed from the intrapelvic region only when it has been established that its presence constitutes a mechanical obstruction or is associated with infection.

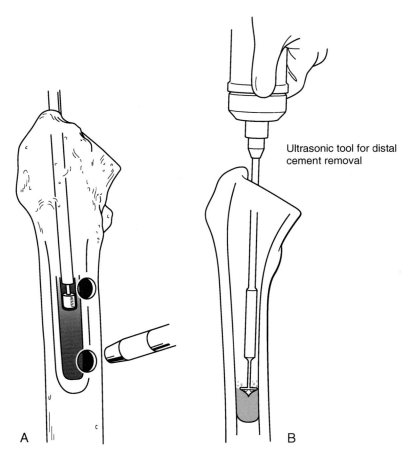

Ultrasonic tool for distal cement removal

A

B

Figure 2. Atraumatic femoral cement removal: **(A)** Controlled perforation technique enhances visualization of the femoral canal and prevents inadvertant perforation of the femur; **(B)** Ultrasonic tools can be used to remove the distal cement cone without damage to bone.

Cementless acetabular components are removed in essentially the same way as metal-backed cemented devices—with curved osteotomes to debond the bone–implant interface. The presence of pegs or screws attached to an acetabular component can complicate the extraction process and necessitates use of special osteotomes or specific instrumentation to dislodge the component. Components with apical holes can be removed with the assistance of an apical hole extraction device. When a broken screw is encountered, a trephine is necessary to remove it. Threaded acetabular components are removed with a specific extraction device.

ASSESSMENT OF BONY AND SOFT-TISSUE DEFICIENCIES

Bony Deficiencies

Although the classification system of bony deficiencies may appear superfluous, it is necessary because it alerts the surgeon to potential technical pitfalls. Furthermore, a classification system of bony deficiencies defines the surgical strategy. Several systems have been described.

Femoral

We use a system that categorizes femoral deficiencies into three types (31) (Fig. 3). A type I femoral deficiency is one in which the corticocancellous content and the cortical

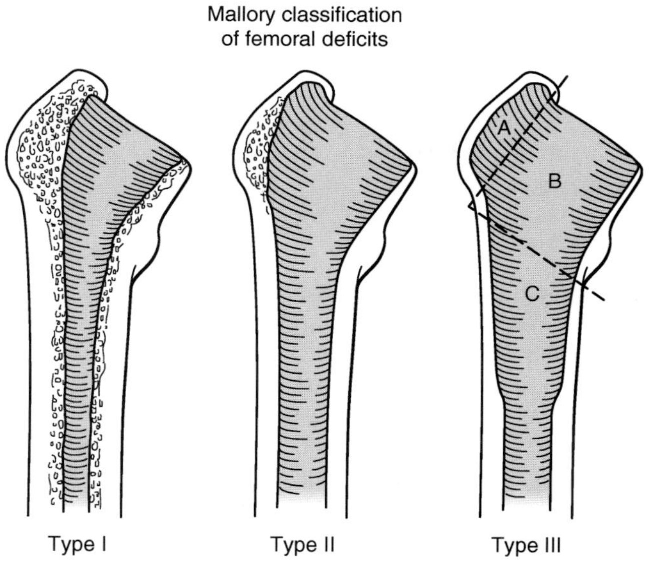

Mallory classification
of femoral deficits

Type I   Type II   Type III

Figure 3. Mallory classification of femoral deficits; Type I-The cortico-cancellous content as well as the cortical structure of the proximal femur remain intact. Type II-The cortical structure is intact, but the cancellous content is deficient. Type III-Both the cortical structure and the cancellous contents are deficient, and can be further defined by zone.

structure of the proximal femur remain intact. A type II deficiency has an intact cortical structure, but the cancellous content is deficient. Type III deficiencies indicate loss of both the cortical structure and the cancellous contents. A type III deficit can be further delineated by zonal deficits involving the cortical structure. Type IIIA zonal deficits are located above the lesser trochanter, Type IIIB deficits are between the lesser trochanter and the isthmus, and type IIIC deficits involve isthmus and distal bone loss.

Acetabular

A classification system for acetabular deficits has been proposed by Paprosky et al. (36) (see Chapter 16). We prefer a modification of this system. A type I acetabulum is one that is essentially intact, but has minor deficits. Type II is indicative of a medial wall or dome deficit with intact anterior and posterior columns. Type III indicates that a deficiency of the anterior or posterior columns exists. Type III can be further subdivided into Type IIIA, which indicates that the anterior column has been compromised by loss of the anterior wall. A type IIIB acetabulum is characterized by compromise of the posterior column caused by loss of the posterolateral aspect of the acetabulum. A Type IIIC acetabulum is characterized by loss of the structural integrity of both the anterior and posterior columns with or without pelvic dissociation.

Soft-tissue Deficiencies

Thorough evaluation of the soft tissues is warranted because revision total hip replacement is associated with a marked increase in dislocation rates (24) and with delayed wound healing. Soft tissue that is well vascularized is essential for wound healing. A tenuous or stretched abductor mechanism is a concern, because if the abductor mechanism is compromised, dislocation is imminent. In such circumstances, prosthetic stability can be enhanced by means of changing the inclination angle to achieve more horizontal placement of the acetabular component. A constrained acetabular component or snap-fit cup with an extended labrum can be helpful when dislocation potential is increased. The effectiveness of such intraoperative technical modifications can be enhanced with modification of the postoperative rehabilitation program to include the use of an orthotic device.

RECONSTRUCTION

Femoral Reconstruction

The mode of fixation in prosthetic selection for a type I femoral deficiency is basically the same as for a primary total hip replacement. Because both the corticocancellous junction and the cortical structures are maintained, a cemented component can be used because microinterlock with the cancellous content can occur. In this situation a cementless device can be used because adequate bone stock is retained. A Type II deficit is complicated by loss of cancellous content, which adversely affects fixation and can directly affect selection of the fixation mode. An *in vitro* study by Dohmae et al. (7) quantified the shear strength of cement–bone interface in primary type I versus revision type II femurs. The authors found that the type II revision femurs had lost 79% of their interface strength as compared to primary femurs. The reduction in strength was attributed to not obtaining a microinterlock between the cement and the bone. Revising a type III deficiency is much more difficult. It involves extensile exposure of the femur, use of long-stemmed prosthetic devices, bone grafting, and adjunct fixation.

The clinical data with respect to outcomes for femoral revision are confusing, the follow-up periods are short, and published reports (Table 1) are flawed by lack of a standardized classification of femoral deficits. Although reoperation rates for type I and II cemented femoral revisions are not especially high, progressive radiolucencies are quite concerning. For example, Kavanagh et al. (25) evaluated the cases of 162 patients who underwent cemented revision and reported a 3.7% reoperation rate due to aseptic loosening after an average of 54 months of follow-up study. However, 64% of cemented femoral components had complete radiolucencies, indicative of impending failure, and 19% of the femoral stems had subsided 2 mm or more. Pellicci et al. (39) reviewed the records of 107 patients who had undergone cemented femoral revisions with an average follow-up period of 41 months. The reoperation rate due to aseptic loosening was 5.5%. An overall mechanical failure rate of 14% was attributed in part to poor bone stock. The authors reexamined these patients an average of 97 months postoperatively and found that 11.7% of the 60 asymptomatic cemented femoral components with no or stable radiolucencies had loosened (40). Meanwhile, Amstutz et al. (1) conducted a follow-up study with 66 patients for an average of 25 months and found an overall reoperation rate of 9% when cement was used. The reoperation rate due to aseptic loosening of the femoral component was 1.7%, and 26% of the femoral components had complete radiolucencies. Callaghan et al. (4) evaluated the cases of 136 patients with an average follow-up period of 43 months and reported a 4.4% reoperation rate due to aseptic loosening of the femoral component and a 13% subsidence rate. Furthermore, progressive radiolucencies were seen in 26% of the cemented femoral components. The radiographic findings reported in these studies raised concerns regarding the efficacy of cement as a fixation mode in revision total hip replacement.

Because of the roentgenographic findings reported with these studies, contemporary cement techniques applied in primary hip arthroplasty were pursued for revision arthroplasty. Rubash and Harris (42) reported the results of 43 cemented revisions in which second-generation cement technology was used. At an average follow-up time of 74 months, radiographic assessment showed a femoral loosening rate of 11% (9% definitely loose and 2% probably loose). The reoperation rate due to aseptic loosening was 2.3% but had climbed to 10.5% when the patients were re-examined a mean of 140 months postoperatively (11). Katz et al. (23) evaluated the cases of 40 patients with a mean follow-up period of 143 months. They found a 9.5% rate of repeat revision for aseptic loosening and a 14.3% definite loosening rate. Weber et al. (49) conducted a

Table 1. Results of clinical studies of cemented versus cementless revision hips: Femoral component

Authors	Publication date	Date prosthesis inserted	Femoral component	Follow-up period (mo)	No. of patients[a]	No. of prostheses inserted	Aseptic re-revision[b]	Subsidence	Fracture	Deep sepsis	Dislocation	Trochanteric nonunion
Cemented revisions												
Kavanagh et al. (25)	1985	1969–78	Var	54	166	135	3.7%	19.0%	5.9%	1.2%	9.0%	13.0%
Amstutz et al. (1)	1982	1970–80	Var	25	66	66	1.7%	NA	8.3%	1.5%	10.6%	7.6%
Pellicci et al. (39)	1982	1973–79	NA	41	107	110	5.5%	NA	NA	1.8%	1.8%	13.0%
Rubash and Harris (42)	1988	1976–80	Var	74	41	43	2.3%	4.7%	4.7%	0.0%	14.0%	6.0%
Estok and Harris (11)	1994	1976–80	Var	140	36	38	10.5%	NA	2.6%	2.8%	2.6%	5.3%
Weber et al. (49)	1996	1976–83	Iowa	77	52	56	5.0%	NA	NA	NA	NA	NA
Katz et al. (23)	1995	1977–83	Var	143	40	47	9.5%	NA	NA	4.2%	6.3%	NA
Callaghan et al. (4)	1985	1979–82	Var	43	136	136	4.4%	13.2%	2.2%	3.4%	8.2%	9.6%
Gross et al. (18)	1995	1983–94	J&J	58	130	130	3.8%	NA	0.0%	3.8%	6.9%	25.0%
Weber et al. (49)	1996	1986–88	Iowa	74	43	49	2.0%	NA	NA	0.0%	16.0%	NA
Gie et al. (15)	1993	1987–89	Exeter	30	56	56	0.0%	39.3%	5.4%	0.0%	0.0%	NA
Slooff et al. (46)	1996	1991–92	Exeter	24	10	10	0.0%	NA	20.0%	0.0%	0.0%	NA
Cementless revisions												
Engh et al. (10)	1988	1980–85	AML, NEB	53	160	127	1.6%	4.0%	NA	0.6%	0.6%	10.4%
Lawrence et al. (29)	1993	1980–86	AML	89	160	174	3.4%	NA	0.6%	1.9%	3.4%	8.6%
Lawrence et al. (28)	1994	1980–86	AML	108	81	83	3.6%	1.2%	2.4%	1.2%	3.7%	1.2%
Mallory (31)	1988	1981–85	MHP, JMP	NA	160	160	5.0%	NA	NA	2.6%	10.0%	NA
Gustilo and Pasternak (19)	1988	1981–85	Bias	34	55	57	7.0%	19.3%	1.8%	4.0%	4.0%	NA
Pak et al. (35)	1993	1982–89	AML	57	113	113	4.4%	NA	NA	0.0%	7.1%	NA
Hedley et al. (21)	1988	1983–87	PCA	21	82	54	3.7%	3.7%	NA	0.0%	7.4%	3.7%
Head et al. (20)	1994	1984–90	MHC	36	106	106	3.4%	4.7%	NA	0.0%	NA	NA
Peters et al. (41)	1995	1985–89	Bias	65	45	49	4.1%	44.9%	24.5%	2.0%	4.1%	10.2%
Mulliken et al. (32)	1996	1987–90	MHP	55	51	52	10.0%	NA	40.0%	0.0%	0.0%	NA
Bargar et al. (2)	1993	1988–90	Custom	30	47	47	2.1%	15.0%	19.0%	0.0%	4.3%	6.4%
Chandler et al. (5)	1994	1989–92	S-ROM	22	29	30	3.3%	NA	NA	3.4%	17.2%	10.0%

The authors have made every effort to accurately represent the data reported in each of the studies. Because of nonstandard reporting associated with the orthopedic literature, this is not always possible. Some percentages have been recalculated to standardize reporting.

[a] Number of patients at follow-up study.

[b] Aseptic re-revision is percentage re-revised because of aseptic loosening.

AML, anatomic locking medullary; J&J, Johnson and Johnson; JMP, Joint Medical Products; MHC, Mallory-Head calcar; MHP, Mallory-Head porous; NA, not available; NEB, New England Baptist; PCA, porous coated anatomic; S-ROM, superior range of motion; Var, variety.

follow-up study with 52 patients with cemented femoral and acetabular components for an average of 77 months and with 43 patients with a cementless acetabulum and cemented femoral component for an average of 74 months. The group with cemented components had an overall femoral reoperation rate of 5% and the group with hybrid components had a reoperation rate of 2%. The femoral loosening rate was 3% for the former group and 6% for the latter. The series presented indicate that contemporary cement technique does improve the reoperation rate when cement is used in type I and type II deficits.

Another approach to improve the corticocancellous content of the femur with type I and type II deficits entails the technique of impaction grafting as popularized by Gie et al. (15). This method involves use of morselized bone chips in combination with a cemented prosthesis to reconstitute bone loss in the proximal femur. The series of Gie et al. showed no reoperations because of aseptic loosening with an average follow-up period of approximately 30 months. However, 39% of the femurs subsided 2 mm or more, but this outcome was expected with this particular type of prosthetic device. Slooff et al. (46) conducted a follow-up study with 10 patients for an average of 24 months and reported 2 (20%) femoral fractures with use of the impaction grafting technique. Although impaction grafting does show promise, there has been limited follow-up information to date. There is also concern that component subsidence or femoral fracture can be a serious consequence of use of this technique.

Cementless fixation for femoral revision is attractive in type I and II femoral reconstruction. There are three types of cementless fixation methods to be considered: distal fixation, proximal filling, and calcar load-bearing fixation (Fig. 4). The proponents of distal fixation emphasize that the proximal bone stock is not adequate for prosthetic support and therefore recommend engaging the prosthesis in the intact distal bone. Clinical series (10,28,29) have shown the results of using the distal fixation mode with a fully porous coated femoral component with average follow-up periods of 4 years or more. Reoperation rates due to aseptic loosening varied from 1.6% to 3.6%, and the rate of radiographic loosening is approximately 1%. Despite the effectiveness of distally fixed prostheses, these series identify concerns with stress shielding and thigh pain. Stress shielding to some degree is found in almost all instances. This raises the question what the potential future for re-revision will be among patients with severe stress shielding and secondary bone loss. Engh et al. (9) reported on a series of patients with pronounced resorption with distally fixed stems larger than 13.5 mm in diameter. They reported the incidence of moderate to severe thigh pain to be as high as 15.5%.

A proximal filling fixation mode relies on maximizing fit and fill to stabilize the prosthesis within the proximal femur. When a proximal filling device is used, the distal portion of the femoral component is used for toggle control (30). Follow-up reports of proximal filling fixation have been less than encouraging. Hedley et al. (21) evaluated 54 porous coated anatomic (PCA; Howmedica, Rutherford, N.J.) stems in patients undergoing revision total hip replacement with an average follow-up period of 21 months. The reoperation rate due to aseptic loosening was 3.7%; however, 9.5% hips were considered radiographically loose. Peters et al. (41) evaluated the Bias femoral component (Zimmer, Warsaw, Ind.) in 45 patients with a mean follow-up period of 65 months. The revision rate due to aseptic loosening was 4.1% with an alarmingly high subsidence rate of 44.9%. In addition, further studies of the Bias prosthesis reported by Gustilo and Pasternak (19) showed that 7% of 57 hips had undergone a reoperation because of aseptic loosening with an average follow-up period of 34 months. Nearly all patients showed radiographic evidence of loosening. Bargar et al. (2), who optimized fit and fill by using a custom femoral component, reported their results with 47 patients at an average follow-up time of 30 months. The reoperation rate due to aseptic loosening was 2%. However, the subsidence rate of 15% and fracture rate of 19% were alarming. Mulliken et al. (32) assessed 52 wedge-shaped, long-stemmed femoral components in a follow-up study for an average of 55 months. The reoperation rate due to aseptic loosening was 10%, and another 14% of replacements were described as radiographically unstable. It can be concluded that there is a high subsidence rate when proximal filling devices are used in revision total hip

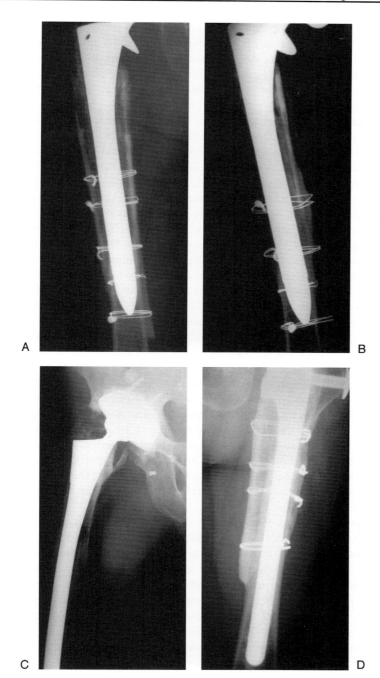

Figure 4. Three common modes of femoral fixation: **(A)** Distal fixation—note proximal femoral reconstruction with graft; **(B)** Distal fixation—note subsequent proximal stress shielding with the distally fixed prosthesis; **(C)** Proximal filling fixation—note subsidence with a proximal filling prosthesis utilized in a compromised femur; **(D)** Calcar bearing fixation—note reconstitution of the femur with a calcar bearing prosthesis.

replacement. The corticocancellous structure is compromised, and therefore a device designed for proximal fit and fill will subside and may eventually fail.

The proximal compression loading attributes of a calcar bearing device promote femoral reconstitution as opposed to proximal stress shielding evidence with distally fixed prostheses. Because of the large platform-loading nature of these prostheses, they inherently resist the subsidence that occurs with proximal filling designs. Head et al. (20) evaluated the Mallory-Head calcar prosthesis (Biomet, Warsaw, Ind.) in 106 patients. These femoral reconstructions were classified as predominantly type III femurs and therefore required supplemental allograft. The follow-up period ranged from 2 to 7 years with an average of 3 years. The revision rate was reported to be 3.4% for this group.

Bone deficiencies involving the proximal femur must be fully appreciated for appropriate use of bone grafting techniques. Type I and Type II femoral deficits may well be managed with impaction grafting. However, type III deficiency, which can be associated with considerable structural bone loss, requires the use of either a bulk structural graft or onlay cortical strut grafts. Gross et al. (18) reported a technique in which bulk-structural graft was used to manage type III deficits. The technique involves cementing a femoral component into a segmental allograft. The femoral component is then press fit into the host bone, and autograft is placed at the graft host junction. Junctional fixation is enhanced with cerclage wire, plates, or screws. When this technique was used to treat 130 patients, who participated in follow-up study for an average of 58 months, a 3.8% reoperation rate due to aseptic loosening was found. An additional 1.2% of the components were radiographically loose, as characterized by nonunion of the graft with the host bone. Chandler et al. (5) conducted a study with 29 patients with long-stemmed femoral components with an average follow-up period of 22 months. The proximal portion of the device was cemented to a proximal allograft and the distal portion was press fit into the host bone. There was a 3.3% rate of reoperation due to aseptic loosening. Although there was initial enthusiasm for bulk proximal allografting, long-term results indicate considerable graft resorption. Onlay cortical strut grafts have been used to augment bony deficiency in type III reconstruction. After combining these strut grafts with distal fixation, Pak et al. (35) conducted a follow-up study with 113 patients for 57 months. Five grafts (4.4%) were revised because of aseptic loosening, and an additional 2 patients (1.8%) were awaiting revision. The authors found that 11 of 18 calcar grafts resorbed. Onlay cortical strut allografts can be used with calcar-bearing method of cementless fixation. Using this method of fixation Head et al. (20) reported a re-revision rate of 3.4% among 106 patients with a follow-up period ranging from 2 to 7 years. The authors found that the calcar load-bearing prosthesis facilitates graft incorporation with subsequent reconstitution of femoral bone stock.

Because type I femoral reconstructions involve essentially primary femurs, no concluding statements can be made about the optimum method of fixation. The cementless versus cemented controversy, which exists in primary hip arthroplasty, applies to type I femoral reconstruction. However, literature review and personal experience suggest that type II and type III femurs are best managed with a cementless mode of fixation. Although distally fixed implants have been shown successfully to reconstruct type I and type II femurs, there is ongoing debate with respect to the degree of thigh pain and the potential for these types of implants to help reconstitute the proximal femur. Proximal filling fixation is flawed by an inability to obtain adequate stabilization in the proximal femur. A high degree of subsidence is found with this type of prosthesis, because of inability of the compromised cortical structure to withstand the radially directed forces. The calcar-bearing prosthesis appears to satisfy the requisites for a stable reconstruction of the femur in revision hip arthroplasty with the ability to promote reconstitution of the proximal femur.

Acetabular Reconstruction

The approach to acetabular reconstruction is dictated by the type of bone deficiency. Type I acetabular deficiency is managed with a procedure essentially the same as primary total hip replacement arthroplasty. However, Type II deficits require reconstruction based on the integrity of the anterior and posterior columns. Most type II acetabular deficits are contained cavitary deficits that can be managed with morselized allograft compacted within the contained deficit. Prosthetic fixation is obtained with an interference fit supported by the anterior and posterior columns. Supplemental fixation, such as peripheral or dome screw fixation, may be necessary. Type IIIA involves compromise of the anterior column but continued integrity of the posterior column and superior dome. A type IIIA acetabular deficit can be managed in much the same way as a type II deficit. In addition to the impacted allograft and adjunct screw fixation, cement can be used. A type IIIB deficit is characterized by compromise of the posterior column with secondary loss of the superolateral aspect of the acetabulum. This deficit requires a structural graft in combination with plate and screw fixation. Depending on the amount of host bone available for fixation of the acetabular component, the component can be supported with either a cementless interface against the host bone or supplementary fixation with cement. A type IIIC acetabular deficit is characterized by loss of structural integrity of the anterior and posterior columns with or without pelvic dissociation. This is a substantial deficit best managed with structural allograft in combination with plates, screws, rings, or cages. Cement or cementless fixation of the acetabular component depends on the amount of host bone available for fixation.

Initial clinical experience with acetabular reconstruction dealt essentially with cemented acetabular components. Reports with long-term follow-up data are lacking and the studies are flawed by the absence of a standardized classification of acetabular deficits (Table 2). Clinical results are best discussed in terms of cement or cementless fixation with separate analysis of acetabular bone grafting. With early or contemporary cementing techniques, the overall results with cemented acetabular revisions show reoperation rates for aseptic loosening as high as 10.5% and progressive radiolucency rates as high as 71%. Weber et al. (49) compared modes of fixation of acetabular components and found a reoperation rate due to aseptic loosening of 9% for cemented fixation compared with 0% for cementless fixation.

The cementless mode of fixation appears to be more effective for managing complex acetabular revisions. However, success with cementless acetabular revision depends on prosthetic design. Experience with threaded acetabular components for revision total hip

Table 2. *Results of clinical studies of cemented versus cementless revision hips: Acetabular component*

Authors	Publication date	Date prosthesis inserted	Follow-up period (mo)	No. of patients[a]	No. of prostheses inserted	Aseptic re-revision[b]	Migration	Deep sepsis	Dislocation
Cemented revisions									
Kavanagh et al. (25)	1985	1969–78	54	162	81	3.7%	9.1%	1.2%	9.0%
Weber et al. (49)	1996	1976–83	77	52	56	9.0%	NA	NA	NA
Callaghan et al. (4)	1985	1979–82	43	136	76	10.5%	9.0%	3.4%	8.2%
Slooff et al. (46)	1996	1979–88	70	80	88	2.3%	5.7%	1.3%	NA
Cementless revisions									
Gerber and Harris (14)	1986	1973–79	85	38	47	8.5%	10.6%	2.1%	10.6%
Mulroy and Harris (33)	1990	1973–79	142	37	46	19.6%	17.4%	2.2%	10.9%
Engh et al. (10)	1988	1980–85	53	160	107	7.5%	15.0%	0.6%	0.6%
Lawrence et al. (28)	1994	1980–86	108	81	43	4.7%	NA	1.2%	3.7%
Hooten et al. (22)	1994	1982–87	46	26	27	18.5%	44.4%	0.0%	NA
Paprosky et al. (38)	1994	1982–88	68	147	147	2.0%	4.1%	0.0%	4.8%
Paprosky and Magnus (37)	1994	1982–91	61	316	316	NA	3.2%	0.0%	2.2%
Silverton et al. (45)	1996	1983–86	100	111	115	0.0%	0.0%	5.0%	3.0%
Schutzer and Harris (43)	1994	1984–88	40	51	56	0.0%	0.0%	0.0%	6.0%
Lachiewicz and Hussamy (27)	1994	1985–90	60	59	60	0.0%	0.0%	1.7%	6.7%
Weber et al. (49)	1996	1986–88	74	43	49	0.0%	0.0%	0.0%	16.0%

The authors have made every effort to accurately represent the data reported in each of the studies. Because of nonstandard reporting associated with the orthopedic literature, this is not always possible. Some percentages have been recalculated to standardize reporting.
 [a] Number of patients at follow-up study.
 [b] Aseptic re-revision is percentage re-revised because of aseptic loosening.
 NA, not available.

replacement is discouraging. Engh et al. (10) evaluated the cases of 160 patients with porous hemispheric and threaded acetabular revision components with an average follow-up period of 53 months. They reported a reoperation rate due to aseptic loosening of 7.5% and a component migration rate of 15%. Lawrence et al. (28) treated 81 patients who underwent acetabular revision with porous hemispherical sockets and participated in follow-up study for an average of 108 months. The investigators found a 4.7% re-revision rate due to aseptic loosening and a 4.7% rate of roentgenographic instability. Combining the results of Silverton et al. (45), Schutzer and Harris (43), Lachiewicz and Hussamy (27), and Weber et al. (49), a total of 280 cementless acetabular components with a follow-up period of 40 to 100 months had no re-revisions due to aseptic loosening. In an effort to avoid bulk allograft, particulate allograft in combination with high hip centers were chosen in some of these studies. Despite such adjustments in technique, these studies showed that the intermediate-term results of cementless acetabular fixation look very promising. To avoid use of a high hip center, some authors recommend use of double-dome or oblong cups to reconstruct large superior deficiencies in a cementless mode. Newman et al. (34) reported results of a multicenter study of 64 patients with an average follow-up period of 44 months. No progressive migration was found, and 97% of the cups had been retained at the time of publication.

Bone loss can greatly influence the outcome of acetabular revision. Structural allografts, which are generally required in a type III acetabular reconstruction, had mixed results. Gerber and Harris (14) reported initial success with structural allografts. They found union and incorporation of the grafts in all of 47 patients who participated in follow-up study for an average of 7.1 years with an 8.5% incidence of aseptic loosening. However, subsequent long-term follow-up data on the same group (33) revealed graft resorption with migration of the acetabular component and subsequent acetabular loosening in 46% of the patients. Hooten et al. (22) reported on 27 patients who participated in follow-up study for an average of 46 months; they had a 19% re-revision rate due to aseptic loosening and a radiographic failure rate of 44%. The authors concluded that structural allografts do not work in the acetabulum and should be used only as a last resort. In contrast, Paprosky et al. (38) outlined a meticulous classification system for acetabular deficits and described specific surgical techniques for managing these deficits. One hundred forty-seven acetabular revisions with deficits of varying degrees were evaluated for an average of 68 months. All failures occurred among the more severe type III deficits. The reoperation rate was 2%, and 4.1% of the acetabular components were considered unstable. Paprosky et al. (37) conducted an additional study involving varying degrees of acetabular deficits in which 316 acetabular components were evaluated for an average of 61 months. There was no migration in cases in which Köhler's line was not violated. In cases in which medial migration had passed Köhler's line, 70% of the components were considered unstable. These authors were optimistic about the ability of the structural graft to unite to the host bone. However, loosening of the acetabular component occurred with cementless fixation. The authors recommended the use of bone cement for fixation of the acetabular component against bulk allograft. The enthusiasm of the authors may have to be tempered by virtue of the fact that these are not 10-year data. Because graft resorption occurs after longer follow-up periods, (14,33) failure may become evident when future evaluation is performed.

Structural allografts in combination with cement fixation and the addition of reinforcement rings has been reported to be a successful revision construct. Garbuz et al. (13) reported successful results with 7 of 8 reconstructions using a roof-reinforcement ring after 7.5 years of follow-up study. Twenty-seven acetabular reconstructions with a reinforcement ring were evaluated by Zehntner and Ganz (51) after an average follow-up period of 7.2 years. A 79.6% probability of survival at 10 years with re-revision as the endpoint was recorded.

As with the femur, there appears to be a growing enthusiasm for impaction grafting techniques in acetabular reconstruction. This technique entails morselized graft as the substructure with cement to fix the prosthetic device. Slooff et al. (46) reported on 88 acetabular revisions with a 2.3% reoperation rate for aseptic loosening after an average of

70 months of follow-up study. The radiographic failure rate for this technique was 6.8%. The combination of morselized compacted allograft with rings, cages, and support devices for type III deficits was proposed by Emerson (8). That experience with such devices, although it has a short follow-up period, may represent a combination that has the potential of becoming durable and stable.

In summary, the success of a revision acetabular procedures is critically dependent on the existing supportive structure of the acetabulum, specifically the anterior and posterior columns, and the medial buttress. When the anterior and posterior columns are intact, cementless fixation is preferred. In the presence of severe anterior or posterior deficiencies, the structural integrity of the acetabulum must be reestablished with the use of bone graft, plates, screws, rings, or cages. Then and only then can prosthetic stability be assured. Cement or cementless fixation is chosen on the basis of the amount of available host bone.

At the conclusion of femoral or acetabular reconstruction, the surgeon must reduce the prosthesis and make final determinations with respect to stability and leg length. The acetabulum optimally should be reconstructed to maintain the anatomic hip center and the femur should be reconstructed to restore its anatomic length. However, if the joint has been reconstructed with a high hip center, the surgeon must make appropriate modifications in the length of the femur. The surgeon can then fine tune leg-length adjustments with modular head and neck units. When dealing with the issue of hip stability versus leg length, one should always opt for stability. Depending on the approach used, the method of closure varies. For example, if a trochanteric osteotomy has been performed, stability may be enhanced by advancement of the trochanteric fragment. If a posterolateral approach has been used, attempts should be made to repair the short external rotators. If the anterolateral approach has been used, meticulous approximation of the myofascial sleeve should be performed. It is also imperative that the surgeon pay particular attention to obtaining hemostasis to avoid development of a serious postoperative hematoma.

POSTOPERATIVE CARE

The postoperative care of patients who have undergone total hip revision arthroplasty is dictated by the extent of the surgical reconstruction performed. Three main factors dictate the postoperative physical therapy and rehabilitation program: the status of the wound, the stability of the arthroplasty, and the integrity of the prosthetic reconstruction. With respect to the status of the wound, one must be cognizant that revision arthroplasty involves a great deal of surgical dissection. If the dissection has progressed rapidly, the patient is prone to development of a hematoma, which may then necessitate return to the operating room for incision, drainage, and evacuation. To avoid postoperative hematoma, the surgeon should consider judicious prophylactic use of anticoagulants and prescribing several days of bedrest until the wound is hemodynamically stable. The stability of the arthroplasty, as determined at the time of reduction, is a critical factor in the determination of the need for a hip abduction orthosis during the initial phase of physical therapy and rehabilitation. Because revision arthroplasty is associated with a high percentage of dislocations, the surgeon should freely recommend a hip abduction orthosis, which may be needed for 8 to 12 weeks postoperatively.

The physical therapist should be apprised of concerns regarding stability and admonish the patient with respect to hip precautions such as prolonged sitting in a chair, techniques for rising from a toilet, climbing stairs, and riding in a car. The physical therapist must be aware of the surgical approach used to perform the operative procedure. If a trochanteric osteotomy was performed, there should be appropriate delay in beginning hip abduction exercises. However, a patient who is operated on with a posterolateral or anterolateral approach may begin hip abduction exercises in the immediate postoperative period. The integrity of the surgical reconstruction is a critical factor in determining the weight-bearing status of the patient postoperatively. When revision arthroplasty necessitates use of large grafts, protective weight bearing is imperative for 3 to 6 months.

CONCLUSION

The primary mission of this chapter is to apprise orthopedic surgeons of the effect of surgical technique on long-term survivorship after revision total hip arthroplasty. Three essential factors correlate with the long-term success of revision total hip arthroplasty. These are host- or patient-related factors, surgical method, and selection of a prosthesis. Reconstructive surgeons are limited in their ability to modify the host factors with which they are presented. However, they have direct control over the surgical technique performed and the prosthesis selected. We have attempted to identify the pertinent variables of the perioperative period that affect the long-term survivorship of the revision total hip arthroplasty. The challenge facing orthopedic surgeons approaching revision total hip arthroplasty is conceptualizing the entire process of the revision operation at the point of initial contact with the patient. It is essential to begin with thorough preoperative planning and carry through each step of the operative procedure realizing that every aspect of the procedure has an effect on the long-term survivorship of the prosthetic reconstruction. Proper execution of the algorithmic approach presented should help to improve the survivorship of the revision total hip arthroplasty.

REFERENCES

1. Amstutz HC, Steven MM, Jinnah RH, Mai L. Revision of aseptic loose total hip arthroplasties. *Clin Orthop* 1982;170:21–33.
2. Bargar WL, Murzie WJ, Taylor JH, Newman MA, Paul HA. Management of bone loss in revision hip arthroplasty using custom cementless femoral components. *J Arthroplasty* 1993;8:245–252.
3. Bischoff R, Dunlap J, Carpenter L, De Mouy E, Barrack R. Heterotopic ossification following uncemented total hip arthroplasty: effect of the operative approach. *J Arthroplasty* 1994;9:641–644.
4. Callaghan JJ, Salvati EA, Pellicci PM, Wilson PD, Ranawat CS. Results of revision for mechanical failure after cemented total hip replacement, 1979 to 1982: a two to five-year follow-up. *J Bone Joint Surg Am* 1985;67:1074–1085.
5. Chandler H. Clark J, Murphy S, McCarthy J, et al. Reconstruction of major segmental loss of the proximal femur in revision total hip arthroplasty. *Clin Orthop* 1994;298:67–74.
6. Dennis DA, Dingman CA, Meglan DA, O'Leary JFM, Mallory TH, Berne N. Femoral cement removal in revision total hip arthroplasty: a biomechanical analysis. *Clin Orthop* 1987;220:142–147.
7. Dohmae Y, Bechtold JE, Sherman RE, Puno RM, Gustilo RB. Reduction in cement-bone interface shear strength between primary and revision arthroplasty. *Clin Orthop* 1988;236:214–220.
8. Emerson RH Jr. G.A.P. reinforcement cage for type III acetabular revision surgery: a preliminary report. Presented at the 1996 Summer Meeting of the Hip Society; 1996 Sept 5–7; Eugene, OR.
9. Engh CA, Bobyn JD. The influence of stem size and extent of porous coating on femoral bone resorption after primary cementless hip arthroplasty. *Clin Orthop* 1988;231:7–28.
10. Engh CA, Glassman AH, Griffin WL, Mayer JG. Results of cementless revision for failed cemented total hip arthroplasty. *Clin Orthop* 1988;235:91–110.
11. Estok DM, Harris WH. Long-term results of cemented femoral revision surgery using second-generation techniques; an average 11.7-year follow-up evaluation. *Clin Orthop* 1994;299:190–202.
12. Frndak PA, Mallory TH, Lombardi AV. Translateral surgical approach to the hip, the abductor muscle "split." *Clin Orthop* 1993;295:135–141.
13. Garbuz D, Morsi E, Gross AE. Revision of the acetabular component of a total hip arthroplasty with a massive structural allograft: study with a minimum five-year follow-up. *J Bone Joint Surg Am* 1996;78:693–697.
14. Gerber SD, Harris WH. Femoral head autografting to augment acetabular deficiency in patients requiring total hip replacement: a minimum five-year and an average seven-year follow-up study. *J Bone Joint Surg Am* 1986;68:1241–1248.
15. Gie GA, Ling RSM, Simon JP, Slooff TJJH, Timperley AJ. Impacted cancellous allografts and cement for revision total hip arthroplasty. *J Bone Joint Surg Br* 1993;75:14–21.
16. Glassman AH, Engh CA. The removal of porous-coated femoral hip stems. *Clin Orthop* 1992;285:164–80.
17. Glassman AH, Engh CA, Bobyn JD. A technique of extensile exposure for total hip arthroplasty. *J Arthroplasty* 1987;2:11–21.
18. Gross AE, Hutchinson CR, Alexeeff M, Mahomed N, Leitch K, Morsi E. Proximal femoral allografts for reconstruction of bone stock in revision arthroplasty of the hip. *Clin Orthop* 1995;319:151–158.
19. Gustilo RB, Pasternak HS. Revision total hip arthroplasty with titanium ingrowth prosthesis and bone grafting for failed cemented femoral component loosening. *Clin Orthop* 1988;235:111–119.
20. Head WC, Wagner RA, Emerson RH, Malinin TI. Revision total hip arthroplasty in the deficient femur with a proximal load-bearing prosthesis. *Clin Orthop* 1994;298:119–126.
21. Hedley AK, Gruen TA, Ruoff DP. Revision of failed total hip arthroplasties with uncemented porous-coated anatomic components. *Clin Orthop* 1988;235:75–90.
22. Hooten JP, Engh CA Jr, Engh CA. Failure of structural acetabular allografts in cementless revision hip arthroplasty. *J Bone Joint Surg Br* 1994;76:419–422.
23. Katz RP, Callaghan JJ, Sullivan PM, Johnston RC. Results of cemented femoral revision total hip arthroplasty using improved cementing techniques. *Clin Orthop* 1995;319:178–183.

24. Kavanagh BF, Fitzgerald RH Jr. Multiple revision for failed total hip arthroplasty. *J Bone Joint Surg Am* 1987;69:1144–1149.
25. Kavanagh BF, Ilstrup DM, Fitzgerald RH. Revision total hip arthroplasty. *J Bone Joint Surg Am* 1985;67:517–526.
26. Klapper RC, Caillouette JT, Callaghan JJ, Hozack WJ. Ultrasonic technology in revision joint arthroplasty. *Clin Orthop* 1992;285:147–154.
27. Lachiewicz PF, Hussamy OD. Revision of the acetabulum without cement with use of the Harris-Galante porous-coated implant: two to eight-year results. *J Bone Joint Surg Am* 1994;76:1834–1839.
28. Lawrence JM, Engh CA, Macalino GE, Lauro GR. Outcome of revision hip arthroplasty done without cement. *J Bone Joint Surg Am* 1994;76:965–973.
29. Lawrence JM, Engh CA, Macalino GE. Revision total hip arthroplastsy: long-term results without cement. *Orthop Clin North Am* 1993;24:635–644.
30. Mallory TH, Head WC. A total hip replacement system: clinical experience and recommendations. *Contemp Orthop* 1988;17:21–28.
31. Mallory TH. Preparation of the proximal femur in cementless total hip revision. *Clin Orthop* 1988;235:47–60.
32. Mulliken BD, Rorabeck CH, Bourne RB. Uncemented revision total hip arthroplasty. *Clin Orthop* 1996;325:156–162.
33. Mulroy RD, Harris WH. Failure of acetabular autogenous grafts in total hip arthroplasty: increasing incidence—a follow-up note. *J Bone Joint Surg Am* 1990;72:1536–1540.
34. Newman MA, Bargar WL, Christie MJ, DeBoer DK, Taylor JK. Multicenter study of acetabular reconstruction using an oblong cup: 2 to 7 year results. Presented at the 64th Annual Meeting of the American Academy of Orthopaedic Surgeons: 1997 Feb 13–17; San Francisco.
35. Pak JH, Paprosky WG, Jablonsky WS, Lawrence JM. Femoral strut allografts in cementless revision total hip arthroplasty. *Clin Orthop* 1993;295:172–178.
36. Paprosky WG, Lawrence JM, Cameron HU. Classification and treatment of the failed acetabulum: a systematic approach. *Contemp Orthop* 1991;22:121–130.
37. Paprosky WG, Magnus RE. Principles of bone grafting in revision total hip arthroplasty: acetabular technique. *Clin Orthop* 1994;298:147–155.
38. Paprosky WG, Perona PG, Lawrence JM. Acetabular defect classification and surgical reconstruction in revision arthroplasty: a 6-year follow-up evaluation. *J Arthroplasty* 1994;9:33–44.
39. Pellicci PM, Wilson PD, Sledge CB, Salvati EA, Ranawat CS, Poss R. Revision total hip arthroplasty. *Clin Orthop* 1982;170:34–41.
40. Pellicci PM, Wilson PD, Sledge CB, et al. Long-term results of revision total hip replacement. A follow-up report. *J Bone Joint Surg Am* 1985;67:513–516.
41. Peters CL, Rivero DP, Kull LR, Jacobs JJ, Rosenberg AG, Galante JO. Revision total hip arthroplasty without cement: subsidence of proximally porous-coated femoral components. *J Bone Joint Surg Am* 1995;77:1217–1226.
42. Rubash HE, Harris WH. Revision of nonseptic, loose, cemented femoral components using modern cementing techniques. *J Arthroplasty* 1988;3:241–248.
43. Schutzer SF, Harris WH. High placement of porous-coated acetabular components in complex total hip arthroplasty. *J Arthroplasty* 1994;9:359–367.
44. Silverton CD, Jacobs JJ, Rosenberg AG, Kull L, Conley A, Galante JO. Complications of a cable grip system. *J Arthroplasty* 1996;11:400–404.
45. Silverton CD, Rosenberg AG, Sheinkop MB, Kull LR, Galante JO. Revision of the acetabular component without cement after total hip arthroplasty: a follow-up note regarding results at seven to eleven years. *J Bone Joint Surg Am* 1996;78:1366–1370.
46. Slooff TJJH, Buma P, Schreurs BW, Schimmel JW, Huiskes R, Gardeniers J. Acetabular and femoral reconstruction with impacted graft and cement. *Clin Orthop* 1996;324:108–115.
47. Sydney SV, Mallory TH. Controlled perforation: a safe method of cement removal from the femoral canal. *Clin Orthop* 1990;253:168–172.
48. Turner RH, Scheller AD Jr, eds. *Revision total hip arthroplasty*. New York: Grune & Stratton, 1982.
49. Weber KL, Callaghan JJ, Goetz DD, Johnston RC. Revision of a failed cemented total hip prosthesis with insertion of an acetabular component without cement and a femoral component with cement: a five to eight-year follow-up study. *J Bone Joint Surg Am* 1996;78:982–994.
50. Younger TI, Bradford MS, Magnus RE, Paprosky WG. Extended proximal osteotomy: a new technique for femoral revision arthroplasty. *J Arthroplasty* 1995;10:329–338.
51. Zehntner MK, Ganz R. Midterm results (5.5–10 years) of acetabular allograft reconstruction with the acetabular reinforcement ring during total hip revision. *J Arthroplasty* 1994;9:469–479.

Evaluating the Painful Total Hip

Revision Total Hip Arthroplasty,
edited by Marvin E. Steinberg and Jonathan P. Garino,
Lippincott Williams & Wilkins, Philadelphia © 1999.

8

Clinical Evaluation of the Symptomatic Total Hip Arthroplasty

Paul N. Smith and Cecil H. Rorabeck

Total hip arthroplasty remains one of the most successful operations devised in terms of relief of symptoms and quality of life enhancement. In considering quality-adjusted life years, total hip arthroplasty compares favorably with other routinely performed major surgical interventions such as coronary bypass operation (15). Notwithstanding the high probability of excellent long-term satisfactory results of total hip arthroplasty, some patients do experience pain at some point after the operation. The report of pain after total hip joint arthroplasty is of itself of sufficient singularity that search for the cause (if any) of the pain is indicated. For a small subgroup of patients the pain is disabling. It is these patients who must be most closely examined for any reason for failure of the prosthesis and for any cause of pain that is remote from the joint replacement. Evaluation of a presumed symptomatic total hip joint replacement involves casting a wide net to include in the process of elimination causes of pain directly related to the total joint replacement and causes of pain that may mimic the pain of a failed total hip joint arthroplasty.

The cornerstone of any such evaluation is a thorough history and physical examination. A patient with a symptomatic total hip joint arthroplasty most often reports pain, but others may cite instability, stiffness, weakness, sensory loss, or even limb-length discrepancy as the root of the problem. Historical inquiry must include evaluation of the patient's general health, problems with the lower back and gastrointestinal and genitourinary tracts, and specific questioning regarding the joint in question. Physical examination must include evaluation of these systems in addition to screening examination of

P. N. Smith and C. H. Rorabeck: Division of Orthopedic Surgery, University of Western Ontario, London Health Sciences Center, London, Ontario, Canada N6A 5A5.

the peripheral vascular supply and innervation. Once a history is taken and a physical examination is performed, investigation with particular reference to serial roentgenograms and other radiologic tests as indicated and appropriate blood tests narrows the focus of the cause of the patient's discomfort.

THE HISTORY

Pain

The location, temporal features of onset, type of pain, and associated features are valuable discriminators in the search for the cause of pain.

Pain: Where Is It?

Pain due to true hip joint disease can present in a variety of guises. Pain may be localized to the groin, buttock, lateral thigh, or trochanteric region. More rarely, pain may be felt in the lower back, but this is far more likely to be caused by concurrent lumbar spondylosis. Pain from the hip may be referred down the thigh to the knee but rarely below the knee. Pain felt to radiate below the knee should invite further inquiry as to the status of the patient's lower back, because it is likely to be a manifestation of a sciatica. In the main, pain clearly localized to the groin or deep buttock is often associated with problems on the acetabular side; however, this is by no means a rule. Thigh pain of itself can be a reason for seeking treatment and can be associated with both well-fixed and failing total hip arthroplasties. It is most commonly seen in problems with the femoral component. Thigh pain has been described in association with well-fixed, stable, uncemented total hip joint arthroplasties and is presumed to be caused by a mismatch in modulus between a stiff implant and less stiff bone. In this scenario it was more an issue in the early-generation uncemented systems and is now far less common in systems of contemporary design. Pain sharply localized to the trochanteric region may be caused by trochanteric bursitis or prominence of trochanteric wires (Fig. 1) or cable.

Pain: When After the Operation?

When the pain began to occur in relation to the operation is an important question. If the pain has been a feature since the time of the initial operation, then infection or failure to obtain component stability at the time of the operation are the likely causes. In the case of infection the patient may have had a history of wound-healing problems following operations, such as prolonged wound discharge or the so-called superficial infection. The patient may have preexisting risk factors for infection, including obesity, diabetes, rheumatoid disease, or immunosuppressant therapy. Although thankfully rare because of the combination of meticulous surgical technique, control of the operating room environment with systems such as laminar flow, and the use of appropriate antibiotics (17) infection is still the most sinister complication of surgical therapy. Infection of total joint replacement is a surgical disaster and even today is only in part surmountable with a combination of surgical débridement and use of antibiotics. Infection usually means the patient needs at least one more surgical intervention and prejudices the end outcome in terms of symptomatic relief of pain and longevity of the prosthetic construct. Infection remains the most important single complication to diagnose and treat as early as possible.

Failure to obtain satisfactory stability of components at the time of arthroplasty is another cause of pain present from the time of operation. The reasons for this problem range from periprosthetic fracture, which can be recognized or unrecognized at the time of the operation, to mismatch between component and bone with too small a component implanted, to just plain poor technique whatever implant system is used. The consequence of this initial instability is more instability because the unstable component will not of

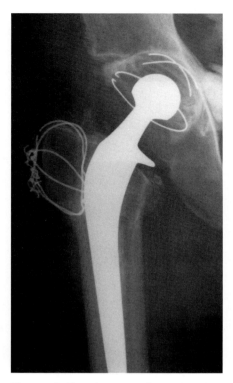

Figure 1. Prominent trochanteric wires caused symptoms of lateral trochanteric pain that necessitated removal of the wire, after which the symptoms totally resolved.

itself become stable. Failure to obtain satisfactory initial stability has been shown with roentgen stereophotogrammetry to be highly predictive of aseptic failure (11).

If a patient has pain after a period of symptom-free function, issues to be considered include aseptic loosening (by far the most common cause), component failure (rare using the materials of today), periprosthetic stress fracture, polyethylene wear, or late infection. Aseptic loosening as the consequence of gradual wear of the prosthetic construct producing vast numbers of polyethylene, cement, and metal wear particles with progressive lysis of periprosthetic bone and eventual destabilizing of the prosthesis is in the main a silent phenomenon. Patients who present with pain due to a total hip prosthesis that has failed because of wear-particle disease usually seek treatment late with severe damage to bone stock. Pain is usually not a feature until structural compromise of the bone–prosthesis composite has already occurred.

Component failure, because of advances in both metallurgy and design, has been almost consigned to the history books. However, one still encounters this problem, often in conjunction with wear particle–induced osteolysis as the initiating factor that removes support from part of the prosthesis. The classic history of sudden onset of pain after a long period of pain-free function implies an acute mechanical event such as fracture of a component or the cement mantle (Fig. 2). Late infection is a rare entity and has been reported in association with dental procedures, distant sites of infection such as cellulitis distal to the implant and with surgical procedures unrelated to the arthroplasty (8). Specific inquiry as to these should be made to rule out the possibility of hematogenous spread of infection as a cause of late-presenting pain.

Pain: When It Occurs and Some Red Herrings

The present situation with respect to a patient's pain is an important issue. Pain due to component loosening is often of the type known as "start up" whereby the patient

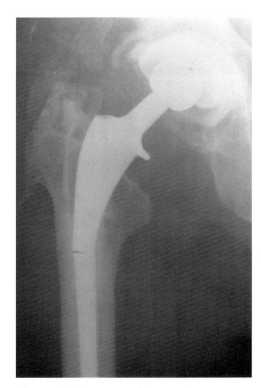

Figure 2. Fracture of femoral stem produced sudden onset of thigh pain after 4 years of symptom-free function.

experiences pain on beginning activity after a period of rest. The pain then gradually recedes to a manageable level. As the component loosening becomes worse, the patient experiences pain that becomes truly activity related, being present at start-up of activity and not receding and remaining constant or even worsening with continued activity. Both types of pain are therefore part of a continuum of component failure and may be experienced at any of the aforementioned sites of pain predilection. Pain around the hip that is activity related can have other causes apart from a failed total hip arthroplasty. Leriche (16) in 1948 described the syndrome of progressive obliteration of the aortic bifurcation. This process begins in an iliac artery and in its final stages produces complete occlusion of the iliac vessels with involvement of the aorta, often up to the level of the renal arteries. The patient experiences pain on walking mainly in the thigh or buttock of a claudicant type. Men experience diminution and later loss of penile erection. Pain with this syndrome also may be caused by diminished blood supply to the sciatic nerve or muscle ischemia.

Activity-related pain also is seen with lumbar spinal stenosis (4). Patients with such pain usually have a history of back problems. The pain they describe often has a neuralgic quality with radiation below the knee associated with dysesthesia, tingling, or numbness. Careful historical inquiry defines a claudicant nature to the pain of spinal stenosis, and care must be taken not to confuse vascular claudication with neurologic claudication. A helpful aphorism is that a person with vascular claudication walks between the light posts (standing during rest), whereas a person with neurologic claudication walks between the park benches (sitting during rest).

As in other aspects of orthopedics, pain that is constant, especially if present at night, is cause for alarm. Infection and less common causes of pain about the hip such as occult malignant disease (21) or stress fracture of the pelvis (18) are the important differentials. The pelvis is a common place for metastatic neoplasia. The hallmark of pelvic tumor is that it presents itself late and is difficult to diagnose on clinical grounds because of an indistinct and inconstant symptom complex. Pain is usually late in the course of the disease and mimics pain due to hip disease. Inquiry as to constitutional symptoms of weight loss, anorexia, fever, and chills is important.

Abdominal disease can provide an interesting red herring in the evaluation of symptomatic total hip arthroplasty. Groin pain can be produced by a number of conditions, including hernia (inguinal, femoral, and obturator), inguinal lymphadenopathy (due to distal skin infection; general viral, bacterial, or tubercular infection; or neoplasia), a pointing psoas abscess, or various gynecologic and genito-urinary disorders. Groin pain should be pursued with specific questions about swelling in the groin, distant sites of infection, and any history of infection, particularly tuberculosis and syphylis. With respect to hernia, femoral and inguinal hernias are associated with swelling in the groin, but an obturator hernia is covered by the pectineus muscle and therefore may not present itself with a lump. In most cases of obturator hernia, the pain is referred to the knee along the genicular branch of the obturator nerve, the so-called Howship-Romberg sign, and any movements of the hip joint are limited by pain. Thus this problem can be very difficult to differentiate from primary hip disease, especially in the acute situation.

Pain: Severity

On purely philosophical grounds, it may be expected that the more severe the pain the patient reports, the more diligent the search for the cause of the pain should be. This is true only in part. Certainly, a patient who is severely disabled by pain should be thoroughly examined and interviewed to ascertain the cause of that pain. However, pain is a subjective entity, and pathologic conditions that produce severe pain and suffering for one person may be tolerated by a second person. In addition, pain often is a late-occurring feature in failure of a total joint arthroplasty. If one waits until pain is sufficiently severe to warrant further investigation, the horse may well have bolted (Fig. 3). It is important to see a painfully symptomatic total hip joint arthroplasty as requiring thorough inquiry and investigation to rule out causes of the pain syndrome, regardless of the degree of pain.

Instability

A patient who has recurrent instability of a total hip replacement is as a rule an extremely unhappy person—rather like a person who buys a car that turns out to be a lemon—and presents a diagnostic and management conundrum to the treating surgeon. Woo and Morrey (23) reviewed the Mayo clinic experience of 10,500 cases of total hip joint arthroplasty. They found the main risk factors predisposing to dislocation are sex of the patient (women predominating in a ratio of 2:1), surgical approach (the posterior approach having about three times the risk of anterior approaches), prior operation, and component orientation (Fig. 4). Retroversion of either acetabular or femoral components is associated with a higher risk of dislocation. Trochanteric nonunion with migration also has been found to increase substantially the risk for dislocation (10) particularly among patients presenting with late dislocation (7).

The timing of dislocation or subluxation is important information. Dislocation in the first month or so after the operation is believed to be the most common presentation. Ali Khan et al. (14) in a study of more than 6,000 arthroplasties found that patients with initial dislocation that presented itself early were less likely to have recurrence than those with dislocation that presented itself late. Frank dislocation, which characteristically requires medical assistance to achieve relocation, must be differentiated from subluxation, which the patient can relocate with a trick maneuver. Clinically, subluxation is much less of an issue, because these patients in the main can live with the problem. However, in many instances subluxation is the harbinger of true dislocation. Once a hip with chronic subluxation goes on to dislocate, dislocation also becomes a chronic problem. The frequency of episodes of instability also is an issue to patients. Frequent incidents are poorly tolerated. Specific inquiry must be made to ascertain the precise position of the patient's hip at the time of dislocation or subluxation to enable deduction of the direction

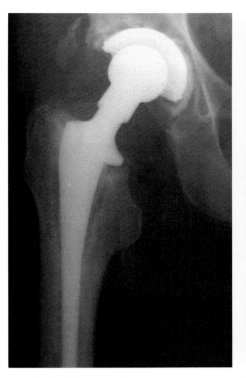
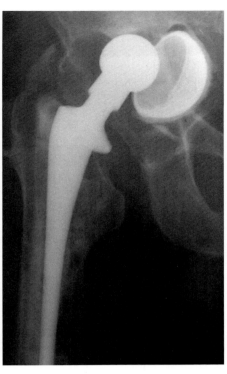

A   B

Figure 3. A 54-year-old man had no symptoms (**A**) when examined 5 years after primary total hip arthroplasty. He did not keep scheduled follow-up appointments but returned with an acute fracture of the acetabulum due to catastrophic wear-debris osteolysis (**B**). He had experienced only intermittent minor hip discomfort in the years before this event. His case is a good example of the need for regular examination of all patients with prosthetic joints.

of instability. Posterior instability is the most common, accounting for about 75% of dislocations. Most of these are associated with the posterior approach. Regardless of the cause, an unstable hip, once relocated should not be painful.

Stiffness

Most patients who have undergone total hip joint arthroplasty achieve a satisfactory range of motion after operation. Exceptions to this rule are rare and encompass a heterogeneous group including those who had poor ranges of motion before the operation, patients who underwent conversion from fusion to arthroplasty, patients who underwent revision, and patients with considerable heterotopic ossification after the operation. It is important to delineate whether stiffness predated the arthroplasty or if it became a feature after the operation. The number of prior hip operations is important to ascertain, as is the precise time sequence of the procedures. Heterotopic ossification is more common among male patients with hypertrophic osteoarthritis. Other risk factors such as Forestier disease and ankylosing spondylitis must be excluded. Of special interest are patients with bilateral arthritis with similarly, bilaterally poor ranges of motion, in particular with serious fixed flexion deformities. Should these patients undergo unilateral total hip arthroplasty, the postoperative range of motion on the side operated on will be dictated by the remaining arthritic hip and therefore be suboptimal. Whether the patient had or has bilaterally stiff hips is therefore important to determine. Once again, patients with stiff hips rarely report pain, and then it is at the extremes of motion.

Limb-Length Discrepancy

Accurate restoration of limb length is one of the goals of a successful total hip arthroplasty. If the patient has a short leg before the operation and has a short leg after the

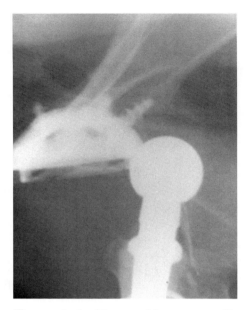

Figure 4. A 47-year-old woman with high-riding congenital dysplasia of the hip underwent total hip arthroplasty. The early postoperative course was complicated by dislocation. Radiographs revealed that the acetabular component had rotated into retroversion about the polar fixation screw. Revision of the cup to an anteverted position solved the problem.

operation, in general this is well tolerated. Most people tolerate length differences of up to 2 cm without the need for a shoe raise. Once the difference is greater than 2 cm, the patient often needs a shoe lift to compensate for the feeling of imbalance. Overlengthening after hip replacement, however, is poorly tolerated, and all patients must be counseled that length restoration is not an exact science and gives way in precedence to establishing a satisfactorily stable prosthetic construct. In some cases, limb lengthening of a small degree is preferable to establish satisfactory soft-tissue tension and protect against dislocation. The exact status of the patient in terms of length before the operation is important to determine in addition to the present situation when a patient is dissatisfied with leg-length inequality. It is essential to find out how that patient manages the length discrepancy and how the discrepancy actually affects the patient. Fortunately, most people dissatisfied because of limb-length inequality can be treated nonsurgically once the situation is fully explained to them. In this situation, a thorough history, physical examination, and sympathetic ear are usually all that is needed.

Weakness and Sensory Loss

Weakness following hip arthroplasty is unusual. The patient is more likely to report a marked limp than specific weakness. Most patients who limp before total hip arthroplasty limp after replacement of the arthritic joint. It is important to define the preoperative status of a patient with either weakness or a limp. It is notable, however, that most patients do not have a marked limp after total hip replacement. The presence of a marked limp after arthroplasty should raise questions about the cause of the problem. A number of possibilities exist, including congenital dislocation, injury to the abductor muscles of the hip, nonunion with migration of the trochanter, failure to reproduce the hip center either on the acetabular or the femoral side, and failure of the prosthetic joint itself. Mainly subclinical injury to the gluteal nerves has been documented in total hip arthroplasty with both the modified anterolateral and the posterior approaches (2) and the transtrochanteric approach to the hip joint (22). A patient with symptomatic weakness or limp should be questioned regarding the time of onset of the limp and whether the limp is in associated with pain. A painless limp is less likely to be caused by failure of the prosthetic joint.

Neurologic complications after total hip joint arthroplasty are rare, with a reported incidence of about 1%, and are in the main transient, most patients recovering by about 1 year postoperatively (2). It is important to document the patient's preoperative and the postoperative neurologic status when confronted with postoperative neurologic loss. Most of these nerve injuries are neuropraxia due to excessive retraction, prolonged abnormal limb positioning, and overzealous leg lengthening. Lengthening of the leg more than 4 cm has been associated with sciatic nerve palsy (9), so neurologic injury must be considered in the light of limb length.

PHYSICAL EXAMINATION

Examination of a patient with a supposedly symptomatic total hip joint replacement begins with observation of the patient as he or she enters the office. The surgeon must closely observe the gait for abnormality such as antalgia, short leg, or Trendelenburg gait. The patient may show evidence of past nerve injury with a foot drop or wear a shoe raise or other assistive orthotic device. Watching the patient enter the office gives an inkling of the problem faced. Most diagnostic hypotheses are formed in the process of taking a thorough history, and the physical examination provides a means of confirming or refuting a number of these hypotheses.

After the history has been taken and with the patient in his or her underwear (it is impossible to examine a patient properly when he or she is fully clothed), first ask the patient to stand. Inspect the patient from the front looking for thigh wasting and obvious pelvic obliquity, which would indicate leg-length difference. A patient with one short leg also has one long leg, and the long leg is often held flexed in gait and in stance to equalize the pelvis. Most scars are laterally based and are obvious to even the casual observer; however, one must check beneath the undergarments especially for anterior scars. If a patient describes groin pain in particular, inspect the groin for any evidence of hernia. A hernia is far more obvious with the patient standing, because many reduce when the patient lies down. Check for evidence of a cough impulse with the patient standing. If you do chance upon a hernia, you can assess it for reduction. Any evidence of old or current infection in the form of sinuses either discharging or healed is important.

From the side note any evidence of hyperlordosis of the lumbar spine. This may be caused by a primary lumbar spinal disorder or by fixed flexion deformity of the hip. From behind the patient note any evidence of gluteal wasting and observe the back for evidence of spinal deformity. After inspecting the spine, palpate the spinous processes and paraspinal muscles and then assess spinal motion for range, rhythm, and comfort. While still behind the patient palpate the posterior iliac spines and iliac crest to again check leg length. If leg-length inequality is found at this stage of the examination, it can be accurately estimated with graduated blocks beneath the patient's foot to level the pelvis. If blocks are not available, use a telephone directory.

The Trendelenburg test should be formally performed at this stage with the patient standing. The precise method of performing this test has been elegantly outlined by Hardcastle and Nade (12). The examining surgeon stands behind the patient to observe the angle of the pelvis, and the patient is asked to stand on one leg. The nonstance hip should be at about 30 degrees of flexion, and the patient can support the stance side only. The pelvis on the nonstance side should elevate if the test result is normal. A positive test result implies inability to elevate the nonstance side of the pelvis, as does inability to maintain position for 30 seconds of stance. This time dependence is important to emphasize; many patients with hip problems can elevate the nonstance side of the pelvis for a short time but fatigue rapidly, and the test result becomes positive after initially being negative. The gait should be reassessed if previous observation has not been adequate to form a conclusion.

The patient is then asked to lie supine. Palpation of painful areas to assess for local tenderness is usually not fruitful; the notable exception occurs in the case of prominent trochanteric wires or true trochanteric bursitis, in which there is considerable tenderness over the trochanter. In rare instances, a patient with thigh pain in the presence of a well-fixed cementless femoral component has thigh discomfort to palpation in the region of the tip of the component. The range of motion of the hip joint is carefully tested. Particular care is taken to perform a Thomas test to evaluate fixed flexion deformity and to establish whether any fixed adduction or abduction deformities are present. Care is taken in examination of the range of motion because it is likely that the pain will be reproduced with examination of the limb. Pain at the extremes of motion of the hip is often a feature of aseptic loosening of a total hip replacement; pain throughout the range is more sinister and may indicate critical bone structural insufficiency or infection. Once the presence or absence of any fixed deformity around the hip is established, formal leg length, both real and apparent, can be measured with a tape measure. It is essential in the presence of a fixed deformity to determine real versus the apparent limb length (13). If a real limb-length discrepancy is found, the site of the shortening—above or below the knee or the trochanter—can be found rapidly by means of eliciting Galleazi's sign and constructing Bryant's triangle.

Provocative maneuvers such as sudden rotation of the hip joint have not in our experience been a reliable addition to examinations of these patients. If there is pain at the extremes of motion, it is usually obvious in routine assessment of the range of motion and further "stress" tests do little apart from stressing the patient further. If a patient has recurrent instability of the hip joint, care must be taken not to perform injudicious maneuvering of the joint. The worst thing one can do is to cause a dislocation in the examining room. If the surgeon wishes to evaluate formally the dislocatability of a total hip replacement, this should be done under fluoroscopic control with appropriate anaesthesia.

Muscle power can be assessed further at this stage. First consider the power of flexion with the patient supine. It is rare to have considerable true weakness in flexion after total hip replacement. Exceptions to this rule are occasionally found among patients who have had release of the iliopsoas tendon to aid in either exposure of the joint or reduction of the prosthesis. Power of the hip abductors can be further assessed with the patient on his or her side, raising the leg, and holding it against resistance. The various causes of hip abductor weakness have already been mentioned; however, we have found that a surprisingly large number of the older population have tears of the abductor insertion. Avulsion of the gluteus medius tendon also has been reported as a cause of pain after hip arthroplasty (Larson JE, Fitzgerald RHF Jr, personal communication). Patients with a failed prosthesis may appear to have weakness, but this is often spurious because they are protecting the joint by reducing the forces through an unsatisfactory construct, whatever the mechanism of failure.

Neurological examination of the lower limbs should be performed to exclude other causes of buttock, thigh, and leg pain. The sciatic nerve (both common peroneal and tibial components), femoral nerve, and obturator nerves are all at risk in hip operations and should be evaluated. Any evidence of a radiculopathy such as dermatomal pain or tenderness and myotomal weakness should be documented. The sciatic and femoral nerve stretch tests may have positive results among patients with radicular abnormalities. Reflexes should be assessed for symmetry and degree. Patients with spinal stenosis often have very little to find at neurologic examinations given the degree of their disability. If a patient has severe disability that on historical grounds appears to be caused by spinal stenosis, a neurologic examination performed immediately after exercise may unmask a neurologic deficit that is not apparent in the rested state. Palpation of the peripheral pulses must not be left out of the examination. One also should palpate the abdominal aorta to exclude aneurysm as part of the Leriche-Morel syndrome.

LABORATORY TESTS

Blood Tests

Complete blood count, erythrocyte sedimentation rate (ESR), and C-reactive protein determination all have been used to a varying degree to complement the clinical features in the evaluation of symptomatic prosthetic total hip joints. The main issue is elimination of the possibility of infection as the cause of the symptoms. Infection of a total joint arthroplasty often is indolent and does not present itself in the classic manner by means of a high temperature or a draining sinus. Most patients with infections of a total hip arthroplasty do not have a reduced hemoglobin level, and the white blood cell count also is likely to be normal. Canner et al. (5) in a series of 52 infected total hips showed that only 15% of patients had leukocytosis and that only 54% had an ESR elevated to more than 30 mm/h. The ESR is elevated normally in the early postoperative period but returns to baseline levels about 3 months after the operation (6). A painful symptomatic total hip replacement in combination with a persistently elevated ESR is good evidence of infection. A normal ESR in this situation, however, does not exclude infection. In addition, a number of patients have intercurrent disease such as rheumatoid arthritis, which of itself causes chronic elevation of ESR.

C-reactive protein is an acute-phase protein normally present in minute amounts in plasma. Among patients with an uncomplicated total joint arthroplasty, C-reactive protein level returns to normal in about 3 weeks (1). Sanzen and Carlsson (20) found that C-reactive protein level was of more value but also complementary to ESR in the diagnosis of infection in a series of proved deep infections. An ESR greater than 30 mm/h was diagnostic of infection for only 50% of patients, whereas only 1 of 23 patients with deep infection had a C-reactive protein level less than 20 mg/L.

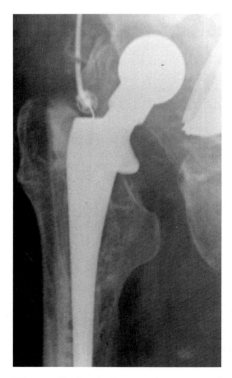

Figure 5. Aspiration arthrogram of the patient in Fig. 3 to rule out sepsis associated with symptomatic total hip arthroplasty. Aspiration showed no evidence of infection, nor did samples of tissue obtained intraoperatively.

Aspiration of the Total Hip Replacement

Preoperative aspiration of a symptomatic total hip arthroplasty may be performed to delineate the presence or absence of infection as a cause of loosening of the prosthesis (Fig. 5). The literature at present is not unanimous in regard to the role of routine aspiration of a symptomatic total hip replacement; however, recent work has helped to clarify the role of this procedure. Roberts et al. (19) performed aspiration on 78 consecutive patients before revision hip operations. Fifteen patients proved to have infection. The investigators found 94% accuracy in comparing the results of aspiration with culture of tissue taken during the operation. In this group the sensitivity was 87% and the specificity was 95%. These surgeons were happy that on the basis of simplicity and reliability, routine aspiration was helpful in the diagnosis of infection. Barrack and Harris (3) reviewed the results of 270 consecutuve hips on which aspiration had been attempted before revision of the prosthesis. They found only 6 hips to have proved infection. Of these 6 hips, only 4 could be successfully aspirated, a total of 10 aspirations being performed on the 4 hips. Cultures of 4 of these aspirates did not grow organisms. The investigators had a 13% false-positive rate for the 254 hips that had been aspirated successfully and did not prove to be infected on the basis of intraoperative cultures. On the basis of these findings and the presence of other features of infection, such as focal lysis, aggressive nonfocal lysis, or periostitis among the patients in the series with proved infection, the investigators did not believe that routine aspiration has a place in the evaluation of symptomatic total hip replacement. They recommended that it be performed on selected patients when the history and radiographs strongly suggest the presence of infection.

SUMMARY

Evaluation of a symptomatic total hip arthroplasty is a process of gradual elimination of a wide range of possible pathologic processes. A surgeon faced with this challenge must keep an open mind as to the cause of the problem and not become tunneled in vision toward only the hip joint, even though in most instances the hip may well be the problem. It is the "curiosities" of such things as abdominal or spinal disorders that mimic the pain syndrome of failed total hip replacement for which the surgeon must continually be on guard. These entities pose the greatest challenge to detect and therefore eliminate from the decision tree. In orthopedic surgery there are few things more unfortunate than revision of a truly blameless arthroplasty for the wrong diagnosis.

In the search for the true cause for a symptomatic arthroplasty the cornerstone is a painstaking history interview. The clues dropped in conversation provide the direction for an informed and directed physical examination. To confirm or deny a provisional diagnosis, or, in situations in which the diagnosis may still be unclear, the next step in the process of elimination is appropriate hematologic, serologic, microbiologic, and radiologic evaluation.

REFERENCES

1. Aalto K, Ostermann K, Peltola H, Rasanen J. Changes in erythrocyte sedimentation rate and C-reactive protein after total hip replacement. *Clin Orthop* 1984;184:118–120.
2. Abitbol JJ, Gendron D, Laurin CA, Beaulieu MA. Gluteal nerve damage following total hip arthroplasty. *J Arthroplasty* 1990;5:319–322.
3. Barrack RL, Harris WH. The value of aspiration of the hip joint before revision total hip arthroplasty. *J Bone Joint Surg Am* 1993;75:66–76.
4. Bohl WR, Steffee AD. Lumbar spinal stenosis: a cause of continued pain and disability in patients after total hip arthroplasty. *Spine* 1979;4:168.
5. Canner GC, Steinberg ME, Heppenstall RB, Balderston R. The infected hip after total hip arthroplasty. *J Bone Joint Surg Am* 1984;66:1393–1399.
6. Carlsson AS. Erythrocyte sedimentation rate in infected and noninfected total hip arthroplasties. *Acta Orthop Scand* 1978;49:287–290.
7. Coventry MB. Late dislocations in patients with Charnley total hip arthroplasty. *J Bone Joint Surg Am* 1985;67:832–841.

8. Cruess RL, Bickel WS, Von Kessler KL. Infections in total hips secondary to a primary source elsewhere. *Clin Orthop* 1975;106:99–101.
9. Edwards MS, Tullos HS, Noble PC. Contributory factors and aetiology of sciatic nerve palsy in total hip arthroplasty. *Clin Orthop* 1987;218:136–141.
10. Etienne A, Cupic A, Charnley J. Postoperative dislocation after low friction arthroplasty. *Clin Orthop* 1978;132:19–23.
11. Freeman MAR, Plante-Bordeneuve P. Early migration and late aseptic failure of proximal femoral prostheses. *J Bone Joint Surg Br* 1994;76:432–438.
12. Hardcastle P, Nade S. The significance of the Trendelenberg test. *J Bone Joint Surg Br* 1985;67:741–746.
13. Ireland J, Kessel L. Hip adduction/abduction deformity and apparent leg length inequality. *Clin Orthop* 1980;153:156–157.
14. Ali Khan MA, Brakenbury PH, Reynolds ISR. Dislocation following total hip replacement. *J Bone Joint Surg Br* 1981;63:214–218.
15. Laupacis A, Bourne RB, Rorabeck CH, et al. The effect of elective total hip replacement upon health-related quality of life. *J Bone Joint Surg Am* 1993;75:1619–1626.
16. Leriche R, Morel A. The syndrome of thrombotic obliteration of the aortic bifurcation. *Ann Surg* 1948;127:193–206.
17. Lidwell O, Lowbury E, Whyte W, et al. Effects of ultraclean air in operating rooms on deep sepsis in the joint after total hip replacement: a randomised study. *Br Med J* 1982;285:10–14.
18. Marmor L. Stress fracture of the pubic ramus simulating a loose total hip replacement. *Clin Orthop* 1976;121:103–104.
19. Roberts P, Walters AJ, McMinn DJ. Diagnosing infection in hip replacements: the use of fine-needle aspiration and radiometric culture. *J Bone Joint Surg Br* 1992;74:265–269.
20. Sanzen L, Carlsson AS. The diagnostic value of C-reactive protein in infected total hip arthroplasties. *J Bone Joint Surg Br* 1989;71:638–641.
21. Swann M. Malignant soft tissue tumour at the site of a total hip replacement. *J Bone Joint Surg Br* 1984;66:629–631.
22. Weber ER, Daube JR, Coventry MB. Peripheral neuropathies associated with total hip arthroplasty. *J Bone Joint Surg Am* 1976;58:66–69.
23. Woo RYG, Morrey BF. Dislocations after total hip arthroplasty. *J Bone Joint Surg Am* 1982;64:1295–1306.

Revision Total Hip Arthroplasty,
edited by Marvin E. Steinberg and Jonathan P. Garino,
Lippincott Williams & Wilkins, Philadelphia © 1999.

9

Radiologic Evaluation

Mari Schenk and Murray K. Dalinka

Various imaging techniques may be used alone or combination in the evaluation of a painful total hip prosthesis. These techniques include plain film radiography, scintigraphy, aspiration and arthrography, ultrasonography, computed tomographic (CT) scanning, and magnetic resonance (MR) imaging. Among these, serial plain film radiography is the initial study of choice because it is both accurate and cost effective. If after clinical evaluation and routine radiography, the cause of pain remains uncertain, additional imaging may be warranted. In this chapter, the role of these imaging techniques is addressed in reference to the diagnosis of specific complications. Because the radiographic appearance and test results vary between cemented and cementless arthroplasty, the two are considered separately in the diagnosis of loosening. Additional information is given regarding two advanced imaging techniques: CT scanning and MR imaging.

LOOSENING

Plain Radiographs

Cemented

Serial plain film radiography is the most accurate method of detecting loosening, which remains the most common cause of failure of cemented hip prostheses (19). The radiographic diagnosis of loosening requires evaluation of implant position, the metal–cement interface, and the cement–bone interface, usually on serial radiographs. Criteria for loosening include implant migration; new metal–cement interface radiolucency; complete, greater than 2-mm cement–bone interface radiolucency; and cement fracture (7,9) (Fig. 1). Harris et al. (9) described the following three categories of *femoral* loosening: (a) definite—component migration or cement fracture; (b) probable—com-

---

M. Schenk and M. K. Dalinka, Department of Radiology, Hospital of the University of Pennsylvania, Philadelphia, Pennsylvania 19104.

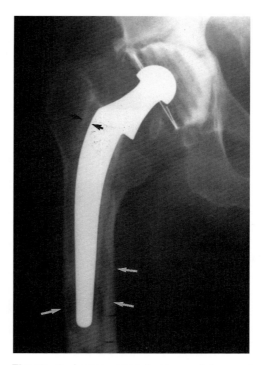

Figure 1. Loose acetabular and femoral components. Radiograph shows a continuous, widened radiolucent zone at the bone–cement interface of the acetabular and femoral components. A metal cement radiolucency (*black arrows*) and varus positioning of the femoral component have developed. The radiolucency with endosteal scalloping (*white arrows*) suggests particle disease along the distal femoral component (zones 3 through 5).

plete radiolucent zone at the bone–cement interface; and (c) possible—radiolucent zone between 50% and 100% of the total bone–cement interface. They (8) also described two stages of *acetabular* loosening, as follows: (a) definite—component migration or cement fracture, and (b) impending—continuous 2-mm bone–cement radiolucency. Hodgkinson et al. (12) correlated the radiographic appearance of the cemented acetabular component with findings at surgical revision and demonstrated that a continuous radiolucent zone, regardless of its width, correlated with loosening 94% of the time.

Implant Migration

Component migration is a reliable indicator of implant loosening. Progressive subsidence, migration, or tilt can be subtle, so direct comparison of radiographs with measurement often is required for diagnosis. For femoral subsidence, the position of a reproducible implant landmark relative to the tip of the greater trochanter or midportion of the lesser trochanter can be compared (Fig. 2A). Assessment of acetabular position includes superior migration, medial migration, and lateral inclination (Fig. 2B).

Metal–Cement Lucency

Radiolucent zones may be present at the metal–cement interface on the initial postoperative radiograph as a result of suboptimal prosthesis cement contact at the time of the operation. If the lucency remains stable, it is not an indicator of loosening (7). If,

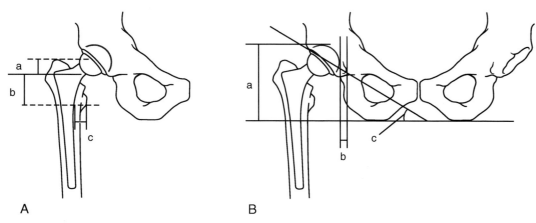

Figure 2. Detection of implant migration. **A:** Femoral subsidence. Measurement from a reproducible landmark on the femoral component (*dotted line*) to the tip of the greater trochanter (*distance a*) or to the midportion of the lesser trochanter (*distance b*). **B:** Acetabular migration. Assessment on serial radiographs of (*a*) superior migration—distance from transischial tuberosity line to top of cup; (*b*) medial migration—distance between the medial margin of the cup and teardrop (*b*), and (*c*) lateral inclination—angle between cup and transischial tuberosity line.

however, a radiolucent zone develops, debonding of the stem from the cement mantle and component migration have occurred. Metal–cement lucency is most common along the superolateral margin of the femoral prosthesis (32) (Fig. 3).

Cement–Bone Interface Lucency

The radiolucent zones along the cement–bone interface of the femoral component are designated by Roman numerals I through VII from lateral to medial on the anteroposterior (AP) view according to the method of Gruen et al. (Fig. 4A) (6). They likely represent a continuum from solid fixation to gross loosening with increasing probability of loosening with increasing thickness and extent of the lucency (23). Lucency at the bone–cement interface that is less than 2 mm in width, discontinuous, and nonprogressive is likely of no clinical significance. A retrieval study of well-fixed cemented femoral components demonstrated that a thin radiolucent zone is usually the result of adjacent bone remodeling with osteoporosis. In rare instances fibrous tissue is seen at the interface, typically along the proximal femur as an extension of the membrane formed at the hip joint (17). Soft-tissue membranes containing macrophages and giant cells consistent with a foreign-body reaction to particulate debris (polyethylene or cement) have been found at the widened interface in loosened femoral components.

The lucent zones along the acetabular component are described according to DeLee and Charnley (4). The acetabulum is divided into thirds and designated with Roman numerals I through III from lateral to medial (Fig. 4B) (4). Unlike on the femoral side, radiolucent zones at the bone–cement interface of acetabular components usually represent fibrous tissue formation (31). The extent of the lucency along the interface of the acetabulum correlates with implant stability. In the study by Hodgkinson et al. (12), 94% of replacements with a complete radiolucency at the interface, 74% with a continuous radiolucency invoving two thirds of the interface, and only 7% with a radiolucency in only one zone (zone I or III) were loose at the time of revision surgery.

Cement Fracture

Cement fracture usually occurs either proximally or distally near the tip of the prosthesis. It is often accompanied by component subsidence and is a reliable indicator of loosening (Fig. 5).

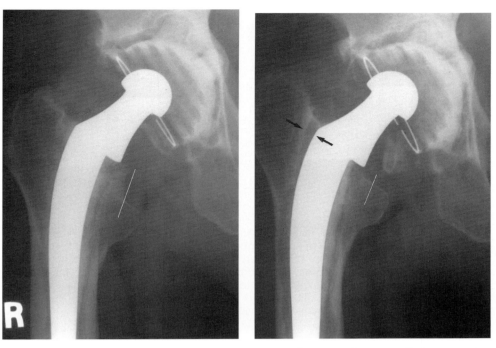

Figure 3. A: Loosened femoral component: metal-cement lucency. **B:** Lucency has developed at the metal-cement interface (*black arrows*). The implant has subsided (decreased distance to mid portion of lesser trochanter (*white line*).

Cementless

Radiographic assessment of cementless implant stability focuses on evaluation of implant position on serial radiographs. A diagnosis of definite loosening requires a progressive change in position of the prosthesis. Unfortunately, serial radiographs are not always available for review. In these cases, less specific signs may be helpful (5). Engh et al. (5) described major and minor signs for assessment of fixation and stability. On the basis of these signs they classified femoral component fixation as stable by bone ingrowth (termed *osseointegration*), stable by fibrous ingrowth, or unstable (Fig. 6).

Stable bone ingrowth prostheses demonstrate no demarcation lines adjacent to the porous coated surface and endosteal hypertrophy (spot welds) at the junction of the

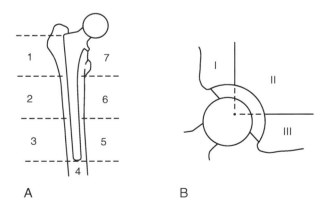

Figure 4. Designation of radiolucent zones. **A:** Femoral zones on the anteroposterior radiograph, according to the method of Gruen et al. (6). **B:** Acetabular zones, described according to DeLee and Charnley (4).

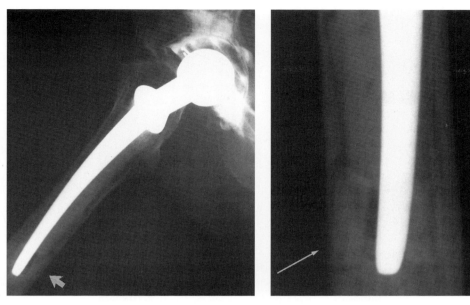

A   B

Figure 5. Loosened femoral component due to cement fracture. **A:** Cement fracture at the tip of the prosthesis (*white arrow*). **B:** Magnified view. Continuous lucency is present at the bone–cement interface.

smooth and porous coated portions of the prostheses (Fig. 7). Variable amounts of stress shielding are seen. If bone ingrowth has occurred, the implant is always stable, although stability may be achieved by fibrous fixation as well. Prostheses that are stable with fibrous fixation show parallel, nonprogressive demarcation lines adjacent to the ingrowth surface. There is either no migration or minimal early migration that stabilizes, usually within the first year. Spot welds are absent. In unstable prostheses, there is progressive migration of the femoral stem or progressive widening of demarcation lines around the prosthesis (Fig. 8). There may be pedestal formation at the tip of the implant, hypertrophy of the calcar, or progressive bead shedding. Many of these signs may be somewhat component specific (5). Mulliken et al. (22) reported on short-term (average 3.7 years) radiographic evaluation and stability of tapered titanium stems. They found spot welds and stress shielding were uncommon and distal endosteal and periosteal cortical hypertrophy were common in clinically stable prostheses.

Implant Migration

The most reliable sign of loosening of either the acetabular or femoral component in cementless total hip arthroplasty is progressive subsidence, migration, or tilt on serial

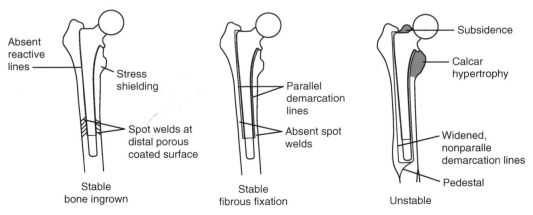

Figure 6. Radiographic features of cementless component fixation and stability as described by Engh et al. (5).

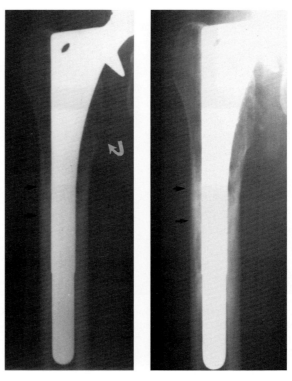

Figure 7. Bone ingrown prosthesis. **A:** Endosteal hypertrophy (spot welds) are present along the distal porous coated portion of the implant (*black arrows*). There is also stress shielding (decreased bone density with cortical thinning; *curved white arrow*). Loose beads are present in zone 7 in this stable implant (*small white arrow*). These were seen on the initial radiograph and were not progressive. **B:** Magnified view.

radiographs. Some degree of subsidence or settling of the femoral component is not uncommon, but it should stabilize at less than 1 cm and generally should not progress beyond 1 year (16).

Demarcation Lines

Thin, parallel radiolucent zones with adjacent sclerotic lines (demarcation lines) may develop adjacent to the porous ingrowth portion of the stem. Demarcation lines are most common proximally and laterally (zone 1) (15) and should stabilize by 2 years (5). Progression in width after 2 years, particularly in the region where spot welds are expected, is a sign of implant instability (5). In a stable, proximally fixed prosthesis, thin demarcation lines may be present along the distal, uncoated portion of the femoral component. When the distal, smooth portion of the stem is not fixed to the adjacent bone, differences in the stiffness of prosthesis and bone result in concentration of loads in the more flexible femur. Thus the bone distal to the implant is more deformed by a given load, causing relative motion between the stem and bone. This motion causes the distal demarcation lines and slight distal canal widening (Fig. 9) (5).

Pedestal Formation

A pedestal is endosteal sclerosis that extends into the medullary canal at the distal tip of the femoral stem. Cortical thickening may occur in conjunction with pedestal formation

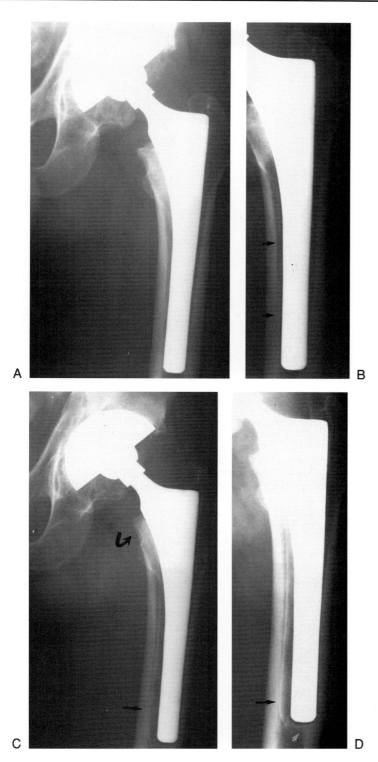

Figure 8. Unstable femoral component. **A:** Anteroposterior radiograph from May 1993 demonstrates parallel demarcation lines (*black arrows*). **B:** Magnified view of **A**. **C:** Follow-up radiograph from September 1996 shows an unstable prosthesis with widened demarcation lines (*straight black arrows*), hypertrophy of the calcar (*curved black arrow*), early pedestal formation (*white arrows* in **D**) and implant migration (subsidence and varus positioning). **D:** Magnified view of **C**.

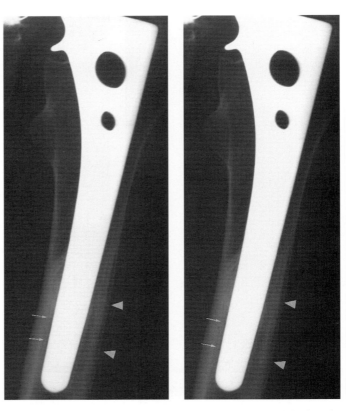

Figure 9. Distal demarcation lines and canal widening in stable prostheses. **A:** Thin demarcation line (*arrow*) distal to a spot weld. Single thin layer of periosteal reaction laterally (*arrowheads*) may be seen in cementless prostheses and should be differentiated from the laminated periosteal reaction of infection as seen in Fig. 11. **B:** Distal canal widening (*white arrows*). Superior pubic ramus fracture is present (*black arrow*).

and both may be seen with either stable or unstable prostheses. Engh et al. described pedestal formation as a minor sign of instability only if demarcation lines along the distal stem were also present (see Fig. 8D). If, on the other hand, the distal stem is fixed to bone (no demarcation lines), loads may be preferentially transferred to the tip in a stable implant. This results in distal pedestal formation and absent or less prominent proximal spot welds (5).

Stress Shielding

Fixed implants carry part of the normal load of bone, resulting in decreased stress on remaining bone or "stress shielding." Bone resorption as a result of stress shielding usually is most prominent in the proximal medial femoral cortex (see Fig. 7A) (32). This phenomenon is more pronounced with greater differences in stiffness between bone and implant. Implant stiffness is determined by both the modulus of elasticity of the stem material (greater in cobalt verses titanium alloy) and the geometric configuration of the stem (greater in larger stems). Stiffer stems transfixed to bone tend to demonstrate spot welds distally at the sites of load transfer and a greater degree of proximal bone resorption (5). Radiographs show decreased density of the bone, cortical thinning, and rounding of the femoral neck (32). Stress shielding usually stabilizes on plain radiographs by 1 to 2 years after the operation (14). However, dual energy x-ray absorptiometry measurements of bone density demonstrate further minor resorptive changes in the proximal femur for up to 5 to 7 years after implantation (15).

Bead Shedding

Loose beads not present on the initial postoperative radiograph likely reflect micromotion between bone and porous surface (5). Early on, some bead shedding may occur with settling of the prosthesis; late or progressive shedding is a sign of implant instability. Heekin et al. (10) found progressive shedding of beads in 10% of acetabular and 15% of femoral components within the first 2 postoperative years. However, after 2 years, progressive shedding was uncommon and if present was associated with acetabular migration and femoral subsidence (10).

Aspiration and Arthography

Cemented

Among patients with persistent symptoms suggestive of loosening but with a radiographically stable prosthesis, aspiration and arthrography may be performed for further evaluation. The overall accuracy, however, is lower than that of conventional radiography. We are rarely asked to perform hip arthrography in the absence of suspected infection.

Attention to arthrographic technique is important for improved accuracy in diagnosing component loosening. To maximize the sensitivity of arthography, a high-pressure technique is necessary in which injection of contrast material is terminated when there is complete filling of the bone–cement interface, the patient reports discomfort as a result of pseudocapsular distention; or there is lymphatic filling. With injection of larger amounts of contrast material, the number of false-negative results can be decreased. The reported increase in accuracy was from 51% (with 5 ml injected) to 92% (with the high-pressure technique) in one series (11). However, if large pseudocapsules or bursae are present, the accuracy of arthrography decreases, presumably as a result of underfilling of the joint. Bursae are smooth outpouchings communicating with the joint that are found in as many as 35% of arthrograms (20). They tend to occur superolateral to the acetabulum among patients with a prior dislocation or adjacent to the trochanter among patients with nonunion of trochanteric osteotomies. Subtraction techniques may be used. They allow easier discrimination of contrast and opaque cement (Fig. 10). In equivocal cases, images obtained after walking may show evidence of loosening not seen on routine images.

In comparison with plain radiography arthrography has more false-positive results for loosening of the acetabular component and more false-negative results on the femoral side. Maus et al. (20) in an attempt to improve the accuracy of arthrography, modified diagnostic criteria on the basis of surgical findings. For the acetabular component, contrast material tracking along at least two contiguous zones (I and II or II and III) or more than 2 mm in width in any one zone constituted a positive result. With this criterion acetabular component loosening was identified with a sensitivity of 97% but a specificity of only 68%. Loosening of the femoral component was defined by contrast material tracking at the implant–cement or cement–bone interface below a line connecting the midportion of the trochanters. Maus et al. (20) reported a sensitivity of 96% and specificity of 92%, although to achieve this sensitivity, they relied on plain radiographic findings when there were large pseudocapsules or bursae.

Cementless

The use of arthrography to evaluate loosening in uncemented components is unreliable. Barrack et al. (2) reported a sensitivity of 57% and a specificity of 60% in examinations of 24 painful uncemented femoral stems and a sensitivity of 29% and a specificity of 89% in examinations of 16 acetabular components. A large number of both false-positive (17% of femoral components) and false-negative results (25% of femoral and 31% of acetabular components) occurred. Contrast material may track at the component–bone interface in the presence of solid fixation, particularly along the femoral component. The lack of contrast material filling the interface does not reliably exclude loosening.

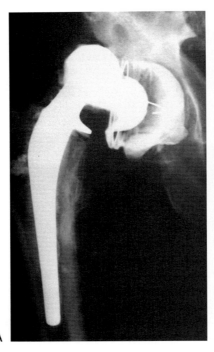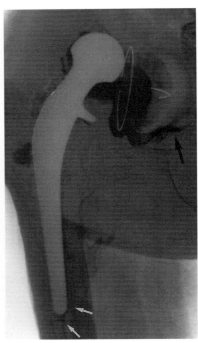

A   B

Figure 10. Loosened femoral and acetabular components: hip dislocation. Arthrogram (**A**) with subtraction technique (**B**) shows contrast
material tracking along the femoral component (*white arrows*) distally to
zone 4 and in zone III (more than 2 mm wide) (*black arrow*) of the
acetabulum. Contrast is more conspicuous and easier to differentiate
from cement on the subtracted image (**B**).

Scintigraphy

Cemented

Technetium bone scanning is not needed in the routine evaluation of a painful total hip
replacement, but may be performed when results of conventional radiography are
inconclusive. Technetium scanning also can be used in combination with leukocyte or
gallium scanning when infection is a consideration. In general, a normal scan result
provides more useful information than an abnormal scan result, because it makes the
diagnosis of loosening or infection unlikely, although not impossible (7,19,32). A
conservative approach has been recommended for patients with completely normal scan
results (7,19).

An abnormal scan can be seen postoperatively for a variety of reasons, including
loosening, infection, fracture, and heterotopic ossification. Utz et al. (31) reported on the
natural history of ^{99m}Tc medronate methylene diphosphonate (MDP) scans obtained
prospectively for 97 patients with asymptomatic cemented total hip replacements. Nine
percent of patients had persistent uptake 1 year after the operation, and even more patients
showed increased activity in subsequent years; the authors attributed this to asymptomatic
loosening.

A ^{99m}Tc bone scan alone cannot be used to differentiate infection from aseptic
loosening. Although diffuse uptake was noted to be suggestive of infection versus focal
uptake for loosening, subsequent studies have not upheld this relation (30). ^{99m}Tc MDP
has been used in combination with indium leukocyte or gallium scans to increase the
specificity for infection. The diagnosis of infection is suggested when greater or
incongruent uptake of indium or gallium is present (Fig. 11). This topic is addressed later.

Cementless

Technetium bone scans appear to be of limited usefulness in the evaluation of loosening
in cementless prostheses. Oswald et al. (24,25) described the natural history of ^{99m}Tc bone

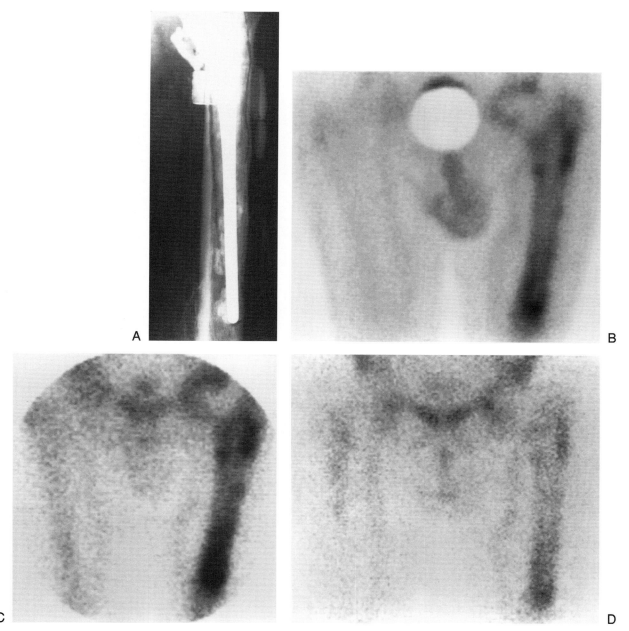

Figure 11. Septic loosening. **A:** Laminated periosteal reaction (*white arrow*). **B:** Technetium-99m medronate methylene diphosphonate (^{99m}Tc MDP) bone scan demonstrates abnormal focal activity both proximally and distally around the femoral component. **C:** Indium-111 white blood cell scan shows greater activity than **B**. Greater activity (^{111}In greater than ^{99m}Tc) or incongruent activity (^{111}In uptake but no ^{99m}Tc uptake) constitutes an abnormal scan. **D:** Technectium-99m sulfur colloid marrow scan shows less activity than **C**; therefore, the ^{111}In activity is caused by infection, not marrow redistribution.

scans in porous coated implants of patients without symptoms and demonstrated that activity is seen around the acetabular component and femoral tip of most patients even as long as 2 years postoperatively. This study suggested that increased flow or increased blood flow activity (after 3 months) on a three-phase bone scan was more suggestive of a complication.

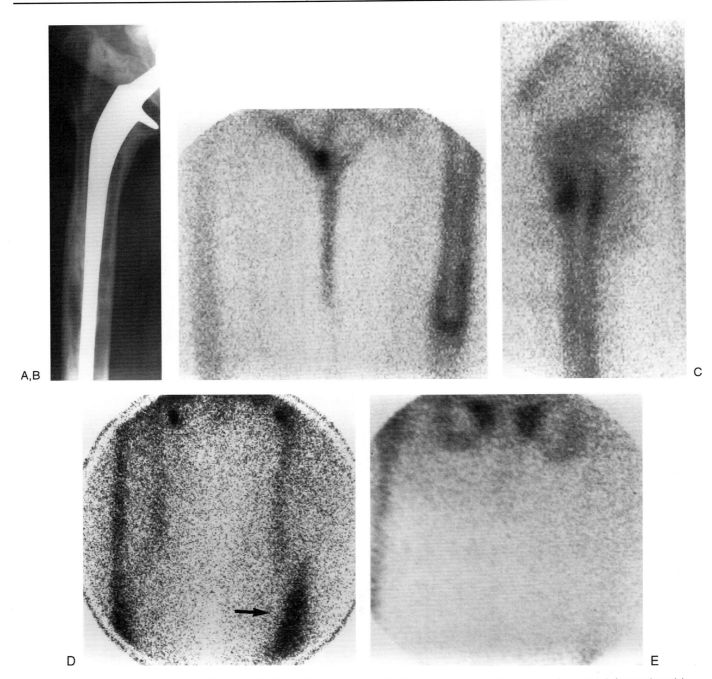

Figure 12. Aseptic loosening. **A:** Metal–cement radiolucency in zone 1 (*arrowheads*). Scalloped radiolucency in zones 3 and 6 suggest particle disease. **B** and **C:** Technetium-99m MDP bone scan. Focal activity is present along the distal femoral implant (**B**) on the anteroposterior view and proximally (**C**) on the lateral view. **D:** Indium-111 white blood cell scan. No corresponding activity on the indium scan of patient with aseptic loosening. **E:** Technetium-99m sulfur colloid bone marrow scan demonstrates congruent activity with the indium scan. The congruent area of activity represents marrow uptake in the distal femur.

Computed Tomography

A "stress" technique has been described for diagnosing loosening of a cemented or cementless femoral component by means of CT scanning. Two cuts, one at the level of the neck of the prosthesis and one at the level of the femoral epicondyle, are obtained with the leg in maximum internal and external rotation. The angle of the prosthesis (long axis of the neck) relative to the transepicondylar line for each position is measured, and two angles are subtracted to determine the rotational angle. A difference of 2 degrees in one study and 4 degrees in a second were criteria for a loose prosthesis. With a rotational angle of 4 degrees, the sensitivity was 67%, specificity was 100%, and accuracy was 75%. This technique helped identify all prostheses that were completely loose at operation but none that were partially loose (27). The reliability of this technique has not yet been confirmed by other investigators.

INFECTION

Plain Radiographs

Plain radiographs are often normal, especially early in the course of infection. As the infection becomes chronic, radiolucencies may develop at the bone–cement or bone–prosthesis interface that are difficult to differentiate from aseptic loosening. Radiographic findings suggestive of infection include rapid development of periprosthetic radiolucency, poorly marginated nonfocal or focal bone destruction, and scalloped endosteal bone resorption. Laminated periosteal reaction is very suggestive of infection but is detected in only 1% to 2% of infected hips (see Fig. 11A). Tigges et al. (29) retrospectively reviewed radiographs of 20 septic hip prostheses and reported findings as follows: normal in 10 instances, nonfocal radiolucencies mimicking aseptic loosening in 4, rapid progression of periprosthetic radiolucency in 2, focal lysis in 2, and periostitis in 2 instances. The investigators found the focal lysis associated with infection difficult to differentiate from particle disease.

Scintigraphy

If the question of infection persists after clinical, hematologic (erythrocyte sedimentation rate, C-reactive protein), and plain radiographic examination, radionuclide imaging may be helpful for further evaluation. A ^{99m}Tc bone scan alone is of limited value because it is nonspecific. Gallium citrate, which accumulates in areas of inflammation and increased bone turnover, may be combined with ^{99m}Tc bone scans to increase specificity. The combined scans are reliable indicators of infection if relative uptake of gallium exceeds that of ^{99m}Tc MDP or the distribution of gallium uptake is different than that of ^{99m}Tc MDP (incongruent). Few false-positive results have been found. However, only approximately one fourth to one third of patients with osteomyelitis have abnormal scans. A normal combined scan therefore does not reliably exclude infection (26).

Indium leukocyte scanning combined with ^{99m}Tc bone scans is commonly used for suspected osteomyelitis in areas of increased bone turnover in the appendicular skeleton. This combination has been less successful in examinations of the marrow-containing skeleton and of patients with joint prostheses. Marrow redistribution is thought to occur after joint replacement operations resulting in increased periprosthetic marrow. Because indium-111 normally accumulates in marrow, discrimination between uptake in normal marrow and infection is difficult, particularly when the marrow distribution is heterogenous. Combining ^{111}In leukocyte scanning with ^{99m}Tc sulfur colloid marrow imaging increases specificity by making use of the fact that increased uptake on both reflects uptake in normal marrow (see Fig. 12). Incongruent images, in which increased leukocyte periprosthetic activity is present in the absence of increased bone marrow sulfur colloid uptake, are positive for infection (see Fig. 11). The combination reportedly increases specificity from 75% (indium alone) to 100% (combination examination) (26). Because indium scanning alone has a high negative predictive value (90%), it may be performed first. When results are normal, no further imaging is needed. If the results are abnormal, sulfur colloid imaging is performed and comparison of the pattern of uptake between the two scans is made.

Limitations of indium scanning include increased uptake in inflammatory arthritides such as rheumatoid arthritis and low spatial resolution, making differentiation of osteomyelitis from adjacent cellulitis sometimes difficult. In these situations, a ^{99m}Tc MDP scan may be performed in an attempt to localize activity to bone. Initial concerns regarding the efficacy of ^{111}In-labeled leukocytes in the setting of chronic infection and antibiotic therapy have not been upheld. Both do not have a considerable effect on the sensitivity of the leukocyte scan (3).

Aspiration and Arthrography

Although O'Neill and Harris (23) in 1984 stated that "aspiration of the joint to diagnose subtle sepsis or identify a specific organism is always indicated prior to surgical revision," the value of routine aspiration has become controversial in more recent literature. The range of reported sensitivity, specificity, and accuracy of the procedure is wide. In 1996, Mulchaney et al. (21) reported a sensitivity of 68%, specificity of 91%, and accuracy of 86% (71 hips). Lachiewicz et al. (18) reported a sensitivity of 92%, specificity of 97%, and accuracy of 96% (142 hips). False-negative and false-positive aspiration findings have been reported. Maus et al. (20) found four normal aspirates among 14 infected prostheses. Barrack and Harris (1) found 32 false-positive results among 254 hips. In the latter series, only patients with clinical or radiographic evidence of infection had a true-positive result at culture. Barrack and Harris (1) concluded that late indolent infection cannot be diagnosed on the basis of aspiration alone. They recommended aspiration be limited to patients with clinical or radiographic signs of infection.

After aspiration, contrast medium is injected under fluoroscopy to verify intraarticular placement of the needle. With injection of contrast medium there may be filling of cavities that communicate with the joint. If the cavities are irregular in contour, they more likely represent infected collections rather than bursae (20). On some occasions, no fluid may be obtained at aspiration despite intraarticular placement of the needle. In these situations saline solution may be injected and aspiration repeated; the efficacy of this practice remains undetermined. Ultrasound scanning may be used to identify loculated fluid within the pseudocapsule or an extracapsular fluid collection in communication with the joint and to subsequently guide aspiration. In rare instances aspiration is unsuccessful because of the presence of periprosthetic heterotopic bone. CT guidance may be used to identify a gap in the heterotopic bone through which to pass the needle into the joint.

OSTEOLYSIS AND POLYETHYLENE WEAR

Particulate wear debris from polymethyl methacrylate (PMMA) or polyethylene from a cementless or cemented prosthesis can stimulate a host foreign-body response, resulting in periprosthetic osteolysis (Fig. 13). Osteolysis typically appears as a focal, well-defined, lytic lesion that tends to enlarge over time. The pattern, location, and extent of osteolysis, however, are variable, which may be related to several factors, including particle size, load, and composition and access of particles to the bone–component interface (33). Zicat et al. (33) found an extensive linear pattern of osteolysis, often associated with symptomatic loosening, surrounding cemented acetabular components, whereas a localized, expansile pattern of osteolysis, usually without symptomatic loosening, occurred in cementless acetabular components. This pattern of expansile osteolysis, which extended away from the implant–bone interface into the cancellous bone, resulted in greater loss of bone stock, with the potential for a more difficult revision operation or fracture (33).

Osteolysis is usually asymptomatic, unless component loosening ensues. In uncemented prostheses, osteolysis is usually not seen until at least 2 years after the operation but increases in prevalence with time. Annual follow-up radiographs are helpful to identify the process before progressive bone loss occurs. Rapidly expanding lesions may necessitate more frequent monitoring. The extent of acetabular bony defects can be difficult to assess on routine AP radiographs alone. Judet views or, when more severe bone loss is present, CT evaluation with image reconstruction can be helpful for evaluation of bone stock before a revision operation.

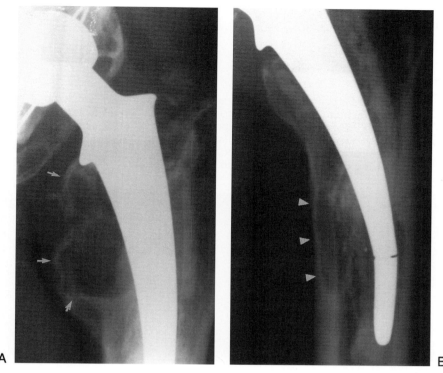

A   B

Figure 13. Osteolysis: particle disease. **A:** Focal expansile osteolysis
(*white arrows*). **B:** Osteolysis with endosteal scalloping (*arrowheads*).

Osteolysis may be associated with radiographic evidence of accelerated polyethylene
wear. Linear polyethylene wear rates for the hip are typically in the order of 0.1 mm/year
(13). Accelerated clinical wear rates likely relate to many factors, including polyethylene
thickness and quality, patient weight and activity level, femoral head size and material,
and modularity of polyethylene acetabular inserts (13). On radiographs wear is appreciated as narrowing of the superolateral margin of the "polyethylene" joint space, that is, an
eccentric position of the femoral head within the cup with superolateral narrowing and
medial widening (Fig. 14). In rare instances asymmetric positioning of the head may be
the result of separation of the polyethylene lining from the metal backing. The liner is
more radiolucent than soft tissue and may be seen as an ovoid lucency within the joint.
Displacement of the liner allows metal-on-metal contact to occur, resulting in shedding of
metal particles into the joint. Deposition of metal particles in synovial tissue can
eventually lead to aseptic arthropathy (metallosis) with increased opacity or thin dense
curvilinear deposits in the joint.

FRACTURE

Insufficiency fractures of the pubic rami, sacrum, or both may occur among patients
with osteopenia from disuse, steroid use, or rheumatoid arthritis after total hip arthroplasty
(THA) (Fig. 15) (28). Increased walking or altered mechanics after the operation may
overload the osteopenic bone, resulting in fracture. Rami fractures typically become
apparent with groin pain that worsens with activity and often is accompanied by a limp.
Sacral fractures usually present with buttock pain and is often accompanied by thigh pain.
These fractures are difficult to identify early in their course (weeks to months) with plain
radiography, appearing as subtle buckling of cortical bone of the rami or a band of
sclerosis in the cancellous bone of the sacrum. Both are readily diagnosed with bone scans
or MR imaging (Fig. 16). The sacral fractures are vertically oriented within the alae and
can be either unilateral or bilateral. A horizontal component may also develop within the

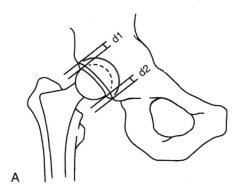

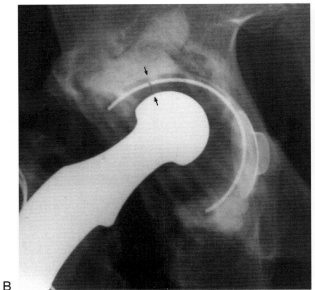

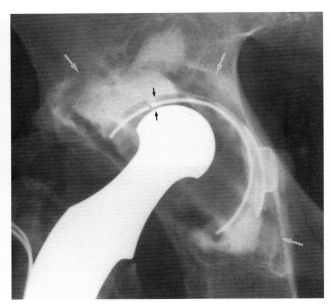

Figure 14. Polyethylene wear. **A:** The distances from femoral head to acetabulum (*d1* and *d2*) in most prostheses should be equal. If d1 is less than d2, there is usually polyethylene wear. **B** and **C:** Progressive decrease in the d1 distance (superior position of the femoral head within the cup) (*black arrows*) caused by polyethylene wear. Osteolysis is present at the bone–cement interface (*white arrows*).

sacral body at the S1-2 level, resulting in the characteristic H-shaped or "Honda trademark" pattern of uptake on ^{99m}Tc bone scans.

Postoperative periprosthetic femoral-side fractures are uncommon and usually develop at the site of stress risers (e.g., at the site of focal osteolysis or a femoral window). Middle-region fractures are frequently associated with loosening of the implant. In rare instances, periprosthetic acetabular fractures occur, often without underlying osteolysis. In addition to routine AP radiographs, Judet views, and possibly CT scans may be necessary for identification and accurate classification of the acetabular fracture.

Computed Tomography

The use of CT imaging in evaluation of hip prostheses is limited because of starburst (beam hardening) artifact, which severely degrades the image and interferes with evaluation of surrounding structures. The artifact is greatest on axial images. Multiplanar image reconstruction with a high-frequency filter (bone algorithm) improves image quality. Potential uses of CT include evaluation of acetabular bone stock before revision operations on patients with osteolysis. It also has a problem-solving role, as with acetabular fracture, or a role in directing aspiration among patients with extensive heterotopic ossification.

Magnetic Resonance Imaging

Joint prostheses may be imaged with magnetic resonance safely without risk of motion or heating. Artifacts caused by magnetic susceptibility of the prosthesis limit evaluation

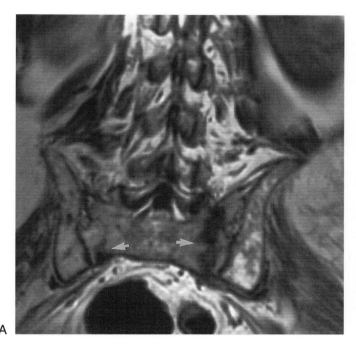

Figure 15. Superior pubic ramus fracture (*black arrow*).

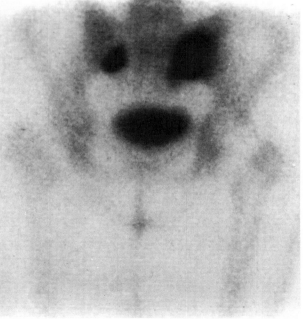

Figure 16. Sacral insufficiency fractures. **A:** T1-weighted coronal magnetic resonance image demonstrates vertical bands of low signal intensity (*arrows*) within the sacral alae (left greater than right) representing sacral fractures in this patient who had undergone total hip arthroplasty (THA). **B:** ^{99m}Tc MDP bone scan of a different patient demonstrates increased uptake within both alae as a result of insufficiency fractures in this patient who had undergone left THA.

of the implant–bone interface but not of periprosthetic soft tissues if imaging parameters are optimized. The implants themselves appear as structures without signal (black). The black signal loss from the prosthesis extends beyond the site of the implant and is bordered in part by a thin, curvilinear line of high signal intensity (Fig. 17). This "blooming" of black signal loss into the surrounding structures is minimized by optimization of independent operator-controlled technical parameters at the time of MR image acquisition. These parameters include high bandwidth, large imaging matrix (256 × 512), multiple refocusing pulses (fast or turbo spin echo sequences), and frequency-encoded direction parallel to the long axis of the implant (30). Stainless steel is associated with severe artifact (probably because of ferromagnetic impurities), whereas titanium is nonferromagnetic and produces less artifact. A potential roles of MR imaging is in the evaluation of soft-tissue fluid collections, deep venous thrombosis, or radiographically occult fractures.

Color Doppler flow imaging with a compression technique is a highly accurate and cost-effective means of evaluating acute deep venous thrombosis of the lower extremity (Fig. 18), but generally cannot be used to assess pelvic veins beyond the distal external iliac vein. MR venography with a two-dimensional time-of-flight technique is valuable in

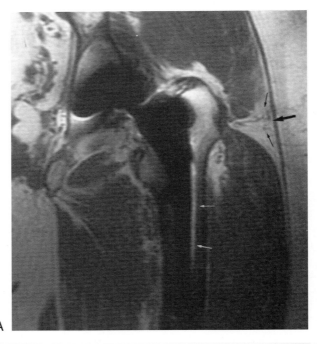

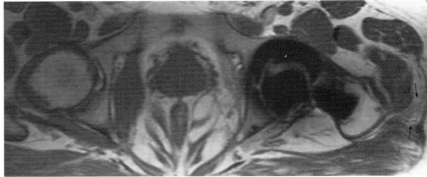

Figure 17. Cementless total hip arthroplasty. Clinical question of soft-tissue abscess superficial to the greater trochanter. T1-weighted coronal (**A**) and axial (**B**) images demonstrate mild stranding of the fat (*black arrow*) but no fluid collection. The prosthesis appears black. The adjacent thin white line is artifact related to metal (*white arrows*).

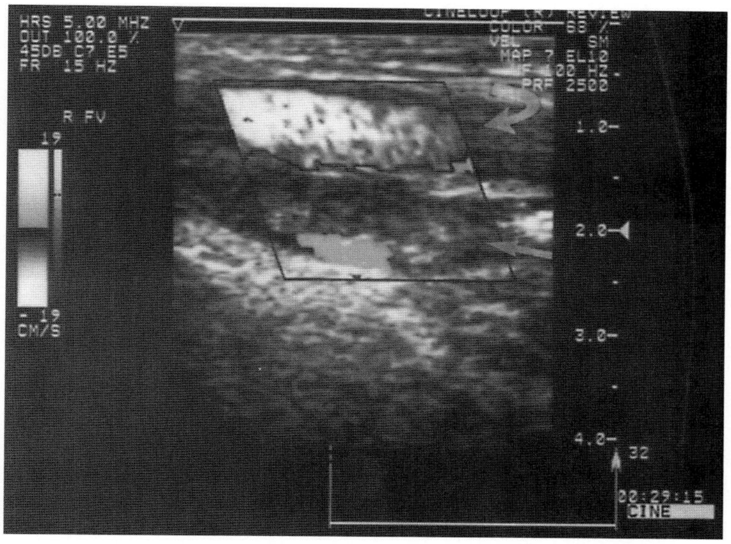

Figure 18. Deep venous thrombosis. Ultrasound scan with color flow imaging demonstrates flow in the superficial femoral artery (*curved arrow*). There is thrombus (*straight arrow*) with minimal flow (*red*) within the superficial femoral vein.

the setting of suspected pelvic or inferior vena caval thrombus. Artifact from the acetabular implant may obscure visualization of the distal external iliac vein on the two-dimensional time-of-flight images but the vein generally can be assessed adequately on axial T1- and T2-weighted images. MR imaging also is effective in evaluation of soft-tissue structures or osseous structures away from the implant.

SUMMARY

The radiographic evaluation of a painful hip prosthesis always begins with conventional radiography, which remains the most accurate and cost effective test. If after clinical evaluation and plain radiographic examination, the diagnosis is still in question, aspiration and arthography or nuclear medicine studies may be used for further evaluation. We do not perform arthrography routinely for suspected loosening or before revision operations but reserve it for the evaluation of infection suspected on clinical or radiographic grounds. In these situations arthrography is performed more to verify intraarticular placement of the needle before aspiration then to identify component loosening. In the scintographic evaluation of a painful arthroplasty, combined ^{99m}Tc sulfur colloid and ^{111}In 111 leukocyte bone marrow scans appear to be most accurate for the diagnosis of infection. If septic versus aseptic loosening is a consideration, a reasonable approach is a combined ^{99m}Tc and ^{111}In scan, in which the greatest value of the test is normal results. If the ^{111}In scan is abnormal, sulfur colloid examination can be performed to increase specificity for infection. The main value of CT, MR, and ultrasound imaging is in a problem-solving role. Attention to technical factors at the time of image acquisition in MR or CT imaging is necessary to minimize artifact from the prosthesis.

In these days of cost containment, one must decide when and how radiography is indicated in the case of patients who have no symptoms after total hip arthroplasty. Everyone agrees that a baseline study should be performed before hospital discharge. Asymptomatic loosening is usually not treated, and osteolysis takes at least 2 years to occur. It seems reasonable and logical to wait at least 2 years for the first postbaseline examination of a patient who has no symptoms.

REFERENCES

1. Barrack R, Harris W. The value of aspiration of the hip joint before revision total hip arthroplasty. *J Bone Joint Surg Am* 1993;75:66–75.

2. Barrack R, Tanzer M, Kattapuram S, Harris W. The value of contrast arthrography in assessing loosening in symptomatic uncemented total hip components. *Skeletal Radiol* 1994;23:37–41.
3. Datz F. Indium-111-labeled leukocytes for the detection of infection: current status. *Semin Nucl Med* 1994;2:92–109.
4. DeLee J, Charnley J. Radiological demarcation of cemented sockets in total hip replacement. *Clin Orthop* 1976;121:20–32.
5. Engh CA, Massin P, Suthers K. Roentgenographic assessment of the biologic fixation of porous-surfaced femoral components. *Clin Orthop* 1990;257:107–128.
6. Gruen T, McNeice G, Amstutz H. Modes of failure of cemented stem-type femoral components. *Clin Orthop* 1979;141:17–27.
7. Harris W, Barrack R. Developments in diagnosis of the painful total hip replacement. *Orthop Rev* 1993;22:439–447.
8. Harris W, McGann W. Loosening of the femoral component after use of the medullary-plug cementing technique. *J Bone Joint Surg Am* 1986;68:1064–1066.
9. Harris W, Penenberg B. Further follow-up on socket fixation using a metal-backed acetabular component for total hip replacement. *J Bone Joint Surg Am* 1987;69-A:1140–1143.
10. Heekin D, Callaghan J, Hopkinson W, Savory C, Xenos J. The porous-coated anatomic total hip prosthesis, inserted without cement. *J Bone Joint Surg Am* 1993;75:77–90.
11. Hendrix RW, Wixson RL, Rana NA, Rogers LF. Arthrography after total hip arthroplasty: a modified technique used in the diagnosis of pain. *Radiology* 1983;148:647–652.
12. Hodgkinson J, Shelley P, Wroblewski B. The correlation between the roentgenographic appearance and operative findings at the bone-cement junction of the socket in Charnley low-friction arthroplasties. *Clin Orthop* 1988;228:105–109.
13. Jacobs J, Shanbhag A, Glant T, Black J, Galante J. Wear debris in total joint replacements. *J Am Acad Orthop Surg* 1994;2:212–220.
14. Kattapuram S, Lodwick G, Chandler H, Khurana J, Ehara S, Rosenthal D. Porous-coated anatomic total hip prostheses: radiographic analysis and clinical correlation. *Radiology* 1990;174:861–864.
15. Kilgus D, Shimaoka E, Tipton J, Eberle R. Dual-energy x-ray absorptiometry measurement of bone mineral density around porous-coated cementless femoral implants. *J Bone Joint Surg Br* 1993;75:279–287.
16. Kiss J, Murray DW, Turner-Smith AR, Bulstrode CJ. Roentgen stereophogrammetric analysis for assessing migration of total hip replacement femoral components. *Proc Inst Mech Eng [H]* 1995;209:169–175.
17. Kwong L, Jasty M, Mulroy R, Maloney W, Bragdon C, Harris W. The histology of the radiolucent line. *J Bone Joint Surg Br* 1992;74:67–73.
18. Lachiewicz P, Rogers G, Thomason C. Aspiration of the hip joint before revision total hip arthroplasty. *J Bone Joint Surg Am* 1996;78:749–754.
19. Lieberman J, Huo M, Schneider R, et al. Evaluation of painful hip arthroplasties. *J Bone Joint Surg Br* 1993;75:475–478.
20. Maus T, Berquist T, Bender C, Rand J. Arthrographic study of painful total hip arthroplasty. *Radiology* 1987;162:721–727.
21. Mulchaney D, Fenelon G, McInerney D. Aspiration arthrography of the hip joint. *J Arthroplasty* 1996;11:64–68.
22. Mulliken B, Bourne R, Rorabeck C, Nayak N. A tapered titanium femoral stem inserted without cement in a total hip arthroplasty: radiographic evaluation and stability. *J Bone Joint Surg Am* 1996;78-A:1214–1225.
23. O'Neill D, Harris W. Failed total hip replacement: assessment by plain radiographs, arthrograms, and aspiration of the hip joint. *J Bone Joint Surg Am* 1984;66:540–546.
24. Oswald S, Van Nostrand D, Savory C, Anderson J, Callaghan J. The acetabulum: a prospective study of three-phase bone and indium white blood cell scintigraphy following porous-coated hip arthroplasty. *J Nucl Med* 1990;31:274–280.
25. Oswald S, Van Nostrand D, Savory C, Anderson J, Callaghan J. Three-phase bone and indium white blood cell scintigraphy following porous-coated hip arthroplasty: a prospective study of the prosthetic tip. *J Nucl Med* 1989;30:1321–1331.
26. Palestro C, Kim C, Swyer A, et al. Total-hip arthroplasty: periprosthetic indium-111-labeled leukocyte activity and complementary technetium-99m-sulfur colloid imaging in suspected infection. *J Nucl Med* 199;31:1950–1955.
27. Reinus W, Merkel W, Gilden J, Berger K. Evaluation of femoral prosthetic loosening using CT imaging. *AJR Am J Roentgenol* 1996;166:1439–1442.
28. Shapira D, Militeanu D, Israel O, Scharf Y. Insufficiency fractures of the pubic rami. *Semin Arthritis Rheum* 1996;25:373–382.
29. Tigges S, Stiles R, Roberson J. Appearance of septic hip prostheses on plain radiographs. *AJR Am J Roentgenol* 1994;163:377–380.
30. Tormanen J, Tervonen O, Koivula A, Juhani J, Suramo I. Image technique optimization in MR imaging of a titanium alloy joint prosthesis. *J Magn Reson Imaging* 1996;6:805–811.
31. Utz J, Lull R, Galvin E. Asymptomatic total hip prosthesis: natural history determined using Tc-99m MDP bone scans. *Radiology* 1986;161:509–512.
32. Weissman B. Imaging of total hip replacement. *Radiology* 1997;202:611–623.
33. Zicat B, Engh C, Gokcen B. Pattern of osteolysis around total hip components inserted with and without cement. *J Bone Joint Surg Am* 1995;77:432–439.

Revision Total Hip Arthroplasty,
edited by Marvin E. Steinberg and Jonathan P. Garino,
Lippincott Williams & Wilkins, Philadelphia © 1999.

10

When Not to Revise the Painful Total Hip Replacement

Michael A. Mont and David S. Hungerford

Although much time is spent by hip surgeons deciding matters of prosthesis selection and technique, the decision-making process of *when* to revise a hip replacement is just as important. This chapter is concerned with this assessment, focusing primarily on when *not* to revise a painful hip replacement. We do not emphasize obvious situations in which pain and revision are logically cause-and-effect responses because these scenarios are covered elsewhere in this book. Obvious situations that necessitate revision of a painful hip include deep infection (see Chapters 26 through 29), recurrent dislocation (see Chapter 32), severely symptomatic aseptic loosening (see Chapters 2 and 3), progressive massive osteolysis (see Chapter 3), and various periprosthetic fractures (see Chapter 34). These topics are covered in this chapter only from the vantage point of when not to revise hip arthroplasties with these problems.

Other painful disorders of the hip deserve mention but would never or only rarely warrant a hip revision (2). These include heterotopic ossification (13) (see Chapter 33), enigmatic thigh pain (1,2,4,6,9), and trochanteric bursitis. A well-taken history, physical examination, and radiographic evaluation should clearly differentiate these problems from inherent hip problems that might necessitate revision (7). When faced with less obvious painful hip replacements it is important to search for alternative sources of pain. Pain around the hip often comes from nerve paresis, pelvic fractures (10–12,14) intraabdomi-

M. A. Mont and D. S. Hungerford: Orthopaedic Department of The Johns Hopkins University School of Medicine; Division of Arthritis Surgery at the Good Samaritan Hospital, Baltimore, Maryland 21239.

nal processes, spinal problems (such as disk disease (8), arthritis, spinal stenosis (3), and metastatic disease), and vascular origins (5). Again, an astute clinician must differentiate nonhip disorders that can cause hip pain from processes inherent in the replacement itself. Most of the time, one can differentiate hip problems from other causes by means of history and physical examination. Special laboratory tests or scans occasionally are necessary.

RISK-TO-BENEFIT RATIO

Although it is difficult to define the concept objectively, the surgeon should try to elucidate the concept of a risk versus benefit analysis to the patient. Sometimes this type of analysis is simple; a relatively active, healthy 32-year old patient with osteonecrosis and a loose stem that has necessitated use of a wheelchair for the previous 2 months clearly needs revision. A 92-year old woman who cannot walk, has a minimally painful loose stem, and has had three myocardial infarctions in the past 6 months would not pass a risk-to-benefit analysis and would not be a candidate for revision.

Factors that increase the benefit of hip revision include scenarios in which there is a likelihood of relieving pain, increasing mobility, increasing strength, and decreasing a limp. Less likelihood of realizing benefit in these areas would lower the benefit of a revision procedure. Factors that increase the risk of surgical intervention include medical conditions, the extent of operation needed, comorbid mobility-limiting diseases, and unreasonable expectations. Conversely, the absence of these limiting factors would decrease the risk of surgical treatment.

SPECIFIC CONDITIONS IN WHICH THE SURGEON MAY NOT WISH TO REVISE ASEPTIC LOOSENING

One common reason for pain is aseptic loosening. Whereas it is often obvious when there is a severely symptomatic, painful, radiographically loose prosthesis requiring revision, at other times the diagnosis is not clear cut. Once a revision for painful aseptic loosening is being considered, discussion between the patient and the surgeon is imperative. The surgeon should outline the specific preoperative plan, including special tests needed (e.g., aspiration), the operative plan, and the expected postoperative course. Because the decision to revise should not be taken lightly, all significant family members who may be involved in the patient's care should be included in the discussion, if possible. The expected outcome should be made clear to the patient; this includes assessment of the likelihood of realizing the benefit from surgical treatment. For example, a patient who has not walked for 6 years and now has a 3-month history of pain from a loose prosthesis may be extremely likely to gain pain relief after successful revision but would be unlikely to walk again. The risks of surgical intervention should be clearly outlined to the patient. They must be informed of the inherent risks of any operation and about the increased risk of excessive blood loss and the prolonged operating time, in considerable excess of primary hip arthroplasty, that the revision usually entails.

Although this might appear to be an obvious statement, the decision to operate should be mutual, based on discussion between surgeon and patient; it should never be made by one party alone. For example, the surgeon may be reluctant to perform revision on a 72-year-old man who has a cardiac ejection fraction of 20%, because of the nearly 10% risk for a perioperative cardiac event. However, this patient might influence the decision by stating that he wants the revision in spite of the increased risk because he absolutely would like the opportunity to be able to walk again and he accepts the increased risks of the operation. The surgeon must then decide whether he or she is equipped to handle the increased risk, both from a technical point of view and in regard to hospital ancillary medical support. Often a patient like this might need to be transferred to a specific facility more equipped to handle the extremely high-risk nature of the operation. By contrast, the surgeon might influence this same patient not to undergo the revision procedure, because the risks of the operation in the specific situation would far outweigh the potential gain.

It is difficult to prescribe a cookbook method for not revising a painful hip, however, certain general guidelines can be considered in the following situations.

Medical reasons. One may choose not to revise a painful hip when medical contra-indications lead to a risk-benefit disproportion that does not favor attempted surgical intervention.

Expectations, psychological factors. Unreasonable expectations on the part of a patient who may not benefit from revision, such as a patient with a modified Harris hip score greater than 70 points, should be a warning to the contemplating surgeon.

Stable or painful condition. A stable painful condition to which a patient has learned to adjust without affecting activities of daily living or otherwise general well-being might be better served without a revision. Such a situation might be that of a patient with a well-fixed porous ingrowth femoral component with mild, chronic thigh pain of uncertain causation. Again, a thorough assessment of the risk-benefit ratio should be made in these scenarios.

Radiographic failure only. Although it is not specifically the subject of this chapter, a nonpainful hip that appears loose does not have to be revised if there is no evidence of progressive bone loss. These patients should be taught about the appearance of their prosthesis and should be examined at regular yearly intervals until the symptoms develop or progressive bone loss is demonstrated.

ALTERNATIVES TO REVISION

Activity Modification

The patient must decide whether there is sufficient disabling pain to warrant another operation. Many of these patients are elderly and are not terribly demanding on their hip and the pain is not a problem for their lifestyle. Often the pain can be controlled to a sufficient degree with various methods used to decrease activity. Patients can use a cane or a crutch for protected weight bearing and often can reduce the pain with this method alone to quite satisfactory levels.

Pain Control

Sometimes, the use of a nonsteroidal antiinflammatory medication on a regular basis is all that is necessary to palliate chronic pain. This can often be maintained long term. Patients undergoing long-term pain control should have periodic checks of renal and liver function, complete blood cell counts for hemoglobin, occasional stool guaiac tests to detect gastrointestinal bleeding, and urinalysis to assess for evidence of microscopic hematuria. Generally as long as there are no gastrointestinal problems associated with taking these medications, use of the drugs can be continued indefinitely.

Physicians are usually reluctant to prescribe narcotic analgesics for long-term management of chronic pain. On one extreme, a patient may be quite comfortable taking one or two narcotic pills a day to become well functioning. Long-term use of medium-dose analgesics once was discouraged. Recent experience with the use of long-acting narcotic analgesics has made this treatment more palatable. For example, the use of morphine (MS Contin) requires taking one or two pills each day that have a relatively long half-life with a long-acting effect. It has not been found to lead to habitual dependence or an elevation in necessary dosage to achieve the same analgesic effect over time. Various other sustained release products, (Oxycontin) have been found to be effective in managing chronic pain.

CASE REPORTS

Case 1

A 41-year-old man undergoes cementless hip replacement through an anterolateral approach. Six months later he is able to walk 3 miles a day but reports stiffness and mild discomfort in his hip when he sits or tries to get out of a chair. At physical examination the patient has a maximum hip flexion of 100 degrees but otherwise satisfactory range of motion with minimal discomfort. Inspection of the radiographs reveals a well-aligned prosthesis with grade III heterotopic ossification (Fig. 1). The patient sees the radiographs with you and wants to know whether revision will be necessary because of this extra bone.

Analysis

We would not revise or explore this hip on the basis of the risk-to-benefit ratio. This patient is able to walk 3 miles a day and has minimal discomfort. The gain from decreasing hip stiffness would be minimal. The risk of an operation to remove heterotopic bone would certainly have to be postponed until 1 year postoperatively with a necessary cold bone scan. This operation should not be contemplated lightly (see Chapter 33).

Case 2

A 56-year-old woman has had a cemented total hip replacement for the past 21 years. She is quite happy with her hip replacement, which remains mildly symptomatic. She returns regularly for annual visits. Over the past 5 years her orthopedic surgeon has pointed out a small cystic area in zone 7 on routine hip radiographs (Fig. 2). This cystic area has not changed radiographically during this time. The patient is concerned about whether she needs to have her prosthesis revised.

Analysis

This is an example of stable, nonprogressive osteolysis. This patient is virtually symptom free, and the osteolysis seen on radiographs has not changed over the past 5

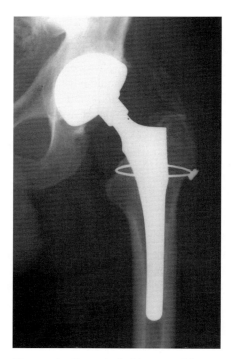

Figure 1. Case 1. A 41-year-old man with mild discomfort and decreased range of motion caused by heterotopic ossification.

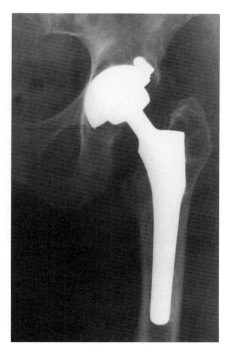

Figure 2. Case 2. A 56-year-old woman with a small area of stable osteolysis and minimal symptoms.

years. The surgeon should recommend continued annual observation unless the symptoms increase or the osteolytic area begins to enlarge.

Case 3

A 72-year-old minimally ambulatory man underwent cementless hip replacement 12 years ago. He returns for a visit when his hip starts hurting him after not seeing an orthopedist for more than 10 years. At radiographic evaluation, massive osteolysis is seen around the acetabular component and femoral stem (Fig. 3). The patient is taken to the operating room, where massive acetabular bone loss is found with no walls or columns intact. The surgeon does not believe there is enough bone stock to place an acetabular component. What should the surgeon do?

Analysis

The surgeon decides not to revise. Resection arthroplasty (Girdlestone procedure) is appropriate, and is performed. The only other possibility is massive structural allografting or use of protrusio rings with allografts and cement, and these two alternatives are deemed too risky for this patient. The surgeon also believes that the benefit derived by this minimally ambulatory patient would not justify a long and extensive revision procedure.

Case 4

A 76-year-old woman undergoes revision hip arthroplasty for pain caused by massive osteolysis of the femur. This procedure requires a massive proximal femoral allograft for reconstruction (Fig. 4). Although there are no gross signs of infection, an intraoperative culture is positive for *Staphylococcus epidermidis*. The patient is treated with 6 weeks of intravenous antibiotics and has an otherwise apparently uneventful postoperative course. Six months postoperatively she is fully ambulatory with minimal hip pain (Harris hip

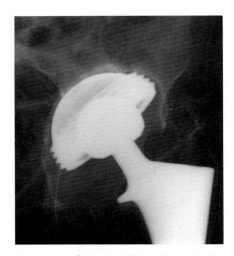

Figure 3. Case 3. Minimally ambulatory patient with massive bone loss around the acetabulum and proximal femur. Treated by means of resection arthroplasty.

score of 84 points). A hip aspiration reveals *S. epidermidis* on cultures. The patient is given an oral antibiotic (ciprofloxacin), which she tolerates well. She elects to live with the minimal pain from her hip (Harris hip score of 82 points). Four years later she is still taking oral antibiotics and remains fully functional with her hip.

Analysis

This patient still has a deep hip infection. The choice is made to retain the prosthesis because of the minimal pain and nonsystemic spread of the infection. The benefit from revising this difficult revision would be minimal with high morbidity from a two-stage reimplantation attempt.

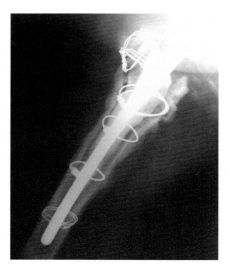

Figure 4. Case 4. A 76-year-old woman with a chronic, low-grade infection after revision. Treated with long-term antibiotic suppression.

CONCLUSIONS

It is important to have a clear understanding of when not to revise a painful hip. The specific cause of pain should be clearly identified. If the pain arises from a situation that might be amenable to a revision operation, it is imperative that a risk-to-benefit analysis concerning the specific need to revise be made by the surgeon and clearly understood by the patient. Unless the cause of the pain has been clearly identified and can be eliminated or improved considerably with revision, it is generally prudent to treat the patient nonoperatively.

REFERENCES

1. Amstutz HC, ed. *Total hip arthroplasty.* London: Churchill-Livingstone, 1992:59–68, 469–472.
2. Berry DJ. Evaluation of the painful total hip arthroplasty. In: Morrey BF, ed. *Reconstructive surgery of the joints.* 1995:1159–1171.
3. Bohl WR, Steffee AD. Lumbar spinal stenosis: a cause of continued pain and disability in patients after total hip arthroplasty. *Spine* 1979;4:168–175.
4. Campbell ACL, Rorabeck CH, Bourne RB, et al. Thigh pain after cementless hip arthroplasty. *J Bone Joint Surg Br* 1992;74:63.
5. DeWolfe VG. Intermittent claudication of the hip and the syndrome of chronic aortoiliac thrombosis. *Circulation* 1954;9:1.
6. Engh CA, Massin PM, Suthers KE. Roentgenographic assessment of the biologic fixation of porous-surfaced femoral components. *Clin Orthop* 1990;257:107–128.
7. Fisher DA. Evaluation of the painful total hip arthroplasty. *Semin Arthroplasty* 1992;3:229.
8. Floman Y, Bernini PM, Marvel JPJ, Rothman RH. Low-back pain and sciatica following total hip replacement: a report of two cases. *Spine* 1980;5:292.
9. Franks E, Mont MA, Maar DC, Jones LC, Hungerford DS. Thigh pain as related to bending rigidity of the femoral prosthesis and bone. *Trans Orthop Res Soc* 1992;38:296 [abstract].
10. Lotke PA, Wong RY, Ecker ML. Stress fracture as a cause of chronic pain following revision total hip arthroplasty. *Clin Orthop* 1986;206:147.
11. Marmor L. Stress fracture of the pubic ramus simulating a loose total hip replacement. *Clin Orthop* 1976;121:103.
12. Mont MA, Maar DC. Ipsilateral femur fractures complicating hip arthroplasty: a statistical analysis of the results based on 487 patients. *J Arthroplasty* 1994;9:511–519.
13. Mont MA, Maar DC, Krackow KA, Jones LC, Jacobs MA, Hungerford DS. Cementless hip replacement for non-inflammatory arthritis after age forty-five. *J Bone Joint Surg Am* 1993;75A:740–751.
14. Oh I, Hardacre JA. Fatigue fracture of the inferior pubic ramus following total hip replacement for congenital hip dislocation. *Clin Orthop* 1980;147:154.

Revising the Aseptic Total Hip

Revision Total Hip Arthroplasty,
edited by Marvin E. Steinberg and Jonathan P. Garino,
Lippincott Williams & Wilkins, Philadelphia © 1998.

11

Preoperative Planning for Revision Total Hip Arthroplasty

Robert L. Barrack

The importance of planning and templating before total hip arthroplasty has been emphasized by a number of authors (10,11,13). Primary hip replacement, however, is generally much more predictable than revision arthroplasty. In primary operations the extent of the procedure is usually apparent after review of conventional plain radiographs, and most patients are treated with instruments, implants, and accessories routinely available in most community hospitals. Intraoperative complications and unexpected findings at the operation are relatively uncommon. Revision total hip arthroplasty, on the other hand, often presents the surgeon with a wide array of complex intraoperative challenges. Preoperative radiographs present a less clear picture of what will be encountered after exposure and removal of implants. Many situations encountered may require use of special instruments, implants, bone grafts, and other accessories that are often not available unless anticipated and ordered days ahead of time. Unavailability of such items often leads to longer operative times and compromise to a less than optimal alternative solution.

Preoperative planning is crucial in the revision situation. Compared with primary arthroplasty, revision hip replacement has been shown to entail a greater degree of surgeon work and risk as reflected by longer operative times, greater blood loss, and a higher complication rate (6). Careful preoperative planning helps to anticipate and prepare for potential complications. It also allows for more specific informed consent by allowing discussion with patients about complications that are particularly likely on the basis of

R. L. Barrack: Department of Orthopaedic Surgery, Tulane University School of Medicine, New Orleans, Louisiana 70112.

planning. Planning also ensures that all material necessary to expeditiously handle the array of potential challenges is readily available. This helps minimize operative time and complication rate and optimize the results of these challenging operations. An organized approach helps to ensure that relevant details will not be overlooked. This begins with general assessment of the patient history, review of systems, and a physical examination. This is followed by review of laboratory results, plain radiographs and other diagnostic tests. The final step is templating plain radiographs to formulate a primary and an alternative plan for the revision procedure.

GENERAL ASSESSMENT

A careful review of the patient's history, review of systems, and physical examination is crucial in arriving at a specific diagnosis before embarking on a revision procedure. An inaccurate preoperative diagnosis is occasionally a cause of failure to relieve symptoms after primary total hip replacement. This is an even more common occurrence in revision surgery. Arriving at an accurate diagnosis based on history, physical findings, and diagnostic tests is discussed in Chapter 8. Specific data obtained from the history and physical examination, however, are important in preoperative planning for the revision procedure.

Most patients undergoing revision hip replacement are older, and many have associated medical problems. Because of this, it is my routine to obtain an internal medicine consultation for virtually all patients. Many patients also are seen by other consultants, such as cardiologists, vascular surgeons, and urologists. It is important to have a mechanism to ensure that consultations are completed and recommendations are addressed, including the results of any further tests that may be ordered. It is helpful in this regard to have a checklist that can be reviewed on a routine basis preoperatively.

Patients with serious cardiovascular problems are often seen preoperatively by an anesthesiologist for assessment of the necessity for additional perioperative monitoring, such as arterial or Swan-Ganz catheters. If it is anticipated that postoperative monitoring is a possibility, it is prudent to schedule an intensive care bed to ensure that adequate staffing is available.

A number of specific items in the history influence preoperative planning. Patients with perioperative fractures or chronic or recurrent dislocations often are transferred from smaller community hospitals to centers that perform a higher number of joint replacements. In such situations it is important to ascertain whether there has been a long period of immobilization before the planned surgical intervention, which is often the case. It also is prudent to obtain preoperative screening for deep venous thrombosis by means of either ultrasonography or venography. If deep venous thrombosis is present, insertion of a Greenfield filter should be considered, because such operations frequently are emergencies and must be performed in spite of the presence of venous thrombosis. Failure to detect a clot and insert a filter can result in a catastrophic intraoperative embolic event.

A number of historical facts suggest the presence of chronic or indolent infection. A history of wound-healing problems with persistent drainage and a history of night pain, constant pain unrelieved by rest, or pain relieved by antibiotic use all suggest infection. In such situations preoperative aspiration is prudent. The results of aspirations, however, are not 100% accurate (5). If aspiration results are normal in the presence of such a history, or if there is an unexplained increase in erythrocyte sedimentation rate or C-reactive protein level, it may be useful to plan to obtain an intraoperative frozen section, particularly if suspicious-appearing tissue is encountered after component removal. It is helpful to notify the operating room and pathologist in advance if it is anticipated that there is high likelihood of submission of tissue for frozen-section histologic analysis. In many hospitals pathologists are unfamiliar with this application of frozen-section analysis. If this is the case, it is useful to provide them with recent publications describing the criteria for examination of tissue during total joint revision (25). Joint fluid is often submitted for Gram stain in such cases as well. Recent evidence indicates that a Gram stain is usually negative even in the presence of infection. A negative Gram stain cannot therefore be taken as strong evidence of the absence of infection. In the presence of infection, a very small percentage of cases actually demonstrate bacteria on Gram stain (12).

Specific historical facts may influence the decision on implant selection. A history of high-dose pelvic irradiation is a relatively strong contraindication to the use of a porous coated cementless hemispheric acetabular component. In such cases a cemented all-polyethylene acetabular component with or without a protrusio ring is an option that should be available. This is probably more frequently an issue in primary joint replacement (19) but is occasionally a factor in the revision situation.

The nature of the pain elicited from the history also influences the preoperative plan. Groin pain typically is attributed to loosening of the acetabular component. If groin pain is present, the entire rim of the component must be exposed and the implant tested for micromotion at the interface with the host bone. Pain in the thigh that is more prominent when getting out of a chair or going upstairs (typical start-up pain) is often attributed to stem loosening. If loosening is not readily apparent after review of sequential plain radiographs, a relatively new preoperative test has been described for detecting occult stem loosening. Dynamic computed tomographic (CT) scanning with the hip in internal and external rotation has been described as a test for loosening of a cementless stem (7). Another option for detection of occult loosening of a cementless or cemented stem is intraoperative use of a torque wrench (18). Surgeons in the past have typically exposed the collar and cement–bone or implant–bone interface and applied a force by hand. A torque wrench can apply several times the force of the surgeon's hand and comes much closer to replicating the out-of-plane force on the component during stair climbing and is more likely to help detect occult loosening.

Patients who have a history of popping, clicking, or a sensation of instability may need special preparation in preoperative planning. If subluxation is suspected on the basis of the patient's history and there is a question whether repositioning of the acetabular component is indicated, it may be advisable to plan fluoroscopic evaluation of the hip before undertaking a revision procedure. This can be done at the time of the operation if there are other indications for revision. If the only indication for revision is a question of instability, fluoroscopic examination on an outpatient basis may be considered. For patients with a history of recurrent dislocation, special implants such as a bipolar or constrained acetabular component may be helpful to have available at the time of the operation (24). Postoperative bracing frequently is indicated, and it may be expeditious to order the brace preoperatively. It is certainly worth discussing with the patient the likelihood of the need for bracing or wearing a pantaloon spica cast postoperatively.

A number of findings at physical examination can influence the preoperative plan. It is helpful to observe the patient's gait with and without any assistive devices. A marked abductor lurch and abductor weakness at manual muscle testing raise the specter of absent or nonfunctional abductor muscles. In the revision situation this may be caused by loss of the abductors through trochanteric migration, osteolysis, or massive proximal femoral deficiency. If the trochanter is present on radiographs and in continuity, preoperative electromyelography may be indicated to determine whether there is abductor muscle paralysis from previous denervation. If there is a history of recurrent dislocation along with the absence of functional abductors, the use of special implants such as constrained liners or a bipolar prosthesis should be considered because the combination of absent abductors and recurrent dislocation is an exceptionally high-risk situation for future instability (24).

Range of motion at physical examination is relevant in planning the operative exposure. In hips that are partially ankylosed or those with marked medial migration or protrusio, a more extensile exposure should be planned including the possibility of trochanteric osteotomy. The level of trochanteric osteotomy and angle of the osteotomy should be planned on the preoperative radiographs. Equipment for trochanteric attachment, including wire tighteners, should be available. If there is a small fragment of trochanteric bone, trochanteric mesh is useful for reattachment. The use of certain cable systems for trochanteric reattachment has been reported to be associated with a high complication rate (28). Patients who are very large may also require a more extensile approach. For patients who are obese and need complex revision, the use of a triradiate exposure has been described (22).

Measurement of limb length is part of the standard physical examination and is relevant for preoperative planning. Limb lengthening frequently occurs in the course of revision hip replacement. If considerable change in length is anticipated on the basis of preoperative assessment, it is helpful to use one of a number of techniques for intraoperative length measurement before component removal and repetition of this measurement after insertion of trials (29,30). Lengthening of more than 2 to 3 cm is associated with a higher risk for nerve palsy. It is generally more of a risk in primary arthroplasty than in revision procedures. This is particularly true if the limb shortening has occurred because of stem subsidence or other mechanisms associated with loosening or change in the position of the components. In such cases the shortening has occurred over a period of years, and typically there is laxity in the sciatic nerve and soft tissues that makes nerve palsy less of a risk than in a typical primary case of dysplasia. Nevertheless, revision occasionally is performed in which a primary arthroplasty was performed at a higher hip center or pseudoacetabulum. When considerable lengthening is anticipated in the process of returning to a more anatomically correct hip center, nerve palsy is a serious risk and use of intraoperative monitoring such as somatosensory evoked potentials is a consideration (21). This must be planned preoperatively, and in most cases a neurologist may want to assess the evoked potential on an outpatient basis preoperatively as a basis for comparison with intraoperative measurements.

Determination of the vascular status of the limb is an integral part of the examination and is relevant for planning purposes. Patients who do not have palpable pedal pulses, who have symptoms of claudication, or who have had a vascular bypass graft should be examined by a vascular surgeon preoperatively. Patients with previous bypass grafts are at risk for clotting of the graft during hip arthroplasty. Alteration of the operative exposure, including trochanteric osteotomy and avoidance of rotation of the femur, has been suggested as a method of minimizing this risk (9).

RADIOGRAPHIC EXAMINATION

Review of a complete set of recent radiographs is crucial in the planning of the revision procedure. The first step is obtaining an adequate series of radiographs. A low anteroposterior (AP) pelvis is used to assess component position and relative limb length. Length is estimated by means of measuring the distance from the interischial line to a fixed point on the lesser trochanter. Radiographic measurements of limb-length discrepancy are correlated with clinical measurements such as use of blocks or tape measurements from the anterior superior iliac spine to the medial malleolus. If there is considerable discrepancy between clinical and radiographic measurements or if there are marked contractures of the hip or knee that may interfere with accurate limb-length assessment, it may be advisable to obtain a scanogram. CT has been described as a useful adjunct in such cases (1).

Judet views are helpful in assessing acetabular bone stock and the extent of the need for allograft bone. A shot through the lateral aspect of the acetabulum is useful for assessing the version of the acetabular component and for templating the acetabulum on the lateral view.

Anteroposterior and lateral views of the femur are necessary for assessing the component and cement that may be present. The length of the film depends on the length of the stem in place. At a minimum it is necessary to visualize the entire extent of the stem and cement (Fig. 1). If a long-stemmed component is in place, it may be necessary to obtain AP and lateral views of the entire femur. In any case, it is necessary to visualize the entire implant and cement and a segment of femur at least two to three stem diameters distal to the extent of the stem or cement (Fig. 1C). When there has been a previous fracture, osteotomy, or any other irregularity of the femur, it is advisable to obtain AP and lateral views of the entire femur. Whereas a shoot through the lateral projection is helpful in assessing the acetabulum component, a Lowenstein lateral view gives more accurate projection of the femur for templating purposes (15). The femoral radiographs should be scrutinized to assess any areas of perforation or excessive thinning of the femur. It is also important to assess the bow of the femur on the lateral radiograph, particularly when use of longer components is anticipated.

In addition to Judet views of the acetabulum, CT scans with three-dimensional reconstructions can be obtained to assess complex acetabular deformities. Although these images were used more commonly in years past, with the availability and more widespread use of oversized

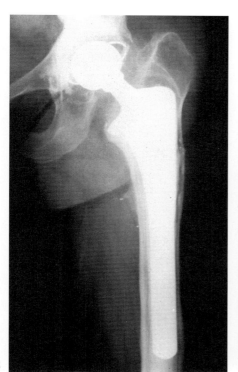
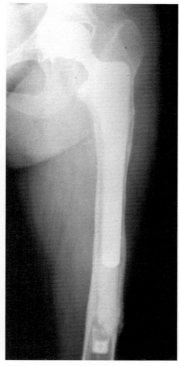
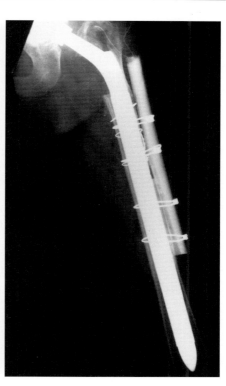

A,B   C

Figure 1. A: Preoperative radiographs of a painful cemented total hip showing the tip of stem. **B:** Longer radiograph reveals extent of cement column with perforation and cement extrusion at tip. **C:** Custom long cementless stem was necessary to bypass defect and obtain stability.

cementless components and protrusio cages, the indications for three-dimensional reconstructions have generally become more narrow. If intrapelvic cement, screws, or components are apparent on plain radiographs, further evaluation of the proximity to vital intrapelvic structures often is useful if removal of the screws, cement, or components is likely during the revision procedure (16). Components and cement that are intrapelvic may displace major vessels such as the iliac artery or vein. In such cases a retroperitoneal approach is a safer option for component removal. Preoperative assessment with an arteriogram is helpful in such a situation (Fig. 2). Newer modalities such as magnetic resonance angiography may be used to assess the proximity of major vessels to intrapelvic implants. This technology however is susceptible to distortion by metal and is more applicable to an all-polyethylene component rather than a metal-backed component.

The presence and extent of heterotopic ossification should be determined on plain radiographs. Formation of grade 3 or 4 heterotopic ossification since the previous procedure may alter the planned surgical approach and necessitate a plan for prophylaxis against re-formation of aggressive heterotopic ossification. Removal of extensive heterotopic ossification often requires a more extensile approach. Because heterotopic bone frequently forms beneath the abductor muscles, trochanteric osteotomy may be necessary to gain access to the heterotopic bone and to obtain adequate exposure. It is necessary to plan a course of prophylaxis preoperatively. Recently recommended protocols involve a single dose of radiation immediately after the operation. Many hospitals in which revision operations are performed may not have the facilities to deliver the radiation therapy, and this must therefore be coordinated well in advance. Recent evidence suggests that an equal dose of radiation administered immediately preoperatively is probably just as effective as postoperative irradiation. If this protocol is elected, the radiation treatment must be carefully coordinated with the subsequent revision procedure. It has been suggested that cementless components and trochanteric osteotomies be shielded (20). It is helpful for the radiation therapist to be provided with a publication with figures explaining the shielding protocol (20).

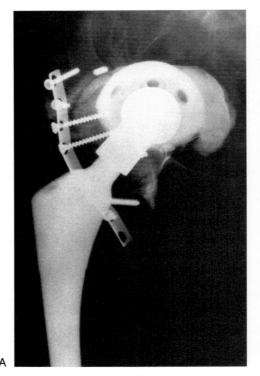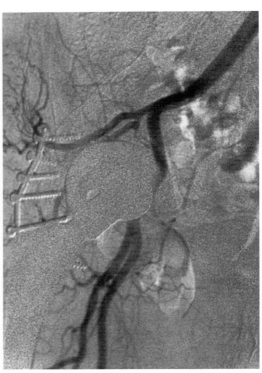

A   B

Figure 2. A: Plain radiograph shows intrapelvic component and cement. **B:** Arteriogram demonstrates displacement of the iliac vessels.

After adequate radiographs have been obtained, it is important to identify as accurately as possible the components that are in place. This is true whether the plan is to remove each component or to leave it in place. It is useful to obtain previous hospital records to verify the manufacturers and sizes of all components. If the surgeon is not intimately familiar with the nuances of the components that are in place, it is helpful to contact the manufacturer or its representative to learn about the special tools that may be available for removing the components. If the components are modular, there may be special tools that facilitate disassembling or reassembling the components. On the acetabular side for instance, a cementless modular component may be well fixed and adequately positioned; however, the liner may be damaged. In such a case, it is important to know how to expeditiously remove the liner and reinsert another one. It is also useful to have some degree of familiarity with the locking mechanism to determine whether another liner that is reinserted is securely fixed. If the locking mechanism is damaged, reinsertion of another liner may not be possible. In such cases it may be necessary to revise the metal shell even though it is well positioned and rigidly fixed. Many early-generation acetabular components had poor locking mechanisms and a low degree of conformity between the liner and acetabular shell. In such cases it may be more prudent to change the acetabular component even if it is well positioned and fixed. This is particularly true if there is evidence of accelerated liner wear or pelvic osteolysis (4). Another alternative is to cement an all-polyethylene component into the existing metal shell, if it has an adequate diameter.

On the femoral side it is important to determine whether the stem has a fixed head or modular head. If the femoral component is of the older, fixed-head variety and there is a chance that the stem will be left in place, it is important to know the head size so that the appropriate size acetabular component can be mated with it. If the head is modular, it is important to have the appropriate extraction tool to remove the head. Head removal is routinely performed to assist in gaining adequate exposure even if the head will subsequently be left in place. Many manufacturers have tools that are unique to their stems that are helpful in removing the head. It is important to know the exact identity of the stem so appropriately sized modular heads are available to replace the head should the stem be left in place. Modular heads cannot be interchanged between manufacturers, and one manufacturer may even have more than one taper size (2). In addition, many manufacturers have recently changed their tapers so that current modular heads are not compatible with earlier designs. Most frequently a longer head component is necessary after the acetabular component is revised. The acetabular component is often placed at a slightly higher hip center, and more length often is necessary to restore tissue tension after operative exposure. For this reason it is important to have longer modular heads available to provide the desirable increase in length and offset. If the longest head is already in place, the options include use of a custom femoral head component of additional length or use of an extra offset acetabular liner (Fig. 3). In recent years extra-offset modular acetabular liners have been become available that can help restore length and offset that cannot be obtained on the femoral side. These extra-offset liners are particularly useful when a well-fixed long femoral stem with a fixed head is in place and the acetabular component requires revision. Availability of an extra-offset liner may obviate trochanteric advancement to increase tissue tension and stability or, worse, revision of a well-fixed monoblock stem strictly to gain more length.

Knowledge of the exact identity of the components in place is important if the components are to be removed. On the acetabular side many modular cementless components have screws that require screwdrivers other than the standard hex head for removal. Many of the screws are titanium and may be stripped at the time of removal. If this occurs it is useful to have a carbide-tipped burr to remove the head and a trephine to retrieve the threaded portion of the screw. Most acetabular components can be removed with a standard set of acetabular curved gouges. A pneumatic torque wrench has been described for removal of a well-fixed acetabular component. Since the original report of the technique, follow-up reports from other centers on the degree of success in use of this instrument have been lacking.

On the femoral side specialized equipment is available for removal of stems in a variety of specific instances. The component type and fixation status must be recognized in

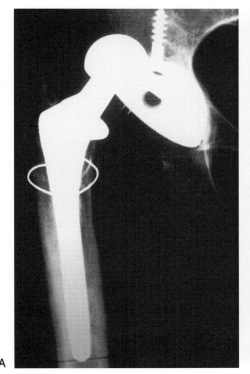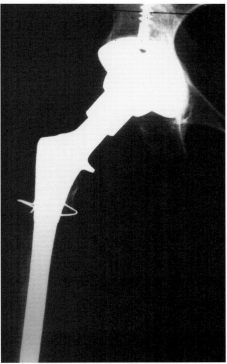

A   B

Figure 3. A: Anteroposterior radiograph shows a dislocated hip with components well aligned and rigidly fixed. **B:** Stability is restored with a custom long modular head.

advance so the appropriate equipment can be available. Many titanium cementless components have a threaded extraction hole in the shoulder of the component that mates to a threaded extraction tool that greatly facilitates removing the component. Many recent-generation modular components also have unique extraction instruments. Stems with modular sleeves or bullets frequently dissociate when the stem is extracted. In such instances use of special tools to retrieve the retained modular piece may save a great deal of operative time and obviate making a cortical window or other invasive procedure that might not otherwise be necessary.

It is useful to know the exact extent of the coating on the femoral component. In a well-fixed component, an extended osteotomy should extend at least to the level of the coating (31). It is also useful to know the surface finish of the non–porous coated portion of cementless stems. Components that are smooth or polished can easily be extracted once the porous implant bone interface is disrupted. Components that have a titanium grit blast may be difficult to remove even after the porous bone-ingrowth interface has been disrupted.

Removing a well-fixed cementless stem requires specific instruments and techniques that must be planned well ahead of time. Special techniques and equipment have been described for removing components such as the Anatomic Medullary Locking (AML; DePuy, Warsaw, Ind.) (17). Radiographic review is usually fairly accurate in determining the fixation status of these stems (15). In general they are more difficult to remove then may be apparent radiographically. The greatest degree of ingrowth is typically at the distal extent of the porous coating. Even small degrees of bone ingrowth present a challenge in component removal. At least two options exist for removing such well-fixed components. An extended osteotomy can be performed down to the distal extent of the coating. Because the best ingrowth typically occurs at this location, it is important that the osteotomy not stop short of the distal extent of the coating. After the lateral window is removed, it is equally important to have available multiple Gigli saws to disrupt the medial ingrowth. The saws are initially placed under the

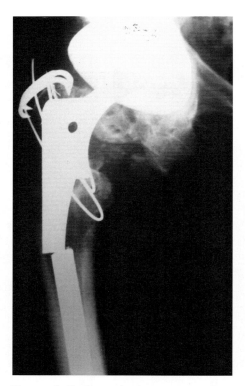

Figure 4. Radiograph demonstrates fractured fully coated cementless stem. The distal ingrown portion of the stem was easily removed with trephines; however, four trephines were required.

collar and slowly progressed from proximal to distal with a sawing motion directly against the implant to disrupt the implant–bone interface. When there is extensive ingrowth the saw frequently breaks after every several millimeters, requiring availability of several saws depending on the length of the porous coated surface.

The other alternative in this clinical scenario is to perform extended osteotomy down to the level where the stem becomes cylindrical (17). The stem can then be transected at this level with a carbide-tipped burr and the proximal portion of the stem extracted. The distal portion of the transected stem is removed with an appropriately sized trephine. Multiple trephines may be needed if there is extensive ingrowth. The trephine cutting blades tend to dull every 5 to 10 mm when cortical bone directly opposed to a metal stem is cut. This technique is equally applicable when a stem breaks, leaving a well-fixed distal cylindrical stem (Fig. 4).

Removing well-fixed cement may require specialized techniques and instruments that must be ordered ahead of time. Special instruments such as ultrasonic cement tools and cement drills and taps may not be kept on hand in many hospitals. It is therefore important to accurately determine the extent of cement removal that will be necessary and to ensure that the appropriate equipment is available to execute the plan.

General review of radiographs includes identification of the components and determination of the component positioning and fixation status, which can then be correlated with intraoperative findings. Fixation status is best determined by means of careful review of sequential plain radiographs. This is followed by planning for the actual implantation of components, which occurs in the process of templating.

TEMPLATING

The mainstay of preoperative planning for revision operations is templating of radiographs. The sequence of steps followed is analogous to that of a primary arthroplasty and follows the same steps as a surgical procedure, which typically starts on the acetabular side. A porous coated uncemented hemispheric component is the most commonly used option for revision operations (26). The acetabular template is placed against the host bone in an attempt to place the inferomedial edge of the component at the teardrop. Because the component must be placed against host bone in the superior dome, some degree of superior displacement may be necessary to achieve maximum host-bone contact. It is usually advantageous to use the largest hemispheric acetabular component to maximize the contact area and bring the center of rotation closer to the anatomic level. This has the additional benefit of ensuring maximal polyethylene thickness. A large-sized template also should be placed on the shoot-through lateral view to assure there is adequate room in the AP dimension of the acetabulum. Excessive reaming without awareness of the AP dimension of the acetabulum can result in reaming away the anterior and posterior walls. It is prudent to template for at least two options on the acetabular side. Most often a smaller component can be placed at a higher hip center with complete bone coverage, or a larger component can be placed closer to the anatomic center with some degree of uncoverage. Both options should be evaluated in the templating process. The center of rotation should be marked so that this can be matched with the femoral side template. The horizontal and vertical distance from the teardrop can be measured and compared with the contralateral normal side to assess the degree that the hip center has been changed both vertically and horizontally.

A high hip center has the advantage of a greater percentage of bone contact in most instances. It has the disadvantage of a lower overall surface area against host bone compared with a larger component. A number of studies have shown that proximal placement of the hip center alone does not appear to impart a biomechanical disadvantage as long as the hip center has moved superiorly rather than superiorly and laterally. A high hip center has an additional disadvantage of a tendency toward instability. If a high hip center is elected, the anterior inferior iliac supine may have to be partially resected to prevent impingement in flexion and internal rotation. Likewise, a portion of the ischium may have to be resected to prevent impingement in extension and external rotation.

The use of a larger component, the so-called jumbo cup, has a number of advantages. The main disadvantage is that there is a greater degree of uncoverage of the component.

Ten to twenty percent uncoverage of the component does not appear to present a clinical problem, although the use of screws for adjunctive fixation is advisable when there are minor degrees of uncoverage or when the rim is not entirely intact. If more than 20% uncoverage is predicted on the basis of templating, it may be advisable to have a structural allograft available. Distal femoral allograft is generally preferred over a femoral head because of its higher strength and larger size. When more than 30% to 40% of the component is to be supported by allograft, other options should be available. This should include the use of an antiprotrusio device or a hemipelvis allograft, both of which would be combined with a cemented all-polyethylene cup (8). Because many hospitals do not keep such equipment on hand, it is important to plan for this possibility. The use of antiprotrusio cages has increased in popularity. This is a useful adjunct to have available for cases of pelvic discontinuity, major medial wall defects, and combined superior-posterior defects (Fig. 5).

When extensive osteolysis is present, careful review of radiographs is necessary to plan appropriately. The extent of bone loss usually exceeds what is apparent on plain radiographs on both the femoral and acetabular sides (14). This normally requires numerous vials of morselized allograft. If the defects are uncontained, they may require structural graft or use of an antiprotrusio cage. Finally, when there is extensive bone loss on the acetabular side, particularly in patients who may be elderly and have low demands, the possibility of resection arthroplasty may be considered. It is important when such extensive bone loss is apparent at preoperative assessment that this be discussed with the patient so that he or she is aware resection arthroplasty may be a possibility.

After the acetabulum-side plan is complete, templating the femoral component is centered on the planned center of rotation. As on the acetabular side, there should be a plan for two if not three potential options. The ultimate goal, as in primary arthroplasty, is to restore hip biomechanics as well as possible. This entails reproducing the length, offset, and center of rotation. Of the three, it is most difficult to reproduce the center of rotation, because the acetabular component must be placed against host bone as the first

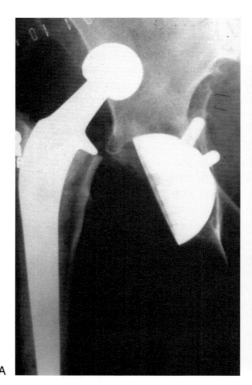
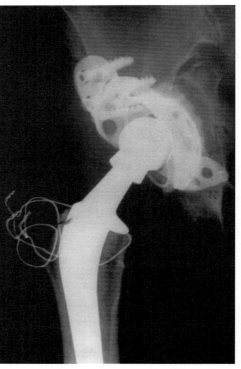

A

B

Figure 5. A: Primary total hip replacement in which posterior and medial walls were reamed away, resulting in pelvic discontinuity with impaction of cementless component. **B:** Bone deficiency and pelvic discontinuity are managed with antiprotrusio cage.

priority. Length and offset can be reproduced consistently with careful planning. Restoring offset is important for stability and abductor strength. An appropriate AP radiograph centered over the hip is required for femoral templating. This is obtained by means of internal rotation of the femur approximately 15 degrees to compensate for the usual amount of femoral anteversion. This brings the femoral neck into a plane 90 degrees from the radiograph and more accurately represents offset and the geometric configuration of the proximal femur. External rotation of the femur has the effect of representing less offset and a smaller triangular area to the metaphyseal portion of the femur (15). If the preoperative side has an external rotation contracture, it may be beneficial to measure the coordinates of the center of rotation on the basis of the acetabular templating, transpose this point to the contralateral normal side, and template the femur on that side. Templating on the normal side, which can be internally rotated, gives a more accurate depiction of the actual dimensions that will be encountered intraoperatively. When there is considerable distortion in length and offset, it is also helpful to template off the contralateral normal side. This situation exists when there is an obvious break in Shenton's line on the operative side but not the nonoperative side. Templating off the pathologic side in such a case reproduces the abnormal length or offset. Templating off the normal side corrects these abnormalities.

Placement of the femoral template varies somewhat on the basis of type of implant chosen. Proximally coated devices must fill the proximal femur and obtain contact with host bone in the proximal metaphyseal portion of the femur. Because host bone is frequently deficient in this area, it is not surprising that proximally coated devices have had an inconsistent track record in revision hip replacement (3). One method of addressing a mismatch between the proximal and distal femoral dimensions in a revision situation is to use a modular prosthesis. Devices such as the S-ROM stem (Johnson & Johnson Orthopaedics, Raynham, Mass.) have had better clinical results than most other proximally coated devices, because the proximal femur can be templated and fit independently of the distal femoral canal.

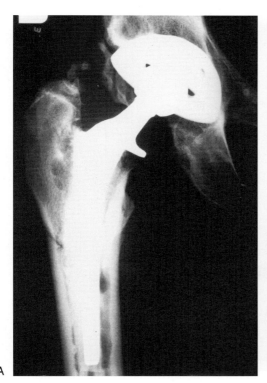
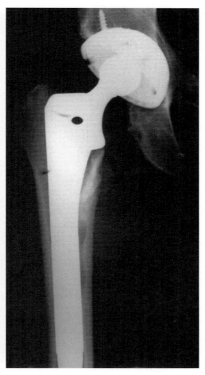

A   B

Figure 6. A: Preoperative radiograph shows femoral loosening and extensive lysis with typical amount of calcar bone loss. **B:** A 15-mm calcar replacement restored length and offset accurately.

Extensively coated devices rely more on distal fixation. The template is placed in the canal in such a manner as to ensure a scratch fit over a minimum of 4 to 5 cm distally. The stem diameter that achieves this at the isthmus is selected, and the template is moved proximally so that a short neck length coincides with the planned center of rotation. The center of rotation may be changed on the basis of the planned degree of lengthening. Because the limb on the revision side is often shorter, the center of rotation should be moved straight superiorly by the amount of lengthening planned. If the templating that fits the canal and contacts the calcar does not provide adequate length or vertical height, a calcar replacement template should be tried. Most systems allow for a 15 to 30 mm increase in vertical height over a standard component by changing to a calcar replacement. In a typical revision operation there is bone loss to the level of the lesser trochanter. Because an average neck osteotomy is about 15 mm above the lesser trochanter, a 15-mm calcar replacement is what is necessary to account for this mild degree of bone loss in many instances (Fig. 6). Bone loss to below the bottom of the lesser trochanter may require a 30 to 40 mm calcar replacement. Greater degrees of bone loss may be addressed in a number of ways. If the stem is cemented, a proximal femoral replacement can be used and the defect essentially replaced with metal. If a cementless component is used, an extensively coated device can simply be left proud. The other alternative is to use a structural allograft composite with either a cemented or cementless stem. In such cases, it is important to try to match the allograft segment to the host bone. The allograft segment should be larger at the isthmus than the host bone to allow cementing of the stem proximally if this is elected. This necessitates measurement of the diameter of the isthmus of the host bone and radiographs of the allograft to ensure that there is adequate diameter to introduce the stem proximally.

The presence of a proximal cortical shell several centimeters long followed by a relatively narrow isthmus presents a situation that is suboptimal for conventional cemented or cementless revision stems (3). In instances of this general description,

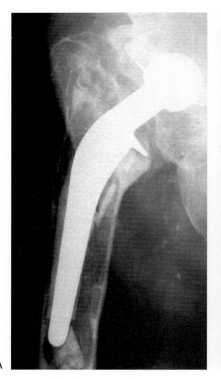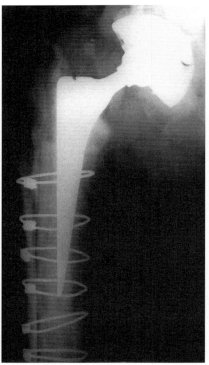

A   B

Figure 7. A: Preoperative radiograph shows proximal cortical shell with narrow distal isthmus. **B:** The condition was managed with impaction grafting with a structural strut graft to reinforce the thin cortical shell laterally.

impaction grafting has been recommended. This technique is discussed elsewhere. For planning purposes, however, impaction grafting requires a host of specialized instruments and accessories. If this option is a serious consideration, extensive long-term planning is necessary, not the least aspect of which is surgeon education. There are several variations of this technique, each of which is accompanied by specialized instruments and implants (Fig. 7).

A stem of sufficient length should be used to bypass any large defects or deficiencies in the proximal cortical tube by at least two to three cortical diameters. It is equally important to perform templating on a lateral radiograph to assess the bow of the femur. Stems greater than 160 to 180 mm in length usually impinge on the anterior cortex if they are straight (Fig. 8). If stem lengths of 200 mm or greater are used, there is a strong likelihood a bowed stem will be necessary to avoid eccentric placement of the stem, if not stem perforation or femoral fracture.

Templating for a cemented stem differs in that there must be a circumferential cement column of at least 2 mm. The cement column generally is more than adequate proximally and only becomes an issue distally near the isthmus. It is difficult to introduce a cemented stem longer than 160 mm without the tip being quite eccentric. For this reason many surgeons try to avoid cementing beyond the isthmus. It is also difficult to plug the canal and obtain pressurization with cemented long stems. Revision of such stems is exceedingly difficult, making this an option used more for salvage operations than for routine revision.

In addition to assessing the anterior bow of the femur, it is important to assess the presence of the varus bow on the AP view. A phenomenon of remodeling into varus has been described after loosening of a femoral stem (23). This can make it difficult to introduce a revision stem without risk for perforation or fracture. This may necessitate either an extended osteotomy or a transverse osteotomy at the apex of the varus bow to allow implantation of a revision stem (Fig. 9). When transverse osteotomy is a possibility, availability of strut grafts and wires or cables is advisable to add rotational stability to the construct. Strut grafts are used frequently when there are areas of extreme cortical thinning, perforations, or deficient areas in the femur from lysis. The use of strut grafts and

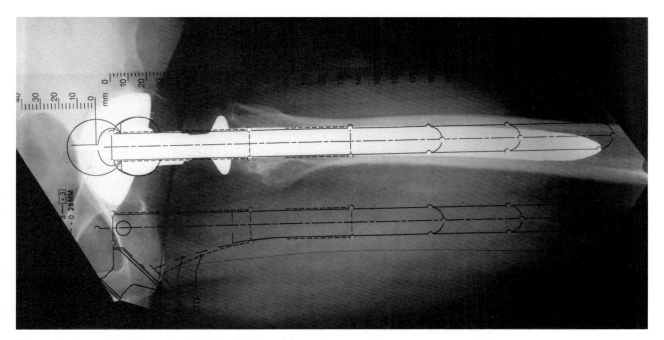

Figure 8. Lateral radiograph of 10-inch (25 cm) bowed cementless stem centered in canal. Overlying template shows that use of a straight stem would have resulted in femur fracture or stem perforation.

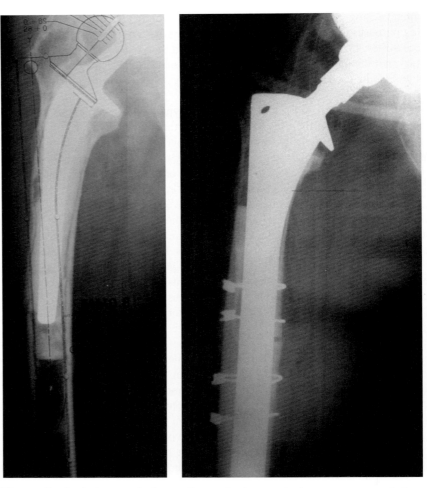

Figure 9. A: Anteroposterior radiograph demonstrates varus remodeling. Template demonstrates that insertion of long stem would not be possible with the current femoral alignment. **B:** Postoperative radiograph shows cementless long stem with strut graft reinforcing the transfemoral osteotomy site at apex of deformity.

morselized graft is so common in revision surgery that it is probably advisable to have these materials available in virtually all revision operations.

CONCLUSION

Revision total hip arthroplasty presents a wide array of challenges to the orthopedic surgeon. A broad spectrum of pathologic conditions are encountered, as are a wide variety of potential solutions. Revision operations are associated with a higher complication rate and longer operative times, which have been documented in a number of studies. This may be inevitable to some degree because of the complexity of many of these operations. Careful preoperative planning can minimize operative time and help the surgeon anticipate many of the potential complications. This minimizes the occurrence of complications and allows patients to be better informed of the risks involved. Such an organized approach increases the likelihood of an optimal result for the patient and a more satisfying experience for the surgeon and operative team.

ACKNOWLEDGMENT

The author wishes to thank Mrs. Gerrie Savage for her tireless efforts in compiling and editing material for this chapter.

REFERENCES

1. Aaron A, Weinstein D, Thickman D, Eilert R. Comparison of orthoroentgenography and computed tomography in the measurement of limb-length discrepancy. *J Bone Joint Surg Am* 1992;74:897–902.
2. Barrack RL. Modularity of prosthetic implants. *J AAOS* 1994;2:16–25.
3. Barrack RL, Folgueras A. Results of revision total hip replacement. *J AAOS* 1995;3:79–85.
4. Barrack RL, Folgueras A, Munn B, Tvetden D, Sharkey P. Pelvic lysis and polyethylene wear at five to eight years in an uncemented total hip. *Clin Orthop* 1997;335:211–217.
5. Barrack RL, Harris WH. The value of aspiration of the hip joint before revision total hip arthroplasty. *J Bone Joint Surg Am* 1993;66:66–76.
6. Barrack RL, Tejeiro W, Carpenter LJ, Hoffman G. Surgeon work input and risk in primary versus revision total joint arthroplasty. *J Arthroplasty* 1995;10:1–6.
7. Berger R, Fletcher F, Donaldson TK, Wasilewski RL, Peterson M, Rubash HE. A dynamic test to diagnose loose uncemented femoral total hip components. *Clin Orthop* 1996;330:115–123.
8. Berry DJ, Muller ME. Revision arthroplasty using an anti-protrusio cage for massive acetabular bone deficiency. *J Bone Joint Surg Br* 1992;74:711–715.
9. Cameron HU. Hip surgery in aortofemoral bypass patient. *Orthop Rev* 1988;17:195–197.
10. Capello WN. Preoperative planning of the total hip arthroplasty. *Instr Course Lect* 1986;35:249–257.
11. Capello WN. Preoperative planning of the total hip arthroplasty. *Instr Course Lect* 1986;35:249–257.
12. Chimento GF, Finger S, Barrack RL. Gram stain detection of infection during revision arthroplasty. *J Bone Joint Surg Br* 1996;78:838–839.
13. D'Antonio JA. Preoperative templating and choosing the implant for primary THA in the young patient. *Instr Course Lect* 1994;43:339–346.
14. D'Antonio JA. Periprosthetic bone loss of the acetabulum: classification and management. *Orthop Clin North Am* 1992;23:279–290.
15. Engh CA. Recent advances in cementless total hip arthroplasty using the AML prosthesis. *Tech Orthop* 1991;6:59–72.
16. Fehring TK, Guilford WB, Baron J. Assessment of intrapelvic cement and screws in revision total hip arthroplasty. *J Arthroplasty* 1992;7:509–518.
17. Glassman AH, Engh CA. The removal of porous-coated femoral hip stems. *Clin Orthop* 1992;285:164–180.
18. Harris WH, Mulroy RD Jr, Maloney WJ, Burke DW, Chandler HP, Zalenski EB. Intraoperative measurement of rotational stability of femoral components of total hip arthroplasty. *Clin Orthop* 1991;266:119–126.
19. Jacobs JJ, Kull LR, Frey GA, et al. Early failure of acetabular components inserted without cement after previous pelvic irradiation. *J Bone Joint Surg Am* 1995;77:1829–1835.
20. Jasty M, Schutzer S, Tepper J, Willett C, Stracher MA, Harris WH. Radiation-blocking shields to localize periarticular radiation precisely for prevention of hererotopic bone formation around uncemented total hip arthroplasties. *Clin Orthop* 1990;257:138–145.
21. Kennedy WF, Byrne TF, Majid HA, Pavlak LL. Sciatic nerve monitoring during revision total hip arthroplasty. *Clin Orthop* 1991;264:223–227.
22. Krackow KA, Steinman H, Cohn BT, Jones LC. Clinical experience with a triradiate exposure of the hip for difficult total hip arthroplasty. *J Arthroplasty* 1991;73:783–786.
23. Kronick JL, Sekundiak T, Paprosky WG. Proximal femoral deformity secondary to loosening and osteolysis: the effect on reimplantation. *J Arthroplasty* 1997;12:226–227.
24. Lombardi AV, Mallory TH, Kraus TJ, Vaughn BK. Preliminary report on the S-ROM constraining acetabular insert: a retrospective clinical experience. *Orthopedics* 1991;14:297–303.
25. Lonner JH, Desai P, Dicesare PE, Steiner G, Zuckerman JD. The reliability of analysis of intraoperative frozen sections for identifying active infection during revision hip or knee arthroplasty. *J Bone Joint Surg Am* 1996;78:1553–1558.
26. Petrera P, Rubash HE. Revision total hip arthroplasty: the acetabular component. *J AAOS* 1995;3:15–21.
27. Ranawat CS. Preoperative planning for total hip arthroplasty. In: Dorr LD, ed. *Techniques in orthopaedics: revision of total hip and knee.* Baltimore: University Park Press, 1984:1–7.
28. Silverton CD, Conlen A, Rosenberg AG. Complications of a cable grip system used for trochanteric osteotomy fixation in total hip arthroplasty. *Orthop Trans* 1995;19(2):304–305.
29. Williamson JA, Reckling RW. Limb-length discrepancy and related problems following total hip joint replacement. *Clin Orthop* 1978;134:135–138.
30. Woolson ST, Harris WH. A method of intraoperative limb length measurement in total hip arthroplasty. *Clin Orthop* 1985;194:207–210.
31. Younger TI, Bradford MS, Magnus RE, Paprosky WG. Extended proximal femoral osteotomy: a new technique for femoral revision arthroplasty. *J Arthroplasty* 1995;10:1–10.

Revision Total Hip Arthroplasty,
edited by Marvin E. Steinberg and Jonathan P. Garino,
Lippincott Williams & Wilkins, Philadelphia © 1999.

12

Surgical Exposures

John J. Callaghan

The complexity of revision total hip arthroplasty has required orthopedic surgeons to be familiar with a number of approaches to the hip. Creativity and new approaches have been required to address the surgical demands the revision situation has created. No greater controversy and disagreement among surgeons who perform reconstructive procedures on the hips of adults exists than deciding which approach is most appropriate for performing the total hip procedure (3,14,17,21,22,25). The following statements of John Charnley (4) and Maurice Mueller (26) are exemplary of this controversy.

> *The most gentle way of retracting the gluteus medius and minimus is by detaching the greater trochanter. In a heavy muscled patient a considerable volume of gluteus medius lies anterior to the greater trochanter. How much of the muscle remains active after anterior exposure without detaching trochanter is unknown. To the damage that retraction may inflict on the gluteus muscles may be added the danger of damaging the nerve supply to the tensor fascia lata.*
>
> *John Charnley*
>
> *If the right instruments are used and if some points of technique during the operation are carefully considered, you will soon be able to do 80 to 90 per cent of total hip replacement without removal of the greater trochanter. The operation is much easier and quicker.*
>
> *Maurice Mueller*

Several basic principles are important in making any approach to the hip. Appropriate patient positioning on the operating table is necessary. Appropriate placement of the incision in relation to patient position is imperative. Fascial planes must be adequately mobilized. The surgeon must maximize exposure with minimal soft-tissue damage. Especially in revision operations, a surgeon must be able to make

J. J. Callaghan: Department of Orthopaedics, University of Iowa College of Medicine, Iowa City, Iowa 52242.

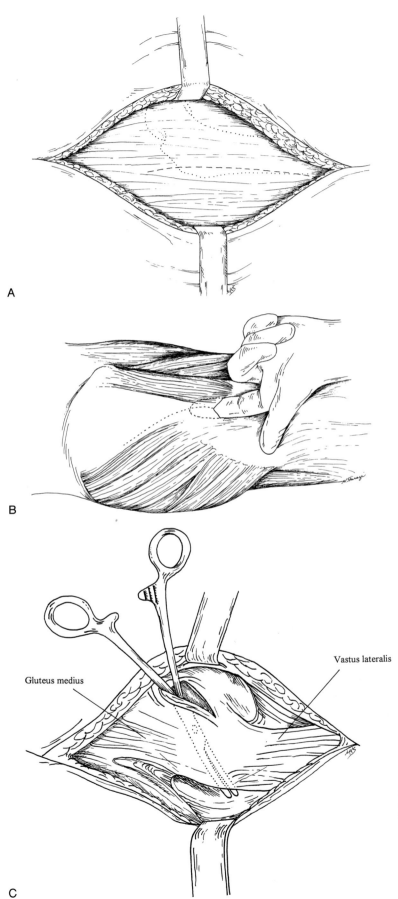

A

B

Gluteus medius

Vastus lateralis

C

Figure 1. When exposing a hip that has undergone a previous operation several steps allow optimal exposure with any approach. **A:** Reflect the adipose soft tissue from the underlying iliotibial band. This also allows closure of the fascia without straggling superficial fat. **B:** Dissect the iliotibial band from the underlying vastus lateralis and gluteus medius muscles. **C:** Expose the anterior and posterior borders of the gluteus medius muscle.

the approach he or she has chosen as extensile as possible, when necessary, to allow better exposure to the pelvis and distal femur. If five basic steps are taken during exposure in the revision situation, many approaches can allow the exposure necessary to remove the previous components and insert the new components while providing minimal soft-tissue and bony damage and allowing reconstruction of the soft-tissue envelope around the hip (Fig. 1). The five following steps provide the basis for surgical exposure in revision operations:

1. The iliotibial band has to be dissected away from the vastus lateralis and gluteus medius muscles. This can present various amounts of difficulty depending on how much scar is present between the iliotibial band and underlying vastus lateralis and gluteus medius fascia. The iliotibial band is adequately reflected from the vastus lateralis muscle posteriorly when the gluteus maximus sling insertion into the linea aspera is identified. The fascia is adequately freed anteriorly when the most medial and inferior borders of the gluteus medius muscle are exposed by means of reflection of the tensor fascia lata muscle anteriorly.

2. The anterior and posterior borders of the gluteus medius muscle must be identified and freed of surrounding scar. Of note is the realization that one third of the gluteus medius muscle is anterior to the hip capsule rather than superior to the capsule.

3. After identification of the anterior and posterior borders of the gluteus medius muscle, any surgical approach requires reflection of the gluteus medius muscle and the greater trochanter. In the case of the posterior approach, the femur and muscles are retracted anteriorly. In the anterolateral approach, the muscles are reflected posteriorly. In the direct lateral approach, the gluteus medius muscle is incised in the vertical direction. In the case of conventional transtrochanteric osteotomy, the gluteus medius muscle is incised with the greater trochanter and reflected superiorly.

4. Capsulotomy or capsulectomy is performed after adequate mobilization of the gluteus medius and minimus muscles.

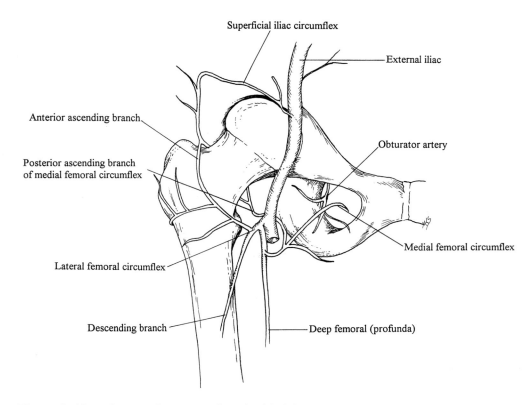

Figure 2. Vascular supply surrounding the hip joint.

5. Skeletonization of the femur from the capsule is undertaken to expose the proximal femur and to mobilize the proximal femur away from the acetabulum.

If these principles are used, various approaches to the hip can be taken to obtain optimal results in revision hip operations.

NEUROVASCULAR ANATOMY OF THE HIP

As with any surgical exposure, in revision hip operations the surgeon must thoroughly understand the course of the nerves and arteries surrounding the hip joint to avoid damage to the neurovascular structures when obtaining exposure and when applying retractors to maintain exposure. The arteries shown in Fig. 2 are the obturator artery, femoral artery, profundus femoral artery, and medial and lateral femoral circumflex arteries. The course of these arteries must be understood. In addition, the course of the nerves surrounding the joint should be thoroughly understood. These include the sciatic nerve, femoral nerve, and obturator nerve (Fig. 3). During hip operations one cannot avoid retraction on the various neurovascular structures. However, understanding their course prevents unintentional retractor placement into one of the structures and excessive retraction on one of the important neurovascular structures.

APPROACHES

The remainder of this chapter describes the standard workhorse approaches in revision operations and in primary operations (posterior, anterolateral, direct lateral, and greater

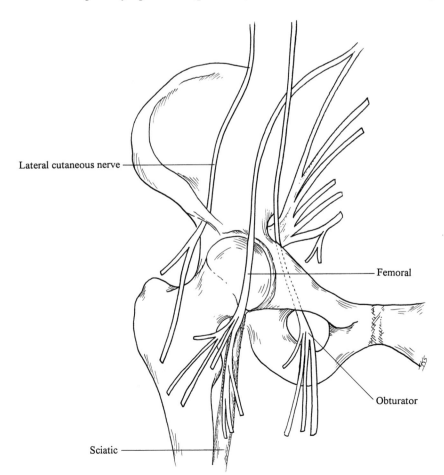

Figure 3. Nerves surrounding the hip joint.

trochanteric osteotomy) followed by three more recently used approaches (extensile direct lateral, greater trochanteric slide, and extended femoral osteotomy). Finally, techniques for exposing the inner wall of the ilium are described.

Posterior Approach to the Hip

Some form of posterior approach is commonly used in both primary and revision situations (8,12,13,20,23,24,28). The classic posterior approach, sometimes called the Southern approach, proceeded over the posterior buttock and greater trochanter. It was developed through the inferior aspect of the gluteus maximus. This approach can make femoral exposure difficult when the femur is placed in the flexed, internally rotated position. For this reason many surgeons, I included, have used a modified approach starting 5 to 8 cm proximal and posterior to the greater trochanter and extending the approach laterally over the greater trochanter and along the lateral shaft of the femur approximately 7 to 10 cm distal to the tip of the greater trochanter. The iliotibial band is identified. Especially among obese patients, the fat overlying the iliotibial band is reflected anteriorly and posteriorly to prevent entrapment of fat during wound closure. After the fascia of the iliotibial band and tensor fascia is incised, the gluteus maximus muscle is spread anteriorly and posteriorly to identify bleeders during dissection. The fat and bursa overlying the posterior external rotator muscles of the hip and greater trochanter and gluteal maximus sling are incised. The posterior border of the gluteus medius is identified as is the piriformis tendon. The gluteus minimus is dissected from the superior capsule, and a retractor is placed between the superior capsule and gluteus medius, superior to the piriformis tendon (Fig. 4). The piriformis tendon, conjoint tendon (superior and inferior gemelli and obturator internus), the obturator externus, quadratus femoris, and gluteus maximus sling are incised (Fig. 5). Perforating vessels from the profundus femoral artery coursing from the linea aspera are ligated. Bleeders that come from the inferior capsule in resection of this "external rotator sleeve" are branches of the medial femoral circumflex artery. The largest and most troublesome branch is actually just adjacent to the obturator externus, as opposed to the common belief that it lies within the quadratus femoris muscle.

After reflection of the external rotator sleeve, the posterior capsule can be incised or excised. The anterior capsule can be excised by means of externally rotating the femur, finding the anterior border of the gluteus medius, and placing a retractor beneath the gluteus medius and minimus superior to the capsule. A second retractor can be placed

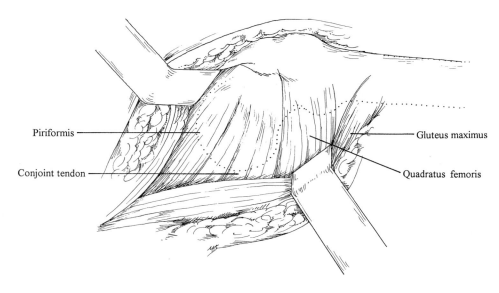

Piriformis

Conjoint tendon

Gluteus maximus

Quadratus femoris

Figure 4. Exposure of the external rotators of the hip through the posterior approach.

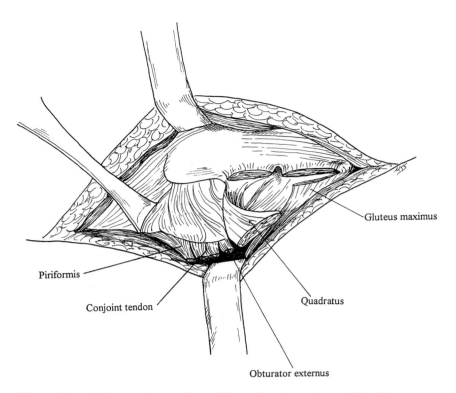

Figure 5. Incision and retraction of the external rotators of the hip.

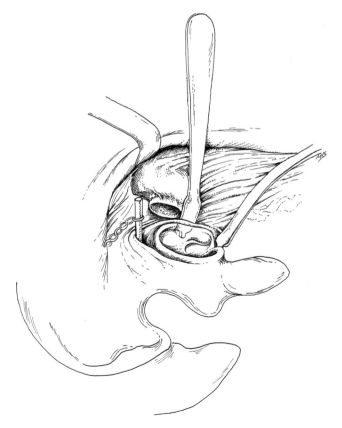

Figure 6. Position of retractors to expose the acetabulum through the posterior approach. Rectus femoris incision can aid in anterior retraction of the femur.

between the capsule and indirect head of the rectus femoris. This retractor is placed over the iliopectineal eminence into the pelvis. A third retractor can be placed inferior to the anterior capsule, and the capsule can be excised from anterior to posterior, avoiding any potential damage to the femoral vessels by pass pointing from posterior to anterior. Inferior bleeding during this dissection arises from the lateral femoral circumflex arteries and vein, which must be ligated.

After a capsulotomy or capsulectomy is performed, the proximal femur should be skeletonized both anteriorly and posteriorly to retract the femur away from the acetabulum (Fig. 6) and to allow internal rotation of the femur to visualize the femoral canal (Fig. 7). A common mistake is to take out the index femoral component before performing all of these procedures because the component provides tensioning of the capsule and orientation to the joint. If one has trouble reflecting the femoral shaft anterior to the acetabulum with a curved retractor placed over the anterior lip of the acetabulum as superiorly as possible, a more extensile exposure can be obtained with incision of the indirect head of the rectus femoris as it inserts over the capsule and anterior superior acetabulum and incision of the posterior border of the gluteus minimus. To expose the acetabulum in this approach, I use a straight cobra retractor in the obturator foramen and resect the transverse acetabular ligament, and place this retractor inferior to the cotyloid notch. A second retractor is placed anterior to the acetabulum usually at the 1 o'clock position and

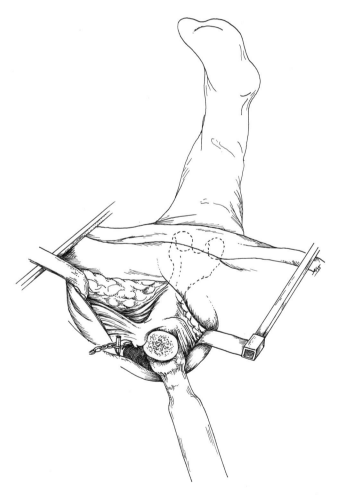

Figure 7. Exposure of the femoral canal by means of flexion and internal rotation of the femur. This requires skeletonization of the proximal femoral canal from the capsule in the revision situation.

optimally over the anterior inferior iliac spine to retract the femoral shaft anteriorly. A Steinmann pin is placed anterior to the 12 o'clock position to retract the gluteus medius anteriorly and superiorly. Finally a bent Hohmann retractor is placed into the ischium and stays anterior to the posterior capsule to not injure the sciatic nerve. The anterior retractors are placed with the femur in flexion and the posterior retractors are placed with the femur in extension to avoid damage to the neurovascular structures.

When possible, closure through the posterior approach includes reattaching the piriformis tendon, conjoint tendon, and gluteal sling to the femoral shaft (Fig. 8). If the capsule is present, this is also reattached in the repair. The sutures are placed through drill holes in the greater trochanter and no. 1 or no. 2 nonabsorbable suture is used. The femur should be internally rotated when the tendons are approximated to not overtighten the external rotator flap; when the patient stands up these sutures will pull out if they are too tight.

To reiterate, the ways to increase exposure through this approach include incising the indirect head of the rectus femoris tendon, incising the posterior part of the gluteus minimus, and fully incising the gluteus maximus sling insertion into the linea aspera. For a tight hip, the iliopsoas tendon insertion into the lesser trochanter can be incised.

Anterolateral Approach to the Hip

The anterolateral approach to the hip is especially useful when there is increased concern for postoperative dislocation. This includes the cases of patients who have mental compromise, those with Parkinson's disease, or those with previous strokes. Care should be taken to preserve the gluteus medius muscle when this approach is used.

Positioning of the patient for the anterolateral approach to the hip is varied. The patient can either be placed supine or bumped with the posterior buttock brought 45 degrees forward. The incision is made posterior to the tensor fascia lata muscle between it and the gluteus medius. Abduction of the leg can help in finding this interval. It is usually located one hand's breadth posterior to the anterior superior iliac spine. I use a gently curved incision for this approach. The incision starts approximately 7 cm proximal to the greater trochanter, slightly anteriorly, and proceeds over the mid to posterior portion of the greater trochanter distally followed by distal extension over the shaft of the femur curving slightly anterior at the distal limb. The tensor fascia lata muscle is reflected anteriorly. The anterior border of the gluteus medius is then identified.

Especially in revision operations, although also in primary operations, the anterior one third of the gluteus medius must be retracted. The anterior border classically is incised from its insertion into the greater trochanter (Fig. 9). I prefer making a 6 cm incision through the belly of the muscle ending at the superior anterior corner of the greater trochanter and reflecting this portion of the gluteus medius anteriorly. This allows

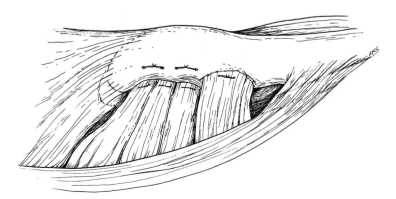

Figure 8. Reapproximation of the external rotators to the femoral shaft.

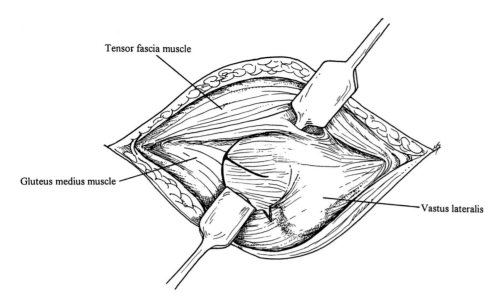

Tensor fascia muscle

Gluteus medius muscle

Vastus lateralis

Figure 9. Anterolateral approach to the hip with the tensor fascia lata muscle reflected anteriorly and a slit in the gluteus medius tendon with posterior retraction of the tendon.

exposure to the anterior capsule of the hip. A retractor is placed superior to the femoral neck to reflect the remainder of the gluteus medius posteriorly. A second retractor is placed inferior to the femoral neck, and a final retractor is placed beneath the indirect head of the rectus femoris and over the iliopectineal line of the pelvis medially. For a tight hip the indirect head of the rectus also is incised. Along with the attachment of the anterior third of the gluteus medius, a portion of the gluteus minimus (with or without a sliver of bone) (5) is detached from the greater trochanter to gain exposure. These tendons are usually retracted by means of placement of large nonabsorbable sutures through their insertions properly to realign the muscles at the time of closure.

An important step of the capsulotomy or capsulectomy through the anterolateral approach is to start the superior limb of the capsule incision as far posterior to the 12 o'clock position as possible and end as far posterior to the 6 o'clock position as possible. This allows the femoral head or femoral prosthesis to be dislocated from the acetabulum and allows retraction of the femoral shaft away from the acetabulum to better expose the acetabulum (Fig. 10). If one is struggling through this approach, more posterior capsular excision or incision should be performed.

To visualize adequately the hip through this approach, it is important to be able to bring the femoral shaft into 90 degrees of external rotation and to be able to bring the foot of the patient up into the groin so as to easily retract the femur. Once again, a straight cobra retractor is placed inferior to the cotyloid notch of the acetabulum. A curved retractor is placed anterior to the acetabulum. A Steinmann pin is placed superior to the acetabulum, and a bent Hohmann Retractor is placed into the ischium. Ischial and obturator foramen retractors are used to retract the femoral shaft away from the acetabulum. The inferior capsule must be excised to allow this exposure of a tight hip. This allows visualization of the acetabulum. The femoral shaft is well visualized by bringing the leg into external rotation and the knee into flexion, which brings the foot into the groin (Fig. 11). When preparing the femoral canal, one should avoid retraction on the posterior aspect of the gluteus medius, because this can contribute to heterotopic ossification. In closure of the anterolateral approach to the hip, the anteriorly reflected anterior one third of the gluteus medius is reattached to the greater trochanter through drill holes by means of heavy, nonabsorbable suture.

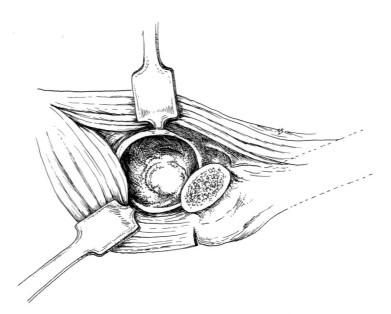

Figure 10. Exposure of the acetabulum through the anterolateral approach to the hip. The exposure is similar when a direct lateral approach is used.

Direct Lateral Approach to the Hip

The direct lateral approach to the hip was originally popularized by Hardinge (10). It has been modified since that time (2,6,7), because Hardinge describes longitudinally going through the posterior 10% to 20% of the gluteus medius muscle and tendon. Today most

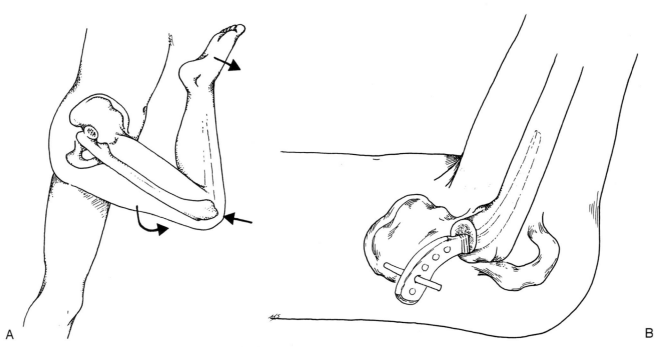

A   B

Figure 11. Adequate capsular release allows the foot to be brought into the groin (**A**) to allow exposure to the femoral canal for cement removal, preparation (**B**), and insertion of the new prosthesis.

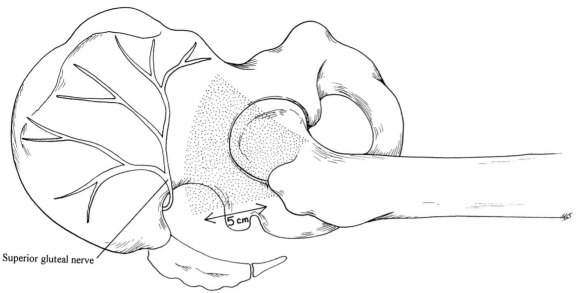

Superior gluteal nerve

Figure 12. Course of the superior gluteal nerve. Longitudinal incision in the gluteus medius muscle should not extend more than 5 cm proximal to the greater trochanter tip.

surgeons perform the approach going half way between the anterior and posterior aspects of the gluteus medius and carrying the incision distally into the vastus lateralis to make a gluteus medius vastus lateralis sleeve (11). The approach is carried out over the center of the greater trochanter starting 7 cm proximally and continuing 7 to 10 cm distally. The interval between gluteus maximus and tensor fascia lata muscle is entered. The anterior and posterior borders of the gluteus medius are identified.

The gluteus medius is incised longitudinally, starting no more than 5 cm proximal to the greater trochanter to avoid damage to the superior gluteal nerve (Fig. 12) (16). The

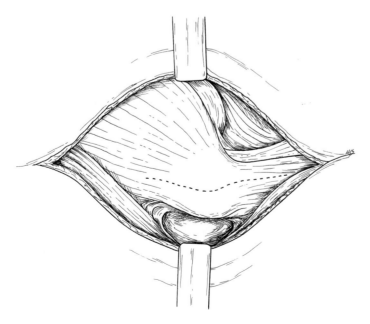

Figure 13. Longitudinal incision through the gluteus medius muscle and vastus lateralis fascia used in the direct lateral approach to the hip.

incision is carried through the gluteus medius and posterior to the gluteus minimus tendon and extended distally 5 to 7 cm longitudinally into the vastus lateralis fascia (Fig. 13). The gluteus medius muscle and gluteus minimus muscle are incised from the greater trochanter, and the vastus lateralis is incised from the anterolateral femoral shaft (Fig. 14). Some surgeons take a small wafer of greater trochanteric bone when incising the gluteus medius.

The gluteus medius–vastus lateralis flap is reflected anteriorly, as is the minimus that has been incised. This allows exposure to the femoral head and anterior capsule similar to that obtained through the anterolateral approach. I consider this a modification of the anterolateral approach if the anterior portion of the gluteus medius is reflected anteriorly rather than posteriorly through the anterolateral approach. The main difference is that the gluteus medius–vastus lateralis sleeve is kept in continuity through the direct lateral approach. The same considerations of superior posterior capsulotomy and inferior posterior capsulotomy are important to adequately retract the femoral shaft away from the acetabulum and gain proper exposure to the acetabulum. The vastus lateralis, gluteus medius, gluteus minimus muscles and vastus fascia are meticulously closed. The gluteus medius and gluteus minimus with or without the wafer of greater trochanteric bone are reapproximated to the greater trochanter through drill holes and use of large, nonabsorbable sutures (Figs. 15 and 16).

The benefit of the direct lateral and of the anterolateral approach is the great postoperative stability achieved with these approaches. The concern of some surgeons, I included, is the potential for the gluteus medius to detach from the greater trochanter with potential for the patient to have a postoperative limp. I have reoperated on patients who had undergone this approach, and no gluteus medius was left at revision (a bald greater trochanter). If this is the case for an elderly patient, one should consider using a constrained acetabular component to prevent postoperative dislocation. Otherwise one can perform tenodesis of the iliotibial band into the greater trochanter to provide some stability.

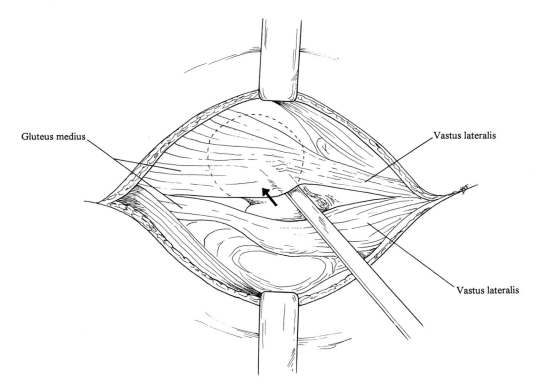

Figure 14. Dissection of the gluteus medius and gluteus minimus from the anterior superior hip capsule and greater trochanter and of the vastus lateralis from the femoral shaft.

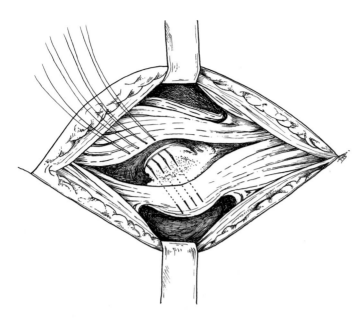

Figure 15. Preparation of the greater trochanter with drill holes to anchor sutures brought through the gluteus medius–vastus lateralis sleeve.

Transtrochanteric Osteotomy Approach to the Hip

Although in the past the transtrochanteric osteotomy to the hip was considered the approach of choice adequately to expose a difficult primary hip and most revision hips, there has been a tendency to avoid this approach because of problems associated with nonunion of the greater trochanter and migration of the trochanter. However, I still consider it an important way of exposing a failed hip replacement, especially when there is curvature of the femoral shaft. The curvature of the femoral shaft usually is a varus bow to the femur caused by remodeling when a femoral stem has loosened.

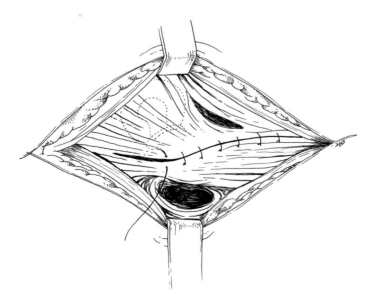

Figure 16. Final reapproximation of the gluteus medius–vastus lateralis sleeve.

The patient can be placed semisupine or in the lateral decubitus position for this approach. The incision is started approximately 7 cm superior to the greater trochanter, proceeds over the middle aspect of the greater trochanter, and is continued distally approximately 7 cm. The incision is carried through the iliotibial band to reflect the tensor fascia muscle anteriorly and the gluteus maximus muscle posteriorly. The anterior and posterior borders of the gluteus medius are identified (Fig. 17). I prefer to identify the vastus lateralis ridge of the greater trochanter and reflect the vastus lateralis distally starting 1 cm proximal to the vastus lateralis ridge. Reflecting the sleeve inferiorly allows one to bring the sleeve over the greater trochanteric wires at the time of wound closure.

I perform the greater trochanteric osteotomy 0.5 cm above the vastus lateralis ridge to enable lateral placement of the greater trochanter at the time of closure (Fig. 18). The osteotomy is performed with Smith-Petersen gouges to provide a crescent-type osteotomy. Chevron osteotomies also have been used (1). In my experience, however, Chevron osteotomies carry at risk for fracture at the time of reattachment of the greater trochanter. They also do not allow any anterior or posterior placement of the greater trochanter, which may be necessary or helpful.

The osteotomy is performed to separate the greater trochanter from anterolateral capsule to maintain the integrity of the gluteus medius and minimus with the greater trochanter bone. The gluteus medius and minimus are reflected medially to the ilium to expose completely the superior capsule. The anterior capsule is easily exposed, and the posterior capsule is exposed through incision of the piriformis muscle and conjoint tendon. A capsulotomy or capsulectomy and skeletonization of the femur are performed.

I prefer to dislocate the femoral component or femoral head anteriorly and bring the leg over the anterior side of the bed in relation to the patient (Fig. 19). Sterile stockinet is placed on the leg to prevent contamination when the leg is brought back onto the operating room table. During the entire procedure the assistant or surgeon in front of the patient must

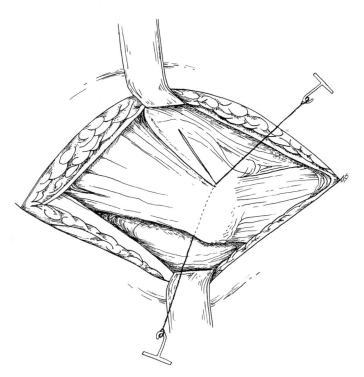

Figure 17. After the iliotibial band is incised, the anterior and posterior borders of the gluteus medius muscle are identified. A Gigli saw can be placed between the gluteus medius and the capsule for exposure in the transtrochanteric approach to the hip.

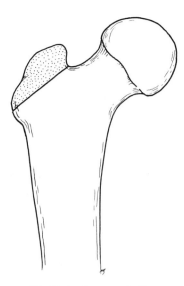

Figure 18. Osteotomy of the greater trochanter exits the lateral cortex superior to the vastus lateralis ridge.

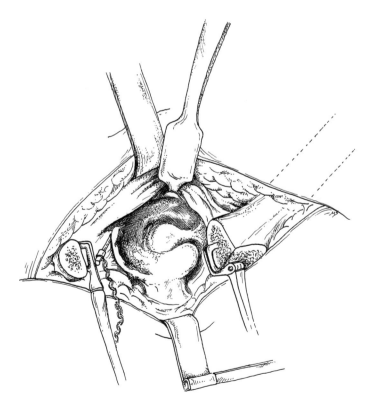

Figure 19. After capsular release the femoral shaft can be retracted away from the acetabulum. A chevron osteotomy has been performed.

prevent the leg from dangling, which prevents stretching of the sciatic nerve. In my operating room, one assistant is always aware of the need to place pressure over the anterior knee to drive the femoral shaft posteriorly. Flexion of the knee also allows relaxation of the sciatic nerve. This approach most adequately allows retraction of the femoral shaft away from the acetabulum and provides optimal visualization of the acetabulum. I use a four-wire technique to reattach the greater trochanter (16-gauge chrome cobalt wire) (Fig. 20).

After the procedure is completed, the hip is located, and the leg is placed on a Mayo stand in wide abduction (approximately 40 degrees). Two wires have been placed through the lesser trochanter and brought anterior and posterior to the femoral shaft. In the cemented situation, two wires have been placed through the lateral cortex of the femoral shaft approximately 5 cm distal to the osteotomy and cemented with the stem. In the uncemented situation, I also place these two wires through the lateral cortex and keep them as lateral as possible to not excessively scratch the uncemented femoral component. These wires are then brought medially to the greater trochanter and over the top of the greater trochanter. The anterior posterior wires are brought through drill holes in the greater trochanter. I first reapproximate the lateral wires going over the greater trochanter to adequately position the greater trochanter in the superior inferior direction. The horizontal wires coming through the lesser trochanter and through drill holes in the greater

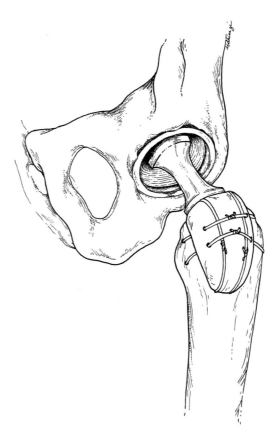

Figure 20. Four-wire technique to reattach the greater trochanter. Two vertical wires are placed through the lateral cortex of the femoral shaft 3 to 5 cm below the vastus lateralis ridge. These wires exit the proximal shaft and proceed around the top of the greater trochanter. Two horizontal wires are placed through the lesser trochanter around the femoral shaft and through the greater trochanter.

trochanter are then reapproximated. I usually advance the greater trochanter at least 1 cm distal to the vastus lateralis ridge where the trochanteric osteotomy was performed. One does not need to tighten excessively the wires because the patient's femur is in wide abduction, and the wires will tighten as the patient brings the leg into adduction, as with any other tension-band procedure. One common mistake with reattaching the greater trochanter either in this situation or with extended osteotomy is to overtighten the wires, which leads to breakage of the wire or fracture of the extended osteotomy segment.

No active abduction is allowed for the first 6 weeks after this procedure. Especially in the revision situation, I prescribe braces for many patients after trochanteric osteotomy and the other approaches I have described. In my own practice, I am unable to decrease my dislocation rate in revision operations to less than 8% or 10%. Few of these hips have recurrent dislocations, but without bracing I believe my rate could be higher.

Additional Extensile Exposures That Allow Maintenance of the Gluteus Medius–Vastus Lateralis Sleeve

I am convinced that maintaining the gluteus medius–vastus lateralis sleeve may prevent some of the problems associated with nonunion and migration of the greater trochanter. Three approaches have been developed for better exposure of the hip in revision operations while the gluteus medius–vastus lateralis sleeve is maintained rather than incising across the sleeve, as is done in traditional greater trochanteric osteotomy. These approaches include extensive gluteus medius–vastus lateralis slitting, as championed by Head et al. (15), the greater trochanteric slide as championed by Glassman et al. (9), and extended femoral osteotomy as championed by Wagner and modified by Paprosky (30).

Extensile Direct Lateral Approach

The extensile direct lateral approach is simply an extension of the direct lateral approach. The gluteus medius is incised longitudinally in its mid or posterior third. This incision is carried distally along the posterior rather than the middle aspect of the vastus lateralis fascia (Fig. 21). The entire vastus lateralis fascia and muscle and the anterior one half or two thirds of the gluteus medius are dissected subperiosteally from the greater trochanter and lateral femoral shaft; this large muscle mass is retracted anteriorly

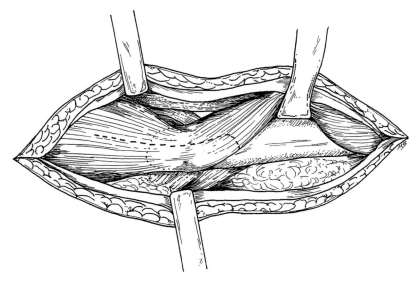

Figure 21. Line of incision through the gluteus medius muscle and posterior to the vastus lateralis muscle in the extended direct lateral approach.

(Fig. 22). The posterior gluteus medius is dissected subperiosteally and posteriorly to allow total exposure of the greater trochanter and lateral femoral shaft if necessary (27). This allows excellent exposure of the femoral shaft and allows one to osteotomize the shaft of the femur or make cortical windows in the femur to more easily remove cement without damaging the femur. Although this approach and extended osteotomy may be considered radical, with more experience in revision surgery, many surgeons consider them the more conservative approach to avoid femoral fracture and excessive perforation of the femoral canal during removal of cement or of secure bone ingrown in uncemented components. After the operation, the gluteus medius is reapproximated from front to back and reattached to the greater trochanter through drill holes. I recommend use of large (no. 5) nonabsorbable suture for reapproximation of the gluteus medius to the greater trochanter. Active abduction should be prevented for the first 6 weeks after the operation.

Greater Trochanteric Slide

A modification of the transtrochanteric approach to the hip is the greater trochanteric slide (9). This approach allows continuity of the gluteus medius–vastus lateralis fascia. A straight lateral incision is performed between the tensor fascia lata and gluteus maximus muscle as with the transtrochanteric approach to the hip. Instead of performing the greater trochanteric osteotomy in a lateral to medial direction between the gluteus medius and vastus lateralis, the osteotomy is performed from posterior to anterior, and the vastus lateralis is incised off its posterior insertion into the linea aspera (Figs. 23 and 24). This allows the greater trochanter to be reflected anteriorly and the gluteus medius and vastus lateralis sleeve to be preserved. The four-wire technique described for trochanteric reattachment can be performed to reattach the greater trochanter. The benefit of this exposure is that in cases of postoperative migration of the greater trochanter, the gluteus medius–vastus lateralis sleeve is maintained for stability. The potential problem with this approach is inability to advance laterally and distally the greater trochanter, although I have been able to do so when using this approach.

Extended Femoral Osteotomy

Especially with the wide use of extensively porous coated femoral components in revision operations, extended osteotomy has gained popularity in revision total hip

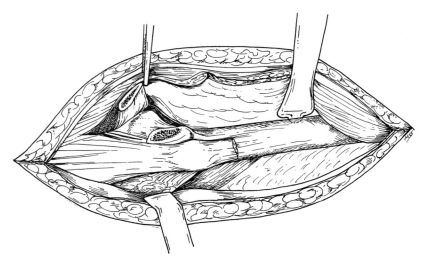

Figure 22. Exposure obtained through the extended direct lateral approach. A sliver of greater trochanter is removed with the gluteus medius–vastus lateralis sleeve.

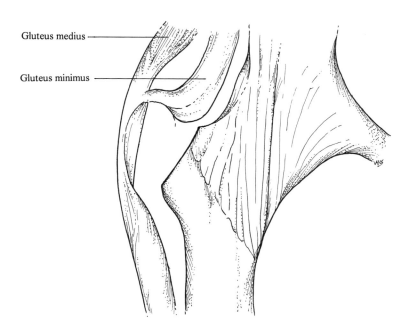

Gluteus medius

Gluteus minimus

Figure 23. Sagittal view of the greater trochanteric slide.

replacement. This approach has been championed by Paprosky and is a modification of a femoral osteotomy performed by Wagner (30). The skin incision is similar to that performed for a transtrochanteric approach to the hip and is midlateral in nature. The tensor fascia lata muscle is retracted anteriorly and the gluteus maximus posteriorly, exposing the gluteus medius–vastus lateralis sleeve. The posterior border of the vastus lateralis is incised from the linea aspera, the perforating branches from the profundus femoris artery are ligated. Especially with the use of extensively coated stems, I prefer to make longer osteotomies in the femoral shaft rather than shorter osteotomies (using slightly longer stems, that is, 8 inch [20 cm] rather than 6 inch [15 cm]) to extend the osteotomy to the most distal cement or to the end of any porous coating (even extensively coated stems). This simplifies removal of cement or porous coated stems and avoids the need to cut across extensively coated stems (which can lead to generation of marked amounts of metal debris).

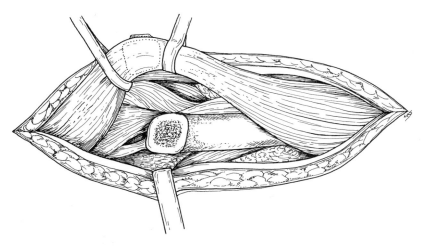

Figure 24. Lateral view of the greater trochanteric slide exposure.

After it is incised from its posterior insertion, the vastus lateralis muscle is reflected anteriorly and its proximal attachment into the vastus lateralis ridge is maintained. The femoral shaft is exposed on its lateral and anterolateral surfaces. If a cemented stem was used at the index operation, the stem is removed before the extended osteotomy is performed. At a minimum, I begin the distal aspect of the extended osteotomy 5 and preferably 7 cm below the vastus lateralis ridge to provide enough lateral femoral shaft for the application of two cables or double Luque wires below the lesser trochanter and around the osteotomized femoral shaft at the time of closure. A ruler is used to marked 7 cm distal to the vastus lateralis ridge along the linea aspera. This may have to be extended distally if one is to carry the osteotomy distal to extensive femoral coating in the uncemented situation or below a well-fixed cemented stem.

A saw is used to make an osteotomy in the posterolateral femoral cortex just anterior to the linea aspera. Care is taken not to direct the saw too anteromedially because the goal is to maintain a U-shaped tube for reinsertion of a prosthesis. My goal is to maintain a 2 to 2.5 cm wide piece of lateral femoral shaft attached to the greater trochanter. At the distal aspect of the osteotomy, which has been measured with a ruler, that is, usually 7 to 8 cm below the vastus lateralis ridge, the saw is used to perform the distal aspect of the osteotomy. Care should be taken not to carry the distal limb of the posterior distal osteotomy distal to this aspect so not to produce a stress riser at the corner of the osteotomy. After the posterior and lateral limbs of the osteotomy have been performed, the anterior part of the osteotomy is performed. Although a thin pencil-tip power instrument can be used to perform the anterior osteotomy, a thin oscillating saw placed through the posterior osteotomy and directed through the anterior cortex is usually sufficient. Care should be taken to preserve the vastus lateralis. I make no attempt at exposing the anterior part of the femoral shaft to visualize the anterior corticotomy. The osteotomy is completed anteriorly with osteotomes, and the gluteus medius, osteotomized fragment, and vastus lateralis are retracted anteriorly (Fig. 25).

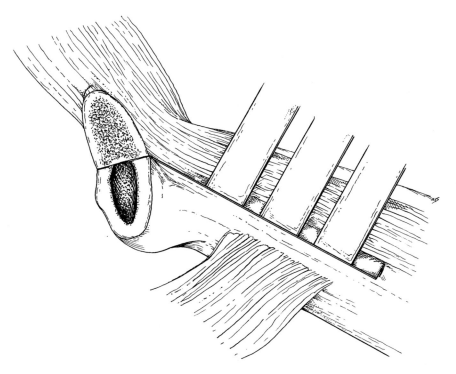

Figure 25. After the extended osteotomy is performed with a saw, the osteotomized bone is reflected anteromedially with osteotomes. I try to preserve two thirds of the proximal medial femoral shaft (note proximal femoral canal) with the distal femur.

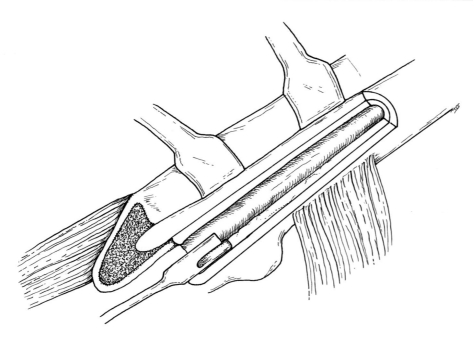

Figure 26. Exposure obtained with extended greater trochanteric osteotomy.

If an extensively coated stem is in place, it is necessary first to expose the proximal femur and to use flexible osteotomes, reciprocating saws, or pencil-sized motorized drills to free the lateral femoral bone from the lateral aspect of the prosthesis. Otherwise the osteotomized fragment will fracture. This approach allows excellent visualization of the femoral canal and exposure of the acetabulum (Fig. 26). In reapproximation of a femoral

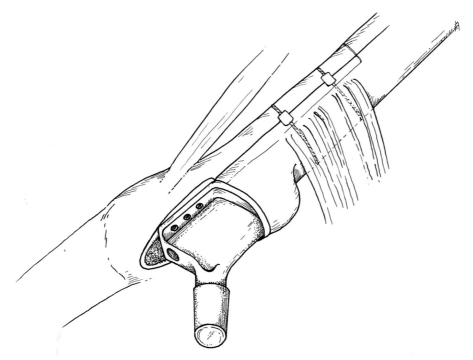

Figure 27. Reapproximation of the osteotomized greater trochanter and lateral shaft with two cables for fixation.

osteotomy, the femur must be internally rotated to allow apposition of the osteotomized fragment onto the remaining femoral shaft. A distal segment of the osteotomized fragment may be removed to allow distal advancement of the greater trochanter. I usually use two cables distal to the lesser trochanter to reattach the osteotomy with the femur in the internally rotated position (Fig. 27). The surgeon should avoid overtightening of the cable because fracture of the osteotomized fragment can occur.

This osteotomy is especially helpful when a femur has remodeled with a varus bow. It prevents the typical anterolateral perforation that can occur in removing cement or drilling for an uncemented prosthesis when a femoral bow is present. I recommend no active abduction for 6 weeks after this osteotomy.

Intrapelvic Approach to the Hip

An intrapelvic approach to the hip may be necessary, especially when cement has protruded through the medial wall of the acetabulum or an uncemented component has protruded through the medial wall. Especially with the use of screws to fix uncemented components, understanding of the intrapelvic vasculature is necessary. Wasielewski et al. (29) Keating et al., (18) and Kirkpatrick et al. (19) described concerns associated with drill placement through the anterior aspect of the acetabulum. The quadrant system described by Wasielewski et al. (29) is especially helpful because surgical anatomic landmarks can be used (Fig. 28).

The quadrant system is devised with the anterior superior iliac spine and ischial tuberosity as the dividing line between the anterior and posterior quadrants and a perpendicular line to this line through the center of the socket providing superior inferior

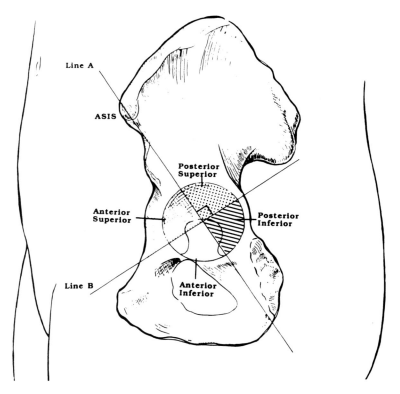

Figure 28. Quadrant system described by Wasielewski et al. (29) to orient screw direction during screw-augmented uncemented acetabular component fixation. Line from the anterior superior iliac spine to the ischial tuberosity separates the anterior from the posterior quadrants. (From ref. 29, with permission.)

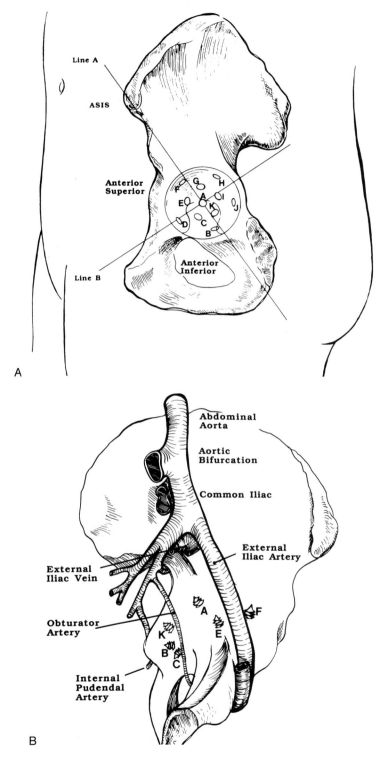

Figure 29. The relation of screws directed into the acetabulum at various sights (**A**) and the medial pelvic vascular structures (**B**) at risk. Anterior superior quadrant screw placement can damage the iliac vessels, and anterior inferior placement can damage the obturator vessels. (From ref. 29, with permission.)

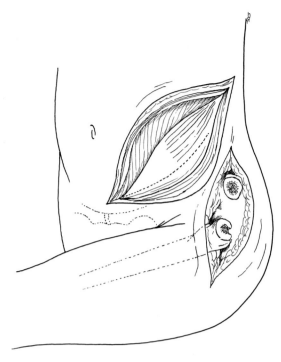

Figure 30. Iliac crest incision to gain access to the medial wall of the pelvis.

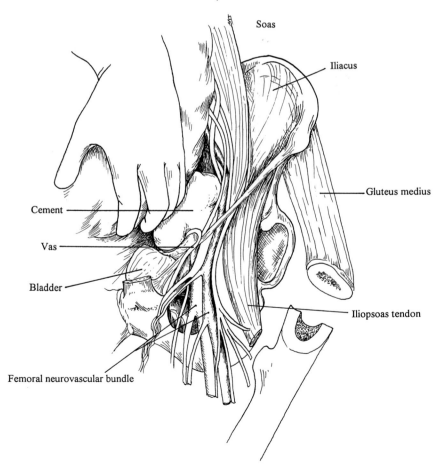

Soas

Iliacus

Gluteus medius

Cement

Vas

Bladder

Iliopsoas tendon

Femoral neurovascular bundle

Figure 31. Exposure of the inner pelvic wall to gain access to cement that has protruded into the pelvis.

quadrant differentiation. Anterior superior quadrant placement of screws and drills can compromise the iliac vessels, and anterior inferior quadrant placement can damage the obturator vessels (Fig. 29). An interesting note is that the optimal purchase of screws is in the posterior superior and posterior inferior quadrants, the safest quadrant for avoiding damage to vascular structures.

Although orthopedic surgeons performing hip operations rarely expose the inner aspect of the pelvis, the approach is not difficult. In my mind, the simplest approach is to use a second incision superior to the anterolateral iliac crest and 3 to 4 cm posterior to the anterior superior iliac spine that continues into the medial groin crease as necessary (Fig. 30). The medial aspect of this incision is demarcated by the femoral artery, which is palpated. The iliacus muscle is incised from the medial aspect of the ilium with the iliacus, psoas tendon, and neurovascular structures reflected medially (Fig. 31). This exposes the quadrilateral plate, and cement can be safely removed from the inner pelvic wall. A Foley catheter should always be placed into the bladder to decompress it and allow adequate medial retraction of the muscle and neurovascular structures.

CONCLUSION

Revision hip operations may require a variety of approaches in a variety of situations for adequate exposure of the acetabulum and femur. More extensile exposures, including extended femoral osteotomies and extensile gluteus medius–vastus lateralis sleeve approaches, have been implemented to avoid damage to the femoral shaft when removing prostheses and to provide adequate visualization for placement of the revised components. Although surgeons who perform revisions should be familiar with all approaches, they should find a single approach with which they are most comfortable to be used in most situations to reproducibly remove components and insert new components. The use of the five basic principles that include dissection of the iliotibial band from the vastus lateralis, identification of the anterior and posterior borders of the gluteus medius, mobilization of the gluteus medius (either through anterior or posterior retraction, trochanteric osteotomy, or a gluteus medius–vastus splitting approach), capsulectomy or adequate capsulotomy, and skeletonization of the femur allows adequate exposure of the acetabulum and femoral shaft in most instances. These five principles are applied no matter what approach is used. In difficult situations the surgeon should always realize that some of the more seemingly radical approaches, such as an extensive medius and vastus splitting approach or extended femoral osteotomy, may actually be the conservative approach to expose a complicated hip.

REFERENCES

1. Berry DJ, Muller ME. Chevron osteotomy and single wire reattachment of the greater trochanter in primary and revision total hip arthroplasty. *Clin Orthop* 1993;294:155–161.
2. Burwell NH, Scott D. A lateral intermuscular approach to the hip joint for replacement of the femoral head by a prosthesis. *J Bone Joint Surg Br* 1954;36:104–108.
3. Carlson DC, Robinson HJ. Surgical approaches for primary total hip arthroplasty. *Clin Orthop* 1987;222:161–166.
4. Charnley J. *Low friction arthroplasty of the hip.* New York: Springer-Verlag, 1979.
5. Dall D. Exposure of the hip by anterior osteotomy of the greater trochanter. *J Bone Joint Surg Br* 1986;30:382–386.
6. Foster DE, Hunter JR. The direct lateral approach to the hip for arthroplasty. *Orthopedics* 1987;10:274–280.
7. Frndak PA, Mallory TH, Lombardi AV. Translateral approach to the hip: the abductor muscle split. *Clin Orthop* 1993;295:131, 135–141.
8. Gibson A. Posterior exposure of the hip joint. *J Bone Joint Surg Br* 1950;32:183–186.
9. Glassman AH, Engh CA, Bobyn JD. A technique of extensile exposure for total hip arthroplasty. *J Arthroplasty* 1987;2:11–21.
10. Hardinge K. The direct lateral approach to the hip. *J Bone Joint Surg Br* 1982;64:17–19.
11. Hardy AE, Synek V. Hip abductor function after the Hardinge approach: brief report. *J Bone Joint Surg Br* 1988;70:673.
12. Harris WH. Extensive exposure of the hip joint. *Clin Orthop* 1973;91:58–62.
13. Harris WH. A new lateral approach to the hip joint. *J Bone Joint Surg Am* 1967;49:891–898.
14. Harty M, Joyce J. Surgical approaches to the hip and femur. *J Bone Joint Surg Am* 1963;45:175–190.

15. Head WC, Mallory TH, Berklacich FM, et al. Extensile exposure of the hip for revision arthroplasty. *J Arthroplasty* 1987;2:265–273.
16. Jacobs LG, Buxton RA. The course of the superior gluteal nerve in the lateral approach to the hip. *J Bone Joint Surg Am* 1989;71:1239–1243.
17. Jergesen F, Abbott LC. A comprehensive exposure of the hip joint. *J Bone Joint Surg Am* 1955;37:798–808.
18. Keating EM, Ritter MA, Faris PM. Structures at risk from medially placed acetabular screws. *J Bone Joint Surg Am* 1990;72:509–511.
19. Kirkpatrick JS, Callaghan JJ, Vandemark RM, Goldner RD. The relationship of the intrapelvic vasculature to the acetabulum: implications in screw-fixation acetabular components. *Clin Orthop* 1990;258:183–190.
20. Kocher T. *Textbook of operative surgery, 4th* ed. London: HJ Stiles, 1903.
21. Krackow K, Steinman H, Cohn BT, Jones LC. Clinical experience with a triradiate exposure of the hip for difficult total hip arthroplasty. *J Arthroplasty* 1988;3:267–278.
22. Light TR, Keggi KJ. Anterior approach to the hip arthroplasty. *Clin Orthop* 1980;152–255.
23. Marcy GH, Fletcher RS. Modification of the posterolateral approach to the hip for insertion of femoral head prosthesis. *J Bone Joint Surg Am* 1954;36:142–143.
24. McFarland B, Osborne G. Approach to the hip: a suggested improvement on Kocher's method. *J Bone Joint Surg Br* 1954;36:364–367.
25. Mostardi RE, Askew MJ, Gradisar IA, et al. Comparison of functional outcome of total hip arthroplasties involving four surgical approaches. *J Arthroplasty* 1988;3:279–284.
26. Mueller ME. Total hip replacement without trochanteric osteotomy. In: *The Hip Society: The hip proceedings of the second open scientific meeting of The Hip Society.* St. Louis: Mosby–Year Book, 1974.
27. Peters PC, Head WC, Emerson RH. An extended trochanteric osteotomy for revision total hip replacement. *J Bone Joint Surg Br* 1993;75:158–159.
28. Shaw JA. Experience with a modified posterior approach to the hip joint. *J Arthroplasty* 1991;6:11–18.
29. Wasielewski RC, Cooperstein LA, Kruger MP, Rubash HE. Acetabular anatomy and the transacetabular fixation of screws in total hip arthroplasty. *J Bone Joint Surg Am* 1990;72:501–508.
30. Younger TI, Bradford MS, Magnus RE, et al. Extended proximal femoral osteotomy. *J Arthroplasty* 1995;10:329–338.

Revision Total Hip Arthroplasty,
edited by Marvin E. Steinberg and Jonathan P. Garino,
Lippincott Williams & Wilkins, Philadelphia © 1999.

13

Component and Cement Removal

William J. Hozack

Component and cement removal in revision total hip arthroplasty can occupy a substantial amount of surgical time for even the best-prepared surgeon. A variety of tools and techniques are available to facilitate this portion of the hip revision procedure, but similar tools and techniques used by different surgeons do not always work equally well. This chapter reviews a variety of choices for surgeons performing revision arthroplasty. While it behooves each surgeon to be familiar with all these techniques, it is also important that each surgeon develop a degree of comfort with the tools and techniques that best suit him or her. The goal of this chapter is to provide a basis for time-efficient yet atraumatic removal of components and cement.

REMOVAL OF THE ACETABULAR COMPONENT

Liner Exchange

The simplest form of acetabular component revision, polyethylene liner exchange, is an alternative available only for modular components. However, liner exchange must be used judiciously. For example, some of the older cementless cup designs were marginal at best (inadequate locking mechanism, poor liner–cup articulation with multiple areas of unsupported polyethylene, nonuniform polyethylene thickness with the hexagonal polyethylene inserts). To replace an older inadequate design with a new polyethylene insert of the same inadequate design would be unwise. The surgeon must check the original operative report for the type of liner in place and consult with the manufacturer for the availability of a replacement.

W. J. Hozack: Department of Orthopaedic Surgery, Thomas Jefferson University, Pennsylvania Hospital, and Thomas Jefferson University Hospital, Philadelphia, Pennsylvania 19107.

Locking mechanisms for the polyethylene liner are different for each component. One must review the specific mechanism for the liner to be exchanged. Whereas wedging a curved osteotome between liner and cup and levering the liner out generally suffices for removal of most liners, a special instrument may be available to minimize damage to the locking mechanism. An alternative technique for removing the polyethylene liner is to use a special threaded extractor device (Fig. 1). The locking mechanism can be damaged by liner extractors. New locking devices can sometimes be ordered from the manufacturer.

Removal of a Cemented Acetabular Component

Disrupting the cement–prosthesis interface is the safest means of removing the acetabular component. Doing so prevents unintentional damage to acetabular bone. The superior aspect of the acetabular component should be exposed and some lateral cement removed with a narrow osteotome. A curved osteotome or acetabular gouge is introduced into the cement–prosthesis interface and gradually surrounds around the acetabular component. With gentle twists of the handle, the acetabular component can be separated from the cement (Fig. 2). Whereas disrupting the cement–prosthesis interface is the safest means of acetabular-component removal, newer cup designs with enhanced cement–prosthesis bonding (precoating, porous coating, textured coating) may frustrate the best attempts to access that interface. Attacking the cement–bone interface is then necessary, again with a curved osteotome. Once the component is separated from the cement, the

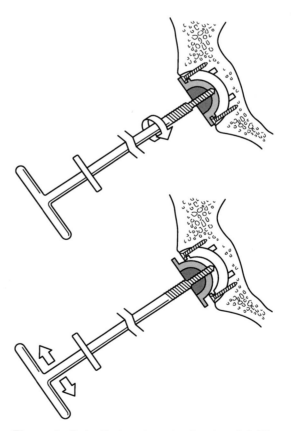

Figure 1. Polyethylene insert extractor. A 0.25-inch (0.6 cm) drill hole is placed through the center of the insert down to the metal, and a threaded polyethylene extractor is inserted into the hole. After it is screwed through the polyethylene, the extractor abuts the metal shell, forcing the liner out.

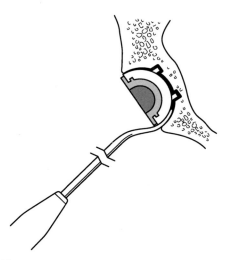

Figure 2. The acetabular gouge can be inserted between polyethylene and cement or between cement and bone. Gentle placement around the edges of the component and cement can loosen them from the underlying bone, allowing removal of the component, cement, or both.

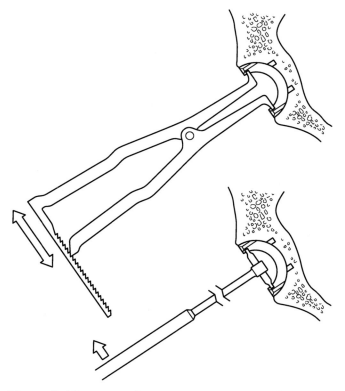

Figure 3. The cementless cup extractors and levers can lock into the metal portion of the cementless acetabular component. A gentle rocking motion allows extraction of the component. Before levering with these tools, it is important to loosening the bone–prosthesis interface with curved acetabular osteotomes.

surgeon grasps the acetabular component with a large cup grasper and gently maneuvers the acetabular component from the acetabular bed. Gentle twists of the curved osteotome facilitate this maneuver.

Removal of a Cementless Acetabular Component

The first step in removal of a cementless acetabular component is full exposure of the margins of the metal shell. The porous coating may extend beyond the margins of the outer metal shell, and proper exposure of the outer confines of this porous coating is essential. A high-speed burr can be used to remove the rim of bone that generally overhangs the acetabular component and its porous coating.

A series of narrow, curved osteotomes are available in the Moreland and other cementless revision sets, and they must be introduced around the edge of the cup. One aims circumferentially around the cup starting with the shortest osteotome and gradually progresses to longer ones. Care is taken to stay close to the bone–prosthesis interface and resist the urge to lever with the tools. Access is gained to areas of the cup where the bone is thickest—ilium, ischium, and pubic ramus—and the anterior and posterior rims are avoided. Once the component is loosened, it can be removed with a large cup grasper.

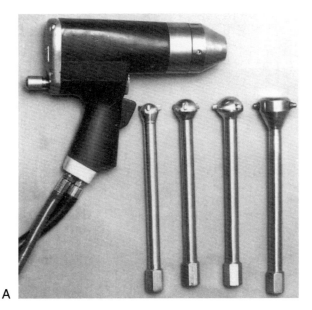

A

Figure 4. A: Photograph of pneumatic impact wrench with drivers of various sizes available for different-sized acetabular components. **B:** A metal cutting burr is used to make holes in the edge of the component. **C:** A driver of the correct size is introduced to sit within the acetabular component, the impact wrench is attached, and torque is applied to loosen the acetabular component. **D:** Nonmodular polyethylene components can be removed through the use of three grooves rather than two. (Modified from ref. 14, with permission.)

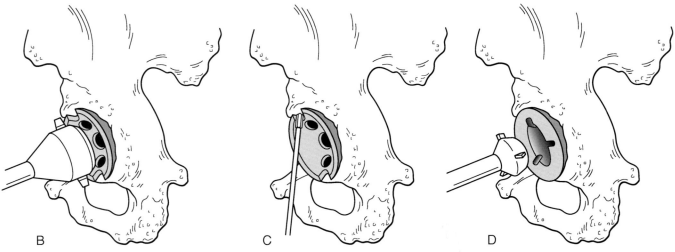

B   C   D

Two special tools are available for use in extracting the acetabular component (Fig. 3). One other alternative may be a cup-out device, as described by Lachiewicz and Anspach (14) (Fig. 4).

REMOVAL OF ACETABULAR CEMENT

Residual cement within the acetabular bed often is poorly fixed to the bone and can be removed with curettage. If the cement is well fixed, fragmentation with a narrow osteotome generally disrupts the cement–bone bond and allows easy extraction. Anchoring-hole cement can cause special problems with extraction. Gentle twisting of the cement with a curette is often successful. I have occasionally removed large anchoring-hole cement plugs with ultrasonic plug-puller tools (Fig. 5).

Components or cement that have passed the iliopectineal line can be considered intrapelvic in location. In most cases, extraction is possible through a standard extensile hip incision, because a thick layer of fibrous pericapsular tissue generally is found around the loose components and cement. The surgeon should resist the urge to remove the intrapelvic component or cement by means of direct, forceful extraction. This could seriously damage vital intrapelvic structures. With gentle traction and a curette to separate the components and cement from the fibrous layer, gradual extraction of the intrapelvic components and cement is possible that leaves the fibrous layer intact.

In rare situations removal of intrapelvic cement or components is not possible through the standard hip approach. One example is intrapelvic cement that has penetrated through a small hole in the bone only to expand behind the hole, making it impossible to remove from the exterior of the acetabulum. One choice is to leave this cement behind, an option only in aseptic cases. However, if removal of the cement and components is necessary, a retroperitoneal approach to the interior wall of the acetabulum can be undertaken (4,9,11,20). During this exposure, the surgeon usually is impressed by the degree of intrapelvic scarring present, often affecting the bladder, ureter, nerves, and iliac vessels. The assistance of a general surgeon is useful for those unfamiliar or uncomfortable with this approach.

REMOVAL OF THE FEMORAL COMPONENT

Cemented Stem Removal

Disruption of the cement–prosthesis interface can be achieved by means of disimpaction of the component with retrograde force if a component has no special surface

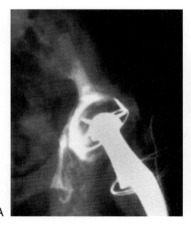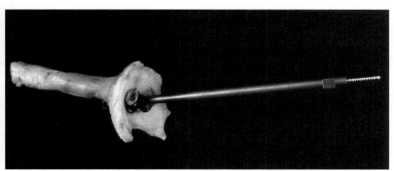

A   B

Figure 5. A: Use of the ultrasonic tools can facilitate removal of anchoring-hole cement plugs, as seen in this radiograph. **B:** In this case, a large anchoring-hole cement plug was removed with a plug-puller device.

treatment. However, before this force is applied, it is critical to remove any overhanging lateral bone or cement. Failure to do so can result in fracture of the greater trochanter. A component that has subsided because of mechanical loosening may have bone overgrowing the collar. This must be removed before component disimpaction.

Extraction of prostheses with enhanced cement–prosthesis interface bonding (precoating, porous coating, textured), can be extremely difficult. Although handheld osteotomes can be used to disrupt the interface, such use runs the risk for bone fracture or perforation. In general, the most effective means of solving this dilemma is to use a thin, high-speed pencil-tip burrs to remove a thin layer of cement at the cement–prosthesis interface. If a collar obstructs access to the medial interface, it may be necessary to remove it with a high-speed carbide drill or a circular saw.

Before the operation, it is important to have an accurate idea of the extent of the cement–prosthesis enhancement. If the enhanced interface extends distally past the metaphyseal flare of the femur, access is restricted with a standard hip approach. In these situations, extended trochanteric osteotomy greatly facilitates exposure of the distal cement–prosthesis interface (19,23). A more radical technique is to transect both femur and femoral component and extract the distal prosthesis with a combination of high-speed burrs and trephines. A femoral window technique has been described (13,21) that can provide access to this area (Fig. 6).

Extraction of the femoral component is relatively straightforward once the cement–prosthesis interface is disrupted. If the component is nonmodular, an extraction force can be applied to the femoral head or collar if present. Components with modular heads can cause special problems, especially if no collar is present. In these situations a universal extraction device can be used (Fig. 7). Special notches on the component must be made to allow the device to attach securely.

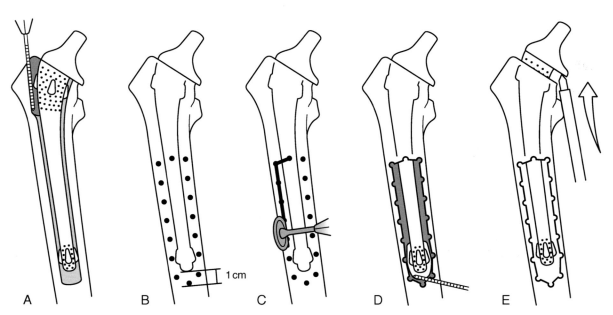

Figure 6. A: Disruption of the proximal cement–prosthesis interface can be accomplished with a high-speed pencil bit. **B:** Outlining the anterior femoral cortical window with drill holes is useful. This window should extend past the tip of the prosthesis by approximately 1 cm. **C:** A high-speed drill or circular saw can be used to make the window. Beveling of the cuts is helpful for replacement of the fragment after removal of the components and cement. **D:** A high-speed pencil bit is used to disrupt the distal cement–prosthesis interface. **E:** Once the proximal and distal cement–prosthesis interface bonding has been disrupted, a carbide bit can be used to extract the prosthesis. (Modified from ref. 21, with permission.)

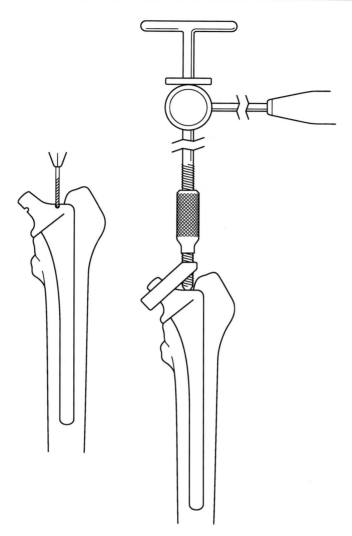

Figure 7. A universal extraction device can be used for modular femoral components. If not already present, special notches must be made on these femoral components using a carbide bit and attachment of the device to the femoral component can allow for extraction.

Removal of a Cementless Stem

The scope and extent of the removal of cementless femoral components depend on the fixation status of the component and the extent of the porous coating. If the femoral component is mechanically loose, as judged radiographically (5), extraction requires mere clearance of the proximal bone overhang and firm disimpaction force by means of any one of the techniques described for removal of cemented femoral components. If the femoral component has bone ingrowth, special instruments and special approaches must be used to remove the implant. The extent of the porous coating also influences the approach to the extraction procedure. If a well-ingrown porous surface is only proximal in extent, disruption of the prosthesis–bone interface can be achieved with standard approaches with or without trochanteric osteotomy. On the other hand, if extensive porous coating is present and bone ingrowth has occurred distally, special approaches such as cortical windows or extended trochanteric osteotomies must be used.

Two techniques can be used for successful removal of a well-ingrown cementless component. The first technique involves graduated exposure depending on the level of

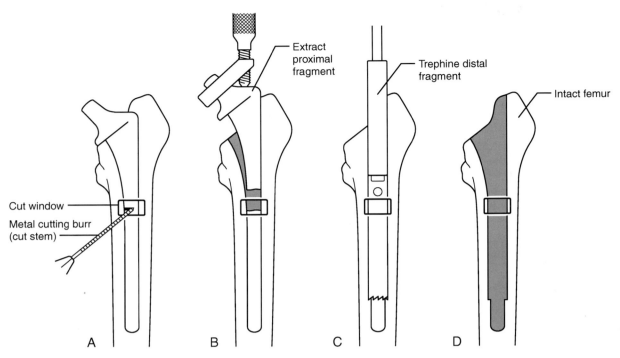

Figure 8. Step-by-step technique for removal of distally fixed porous coated femoral component. (Modified from ref. 8, with permission.)

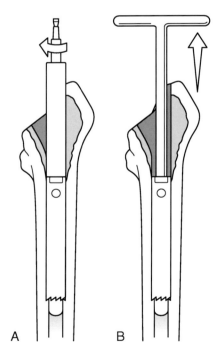

Figure 9. After removal of the proximal uncemented femoral component, the distal conical section can be removed with hollow trephines. A trephine of proper size overdrills the distal segment. Then, because the reamer generally entraps the femoral component, a T-bar attachment and mallet can be used to extract the femoral stem from the canal.

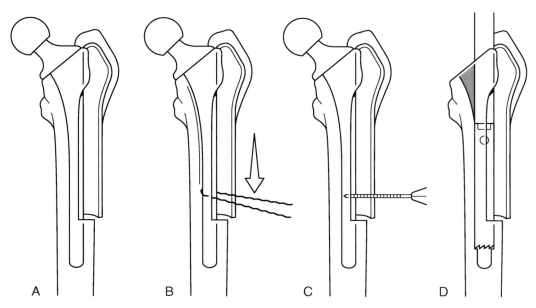

Figure 10. A: Extended trochanteric osteotomy is used to expose the proximal aspect of the femoral component. **B:** A Gigli saw is used to disrupt the bone–prosthesis interface. Multiple Gigli saws may be necessary. **C:** If distal bony ingrowth prevents removal of the stem, a metal-cutting high-speed burr is used to transect the stem for removal of the proximal segment. **D:** Trephining of the distal stem allows extraction of that segment. (Modified from ref. 24, with permission.)

fixation of the porous coat (8). The proximal porous coat (primarily metaphyseal in extent) can be interrupted with thin flexible osteotomes or a thin high-speed pencil-tip burr. Access to the medial portion of the prosthesis is the most difficult and can be hampered by a collar, which can be removed with a metal-cutting high-speed bit.

If the porous coating extends distally into the diaphysis, use of flexible osteotomes is potentially dangerous. In these situations, a cortical window is made in the femur at the point where the proximal tapered and distal conical portions of the stem intersect (Fig. 8). The stem is transected with a high-speed, metal-cutting bit through this cortical window. The proximal portion of the femoral component is removed by means of the standard technique described for a proximally porous coated stem. The remaining distal stem is removed with trephines, which can overdrill the distal stem thereby disrupting the prosthesis–bone interface (Fig. 9). An extraction device can then be attached to the trephine to effect removal of the femoral component.

As an alternative an extended trochanteric osteotomy, as described by Younger et al. (24), is used with the distal extent of the osteotomy placed at the junction of the tapered and cylindrical portions of the femoral component. Once the osteotomy exposes the femoral component, a Gigli saw is used to disrupt the proximal prosthesis–bone interface. If the stem is still secure, the prosthesis is transected and removed as described earlier (Fig. 10).

CEMENT REMOVAL OF FEMORAL

One alternative to the potentially formidable task of cement removal is recementing of a femoral component into the preexisting cement mantle. This technique has been used by several authors (1,16,17) with excellent results. Situations in which the cement-to-cement approach should receive serious consideration include revisions for instability or leg-length inequality or isolated acetabular revisions in which femoral cement technique is adequate. Another indication for this technique is when the need for increased exposure requires femoral component removal without removal of the femoral cement mantle.

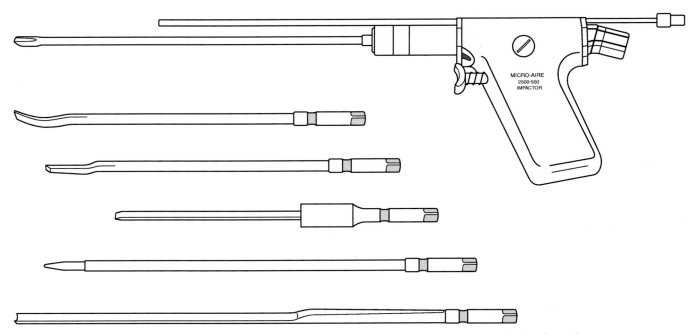

Figure 11. The Micro-Aire pneumatic power system (Zimmer, Warsaw, Indiana) can be used in a manner similar to use of standard hand tools.

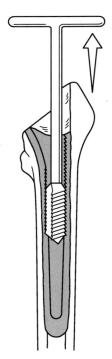

Figure 12. Tapping the cement tap into the femoral cement mantle may allow extraction of the femoral cement if the cement–bone interface is weak.

If the cement has to be moved, removal is best approached in three stages, as follows: stage 1—metaphyseal cement above the lesser trochanter; stage 2—diaphyseal cement below the lesser trochanter but proximal to the cement plug; and stage 3—distal plug cement.

The workhorses for femoral cement removal are hand tools. A variety of other tools and techniques are available but should be viewed as complementary to hand instruments, not as replacements for them. These include high-speed drills, ultrasonic tools, and the segmental extraction technique of cement removal. A special pneumatic hand-tool system also is available (Fig. 11). Occasionally the entire cement mantle is loose within the canal. In these situations, a tool can be anchored into the mantle and the entire mantle removed with a single disimpaction force (6,7,12). A metal tap can be threaded into the cement (Fig. 12), or an ultrasonic plug puller can be anchored. If only some of the cement is removed with the first disimpaction, the steps can be repeated as needed. The success of this technique depends on a greater mechanical bond between instrument and cement than between cement and bone. Unfortunately, this technique is rarely an option.

Metaphyseal cement tends to be bulky, and the bone tends to be thin and weak. Although hand instruments are needed in this stage of cement removal, initial debulking of the cement with a high-speed burr is helpful. The cement should be split longitudinally

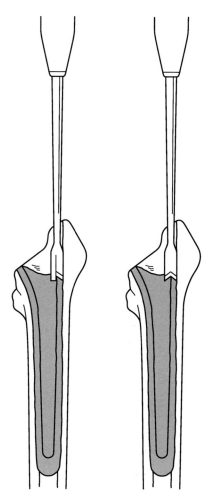

Figure 13. Proximal metaphyseal cement can be split with special T or V osteotomes. Sharp taps are necessary, but care must be taken to avoid splitting the metaphyseal bone.

with osteotomes into three or four segments (Fig. 13). Sharp taps are necessary to split the cement, but care must be taken to avoid splitting the metaphyseal bone. An ultrasonically or pneumatically driven osteotome can be used to make the longitudinal splits, avoiding the force needed to crack the cement manually (6,7,12). A curette is used to separate cement from bone, and the cement fragments are retrieved with a pituitary rongeur. A fibrous membrane is generally apposed to the bone and should be curetted away before the next stage. At this time, it is critical to remove cement and bone from the trochanteric bed to allow direct longitudinal access to the diaphyseal part of the femur. Failure to do so can lead to perforation of the lateral cortex of the femur during attempts to remove the distal cement.

Diaphyseal cement should be removed in the following sequence in 1 to 2 cm increments, as follows:

1. Split the cement mantle circumferentially with osteotomes.
2. Chip the cement away from the bone with a sharp curved osteotome. Keep the curved osteotome at the cement–bone interface for best efficacy (Fig. 14).
3. Use a curette or pituitary rongeur to remove the loose cement and fibrous membrane.
4. Irrigate the canal and then dry it to restore proper visualization.

Removal of distal plug cement can be tedious and frustrating. Hand tools are often inadequate. It is important to evaluate the preoperative radiographs to determine the extent and nature of the cement plug. How long is it? Does it pass the isthmus of the femur and

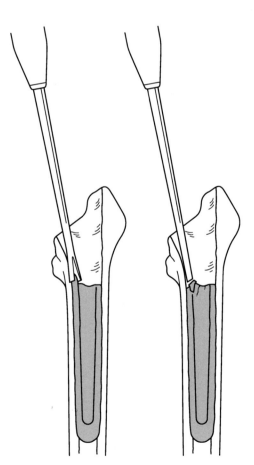

Figure 14. Sharp cement osteotomes and gouges introduced at the cement–bone interface can chip away the diaphyseal cement after splitting of a cement mantle with T- or V-shaped osteotomes.

then expand? Is it well bonded to bone or is the cement–bone interface loose? Can an instrument be passed between the plug and the endosteal bone or does the cement plug completely obliterate the canal?

If a space exists between the distal plug and the endosteal bone, a thin hook curette can be inserted past the plug and rotated 90 degrees. An extraction force can then remove the plug. If no space exists for the hook curette but the cement–bone interface is weak, the plug can be removed in one of three ways. First a sharp osteotome can "work" the bone–cement interface and with gentle twists fully free-up the plug. The plug can then be grasped with pituitary forceps. A hole can be drilled into or through the plug, and a threaded extractor or hook can be used to remove the cement. As an alternative, the ultrasonic plug puller can be used as described earlier to engage and disimpact the loose cement plug (Fig. 15).

The most troublesome situation occurs when the distal cement plug is well fixed and fills the canal completely. In this situation, hand tools alone are insufficient, and power instruments are necessary to remove the distal cement plug. The general principle is to drill a hole through the distal plug to convert it to a cement mantle similar to that in the proximal diaphyseal area. The rest of the cement can then be excised in the manner previously described for the diaphyseal cement-removal stage. Reverse hook curettes should be used to remove all residual cement.

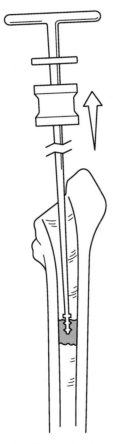

Figure 15. An ultrasonic plug puller can be inserted in the cement plug, and the cement plug can be disimpacted with a small 1-lb (0.45 kg) weight. This technique works only if the cement–bone interface is weak. This technique should not be used if the cement plug expands past the isthmus of the femoral canal.

Drilling through the cement can be accomplished with several tools—conventional drills, high-speed burrs, or ultrasonic drills. Conventional drills are used through graduated centering cones to guide the drill through the approximate center of the distal plug. Unfortunately, the femoral curvature makes drilling much more precarious than can be shown diagrammatically. In these situations, extended exposure of the femur should be undertaken, and controlled perforation of the femoral bone should be performed to ensure proper orientation of the drills within the canal (24). Controlled perforation involves subperiosteal stripping of the vastus lateralis off the femur and the creation of 9 mm round holes in the shaft of the femur with a high-speed burr (22). This portal should be placed just proximal to the distal plug, allowing the surgeon direct visualization of the drill as it enters the distal plug. Illumination and irrigation of the canal can be accomplished through the portal. Additional controlled perforations can be made as needed. During the reconstruction phase of the revision procedure, these defects must be bypassed by the new femoral component (15). High-speed burrs can be used for drilling of the distal cement plug. They tend to be more efficient at cement removal than the conventional drills and are relatively safe if guided with the controlled perforation technique (10). If improperly guided, high-speed burrs can remove bone rather than cement with no tactile feedback to the surgeon using the tool. Facility with high-speed instrumentation is definitely based on experience. Fluoroscopic control of the drilling process has been used but is cumbersome, time consuming, and less safe than the controlled perforation technique.

Ultrasonically driven tools can be used to drill through the distal cement plug (2,3,6,7,12). The main advantage of this approach is that tactile and auditory feedback is provided by the instrumentation, allowing an experienced surgeon to differentiate bone from cement. The ultrasonic tool can be guided gently through the distal plug to avoid damage to the surrounding bone. Four disk drills (7 mm, 9 mm, 11 mm, 13 mm in diameter) are available to perforate the distal plug. They are used sequentially with copious irrigation to push through the distal plug to enlarge the hole as the disk drills increase in size. After the largest disk drill possible is used, residual cement is removed with the hand tools as described earlier.

Distal cement plugs that extend past the isthmus and around the curvature of the femur pose special problems of removal. Complete removal of the cement plug may not be necessary. If a new cemented component is to be implanted, the distal cement can act as a cement restrictor. If a new cementless component is to be implanted, removal of cement need be undertaken only to the level of the tip of the new stem. Drilling through an extended distal cement plug from the proximal end of the femur is likely to result in either perforation or eccentric cement removal, which encourages bone perforation during insertion of the new femoral stem. In these situations, extended trochanteric osteotomy exposure with the distal aspect of the osteotomy near the apex of the curvature of the femur is the best approach. Drilling of the cement mantle can then be performed in a more controlled manner.

REFERENCES

1. Archibald DA, Protheroe K, Stother IG, Campbell A. A simple technique for acetabular revision: brief report. *J Bone Joint Surg Br* 1988;70:838.
2. Brooks AT, Nelson CL, Hofmann DE. Minimal femoral cortical thickness necessary to prevent perforation by ultrasonic tools in joint revision surgery. *J Arthroplasty,* 1995;10:359–362.
3. Callaghan JJ, Elden SH, Stranne SK, Fulghum CF, Seaker AV, Myers BS. Revision arthroplasty facilitated by ultrasonic tool cement removal. *J Arthroplasty* 1992;7:495–500.
4. Eftekhar NS, Nercessian O. Intrapelvic migration of total hip prosthesis. *J Bone Joint Surg Am* 1989;71:1480–1486.
5. Engh CA, Bobyn JD. Biological fixation in total hip arthroplasty. Thorfare, NJ: Slack, 1985:89–107.
6. Frankel A, Hozack WJ. Ultrasound for revision hip arthroplasty. *Curr Opin Orthop* 1993;4:43–45.
7. Gardiner R, Hozack WJ, Nelson CL, Keating EM. Revision total hip arthroplasty using ultrasonically driven tools, *J Arthroplasty* 1993;8:517–521.
8. Glassman AH, Engh CA. The removal of porous-coated femoral hip stems. *Clin Orthop* 1992;285:164–180.
9. Grigoris P, Roberts P, McMinn, DJW, Villar RN. A technique for removing an intrapelvic acetabular cup. *J Bone Joint Surg Br* 1993;75:25–27.
10. Harris WH, Oh I. A new power tool for removal of methylmethacrylate from the femur. *Clin Orthop* 1978;132:53–54.

11. Head WC. Prevention of intraoperative vascular complications in revision total hip replacement arthroplasty. *J Bone Joint Surg Am* 1984;66:458–459.
12. Klapper RC, Caillouette JT, Callaghan JJ, Hozack WJ. Ultrasonic technology in revision joint arthroplasty, *Clin Orthop* 1992;285:147–154.
13. Klein AH, Rubash HE. Femoral windows in revision total hip arthroplasty. *Clin Orthop,* 1993;291:164–170.
14. Lachiewicz PF, Anspach WE. Removal of a well fixed acetabular component: a brief technical note of new method. *J Bone Joint Surg Am,* 1991;73:1355–1356.
15. Larson JE, Chao EYE, Fitzgerald RH. Bypassing femoral cortical defects with cemented intramedually stems. *J Orthop Res* 1991;9:414–421.
16. Lieberman JR, Moeckel BH, Evans BG, Salvati EA, Ranawat CS. Cement-within-cement revision hip arthroplasty. *J Bone Joint Surg Br* 1993;75:869–871.
17. McCallum JD, Hozack WJ. Recementing a femoral component into a stable cement mantle using ultrasonic tools. *Clin Orthop* 1995;319:232–237.
19. Peters PC, Head WC, Emerson RH. An extended trochanteric osteotomy for revision hip replacement. *J Bone Joint Surg Br* 1993;75:158–159.
20. Petrera P, Trakru S, Mehta S, Steed D, Towers JD, Rubash HE. Revision total hip arthroplasty with a retroperitoneal approach to the iliac vessels. *J Arthroplasty* 1996;11:704–708.
21. Pierson JL, Jasty M, Harris WH. Techniques of extraction of well-fixed cemented and cementless implants in revision total hip arthroplasty. *Orthop Rev* 1993;22:904–916.
22. Sydney SV, Mallory TH. Controlled perforation: a safe method of cement removal from the femoral canal. *Clin Orthop* 1990;253:168–172.
23. Younger TI, Bradford MS, Magnus RE, Paprosky WG. Extended proximal femoral osteotomy: a new technique for femoral revision arthroplasty. *J Arthroplasty* 1995;10:329–338.
24. Younger TI, Bradford MS, Paprosky WG. Removal of a well-fixed cementless femoral component with an extended proximal femoral osteotomy. *Contemp Orthop,* 1995;30:375–380.

Revision Total Hip Arthroplasty,
edited by Marvin E. Steinberg and Jonathan P. Garino,
Lippincott Williams & Wilkins, Philadelphia © 1999.

14

Selection of Acetabular Component

Leo A. Whiteside

Failed acetabular components are accompanied by variable amounts of bone loss, distortion of anatomy, and change in acetabular position. The process also is accompanied by changes in the supporting capsule, ligaments, and muscles. All of these changes must be considered in selection of the next acetabular component. Although leaving the acetabular position unchanged often is convenient, it is not always the best biomechanical choice. A high hip center after revision total hip replacement leads to abnormal forces on both the femoral and acetabular components and may be associated with high rates of loosening (12,26). However, lowering the acetabular center often requires bone grafting and other techniques that have high failure rates (1,10). Acetabular components that accommodate or obviate this bone grafting are attractive, but many do not have proven long-term results and must be approached with caution.

One of the most important concerns with revision of the acetabular component is avoiding osteolysis of the already compromised bone stock in ensuing years. Factors involved in development of osteolysis include motion of the polyethylene liner within the metal shell, wear of the backside of the polyethylene component, articular surface wear, configuration of the porous coating on the shell, presence of screws and screw holes, support of the polyethylene liner by the metal shell, and sealing of the interface between the polyethylene liner and the metal shell (2,4,9).

In rare instances, muscle and ligaments have been so badly damaged that stability of the hip cannot be restored. In these instances special considerations must be made in choice of the acetabular component on the basis of stability. All the anatomic and pathologic characteristics of the hip and mechanical features of the new acetabular component must

L. A. Whiteside: Biomechanical Research Laboratory, Missouri Bone and Joint Center, Barnes–Jewish West County Hospital, St. Louis, Missouri 63141.

be considered as the revision operation is planned. Choosing implants on the basis of their design and materials often is the most difficult problem for the surgeon, because it requires knowledge of the mechanical details of implants and understanding of the function of biomaterials. This chapter is designed to help the surgeon choose a well-designed implant that addresses the pathologic characteristics of the hip.

ANATOMIC CHARACTERISTICS

Anatomic characteristics of the acetabulum after removal of a failed total hip replacement vary from a condition similar to that of a primary hip replacement to one involving considerable loss of bone stock, ligament support, and muscle function. The surgeon should choose an acetabular component that can be attached reliably to the bone, can restore acceptable position of the hip center, and can create a stable articulation in the face of compromised bone, ligaments, and muscles around the hip. A number of studies have demonstrated the superiority of porous ingrowth acetabular components over cemented components, especially in revision total hip arthroplasty. I therefore favor the use of uncemented acetabular components whenever possible. This requires intimate contact with a sufficient quantity of structurally sound, viable host bone. If this cannot be achieved, cemented components may be needed. These can be used in conjunction with various types of metal acetabular reinforcement rings and cages, with morsellized graft, and with large, structural allografts. See Chapters 16, 17, and 20 for discussion of cemented acetabular components.

Failure of the acetabular component nearly always destroys the subchondral bone and some of the underlying cancellous stock, but in mild cases the outer cortical walls remain intact. When these major supporting walls are intact, a standard uncemented hemispheric acetabular component can be used, but press fit usually is compromised, so augmented fixation with screws usually is necessary. Because the subchondral and cancellous bone stock is damaged, the outer cortical support must be engaged by the metal shell, thus requiring larger sizes, especially for large men.

If the circumference of the acetabular rim is maintained, a large, hemispheric component can usually achieve stable seating, but screws are almost always needed because rigid frictional fit cannot be obtained through the fragile peripheral cortical bone structure. Outer diameters of 74 mm occasionally are needed to achieve adequate press fit in these circumstances, and cancellous screw fixation through the dome is an important part of the surgical procedure (Fig. 1). Central wall destruction usually is not an indication for use of more advanced hardware.

Destruction of the anterior acetabular wall does not usually necessitate augmented fixation through a flange on the cup rim, nor does it usually require use of augmented cups, cement restrictor cages, or other advanced fixation techniques. If the anterior wall is missing, a standard uncemented hemispheric acetabular component can be fixed securely to resist axial loading, and shear loads can readily be managed with screws.

If the posterior wall is missing, more advanced augmentation options may be necessary. Because acetabular loads are directed superiorly and posteriorly in most load-bearing conditions (6,7), posterior wall damage necessitates that the component be supported until healing of the posterior bone graft can occur. Loss of the entire anterior and central walls usually results in the same choice of acetabular component as does major posterior wall damage. Often in these cases, the acetabulum has not migrated far superiorly, and an acetabular component with augmented rim fixation is sufficient (Fig. 2A). This component is placed against the shallow, incompetent acetabular bone stock and held with dome screws to control shear loads. Fixation is augmented with rim screws to resist tilting (Fig. 2B). If the acetabular component can be solidly abutted against a partially intact iliac dome, adequate fixation can be obtained with this style of component, and regrowth of grafted bone stock can be expected to provide long-term support.

Proximal bone destruction and shortening of the iliac column raise the hip center and cause unacceptable hip joint mechanics if the center of rotation approaches the level of the sciatic notch (8,12,26). Although use of small acetabular components has been advocated

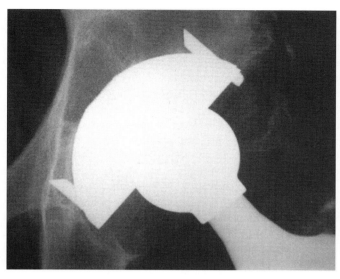
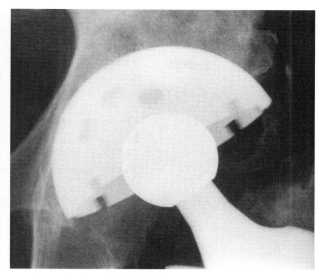

A   B

Figure 1. A: Preoperative radiograph shows a failed acetabular component with central osteolysis but an intact peripheral rim. **B:** Postoperative radiograph shows the same patient as in **A** with a revised acetabular component. Peripheral contact was maintained, and adequate fixation was achieved without bone screws.

for management of a high hip center (18), the iliac wing rarely is incapable of supporting normal loads in the hip. The abnormal mechanics resulting from the compensatory extra length of the femoral neck also overloads the femoral component (22). Most experts in reconstructive surgery of the hip do not recommend this approach but advocate various methods to lower the hip center (14,17). Probably the most common method to accomplish this change in position is to use a very large acetabular component with a diameter as large as 76 mm. When the anterior and posterior walls are deficient, this large component can place the acetabular center 1 to 1.5 cm lower than its prerevision position. This component usually is sufficient to restore hip mechanics to a condition acceptable for

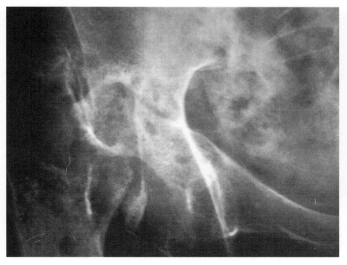
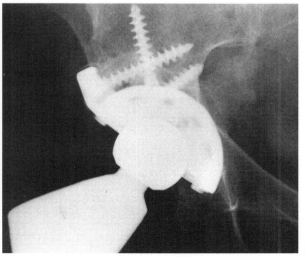

A   B

Figure 2. A: Preoperative radiograph shows a hip with fairly severe bone destruction. Anterior and posterior wall support has been lost but without severe proximal migration. **B:** Postoperative radiograph shows the same patient as in **A**. A Healey acetabular component (Biomet, Warsaw, Ind.) has been seated firmly against the partially deficient iliac dome and held with dome screws augmented with rim screws. The effect of the rim screws is to prevent tilting toward horizontal.

the restricted activity level of most patients who have undergone hip revision. When proximal migration of the acetabular component occurs but the anterior and posterior walls remain reasonably intact, use of an oblong component may be indicated (19). These components engage the iliac bone stock proximally but are small enough from anterior to posterior that they may be inserted without removing the intact anterior or posterior acetabular wall (Fig. 3).

Occasionally the supporting bone stock of the acetabulum is so severely disrupted that none of the techniques works that rely on proximal abutment of the cup against the iliac dome. The acetabular bone stock assumes a planar configuration or may be so severely disrupted that continuity between the ilium, ischium, and pubis is disrupted (pelvic dissociation). In these instances the acetabular component must be supported by a bridge between ilium and ischium to prevent medial migration of the implant and disruption of the construct. None of the components available for this application achieves permanent intrinsic stability of the acetabular component. They do allow the surgeon to erect scaffolding that supports a bone graft to achieve reconstitution of acetabular bone stock. The Burch-Schneider cage (Sulzer, Baar, Switzerland) represents the classic prototypical reconstructive device. This simple device can be rigidly attached to the ilium while engaging the ischium and supports the implant above and below (Fig. 4). The bone graft is packed into the cavity behind the cage, and the acetabular component is cemented into the central cage. The graft heals to form permanent support for the acetabular component. The success rate for this method has been good, and the acetabular cage with allograft and cemented cup remains a good choice for a severely disrupted acetabulum (13). Other options have become available to manage a massively deficient acetabulum. The GAP component (Osteonics, Allendale, N.J.), which has plates that can be formed to fit the iliac wing and a hook for engaging the inferior border of the acetabulum, provides a similar solution to this problem but adds versatility and convenience to the procedure (Fig. 5).

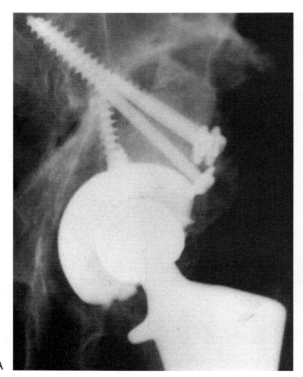
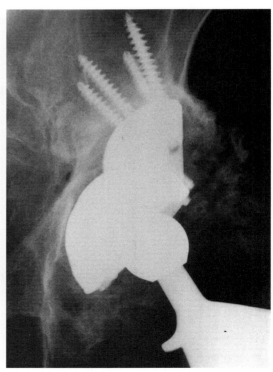

A

B

Figure 3. A: Preoperative radiograph shows a deficient acetabulum with a failed iliac allograft. **B:** Postoperative radiograph shows the same patient as **A**. An oblong, augmented acetabular component (MARS; Biomet, Warsaw, Ind.) is used to fill the defect and to displace the hip center toward its normal position.

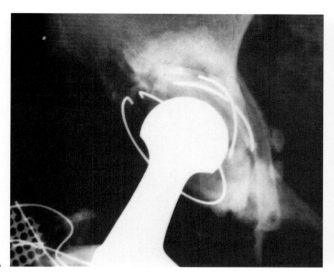 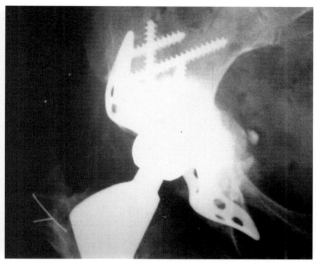

A
B

Figure 4. A: Preoperative radiograph shows a failed cemented cup in extremely poor bone stock. **B:** Postoperative radiograph shows the same patient as in **A** in whom a Burch-Schneider cage was used. The inferior flange does not engage the ischium, but inferior purchase was achieved farther proximally.

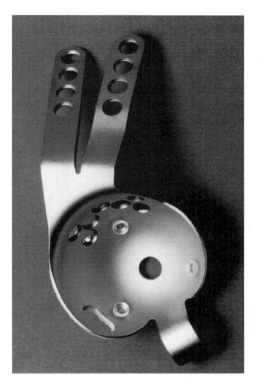

Figure 5. Photograph shows the GAP acetabular component. This component provides malleable plates that are applied against the iliac wing and a hook to attach to any remaining inferior acetabular bone bridge. This implant allows the iliac bone stock to be partially reconstructed with bone graft. The polyethylene liner is cemented into the metal shell.

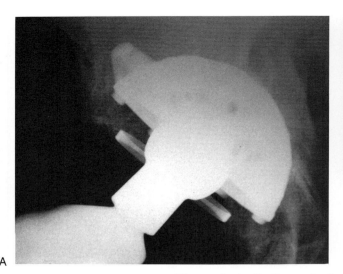
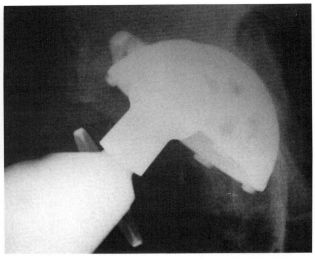

A   B

Figure 6. A: Radiograph shows a hip with a constrained acetabular component. A polyethylene rim around the femoral head and neck prevents dislocation. The metal ring inside this polyethylene rim adds tensile strength to the rim. **B:** Radiograph shows the same component as in **A** after the constraining mechanism failed and the hip redislocated.

Stability of the hip joint is a special concern in revision total hip arthroplasty. Because augmented rim polyethylene components add virtually no risk to the procedure and markedly decrease the dislocation rate (5) some experts suggest that this is the appropriate choice for all revision hip procedures. In extremely rare instances the supporting capsule and muscles of the hip have been damaged so badly by the pathologic process that stability cannot be achieved with conventional revision techniques. Patients with loss of the greater trochanter, massive proximal femoral allograft, chronic or recurrent dislocations, and neurologic conditions should be considered possible candidates for use of constrained acetabular components (3). These patients are rare, and constrained acetabular components should be used sparingly and with caution (Fig. 6).

DESIGN

Design features of acetabular components are important determinants of early fixation and late wear. Design features that are related to fixation of the component to bone are foremost in the minds of most surgeons. Dome screws are the mainstay of fixation, and attempting to fix the acetabular component without this basic feature is unrealistic in most revision total hip operations. Early stabilization and fixation of the acetabular component usually are tenuous. In most revision hip operations, the implant must be secured with screws. The screw holes in the shell can be an important issue associated with wear and osteolysis. Adequate support of the polyethylene is important to minimize the stress of weight bearing and to minimize wear on the polyethylene. Large, closely spaced holes diminish support of the polyethylene and place a great deal of stress on the backside and articular surface of the polyethylene (16). This error in design eventuates in considerable wear and failure. Very thick metal shells have small inner diameters and therefore less surface area in which to place holes. If those holes are enlarged to allow angulation of the screws, even less support is available for the polyethylene. Thin shells with widely spaced screw holes should be chosen when possible.

The locking mechanism of the polyethylene liner in the metal shell is important initially to prevent dissociation of the liner from the metal shell. Later it maintains rigid apposition of the polyethylene component to the metal shell to eliminate pumping and wearing mechanisms in the joint. A rigid peripheral press-fit locking mechanism is especially important in these components and is the only means to ensure durability for millions of cycles (Fig. 7).

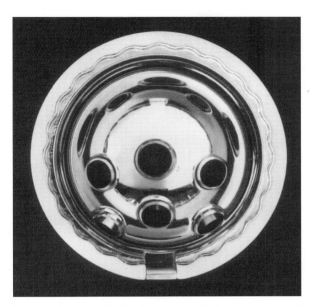

Figure 7. The Reflection acetabular component (Smith & Nephew, Memphis, Tenn.) is typical of several acetabular components that have a reliable, tested, peripheral locking mechanism that eliminates backside wear and destruction of the polyethylene.

Unfortunately, many acetabular components do not fulfill the basic design requirements of metal support and rigid fixation of the polyethylene liner, but with careful inspection of the locking mechanism one usually can identify the implants that are likely to perform well. If the metal shell and plastic liner can be fully interlocked by hand, and if the locking mechanism entails a flimsy peripheral press-fit mechanism, it is not likely that micromo-

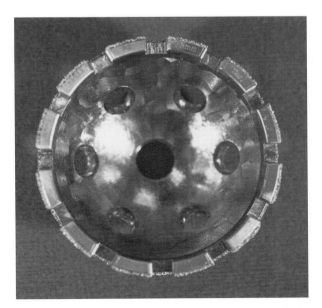

Figure 8. The MicroSeal acetabular shell (Whiteside Biomechanics, St. Louis, Mo.) has screw holes that are widely spaced so that the polyethylene is supported adequately.

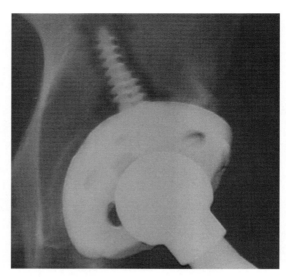

Figure 9. Radiograph shows an osteolytic cyst around a screw. Reactive joint fluid that flows from the joint cavity behind the polyethylene and out the screw holes can cause severe bone destruction.

tion will be controlled adequately. Early destruction of the polyethylene component also can occur if the component is not adequately supported by the metal shell. Full congruency between the polyethylene component and the metal shell is essential to prevent backside wear. The holes should be spaced widely to minimize stress on the polyethylene (Fig. 8). Without these features to protect the polyethylene liner, early wear and rapid breakdown of the articular surface are likely to occur.

An additional feature of acetabular components that is especially important in revision operations is the ability to seal the bone stock from joint fluid and debris. Just closing off the holes is an unacceptable alternative because press-fit fixation alone is seldom sufficient to hold the acetabular component. Screws that enter the already deficient bone stock of the acetabulum act as a conduit for osteolytic joint fluid and worsen the risk for bone destruction (Fig. 9). Sealing the interface between the metal shell and polyethylene liner offers a solution to this dilemma. The peripheral rims of the cup and liner form a water-tight seal, so screw fixation of the metal shell presents no risk of potentiating osteolysis (9). As designs evolve, fewer pitfalls remain, and more solid solutions arise to produce a durable acetabular reconstruction. Nevertheless, finding all the essential features of a successful implant in one of the commercially available products requires wise and careful shopping.

POLYETHYLENE QUALITY

Polyethylene quality is one of the most important features of revision acetabular components but one of the factors least considered when the actual component is chosen. Extensive information is available to lead surgeons to a good choice for the patient. One of the first responsibilities of a surgeon in choosing a revision acetabular component is to evaluate the quality of the polyethylene. Polyethylene that contains calcium stearate is subject to progressive deterioration caused by fusion defects in the material. How the calcium stearate particles cause these fusion defects is not clear, but it is a well-documented fact that the defects they cause lead to delamination and high wear rates (21,23,25). Other special processing methods, such as those used in producing Hylamer polyethylene (DePuy, Warsaw, Ind.), result in severely crystallized, embrittled material that is permeated with fusion defects (11). Photomicrographic evidence of polyethylene that is highly uniform and free of fusion defects should be available and confirmed by the surgeon (Figs. 10 and 11).

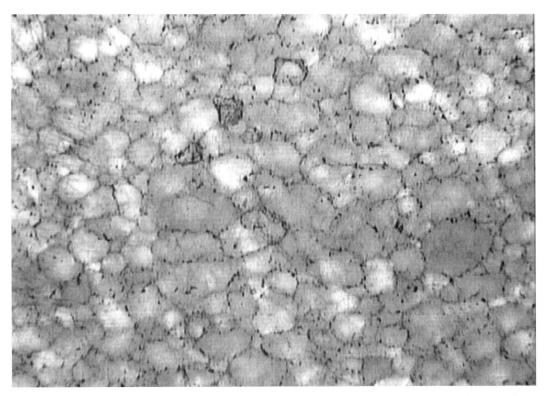

Figure 10. Photomicrograph shows Hylamer polyethylene with severe fusion defects and crystallization. These microscopic defects predispose the material to delamination and early failure.

Figure 11. Photomicrograph shows calcium stearate–free polyethylene with no detectable fusion defects at light microscopic examination. Use of this type of material is virtually free of risk for delamination.

Sterilization of polyethylene with gamma irradiation in air increases the number of free radicals that progressively oxidize, leading to chemical and mechanical degradation of the polyethylene. This is a gradual process that is especially treacherous because it takes years to develop and cannot be evaluated adequately with short-term laboratory bench tests (20). However, gamma sterilization in an inert environment or in a vacuum markedly diminishes production of these free radicals and allows an increase in cross linking, which may improve its wear. Low-stearate or stearate-free polyethylene sterilized with ethylene oxide or gas-plasma methods is highly reliable material. It is strong, wear resistant, and inert (15). Use of these materials does not cause an increase in cross linking or free radical formation. Progressive oxidation, chain scission, and embrittlement do not occur during decades of clinical service (24). Results of long-term comparative clinical studies are available to substantiate the clear superiority of gas-sterilized polyethylene over that treated with conventional methods of gamma irradiation (24). Additional studies are needed to validate claims of superiority for polyethylene irradiated in an inert atmosphere. Surgeons have fairly clear choices regarding technology available for polyethylene. They should exert their influence to ensure use of the best possible material for long-term durability. Low stearate (or stearate-free), gas sterilized polyethylene currently is the best clinical choice.

REFERENCES

1. Armstrong RA, Whiteside LA. Results of cementless total knee arthroplasty in an older rheumatoid arthritis population. *J Arthroplasty* 1991;6:357–362.
2. Berry DJ, Barnes CL, Scott RD, Cabanela ME, Poss R. Catastrophic failure of the polyethylene liner of uncemented acetabular components. *J Bone Joint Surg Br* 1994;76:575–578.
3. Cameron HU. Use of a constrained acetabular component in revision hip surgery. *Contemp Orthop* 1991;23:481–484.
4. Chen PC, Mead EH, Pinto JG, Colwell CW. Polyethylene wear debris in modular acetabular prostheses. *Clin Orthop* 1995;317:44–56.
5. Convery FR, Minteer-Convery M, Devine SD, Meyers MH. Acetabular augmentation in primary and revision total hip arthroplasty with cementless prostheses. *Clin Orthop* 1990;252:167–175.
6. DeBrunner HU. Studien zur Biomechanik des Huftgelenkes, I: Ein neues Modell fur die Berechnung der Huftbelastung. *Z Orthop* 1975;113:377–388.
7. Greenwald AS, O'Connor JJ. The transmission of load through the human hip joint. *J Biomech* 1971;4:507.
8. Kelley SS. High hip center in revision arthroplasty. *J Arthroplasty* 1994;9:503–510.
9. Khalily C, Tanner MG, Williams VG, Whiteside LA. Effect of locking mechanism on fluid and particle flow through modular acetabular components. *J Arthroplasty* 1998;13:254–258.
10. Mulroy RD, Harris WH. Failure of acetabular autogenous grafts in total hip arthroplasty. *J Bone Joint Surg Am* 1990;72:1536–1540.
11. Muratoglu OK, Imlach H, Estok D, et al. Analysis of eight retrieved Hylamer acetabular components. *Trans Orthop Res Soc* 1997;22:852 (abstract).
12. Pagnano MW, Hanssen AD, Lewallen DG, Shaughnessy WJ. The effect of superior placement of the acetabular component on the rate of loosening after total hip arthroplasty. *J Bone Joint Surg Am* 1996;78:1004–1014.
13. Peters CL, Curtain M, Samuelson KM. Acetabular revision with the Burch-Schneider antiprotrusio cage and cancellous allograft bone. *J Arthroplasty* 1995;10:307–312.
14. Radogevic B, Zlatic J. An L-shaped bone graft for acetabular deficiency. *J Bone Joint Surg Br* 1990;72:152–153.
15. Ries MD, Weaver K, Rose RM, Gunther J, Sauer W, Beals N. Fatigue strength of polyethylene after sterilization by gamma irradiation or ethylene oxide. *Clin Orthop* 1996;333:87–95.
16. Rosner BI, Postak PD, Greenwald AS. Cup/liner conformity of modular acetabular designs. *Orthop Trans* 1995;19:469–470 (abstract).
17. Rossen J, Schatzker J. The use of reinforcement rings to reconstruct deficient acetabula. *J Bone Joint Surg Br* 1992;74B:716–720.
18. Schutzer SF, Harris WH. High placement of porous-coated acetabular components in complex total hip arthroplasty. *J Arthroplasty* 1994;9:359–367.
19. Sutherland CJ. Early experience with eccentric acetabular components in revision total hip arthroplasty. *Am J Orthop* 1996;25:284–289.
20. Sutula LC, Collier JP, Saum KA, et al. Impact of gamma sterilization on clinical performance of polyethylene in the hip. *Clin Orthop* 1995;319:28–40.
21. Tanner MG, Whiteside LA, White SE. Effect of polyethylene quality on wear in total knee arthroplasty. *Clin Orthop* 1995;317:83–88.
22. Trakru S, Rubash HE. Early aseptic loosening of precoated femoral components in hybrid total hip arthroplasty. *Orthop Trans* 1996;XX:312.
23. Walker PS, Blunn GW, Lilley PA. Wear testing of materials and surfaces for total knee replacement. *J Biomed Mater Res* 1996;33:159–175.
24. Williams IR, Mayor MB, Surprenant HP, Sperling DK, Currier JH. The impact of sterilization method on

the clinical damage of UHMW polyethylene knee components. Poster presentation at the 64th Annual Meeting of the American Academy of Orthopaedic Surgeons; 1997, Feb. 13–17; San Francisco.

25. Wrona M, Mayor MB, Collier JP, Jensen RE. The correlation between fusion defects and damage in tibial polyethylene bearings. *Clin Orthop* 1994;299:92–103.
26. Yoder SA, Brand RA, Pedersen DR, O'Gorman TW. Total hip acetabular component position affects component loosening rates. *Clin Orthop* 1988;288:79–87.

Revision Total Hip Arthroplasty,
edited by Marvin E. Steinberg and Jonathan P. Garino,
Lippincott Williams & Wilkins, Philadelphia © 1999.

15

Selection of Femoral Component

John M. Cuckler

The selection of the optimum femoral component for revision total hip arthroplasty is essentially the result of careful preoperative planning, which is the most important aspect of revision surgery. Careful consideration of preoperative radiographs and consideration of the clinical situation and needs of the patient produce the proper selection of femoral component, particularly as experience is gained by the surgeon in revision arthroplasty.

DEFINITION OF THE CLINICAL PROBLEM

Selection of the femoral component should be based on careful review of the radiographs of the failed implant. A 14 × 17 anteroposterior (AP) radiograph of the hips and pelvis allows determination of limb-length discrepancy and provides information on the appropriate offset of the revision stem and neck length. It also allows consideration of acetabular revision needs if appropriate. The surgeon can use the femoral head diameter of the existing component, which should be available from the original operative record, to determine the magnification factor of the radiograph.

Two additional radiographs are necessary for examination of bone-stock deficiency, which may affect choice of the revision component. AP and lateral views, also 14 × 17 inches, should be obtained of the femur. Additional views should be obtained if the entire femoral component and distal cement column are not visualized on these radiographs. These radiographs allow the surgeon to determine the appropriate length of the revision component and allow choice of the more appropriate fixation method. In addition, the possible necessity for a bowed stem and the extent of proximal bone loss can be evaluated

---

J. M. Cuckler: Division of Orthopaedic Surgery, University of Alabama at Birmingham, Birmingham, Alabama 35294.

with these radiographs. Templates of the proposed revision stem should be used to confirm the adequacy of the component for the reconstruction. Classification of femoral bone loss, as with the scheme proposed by D'Antonio et al. (5) is not as important as identifying the extent of bone loss and the anticipated solution. Other factors that may affect stem selection can also be considered at this time. Extended trochanteric slides, cortical windows, and femoral fractures or defects (either preoperative or intraoperative) influence selection of the revision femoral component. The surgeon is well advised to select a revision component that allows sufficient adaptability in the event of intraoperative misadventures such as fracture, canal perforation, or other mechanisms that may further compromise bone stock.

ASSESSMENT OF FIXATION NEEDS

The surgeon must decide between cemented and cementless fixation on the basis of existing bone quality and the needs of the patient. The fixation used influences selection of the femoral component.

Cemented Fixation for Revision Total Hip Arthroplasty

Cemented fixation is indicated for patients with limited life expectancy and activity expectations. Although some authors have reported excellent intermediate results with the use of bone cement for femoral revision operations (12,18), other reports in the orthopedic surgery literature indicate disappointing intermediate results with mechanical or radiographic loosening rates approaching 40% after 5 years of follow-up study (13,20). In my practice, polymethyl methacrylate (PMMA) fixation is reserved for patients with less than a 5 to 10 year life expectancy and low activity expectations. Other relative indications for cemented fixation include the existence of severe metabolic bone disease, such as osteopenia syndromes, osteomalacia, and Gaucher's disease. Cemented fixation ideally should be used when there is relative preservation of femoral bone stock. If there is a history of infection, antibiotic impregnation of the PMMA may afford increased likelihood of success (21). However, cemented fixation is relatively contraindicated in the presence of femoral fracture or other defects in the cortex of the femur that may make containment of the bone cement difficult.

Cementless Fixation for Revision Total Hip Arthroplasty

The ability of a cementless implant to achieve femoral component stability in revision total hip arthroplasty, particularly in revision of a failed cemented component, is now well established (10,15,19). Particularly when loss of the cancellous bone of the femur exists or when bone stock reconstitution or healing is necessary, as with fractures around loose femoral stems, cementless fixation appears to be superior at intermediate follow-up periods compared with cemented fixation. However, results with different components vary considerably. Relative youth (life expectancy greater than 5 to 10 years) and moderate to high activity expectations constitute relative indications for use of cementless revision stems in my practice.

Compaction Grafting Technique

The technique of compacting cancellous allograft bone within the femoral canal followed by cemented fixation of a polished, wedge-shaped stem had been advocated by Gie et al. (6). Intermediate follow-up results appear promising, but wide acceptance of the technique should await confirmation of the results by others. The use of this technique has implications with regard to selection of the femoral component if the technique of the originators is followed. Because the technique is still evolving and the results not yet sufficiently confirmed, this method is not discussed herein. Femoral impaction grafting is discussed in detail in Chapter 19.

IMPLANT SELECTION

Material

Only two alloys are used for revision femoral stems, cobalt chrome molybdenum (CoCrMo; American Society for Testing and Materials-[ASTM] F75), and titanium–6 aluminum–4 vanadium (Ti6Al4V). Other alloys such as stainless steel do not appear to provide sufficient fatigue strength, and some newer titanium alloys are still in development for the U.S. market. CoCrMo alloy can be characterized as a relatively stiff and hard material compared with titanium alloy implants (2). Although the increased stiffness (modulus of elasticity) of CoCrMo has led some surgeons to express concern over clinical results such as stress shielding and thigh pain, there are surprisingly few clinical data to substantiate this concern. Stress shielding and thigh pain are probably more related to implant design factors such as diameter, extent of porous coating, and proximal canal fill than the material of the implant.

Fretting corrosion and fretting wear can compromise the long-term performance of the revision procedure when modular stems are used. Both Ti6Al4V and CoCrMo implants are subject to fretting corrosion and wear under proper conditions (7). Modular junctions such as those found in the Morse-type taper of the femoral head or at the junction of modular stems are common sources of fretting corrosion, but the corrosion is probably more a function of the quality of the modular junction fit and design than the materials themselves. Ultimately, the surgeon is advised to select the stem not so much for material qualities as for the clinical needs of the revision situation. The algorithm for selecting the fixation mode for the revision stem is shown in Fig. 1.

Cemented Revision Stem Design

Cobalt chrome alloy is the preferred material for cemented revision stems in my practice. The high fatigue strength of wrought or forged CoCrMo coupled with the inherent hardness of the material and stiffness of the alloy in effect stress-protect the cement mantle while allowing stems of sufficiently small diameter to produce a 2 to 3 mm cement mantle. Texturing of the surface of the stem, by means of ceramic bead blasting and macrotexturing with divots or grooves can further enhance fixation of the implant–

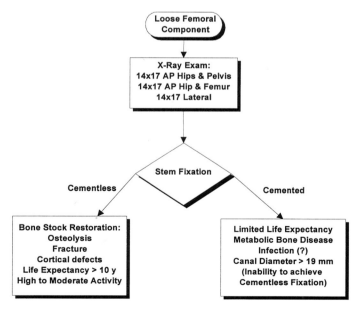

Figure 1. Stem fixation algorithm.

PMMA interface. As an alternative, PMMA precoating can enhance bonding of the stem to the adjacent cement mantle (9). However, the effect of surface finish on component loosening and failure is being reevaluated.

The length of the cemented revision stem should be sufficient to bypass any cortical defects by at least two cortical diameters at the level of the defect (1). In general, however, efforts should be made to confine the length of the cemented revision stem to just short of the isthmus of the femur. Stems that extend beyond the isthmus have to be curved to avoid perforation of the anterior cortex of the femur. Achieving fixation of a cement plug will be quite difficult because of progressive enlargement of the femoral canal beyond the isthmus.

Proximal and distal centralizers for cemented stems have been suggested to improve the symmetry of the cement mantle to optimize the long-term results of cemented fixation. However, no clinical data exist to confirm this hypothesis. The revision surgeon is further cautioned that use of a distal centralizer at or near the isthmus may make complete seating of the implant difficult or impossible. Trial reduction with the actual implant and centralizer should be considered to avoid this problem. I prefer to avoid the use of distal centralizers in cemented stems approximately 200 mm long or longer.

Porous Ingrowth Revision Stem Design

The absolute requisite for cementless revision operations is achievement of stability at the bone–implant interface at the completion of the procedure. This requires selection of a stem that achieves cortical contact to provide stability and achieve bone ingrowth. In some situations, use of a modular stem may be advantageous to achieve the cortical fit necessary, although the surgeon needs to consider carefully the potential disadvantages of the modular designs. An algorithm for selection of a cementless stem is shown in Fig. 2.

The selection of implant alloy (CoCrMo versus Ti6Al4V) is probably less important than the implant design. Both alloys suffer approximately a 66% decrease in fatigue strength (compared with wrought or forged alloy) because of the porous coating sintering process (23). However, the fatigue strength reduction of porous ingrowth revision stems has not been reported to result in a high rate of clinical failure.

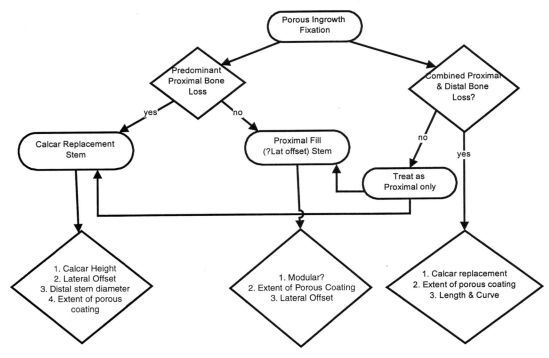

Figure 2. Selection of cementless revision stem.

The extent of porous coating has to be based on an assessment of the bone-stock compromise and the ability of the stem to achieve contact with vascularized host bone of sufficient strength to allow stress sharing between implant and bone. When severe compromise of the proximal (metaphyseal) bone stock exists, a distally coated stem is recommended to achieve fixation. Lawrence et al. (7) suggests on the basis of their clinical experience that 5 cm of scratch fit between porous coating and cortical bone is necessary for stability of the implant. On the other hand, Cameron (3) reported excellent results with the S-ROM proximal filling modular prosthesis (Joint Medical Products, Stamford, Conn.) even in the face of considerable metaphyseal bone loss. Users of other proximally coated revision stems have not reported results as successful as Cameron's, perhaps because of decreased proximal fill relative to the S-ROM prosthesis (8,11,16). This experience has influenced the trend toward more distal and extensive porous coating in revision operations as the design factor more likely to produce long-term stability and success of the procedure.

Modular stems allow the surgeon intraoperative adaptability with regard to the goal of achieving proximal and distal cortical contact, varying the length of the stem, or using bowed stems when extension of the stem beyond the isthmus is necessary. Modular designs can be grouped into two basic types of body designs. The S-ROM design entails a proximal triangular sleeve component through which a stem of varying diameter, length, and offset is inserted. The S-ROM stem also has flutes distalally to enhance rotational stability. It is slotted in the coronal plane to reduce distal stiffness. Other modular designs, such as the Mallory-Head modular revision stem (Biomet, Warsaw, Ind.) have a variety of proximal stem bodies to attach to distal stems with a Morse-type taper and taper bolt junction. The stems for this system are available with variable extents of porous coating, or flutes, and have distal coronal slots. At this time, however, no advantage to modular designs has been demonstrated with regard to clinical outcome. The intraoperative advantages of easy variation of stem length, diameter, and proximal body size explain the popularity of these designs.

The length of the porous stem should be determined according to similar principles for a cemented stem. The tip of the stem should bypass by two cortical diameters the most severe distal defect. For instance, if an extended trochanteric slide is planned to obtain exposure of a distal cement column, the length of the revision stem should extend at least twice the diameter of the femur at the lower extent of the slide to minimize risk for postoperative fracture. If the necessary length of stem extends beyond the midpoint or isthmus of the femur, a curved stem is necessary to avoid penetration of the anterior cortex of the femur. Thus the templating process determines both anticipated stem diameter and length of stem necessary. The surgeon is well advised to have longer stems available in the event of unanticipated problems such as intraoperative fracture. Modularity offers particular advantages with regard to stem length and diameter adjustment.

Another essential consideration during templating is restoration of limb length and lateral offset. If acetabular revision is anticipated, the surgeon should estimate the expected diameter and position of the revised socket and mark on the AP radiograph of the pelvis and hips the anticipated center of rotation of the new acetabulum. This allows determination of the expected neck length and lateral offset necessary to restore stability to the hip and optimize abductor function of the hip. When porous coated devices are used in revision operations, the surgeon must simultaneously achieve stability of the implant through cortical contact of the prosthesis with the femur while choosing a proximal stem design that restores offset and limb length. Lateral offset designs, which extend laterally the central axis of the femur away from the midline of the pelvis (midsagittal plane), frequently are useful. The surgeon should avoid when possible the use of skirted femoral head components, because extended length femoral heads reduce the range of motion of the reconstructed hip, possibly increasing risk for postoperative dislocation (14). In addition, skirted femoral heads may produce increased risk for fretting corrosion of the modular head–neck junction, which may produce accelerated third-body wear of the acetabular component (22). In considering the proximal stem design, the surgeon is generally well advised to assume more loss of proximal bone may be encountered during the operation than is evident on preoperative radiographs, thus necessitating use of calcar or proximal femoral replacement devices.

Femoral Head Selection

Three decisions must be made before revision operations with regard to femoral head selection—length, material, and diameter. Femoral head diameter may be constrained to the inside diameter of the acetabular component if revision of the acetabulum is not anticipated. Exchange of the acetabular liner is not required or possible in the instance of nonmodular metal-backed sockets. The surgeon is cautioned to be aware of implants such as the Bechtol hip (Smith and Nephew Richards, Memphis, Tenn.), which have a 25.4-mm femoral head and thus should not be matched with 26-mm femoral heads if the acetabulum is well fixed. Fortunately, such devices are becoming increasingly rare, and most failed implants encountered have acetabular inside diameters of 22, 26, 28, or 32 mm.

Length of the femoral head can be estimated with preoperative templating. The surgeon should try to avoid skirted femoral heads to minimize risk for impingement and subsequent dislocation and to minimize risk for fretting corrosion. The choice of diameter of the femoral head should be based on the realization that the volume of wear debris produced correlates directly with the diameter of the femoral head, that is, the larger the head, the greater is the expected debris production (17).

Ceramic femoral heads composed of alumina (Al_2O_3) or zirconia (ZiO) may offer considerable wear reduction compared with CoCrMo alloy femoral heads (4). These ceramic materials are extremely hard and therefore resist scratching by third-body wear debris. The smoothness of ceramic femoral heads also reduces wear caused by friction or transfer mechanisms. However, the decreased tensile strength of ceramic materials places limitations on size and length and increases the importance of precision of the manufacturing process with regard to the Morse-type taper junction. In my practice, ceramic femoral heads are reserved for young patients with greater than 10 year life expectancy and moderate to high activity expectations.

TEMPLATING AND PREOPERATIVE PLANNING

Templating before revision arthroplasty is essential to identify the design, fixation method, and length of implant necessary to restore hip function in the setting of a failed prior implant. The additional advantage of preoperative templating is that the surgeon has the opportunity to study, in the quiet of his or her office, the available radiographic views of the failed implant, allowing time to identify possible problems that may be encountered during the revision procedure. The surgeon should be able to plan for all contingencies during the procedure and have the appropriate instruments and implants available to solve any intraoperative difficulties. A suggested algorithm for preoperative templating is shown in Fig. 3.

Good-quality radiographs are essential to preoperative planning and templating. The radiographs should show the most distal extent of cement in the femoral canal on both AP and lateral views. The AP view of the pelvis and both hips allows consideration of the effects of acetabular revision on limb length, acetabular center of rotation, and offset necessary to reconstruct hip function. The femoral head of the existing component may be used to calculate the precise magnification factor inherent in the radiographs and assure precise determination of the dimensions of the revision implants to be used.

Length of the femoral component is determined with bone-stock considerations, such as distal osteolysis, the distal extent of a cortical window or extended trochanteric slide, and the extent of distal stem judged necessary to obtain stable fixation (whether cemented or cementless fixation is chosen). If the length of the stem needed reaches to or beyond the isthmus of the femur, a curved stem is necessary. Lateral templates should be used against a leg-down or true lateral view of the femur to assure proper fit of the implant within the

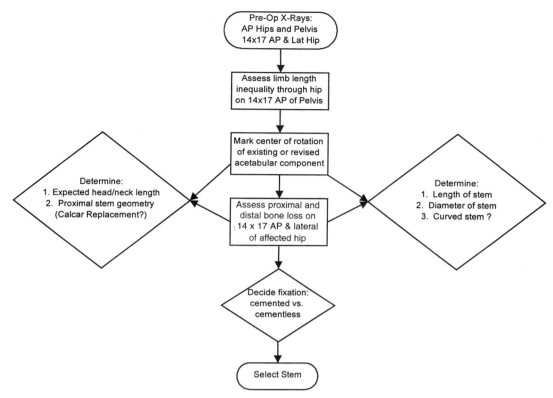

Figure 3. Preoperative templating.

anatomic configuration of the femur. The stem selected should bypass cortical defects by at least two cortical diameters at the level of the defect.

The preoperative radiographs should be marked with a wax pencil to indicate the site of cortical windows, the expected position of the tip of the stem, and the expected diameter, length, and if appropriate, proximal stem size and location for intraoperative reference. Neck length may be estimated preoperatively on the basis of planned acetabular revision and the need for offset restoration. If lateral offset is not restored with the selected implant, consideration should be given to an alternative stem with increased lateral offset.

CASE STUDIES

Three case studies are provided to serve as examples in the decision-making process for stem selection and choice of fixation and as examples of the accuracy with which preoperative templating can facilitate the revision procedure. All patients had participated in at least 3 years of follow-up study and had successful early outcomes.

Case 1

In Fig. 4A the preoperative radiograph of a 58-year-old man demonstrates a cementless total hip replacement implanted 10 years earlier. The femoral head is fractured and nonmodular. Substantial osteolysis surrounds the acetabular component, which also shows catastrophic wear of the polyethylene liner and migration into a vertical position. The extensively porous coated femoral stem appears well fixed. There is osteolysis of the greater trochanter. The intended femoral stem template indicates selection of a modular calcar replacement cementless stem. Cementless fixation was selected because the patient was quite active and healthy, although cemented fixation also can be used. The modular

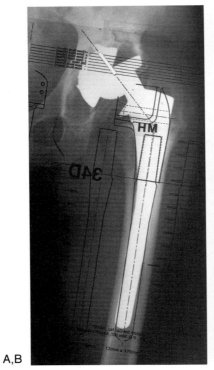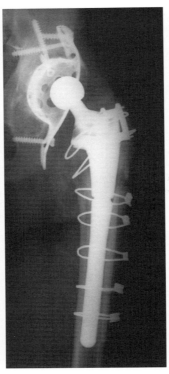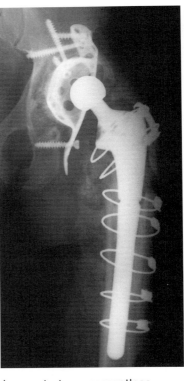

Figure 4. A: Preoperative radiograph of a 58-year-old man demonstrates a cementless total hip implanted 10 years earlier. **B:** Same patient 1 year after revision. **C:** Same patient 2 years after revision.

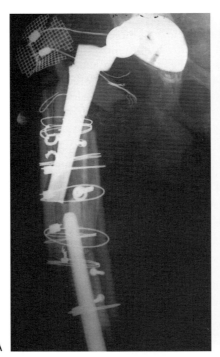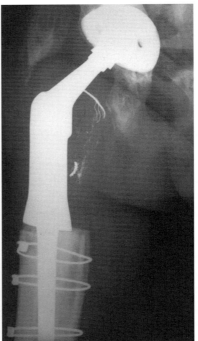

Figure 5. A: Preoperative radiograph of 42-year-old woman who underwent four prior hip operations for management of hip arthritis associated with Gaucher's disease. **B:** Radiograph shows a cemented proximal femoral replacement device.

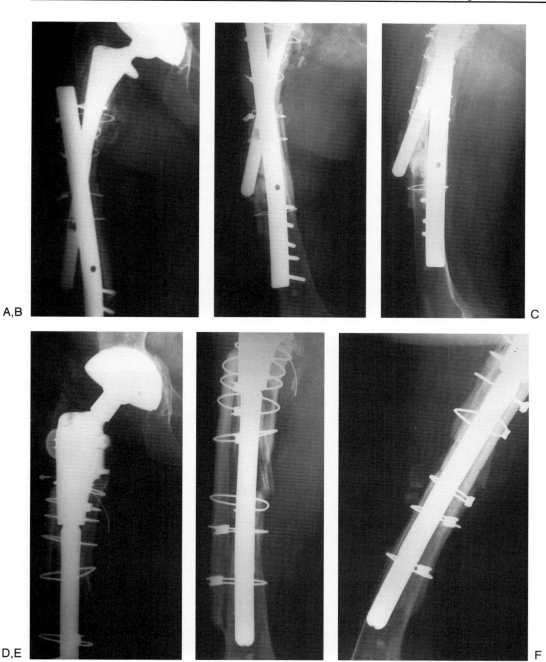

A,B

C

D,E

F

Figure 6. A: Radiographs of a 73-year-old woman who had undergone prior revision complicated by perforation and subsequent fracture of the femur. **B:** Radiograph shows extruded cement, protruded stem tip (**C**), and failed internal fixation. **D:** Views 3 years after revision. **E:** The fracture has united, and the cortical allograft appears incorporated (**F**).

stem allowed use of a smaller distal stem diameter than could have been achieved with a nonmodular design, which therefore allowed conservation of femoral bone stock. Use of a protrusio ring with a cemented all-polyethylene cup restored lateral offset without use of a skirted femoral head. The preoperative plan was to perform an extended trochanteric slide to remove the well-fixed femoral component. The end of the revision stem has extended two cortical diameters beyond the distal extent of the extended trochanteric slide. Fig. 4B and 4C show the same patient at 1 and 2 years postoperatively. An onlay cortical allograft strut was used to augment the proximal femur where osteolysis was encountered and appears to have incorporated. Operative time was 150 minutes; the 2-year postoperative Harris hip score was 86.

Case 2

Figure 5A shows the preoperative radiograph of a 42-year-old woman who had undergone four prior hip operations for management of hip arthritis associated with Gaucher's disease. A poorly conceptualized attempt at revision of the failed cemented total hip at another institution shows the hip dislocated when the cementless implant (which had been cut intraoperatively when the surgeon discovered that the presence of an intramedullary stem from a revised knee prevented full seating of the prosthesis) migrated within the proximal allograft. The allograft had failed to unite to host bone in the absence of a stable mechanical construct at the graft–host interface. When she sought treatment, the patient's medical status had stabilized with respect to Gaucher's disease. The patient was counseled with regard to the alternative of proximal femoral allograft replacement of the femur versus proximal femoral prosthetic replacement. After long discussion, the surgeon and patient decided that immediate stable fixation was preferable to attempted bone-stock restoration with a massive proximal allograft. Because of the patient's metabolic bone disease and because fixation of the implant in the distal femur was deemed extremely difficult given the extent of proximal bone loss, a cemented proximal femoral replacement device was chosen (Fig. 5B). The patient underwent a knee arthrotomy as part of the revision procedure to disimpact the intramedullary stem of the knee component. A total hip replacement orthotic device (brace) was used for 6 months postoperatively to ensure stability of the implant and prevent dislocation. The patient had excellent hip function 3 years postoperatively with a mild limp, no pain, and a Harris hip score of 92.

Case 3

Figure 6A shows the presenting radiograph of a 73-year-old woman who had undergone a prior revision complicated by perforation and subsequent fracture of the femur. Figures 6B and 6C are additional radiographs demonstrating extruded cement, the protruded stem tip, and failed internal fixation. This example presents the challenge of a femoral fracture with nonunion, severe loss of bone stock, and marked osteopenia. Because healing of the femoral fracture was necessary, cementless fixation was chosen in spite of the observed osteopenia. A curved stem was judged necessary to extend the length of the femoral component beyond the isthmus. Onlay cortical allograft struts were used to enhance the stability of the reconstruction, and a calcar replacement stem was used to gain limb length. A modular stem was chosen to assure excellent distal fit of the stem to stabilize the femur. To avoid distraction of the femur at the fracture site, however, a fluted, rather than extensively coated stem was chosen to assure impaction at the fracture site. Cancellous graft was placed around the comminuted portion of the fracture site to ensure healing. Figures 6D–F show the appearance 3 years after revision. The patient had no pain and no disability that she perceived relative to the hip. The fracture united, and the cortical allograft appeared incorporated. Postoperatively the patient was treated with a fracture brace with a pelvic band to assure stability and healing.

SUMMARY

The single most essential step in selection of a femoral component for hip revision is the preoperative planning process, in particular templating of the chosen femoral stem against preoperative radiographs. The surgeon must also plan for unexpected events such as more extensive bone loss, intraoperative fracture, and perforations of the femoral cortex. Ideally, the stem selected should be one with which the surgeon has had experience in simpler, more straightforward operations. It is necessary that the stem system selected have stems both larger and longer than predicted from templating to address unanticipated intraoperative problems. Complete familiarization with instrumentation, options, and limitations of the system is important to the confidence of the surgeon and the facilitation of the procedure.

Fixation should be selected according to the needs of the patient. Consideration of bone stock, including the presence or absence of metabolic bone disease, and the life expectancy and activity expectations of the patient guide the decision between cemented and cementless fixation. In general, for patients with a life expectancy of less than 10 years, relatively intact femoral anatomic features, and low activity expectations, cemented fixation will suffice. Addition of antibiotics to cement in revision operations or in operations on patients with a history of (inactive?) infection should be considered. However, when bone-stock restoration, fracture or cortical defect healing, or substantial loss of cancellous or cortical femoral bone exists, cementless fixation appears in the intermediate follow-up period to be substantially superior to cemented fixation. The cementless device chosen must contact sufficient cortical bone for stability and ultimate fixation. This principle guides selection of the design of the stem, the possible need for modularity, and the extent of porous coating.

The revision surgeon must anticipate the need for increased neck length and offset to restore limb length and hip stability and must carefully evaluate the appropriateness of the chosen design during the templating process. If possible, the surgeon should avoid use of skirted femoral heads to restore neck length to avoid reduction in range of motion of the hip and minimize the risk of fretting corrosion of the Morse taper.

At the conclusion of the revision procedure, the surgeon can accept only excellent stability at the bone–implant interface, regardless of fixation or stem chosen. In addition, the revised hip must demonstrate absence of subluxation or dislocation throughout the usual range of motion of the prosthetic hip joint, and ideally restoration of limb length and abductor offset. Careful preoperative planning and templating assure success in the quest for these difficult goals.

REFERENCES

1. Burstein AH, Currey J, Frankel VH, Heiple KG, Lunseth P, Vessely JC. Bone strength: the effect of screw holes. *J Bone Joint Surg Am* 1972;54:1143–1156.
2. Callaghan JJ. The clinical results and basic science of total hip arthroplasty with porous-coated prostheses. *J Bone Joint Surg Am* 1993;75:299–310.
3. Cameron HU. The two- to six-year results with a proximally modular noncemented total hip replacement used in hip revisions. *Clin Orthop* 1994;298:47–53.
4. Cuckler JM, Bearcroft J, Asgian CM. Femoral head technologies to reduce polyethylene wear in total hip arthroplasty. *Clin Orthop* 1995;317:57–63.
5. D'Antonio J, McCarthy JC, Bargar WL, et al. Classification of femoral abnormalities in total hip arthroplasty. *Clin Orthop* 1993;296:133–139.
6. Gie GA, Linder L, Ling RS, Simon JP, Slooff TJ, Timperley AJ. Impacted cancellous allografts and cement for revision total hip arthroplasty. *J Bone Joint Surg Br* 1993;75:14–21.
7. Gilbert JL, Buckley CA, Jacobs JJ. In vivo corrosion of modular hip prosthesis components in mixed and similar metal combinations: the effect of crevice, stress, motion, and alloy coupling. *J Biomed Mater Res* 1993;27:1533–1544.
8. Gustilo RB, Pasternak HS. Revision total hip arthroplasty with titanium ingrowth prosthesis and bone grafting for failed cemented femoral compontent loosening. *Clin Orthop* 1988;235:111–119.
9. Harris WH. Is it advantageous to strengthen the cement–metal interface and use a collar for cemented femoral components of total hip replacements? *Clin Orthop* 1992;285:67–72.
10. Head WC, Wagner RA, Emerson RH Jr, Malinin TI. Revision total hip arthroplasty in the deficient femur with a proximal load-bearing prosthesis. *Clin Orthop* 1994;298:119–126.
11. Hedley AK, Gruen TA, Ruoff DP. Revision of failed total hip arthroplasties with uncemented porous coated anatomic components. *Clin Orthop* 1988;235:75–90.
12. Katz RP, Callaghan JJ, Sullivan PM, Johnston RC. Results of cemented femoral revision total hip arthroplasty using improved cementing techniques. *Clin Orthop* 1995;319:178–183.
13. Kavanagh BF, Ilstrup DM, Fitzgerald RH Jr. Revision total hip arthroplasty. *J Bone Joint Surg Am* 1985;67:517–521.
14. Krushell RJ, Burke DW, Harris WH. Range of motion in contemporary total hip arthroplasty: the impact of modular head-neck components. *J Arthroplasty* 1991;6:97–101.
15. Lawrence JM, Engh CA, Macalino GE, Lauro GR. Outcome of revision hip arthroplasty done without cement. *J Bone Joint Surg Am* 1994;76:965–973.
16. Malkani AL, Lewallen DG, Cabanela ME, Wallrichs SL. Femoral component revision using an uncemented, proximally coated, long stem prosthesis. *J Arthroplasty* 1996;11:411–418.
17. McKellop H, Lu B, Benya P. Friction, lubrication and wear of cobalt-chromium, alumina, and zirconia hip prostheses compared on a joint simulator. *Trans Orthop Res Soc* 1992;17:402 (abstract).

18. Mulroy WF, Harris WH. Revision total hip arthroplasty with use of so-called second-generation cementing techniques for aseptic loosening of the femoral component: a fifteen-year average follow-up study. *J Bone Joint Surg Am* 1996;78:325–330.
19. Paprosky WG, Krishnamurthy A. Five to 14-year follow up on cementless femoral revisions. *Orthopedics* 1996;19:765–768.
20. Pellici PM, Wilson PD Jr, Sledge CV, et al. Long term results of revision total hip replacement: a follow-up report. *J Bone Joint Surg Am* 1985;67:513–516.
21. Tsukayama DT, Estrada R, Gustilo RB. Infection after total hip arthroplasty: a study of the treatment of one hundred and six infections. *J Bone Joint Surg Am* 1996;78:512–523.
22. Urban R, Jacobs J, Gilbert J, Galante J. Migration of corrosion products from modular hip prostheses. *J Bone Joint Surg Am* 1994;76:1345–1359.
23. Yue S, Pilliar RM, Weatherly GC. The fatigue strength of porous-coated ITit-6%Al-4%V implant alloy. *J Biomed Mater Res* 1984;18:1043–1058.

Revision Total Hip Arthroplasty,
edited by Marvin E. Steinberg and Jonathan P. Garino,
Lippincott Williams & Wilkins, Philadelphia © 1998.

16

Acetabular Bone Grafting: Structural Grafts

Wayne G. Paprosky and
Todd D. Sekundiak

Because of the increasing prevalence of primary total hip arthroplasty and the wider age distribution of patients, the number and complexity of revision arthroplasties is increasing. With the demands on arthroplasties increasing and the length of time these arthroplasties are in place, failures most commonly occur from wear, osteolysis, or aseptic loosening. Despite the improved technique of insertion and the quality of product inserted, the global prevalence of total hip arthroplasties also leads to failures from infection, recurrent dislocation, periprosthetic and prosthetic fracture, component incompatibility, and recurrent dislocation. The *in situ* process of component failure and iatrogenic removal of this failed component can lead to massive bone loss that prevents the surgeon from inserting a component in the routine primary way.

A multitude of techniques have been described for acetabular revision. These have included cemented cups, press-fit and porous coated components, bilobed components, threaded cups, bipolar stems, reconstruction, and antiprotrusio cages, all with or without bone graft. With minor bone defects, excellent results have been obtained with press-fit porous ingrowth implants (7,24). The use of these press-fit components in isolation has been precluded in larger acetabular defects. Cemented acetabular revisions generally have led to unacceptably high failure rates in long-term follow-up studies (21). The concom-

W. G. Paprosky: Department of Orthopedic Surgery, Rush-Presbyterian-St. Luke's Medical Center and Central DuPage Hospital, Chicago, Illinois 60612.
T. D. Sekundiak: Section of Orthopaedic Surgery, University of Manitoba, St. Boniface Hospital, Winnipeg, Manitoba, Canada, R2H 3C3.

itant use of impacted morselized allograft has lead to promising results in less severe defects (25). Acetabular reconstruction with threaded and bipolar cups has proved unsuccessful (15,18).

Acetabular bone grafting has been used to augment components in the revision setting and has shown generally good results (2,6,7,24). It serves multiple functions. It can provide initial stability for the acetabular component. The long-term goal is to restore patient bone stock that will prolong the length of fixation of the component and reduce the difficulty of possible future revisions. Autogenous bone graft has the advantages of improved osteoinductive potential and decreased risk for disease transmission (5). Unfortunately, the amount of graft available is limited. Allogeneic bone or bone substitutes are left as an alternative. Morselized graft can be impacted into contained defects that then can be substituted for host bone (10). Structural grafts can reconstitute rim or column defects and restore normal bone architecture (4).

With porous ingrowth cups, the allograft provides initial support until this is supplanted by actual ingrowth of host bone into the component (4). Ultimately with cemented components, stability must be transferred to host bone (25). If this is not possible, components must be supported by ancillary cages, or the graft must be large enough to prevent complete revascularization and ultimate graft failure (11,22,23,27). Use of graft in both these situations can allow placement of a cup in a more normal anatomic position that may prevent excess stress on the components and allow better joint function.

Differences in philosophies as to how acetabular component fixation should be achieved determine the type and need for acetabular allografting in the revision setting. In this era of fiscal constraint and informed consumerism, unjustified use of allograft no longer is tolerated. The surgeon is accountable for the increased monetary cost, risk for infection, operating time, and survivability of the component in determining the need for acetabular allograft in the revision setting. To be efficient, the surgeon must anticipate possible and probable difficulties with revision arthroplasty and therefore must have a preoperative plan based on the defects presented. This requires determination of the type of components, need for allografting, and equipment for removal and insertion of the components.

We have raised concerns with the American Academy of Orthopaedic Surgeons classification of acetabular defect because its descriptive nature fails to provide adequate criteria for classification and recommendations for reconstruction (6). We therefore prefer to use our own classification in determining when and where acetabular allograft should be used along with the reconstructive procedure in total (4) (Table 1).

Structural allografts are not required for less severe defects. We have presented the results of 125 acetabular revisions reconstructed with a porous ingrowth cup that were

Table 1. *Classification of acetabular defects*

Defect type	Superior migration[a]	Ischial lysis[b]	Medial migration[c]	Tear-drop lysis[d]
I	Insignificant	None	None	None
IIA	Insignificant	Mild	Grade I	Mild
IIB	Insignificant to significant	Mild	Grade II	Mild
IIC	Insignificant	Mild	Grade III	Moderate to severe
IIIA	Significant	Moderate	Grade II+ or III	Moderate to severe
IIIB	Significant	Severe	Grade III+	Severe

[a] Insignificant, less than 3 cm above superior transverse obturator line; significant, more than 3 cm above superior transverse obturator line.
[b] Mild, 0 to 7 mm below superior transverse obturator line; moderate, 7 to 14 mm below obturator line; severe, 15-mm lysis.
[c] Grade I, lateral to Kohler's line; grade II, migration to Kohler's line; grade II+, medial expansion of Kohler's line into pelvis; grade III, migration into pelvis with violation of Kohler's line; grade III+, marked migration into pelvis.
[d] Mild, minimal loss of the lateral border; moderate, complete loss of lateral border; severe, loss of lateral and medial borders.

either a type I or type II acetabular defect. By definition, these acetabula have at least 70% of host bone in contact with the acetabular cup. Cup fixation did not require augmentation, and use of morselized graft was solely for reconstitution of bone stock (20). After an average follow-up period of 6.6 years, all cups are stable with no radiographic or clinical evidence of aseptic loosening. Two revisions failed from septic processes, but all other patients continued to function well with an average Harris hip score improvement from 36 preoperatively to 86 at final follow-up examination.

Use of structural allograft is reserved for revisions in which extensive bone loss precludes use of alternative means of reconstruction. The use of structural allograft was initially supported by Jasty and Harris (12) when press fitting of cups was not possible. They later advised against use of allografts quoting a failure rate of 47% (13). Paprosky et al. (19) and Gross et al. (9) had better results but had stringent selection criteria in determining use of allografts and performing the insertion.

PREOPERATIVE PLANNING

The need for a structural allograft is determined preoperatively by templating. Use of specialized radiographs and computed tomographic (CT) scans has been advocated to assess acetabular bony defects and the likelihood of needing an allograft. These techniques can be cumbersome and difficult to evaluate. On an anteroposterior radiograph of a pelvis, the four radiographic criteria of hip center migration, degree of ischial lysis, presence of teardrop destruction, and extent of Kohler's line disruption can be determined simply. These criteria can then be quantitated to determine the structural integrity of the walls and columns of the host acetabulum. With knowledge of the extent of bone loss and the amount of host bone remaining, the type of acetabular reconstruction can be estimated. This is the basis of our classification of acetabular defects (4) (see Table 1).

The superior migration of the hip center determines the degree of involvement of the confluence of the anterior and posterior columns and its ability to support a new component. As migration progresses more superolaterally, more posterior column is involved; superomedial migration involves more of the anterior column. Ischial lysis determines the degree of posteroinferior wall and column involvement, and teardrop lysis determines the extent of anteroinferior wall and column involvement. The integrity of Kohler's line is used to assess the amount of medial wall involvement. When all of these sectors of involvement are combined, the degree of bone loss can be determined and estimated.

If the hip center has migrated 3 cm from the superior transverse obturator line or more than 2 cm from the normal hip center, ischial lysis is mild (0 to 7 mm) to moderate (8 to 14 mm), teardrop lysis is mild (minimal loss of the lateral border of the tear drop) to moderate (complete loss), and Kohler's line disruption is at least grade II (migration of the cup to Kohler's line but not through) to II+ (migration through Kohler's line but with expansion of the medial wall), one is dealing with a minimum type IIIA acetabular defect. If ischial lysis has become severe (more than 15 mm of involvement), tear-drop lysis involves the medial portion, and Kohler's line violation has progressed to a grade III or III+ (migration of the component into the pelvis), a type IIIB defect is present.

By determining that a type IIIA defect is present, we have estimated that at least 50% of host bone is remaining and there exists the possibility of obtaining ingrowth of a porous cup into the host acetabulum. With a type IIIB defect, the degree of radiographic alteration is so severe that a minimum of 50% host bone is lost and the columns cannot support the use of a press-fit cup in the acetabulum. Attempts at obtaining ingrowth of a porous ingrowth cup with a type IIIA defect without use of an allograft is possible but associates with a higher loosening rate than with lesser defects. To aid initial stability and to reconstitute overall bone stock, a structural allograft is suggested to substitute for the deficient wall and column. With a type IIIB defect, the peripheral wall and column defects are so massive that the allograft will not be able to reconstitute the rim, and press fitting a cup will not be successful. Even if rim fit is possible, a porous implant is not recommended because the area of contact with the host bone is decreased to such a degree that sufficient ingrowth rarely takes place. Hemipelvis allograft transplantation is recommended with an implant cemented into the allograft.

OPERATIVE TECHNIQUE

The operative technique begins with full preoperative planning. The appropriate graft has been selected, and harvesting should comply with the guidelines recommended by the Musculoskeletal Council of the American Association of Tissue Banks (16). A postero-lateral approach is standard for this procedure. This allows complete visualization of the acetabular rim, both the anterior and posterior aspects and the iliac wing and ischium proximally and distally. Débridement of the acetabular pseudocapsule is pursued until exposure of the acetabular rim is complete. Posterior dissection must proceed in a subperiosteal manner to protect the sciatic nerve. A posterior flap of pseudocapsule is maintained as a protective layer for the sciatic nerve. This flap can be used as retraction point for self-retaining retractors. In large defects, anterior dissection must proceed judiciously because the femoral neurovacular bundles or branches of the bundle can be encountered. Adequate anterior dissection is essential to remove scarred reactive capsule and allow anterior displacement of the femur. This provides adequate exposure of the acetabulum for removal and insertion of components. Components, cement, and debris are removed. At this stage, final determination of the acetabular defect is made. If visualization is not adequate, an extended trochanteric femoral osteotomy can be used at any point during the procedure (26).

With severe type IIIB defects, the options for reconstruction are obvious. With type IIIA or severe type II defects, the ability of the host to support a press-fit acetabulum is undetermined until reaming proceeds and attempts at trial component insertion are completed. Reaming proceeds until contact occurs with some point of the medial wall and the remaining peripheral rim. Reaming should be minimal and is performed to obtain the best sphere without producing further structural bone loss.

Acetabular defects are not always self-evident. Trial shells are indispensible in determining whether a press-fit component will be successful. On trials of the component, the surgeon must assess the size and location of the peripheral and contained defects and the ability of the host bone to support the component. At this stage, the surgeon can finalize the mode of reconstruction required. If structural allograft is considered, dissection both superiorly and inferiorly is needed for placement of the graft. Dissection always proceeds subperiosteally from the remaining acetabular rim to avoid neurovascular compromise. Superior dissection lifts the abductor musculature for access to structural bone for fixation of the graft. The superior gluteal neurovascular bundle is avoided with subperiosteal dissection and avoidance of the greater sciatic foramen.

Throughout the operation and especially before further reconstruction, it is essential to rule out the existence of pelvic discontinuity. Pelvic discontinuity in revision arthroplasty occurs from a chronic degenerative process not from acute trauma. The discontinuity can be obscured by osteolytic fibrous tissue, and its insidious presence may be confirmed only at the time of reaming. Reaming débrides the acetabulum further and removes nonstruc-tural bone excrescences that may mask the discontinuity. Avoiding full exposure and exploration of the defect blinds the surgeon to the possibility of discontinuity and leads to catastrophic early failure of the reconstruction. If present, the discontinuity must be stabilized before the reconstruction. With a type IIIA defect, a pelvic reconstruction plate is used to bridge the discontinuity initially. Then reconstruction of the acetabular defect with the structural allograft proceeds. This same type of stabilization can be used with a type IIIB defect, although use of a reconstruction cage has supplanted use of a structural allograft. For most discontinuities, stabilization is required only along the posterior column. When the initial dissection is extended posteriorly, the plate can be fashioned to the posterior column and transfixed to the remaining column, superior acetabular dome and iliac wing and inferiorly to the ischium.

Type IIIA Defect

Initial acetabular reaming is used to size the defect, size the remaining host acetabulum, and size the amount of allograft required. To attempt to use a structural allograft with a press-fit component, at least 50% of the host acetabulum should be present to support the acetabular shell. Trial acetabular inserts are essential to assess the defect present and the viability of obtaining a press fit. The allograft is relied on to augment bone stock and augment initial stability but cannot be relied on to obtain initial stability. If a trial acetabular shell cannot provide gross stability without the graft, an alternative method of reconstruction must be chosen.

Once the acetabular trial is in place, the allograft is selected to reconstruct the defect while allowing placement of the acetabular shell. The graft must span the defect, allow fixation onto the iliac wing, and incorporate the shape of the acetabular shell, and not be weakened by the sculpting process. Because of these multiple criteria, bone of sufficient structural caliber is required, and distal femur therefore is chosen. The medial and lateral femoral condyles act as extensions that reproduce the deficient anterior and posterior columns. Their confluence reconstitutes the superior dome, and the distal femoral diaphysis acts as an extension to anchor the graft to the host iliac wing.

Initial sculpting of the graft is aimed at debulking its mass. A female reamer or an oscillating saw is used to remove excess anterior, lateral, and medial bone from the graft. A female reamer 2 mm larger than the last acetabular reamer is selected and placed distal to the graft. The reamer is directed proximally to remove enough anterior bone to remove the anterior femoral flare without producing a notch (Fig. 1). Symmetric bone should be removed from the medial and lateral sides to prevent weakening of the graft. This reaming or cutting is best performed with the bone in a vise.

The graft is cut along the midcoronal axis of the femoral shaft to a point proximal to the femoral condyles. The cut is completed in an oblique, posterior, and distal direction to the femoral condyles. The remaining anterior proximal shaft is cut to 4 to 5 cm. This acts as a proximal flange for fixation of the graft to the remaining host ilium. The length and shape of the graft are modified in this upside down 7 configuration to allow the graft

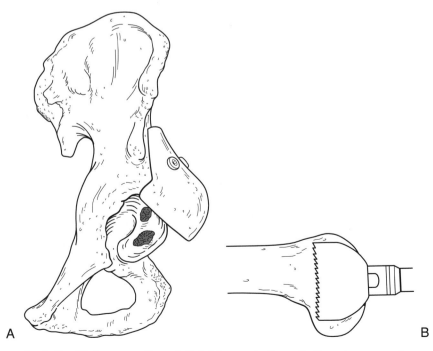

A   B

Figure 1. A: Sagittal perspective of distal femoral allograft. Female reamer is used to remove bulk of distal femoral graft. **B:** Anterior perspective of distal femoral allograft secured to pelvis and occupying acetabular defect.

to buttress the remaining anterior and posterior columns, superior dome and iliac wing. The graft can be oriented more anteriorly or posteriorly to compensate for individual bone-loss patterns. With the graft shaped in this way, no rocking or point loading should be present. Supplemental screw fixation is needed to provide compression to prevent migration of the graft. Before screw insertion, a stable interference fit between the host and the graft is essential to prevent early failure. Temporary fixation of the graft is achieved with two Kirschner wires.

The graft is fixed with three or four 6.5-mm cancellous screws with washers. The screws are placed in an oblique manner along the same plane as normal hip loading. This allows compression at the graft–host junction and possible settling of the graft into its most stable position. Screws are directed proximally and medially through the femoral diaphysis of the graft and into the remaining superior iliac wing of the host. If screws are placed too proximally, host bone of insufficient structural integrity will be encountered. If, however, the screws are placed too distally, they will intrude into the acetabular space (Fig. 2).

Once the graft is solidly fixed to the pelvis, the graft is reamed to accept the uncovered dome of the acetabular shell. Small acetabular reamers are used to produce a rounded defect in the graft to accept the component. Reaming size progresses to the last size of acetabular reamer used in the initial sizing. If the graft is excessively bulky, a saw is used initially to remove some of the excess bone. When reamers are used, it is essential not to allow them to migrate off their initial path because excess bone can be removed from the graft, causing it to weaken. Worse yet, large reamers can remove bone from the anterior or posterior columns of the host, producing a more severe acetabular defect. Reaming must continue to ensure that the maximum host bone is in contact with the acetabular shell without weakening the graft or the host. Underreaming by 1 to 2 mm is suggested to allow the porous coated shell to be press fit into the reconstructed acetabulum.

A trial is suggested to ensure that press fit is obtainable. If the trial component cannot be seated into the host acetabulum at this stage, the graft is likely too large because reaming did not continue to the medial wall of the host acetabulum. Aggressive impaction of the trial component can explode or fracture the allograft construct. If reamers have

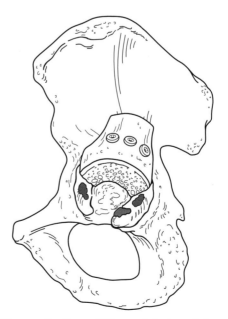

Figure 2. Type IIIA acetabular defect reconstructed with distal femoral allograft. More than 50% of host bone remains for acceptance of a press-fit component.

wandered during the allograft shaping, the acetabular cavity can be made elliptical, and a larger trial is needed to obtain press fit. The host–graft intraacetabular junction and any other contained defects can be impacted with morselized graft before seating of the actual acetabular component. Impaction grafting at these junctions aids in further stabilizing the graft and ensures maximum contact with the cup to improve its stability.

The acetabular component must be stable at insertion (Fig. 3). If motion can be produced by means of manipulation of the component, the graft must be redone, or consideration must be given to acetabular transplantation. The acetabular component recommended contains peripheral screws, which parallel the forces at the hip joint and allow initial early settling. Early migration of a cup is possible without compromise to its stability if peripheral screws are used (20).

Type IIIB Defect

Sizing of the acetabular defect with acetabular reamers gives a hemispheric shape to the remaining bone for acceptance of the transplant and sizes the acetabular defect and the remaining rim diameter. With classification of the defect as type IIIB, it has been determined preoperatively and intraoperatively that less than 50% of host bone is remaining within the acetabulum and that press fitting an acetabular component is accompanied by a high failure rate. An ipsilateral hemipelvic allograft is obtained from a tissue bank to reconstruct the deficient acetabulum. Graft, if possible, should be from a young man to ensure that it is strong enough to accept screw fixation and prevent late collapse and failure. Grafts from male donors also are likely to be large enough to bridge the defect.

Exposure of the posterior column, lateral aspect of the ilium, and the ischium is required for fixation of the graft. It is performed in a subperiosteal manner to protect the sciatic nerve posteriorly and inferiorly and the superior gluteal neurovascular bundle superiorly.

The aim in preparing the graft is to produce a tongue-and-groove mortise that ensures intimate contact of the graft bone to the host. This allows transfer of the load from the graft

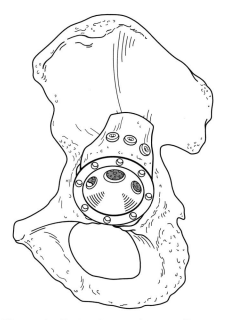

Figure 3. Porous coated press-fit component has been inserted into reconstructed type IIIA acetabulum. Acetabulum has been underreamed by 1 to 2 mm to give initial stability to the component.

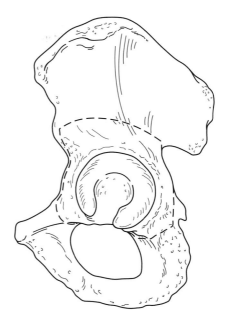

Figure 4. Allogeneic hemipelvic transplant initially cut along marked lines for acceptance into host acetabulum.

to the host, which may aid in biologic incorporation and improve longevity. The acetabular allograft is shaped to buttress the host bone. The superior pubic and ischial rami of the graft are cut at a point distal to the acetabular portion with a length remaining to fill the defects in the host pelvis and buttress the remaining pubic and ischial rami of the host pelvis (Fig. 4). The iliac wing of the graft is cut in a curvilinear manner from the greater sciatic notch to the anterior inferior iliac spine (see Fig. 4). This gives ample room for the graft to accept fixation without the bulk of excess bone and the concern of entering the joint cavity. The iliac flange can be customized in size and shape to allow best positioning of screws for purchase in the iliac crest host bone. Initial trialing of the graft for fit and modification of the preliminary cuts is performed. Initial cuts should be conservative to maintain as much structural bone as possible and avoid the possibility of undersizing the graft. This can lead to poor fixation, poor stability, and early failure.

The tongue-and-groove mortise is made on the medial aspect of the graft by developing a groove in the inner table of the graft at a point where contact is made with the superior acetabular rim of the host (Fig. 5). A high-speed cylindrical burr or female reamer sized 2 mm larger than the last male reamer used in the host acetabular defect is used to score the medial side of the graft. This produces a hemispheric defect 1 to 1.5 cm deep that

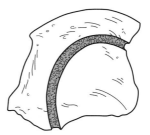

Figure 5. Medial aspect of transplant has been scored with a female reamer to provide an interference fit with the remaining host acetabular rim.

accepts the remaining rim of host acetabulum. The position of the groove is marked by means of templating the graft to the host bone and typically extends from the anterior inferior iliac spine to the ischium. The cylindrical burr is used to sculpt the groove in the graft to accept the irregularities in the host rim and to ensure that there is a tight tongue and groove fit. The medial portion of the graft should not be thinned to allow compromise of the articular surface or outer table because this leads to loss of structural integrity and the possibility of graft fracture. The graft is seated in position, and manipulation of the graft in all planes determines the most stable position.

Reconstruction cages present surgeons with more options. The role of these devices has not been clearly defined, and different surgeons have been using them for different types of defects. The anatomic features of the cage are as varied as the manufacturers. Cages such as the Müller (17) (Sulzer Orthopaedics, Inc., Austin, TX) acetabular reinforcement ring cannot bridge severe type III defects and therefore we do not use them. The Burch-Schneider antiprotrusio cage (Sulzer Orthopaedics, Inc., Austin, TX) allows fixation proximal and distal to the acetabular defect and provides greater ability to customize the cage to the appropriate defect (3) (Fig. 6). Other newer devices, such as the GAP cup (Osteonics, Allendale, N.J.) and the antiprotrusio cage (DePuy, Warsaw, Ind.), are similar in design. It is essential to understand that these cages act as supports for the bony reconstruction, which must precede placement of the cage. The method of reconstruction behind the cage can be as varied as the design of the cage itself.

Use of a cage allows the surgeon to customize the graft to more accurately fit the defect. Use of the cage also prevents heavy reliance on a bone bank to provide an accurately sized graft for reconstruction. Grafts can be trimmed and customized to fit the actual defect. When there is more independent posterior or anterior column defect, the graft can be split in a vertical direction. This allows the remaining host bone to accept load and decrease the amount of load on the allograft. Splitting the graft decreases its overall mass and decreases the peak loads it can carry. The graft is therefore supported by a reconstruction cage that fits into the defect and acts as a bridge between the ischium, graft, and ilium. Fixation of the graft can be optimized with screws through the cage and into the graft. This technique should be considered only when there is remaining host column to provide structural support for the cage. If there is no column, the entire hemipelvic allograft should be used.

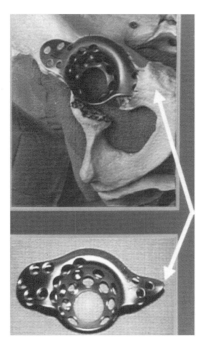

Figure 6. Burch-Schneider antiprotrusio cage positioned into defect. If inadequate bone is present for screw fixation inferiorly, the cage can be impacted into the ischial endosteal compartment.

The graft seated in position is gently impacted and locked into its final position. An acetabular reamer with an attached wooden handle or a trial acetabulum with an insertion handle is used to impact the graft in place without producing peak stress concentrations, which may fracture the host or graft bone. The graft should be stable enough that no gross motion occurs with gentle manipulation. Temporary fixation can be achieved with two Kirschner wires if needed. Final fixation proceeds with 6.5-mm, partially threaded, cancellous screws and washers (Fig. 7). They are placed in the iliac wing just superior to the acetabular dome of the graft. Screws are directed in the direction of load, superior and medial, to allow collapse and migration. This optimizes host–graft contact for early union. Screw placement should aim for the remaining host's confluence of acetabular columns with as wide anterior and posterior placement as possible (see Fig. 7). Screws placed too far superiorly obtain weaker fixation as the iliac wing thins in its inner and outer tables. It is optimal to use three to four screws that each obtain bicortical purchase into the host ilium. No manipulation from any force vector should produce motion at this time.

Graft acetabular preparation proceeds by means of sequential reaming to remove cartilage and to minimally ream subchondral bone. Reaming should not proceed through subchondral bone because this weakens the graft. Reaming should not begin until fixation of the graft is complete. Small cement anchor holes can be placed but should not violate the medial cortical table of the graft. This weakens the graft and places cement at the host–graft interface, which may prevent union of the graft to the host.

If a reconstruction cage is considered, preparation of the acetabular shell proceeds in a similar manner. Reaming need not be as aggressive as with a type IIIA defect. Reaming is only to shape the graft so it can accept the outer diameter of the reconstruction cage. Any remaining defects or host–graft junction points are impacted with morselized allograft with the last acetabular reamer in reverse or a finishing reamer. It is important to impact the graft manually because this prevents the graft from being crushed and losing its structural integrity. The same size reconstruction cage is used as the last acetabular reamer. The cage is then placed by toeing-in the inferior or superior extensions and seating

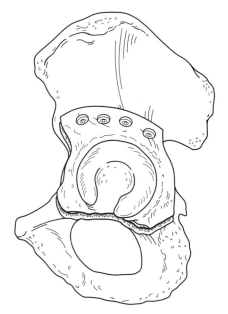

Figure 7. Hemipelvic transplant has been seated into host acetabulum. Interference fit has been obtained at graft–host junctions. Fixation is augmented with 6.5-mm cancellous screws.

the cup in position. Exposure is essential to optimize positioning of the cage and may require further superior or inferior dissection to obtain fit. A sharp retractor superior into the outer table of the ilium is used to retract the abductor mass anteriorly and superiorly for placement of the extensions. Placement of the cage is a compromise between best fit and best orientation of the acetabulum. The aim is to achieve the most appropriate anatomic position of the cage, but fixation and stability are the most critical factors. Multiple trial and moldings are required to ensure the cage maximizes surface contact with the bony surfaces. For this reason, we suggest use of a malleable cage to allow diversity of pelvic defects and shapes.

Stability of the cage is obtained by means of press fitting against the acetabular allograft and the remaining host acetabular rim, iliac wing, ischium, or pubis. Extensions exist on most cages that allow augmentation of stability and fixation through the iliac wing, ischium, or pubis. The cage therefore must be contoured to achieve the best apposition with the bone. Once inserted, the cage should not be rocking or grossly mobile because of a point of contact of the cage to the bone. The cage should buttress the largest surface area of remaining pelvis to achieve best stability.

Fixation proceeds with initial placement of dome screws to ensure that the cage is in maximum contact with the superior portion of the graft and the remaining host acetabulum. Multiple dome screw holes in the cage allow fixation of the cage to the remaining host acetabulum and graft acetabulum. Inferior fixation may occur by means of wedging the inferior extension into the ischium or hooking around the inferior margin of acetabulum. We use screws, if possible, that extend through the inferior extension of the cage and into the anterior aspect of the ischium. Superior fixation is augmented by means of screw placement into the iliac wing. The pelvic tables thin and become nonstructural as one proceeds more superiorly. Screws should be placed close to the acetabulum to exploit the most structural bone. For concomitant pelvic discontinuities, a minimum of two bicortical screws are essential to bridge the defect on each side.

Trial reduction with a cup in the cage or acetabular graft proceeds. Because the trial is mobile, stability is difficult to assess, but leg length and offset are appreciable. Cementing of the cup into the acetabulum or cage entails the same techniques as with other acetabular cementing techniques. Cup placement is determined by the orientation needed for stability with trialing. The cup commonly is uncovered posterosuperiorly. Cement is placed posteriorly to the cup to provide a buttressing effect. If the cage or graft is excessive anteriorly and causing impingement, a saw or power burr can be used for resection. Rarely does a hooded component provide improved stability, but it can be used when the cage is excessively vertical or retroverted. If stability is inadequate because of complete abductor loss or muscular imbalance, a constrained acetabular liner may be used. The long-term sequelae of use of this device are undetermined.

POSTOPERATIVE CARE

For patients who undergo reconstruction with distal femoral allografts, weight bearing remains toe touch for 3 months and then one-third weight bearing for an additional month. Patients then proceed to full weight bearing. A hip abduction brace is used for the initial 3 months. Prophylactic antibiotics are given for 48 hours. Routine hip strengthening proceeds after this initial protective period. Radiographic and clinical follow-up examinations are performed 6 weeks and 3 and 6 months after the operation, and then annually.

Postoperative rehabilitation for the acetabular allografts consists of protected weight bearing for 6 months with use of a hip-knee-ankle-foot orthosis for the initial 4 months. Touch weight bearing continues for the first 4 months. Progressive weight bearing continues for an additional 1 to 2 months. All patients should wear a brace because of poor soft-tissue tension, multiple previous operative procedures, and extensile exposure. With adequate abductor musculature, the knee-ankle-foot extension can be eliminated. Prophylactic antibiotics are continued for 5 days. Radiographic and clinical assessment is made every 1 to 3 months, biannually for 2 years, and then annually.

Thromboembolic prophylaxis proceeds as for any arthroplasty. Patients take low-molecular-weight heparin 24 hours after the operation and then warfarin to maintain an international normalized ratio of 1.3 to 1.5 for 4 weeks.

RESULTS

Type IIIA Defects

We have reviewed distal femoral allograft reconstructions with a minimum follow-up period of 7 years. All reconstructions were performed with a porous coated acetabular shell. Twenty-nine of 30 patients were available for final clinical and radiographic follow-up examinations. The follow-up period averaged 10.1 years. One early radiographic failure had been reported previously. This acetabular component showed more than 4 mm of superior migration during the initial 6 months with no further migration after a follow-up period of 9 years. No other failures occurred. Of all 48 distal femoral allografts inserted between 1982 and 1992 for type IIIA defects, three failures occurred, the one mentioned earlier remaining *in situ*. The other two failures occurred with a cemented acetabular shell and a threaded cup. No late complications developed, but polyethylene wear had progressed at an average of 0.06 mm/year.

Type IIIB Defects

We reported on 20 whole acetabular transplant allografts performed for severe type IIIB defects (3). Patients had received diagnoses of primary osteoarthritis in 11 instances, trauma in five instances, and rheumatoid arthritis, gunshot wound, developmental dysplasia, and radiation necrosis in one instance each. At the most recent follow-up examination, 17 patients were available (14). Garbuz et al. (8) previously reported on a

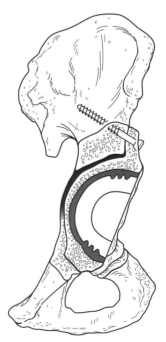

Figure 8. Coronal view of hemipelvic transplantation for type IIIB defect. Intimate host–graft contact ensures stability of graft. Screws are placed in the direction of hip-loading forces. Screw placement is optimized in remaining structural bone.

series of 11 acetabular transplants with a 2-year success rate of 71%. The average radiographic and clinical follow-up was 33 months.

All patients underwent reconstruction with a whole acetabular transplant allograft and a cemented acetabular component with the technique previously described (Fig. 8). All grafts had radiographic evidence of union at 2 years, one union being confirmed by means of bone biopsy. Early migration of the graft was evident in most instances. Migration averaged 1 to 2 mm. One graft migrated 4 mm over 36 months and ultimately failed. Three failures occurred—two caused by sepsis and one by graft resorption and migration. Most grafts showed some continual minor lateral resorption. According to the modified D'Aubigne and Postel pain and walking score, patients improved from 3.7 preoperatively to 8.9 at last follow-up examination.

The most common complication was instability, six patients experienced dislocation. Five patients were treated successfully with a brace, and one patient needed revision to a constrained cup. Two dislocations occurred anteriorly from excessive anteversion of the resultant cup, one from patient noncompliance, and three others from poor musculature, multiple previous operative procedures, and a history of recurrent dislocation. Consideration to the aforementioned constrained acetabular liners is given if abductor muscles are absent or stability is not within a safe range.

Infection occurred among four patients; two were treated with local débridement and antibiotics. One patient had a recurrence of a previously present gram-negative infection. He was treated with suppressive antibiotics and had no symptoms despite radiographic evidence of graft failure. The last infection necessitated resection arthroplasty as curative treatment. Berry et al. (1) reviewed two-stage reconstructions after failure of hip replacements due to infections and found the infection rate to parallel those in other studies in which revisions were performed without allografting. They concluded that the concern is unfounded that the presence of allografts leads to a high rate of infection.

CONCLUSIONS

We continue to evolve the process of acetabular revision. Attempts to reconstruct a failed acetabulum with cement have shown poor long-term results. Attempts have led to the use of threaded cups and complete abandonment of reconstructing the acetabulum with the use of a bipolar prosthesis (15,18). All attempts have lead to failures. Reconstruction with impacted morselized allograft and cemented cups has led to some promising results, although defect size has been mixed (25). Use of a high hip center and an ingrowth cup shows promise in the treatment of selected patients and has been an alternative chosen because of the high failure rate with acetabular allografts (13).

We continue to support the use of allografts in the management of selected acetabular defects. Through experience we have quoted failure rates with distal femoral allografts to be 6% and 64% after 6.1 years of follow-up study (19). The difference in failure rate is attributable to the fact that success depends not only on the type of graft but also on the type of acetabular defect. The identical technique gave the aforementioned different results because the defects were type IIIA versus type IIIB. Although retrospective and not randomized, the failure rate for reconstructions without structural allografts for type IIIA defects has been shown to be much higher, 18.5% after 6.6 years of follow-up study (2).

We are still faced with the dilemma of what to do with severe acetabular type IIIB defects. Bone loss is massive, reconstruction is difficult, and the postoperative course is tenuous. We recommend use of a hemipelvic transplant. After average follow-up periods of 33 months, failure rates are approximately 18% (14). This is not optimal but is acceptable in view of the situation. We are continuing to tune our reconstruction to bring survivability of these constructs to a longer term. Garbuz et al. (8) concurred with our results and reported good results with the use of cemented acetabular components and large segmental allografts provided that strict adherence to technical aspects of graft placement and fixation are observed.

Use of a reconstruction cage to augment a hemipelvic allograft may show promise in protecting the graft but not totally shielding it from normal hip stresses. The cages may allow the surgeon to debulk and customize the graft to optimize the fit and amount of load transmitted to the host bone. This could stimulate osteogenesis and improve longevity of the construct. More current is the monetary concern over large structural allografts. The reconstruction cage may prevent reliance on scarce hemipelvic allografts and allow other types of graft to substitute. The surgeon also can modify the graft for variably sized defects without reordering graft for each patient. These proposals are speculative without confirmed benefits of one method over the other. It is essential, however, that the graft span the defect. In many type IIIB defects, only an entire hemipelvic allograft is capable of spanning the defect and providing support for the acetabular component.

Surgeons must accept these technically demanding features if the reconstruction is to be undertaken. They also must accept the higher complication rate with the use of structural allografts, because these patients have severe bone loss with severe soft tissue compromise after multiple previous operative procedures. Surgeons also need to be efficient in the operating theater to ensure that the optimal procedure is performed for the least cost and with minimal risk to both hospital and patient. No longer can the use of bulk graft be accepted for lesser defects when the use of porous coated press-fit implants has been shown to have very acceptable long-term results.

We recommend use of distal femoral allografts for type IIIA acetabular defects when more than 50% host bone is available for biologic fixation. If more than 70% of host bone is available for biologic fixation, then the need for structural allografting should be questioned. The acetabulum must be able to support the shell in isolation, and the graft acts to augment this fixation. With placement of the graft and shell to accept normal physiologic hip loads, failures should be minimized.

For type IIIB defects in which the acetabulum cannot support the use of a porous acetabular shell, the options are few, the follow-up period short, and the argument less controversial. Less than 50% of host bone is available for fixation of an implant, which makes options limited. Our short-term results with whole acetabular transplants indicate a success rate of about 82% at 3 years. The use of reconstruction cages has met with a failure rate of 24% at 5 years (2). Unfortunately, direct comparison of results is difficult because there is no unanimity on classification of the acetabular defects and the types of reconstruction that follow use of reconstruction cages is as different as the number of cages manufactured. With newer design features for the cages, their uses are expanding. We continue to support use of a reconstruction cage to aid in load transfer from the structural allograft to the host and to aid in fixation.

The technique of acetabular structural allografting is demanding, costly, and risky to all involved. Results are encouraging but still suboptimal compared with those of revisions for lesser defects. Undertaking this endeavor should be sought by those who have the resources to deal with the procedure, the rehabilitation, and the complications.

With adherence to a strict protocol in the preoperative, operative, and postoperative phases, use of structural allograft in revision acetabular arthroplasty can promote success. The selection of graft depends entirely on the type of defect being reconstructed. Attempts to use graft when not indicated will lead to disastrous consequences with early failure, infection, difficult reconstruction, or at the very least monetary waste. Structural allografting can be the most viable option in other situations; even when it fails, the presence of the graft has been reported to improve host bone stock and facilitate subsequent re-revision.

REFERENCES

1. Berry DJ, Chandler HP, Reilly DT. The use of bone allografts in two-stage reconstruction after failure of hip replacements due to infection. *J Bone Joint Surg Am* 1991;73:1460–1468.
2. Berry DJ, Müller ME. Revision arthroplasty using an anti-protrusio cage for massive acetabular bone deficiency. *J Bone Joint Surg Br* 1992;74:711–720.
3. Bradford MS, Paprosky WG. Total acetabular transplant allograft reconstruction of the severely deficient acetabulum. *Semin Arthroplasty* 1995;6:86–95.
4. Bradford MS, Paprosky WG. Acetabular defect classification: a detailed radiographic approach. *Semin Arthroplasty* 1995;6:76–85.

5. Czitrom AA, Gross ARE, Langer F, et al. Bone banks and allografts in community practice. *Instr Course Lect* 1988;37:13–24.
6. D'Antonio J, Capello WN, Borden LS, et al. Classification and management of acetabular abnormalities in total hip arthroplasty. *Clin Orthop* 1989;243:126–137.
7. Dorr LD, Wan Z. Ten years of experience with porous acetabular components for revision surgery. *Clin Orthop* 1995;319:191–200.
8. Garbuz D, Morsi E, Gross AE. Revision of the acetabular component of a total hip arthroplasty with a massive structural allograft: study with a minimum five-year follow-up. *J Bone Joint Surg Am* 1996;78:693–697.
9. Gross AE, Allan DG, Catre M, et al. Bone grafts in hip replacement surgery: the pelvic side. *Orthop Clin North Am* 1993;24:679–687.
10. Heekin DR, Engh CA, Vinh T. Morselized allograft in acetabular reconstruction: a postmortem retrieval analysis. *Clin Orthop* 1995;319:184–190.
11. Hooten JP, Engh CA Jr, Engh CA. Failure of structural acetabular allografts in cementless revision hip arthroplasty. *J Bone Joint Surg Am* 1994;76:419–422.
12. Jasty M, Harris WH. Salvage total hip reconstruction in patients with major acetabular bone deficiency using structural femoral head allografts. *J Bone Joint Surg Br* 1990;72:63–67.
13. Kwong LM, Jasty M, Harris WH. High failure rate of bulk femoral head allografts in total hip acetabular reconstruction at 10 years. *J Arthroplasty* 1993;8:341–350.
14. Macdonald SJ, Paprosky WG, Krishnamurthy A, Bradford M. Acetabular transplants in revision total hip arthroplasty: when there are no alternatives. Presented at the 63rd Annual Meeting of the American Academy of Orthopaedic Surgeons; Feb. 22-26, 1996: Atlanta.
15. More RC, Amstutz HC, Kabo JM, et al. Acetabular reconstruction with a threaded prosthesis for failed total hip arthroplasty. *Clin Orthop* 1992;282:114–122.
16. Mowe JC, ed. *Standards for tissue banking.* Arlington, Va: American Association of Tissue Banks 1988.
17. Müller ME. Acetabular revision. In: *The hip: proceedings of the meeting of the Hip Society.* St. Louis: Mosby, 1981:46–56.
18. Namba RS, Clarke A, Scott RD. Bipolar revisions with bone-grafting for cavitary and segmental acetabular defects. *J Arthroplasty* 1994;9:263–272.
19. Paprosky WG, Perona PG, Lawrence JM. Acetabular defect classification and surgical reconstruction in revision arthroplasty: a 6 year follow-up evaluation. *J Arthroplasty* 1994;9:33–44.
20. Paprosky W, Sekundiak T, Kronick J. Porous ingrowth acetabular cups with peripheral screw placement: a solution to the deficient acetabulum. Presented at the 52nd Annual Canadian Orthopaedic Association Meeting: May 31, June 4, 1997, Hamilton, Ont.
21. Petera P, Rubash HE. Revision total hip arthroplasty: the acetabular component. *J AAOS* 1995;3:15–21.
22. Peters CL, Curtain M, Samuelson KM. Acetabular revision with the Burch-Schneider antiprotrusio cage and cancellous allograft bone. *J Arthroplasty* 1995;10:307–312.
23. Rosson J, Schatzker J. The use of reinforcement rings to reconstruct deficient acetabula. *J Bone Joint Surg Br* 1992;74:716–720.
24. Silverton CD, Rosenberg AG, Sheinkop MB, Kull LR, Galante JO. Revision total hip arthroplasty using cementless acetabular component: technique and results. *Clin Orthop* 1995;319:201–208.
25. Slooff TJJH, Buma P, Schreurs BW, Schimmel JW, Huiskes R, Gardeniers J. Acetabular and femoral reconstruction with impacted graft and cement. *Clin Orthop* 1996;323:108–115.
26. Younger TI, Bradford MS, Magnus RE, Paprosky WG. Extended proximal femoral osteotomy: a new technique for femoral revision arthroplasty. *J Arthroplasty* 1995;10:329–338.
27. Zehntner MK, Ganz R. Midterm results (5.5–10 years) of acetabular allograft reconstruction with the acetabular reinforcement ring during total hip revision. *J Arthroplasty* 1994;9:469–479.

Revision Total Hip Arthroplasty,
edited by Marvin E. Steinberg and Jonathan P. Garino,
Lippincott Williams & Wilkins, Philadelphia © 1999.

17

Acetabular Bone Grafting: Impacted Cancellous Allografts

Tom J. J. H. Slooff,
Jean W. M. Gardeniers,
B. Willem Schreurs, and Pieter Buma

Total hip arthroplasty, cemented and cementless, fails in time through multiple failure mechanisms. In most instances failure is caused by aseptic loosening, a slow but progressive process that often is accompanied by loss of bone stock. These lesions may result in enlargement of the acetabulum with superolateral and medial migration of the socket. Choices have to be made in regard to how to deal with loss of bone stock, how to stabilize the new implant, and how to restore hip mechanics. Surgical options have been using more cement (22), metal reinforcement (1), larger implants (17), structural (9), or morselized (19,21) grafts and resection arthroplasty. Although controversies still exist about the management of choice of these bone-stock deficiencies, we prefer a biologic method with tightly impacted cancellous allografts in direct contact with bone cement. We report on the results of this reconstruction in acetabular revision at our center with an average follow-up period of 12 years.

BACKGROUND

In medical practice bone transplantation has a long history. In the early years of surgical treatment, bone transplantation was not an accepted technique. It was

T. J. J. H. Slooff, J. W. M. Gardeniers, B. W. Schreurs, and P. Buma: Orthopaedic Department, University Hospital Sint Radboud, 6500 HB Nijmegen, The Netherlands.

considered an experimental approach with an unpredictable outcome. A breakthrough came in 1947 when techniques (4,24) were developed for preserving and storing allograft bone at −20°C. Although it soon became clear that allografts would not be as successful as autogenous grafts, it became clinically possible to use allografts on a larger scale. During the 1960's, the clinical use of massive allografts became generally accepted to replace parts of the skeleton that had been lost through trauma or tumor (15). Another important clinical application of bone grafts began in 1970's—the repair of osseous defects in association with primary and revision hip arthroplasty. Initial reports (10,14) on acetabular reconstruction with morselized and structural bone grafts set the standard in this field. Regardless of the type of graft used, essential factors that influence the incorporation process are the stability of fixation of the graft, the amount of contact between host and graft, the strain pattern within the graft, and the vascularity of the host bed. The size of the graft also has been found to play an important role in the graft incorporation process (11). This is in accordance with our clinical and experimental experience. Therefore we make the distinction between large-fragment and small-fragment grafts. Large-fragment grafts, such as massive cortical and corticocancellous structural grafts, incorporate incompletely, irregularly, and slowly (6,23). The incorporation process is confined to the outer few millimeters, leaving a more centrally located core permanently necrotic. In time this may cause failure of the graft because of fracture and resorption (13). Impacted cancellous chip allografts allow rapid vascular invasion through the open structure and therefore enable more rapid, complete, and uniform incorporation without mechanical weakening. We have found that grafting with impacted allograft chips does not have the disadvantages of structural allografts. Since the late 1970's the technique of impaction grafting combined with cement fixation of the prosthetic components has been our treatment of choice for restoring bone-stock loss in failed hip arthroplasties on the pelvic side. Since the 1980's a similar technique has been used on the femoral side. The acetabular technique is a modification of the techniques developed by Hastings and Parker (14) and McCollum et al. (12). Morselized, cancellous, small-fragment chips are used. These chips are impacted tightly in the enlarged and distorted acetabular cavity, and cement is applied directly on the graft before the acetabular component is inserted. In medial and peripheral segmental defects, containment is achieved by means of reconstructing these defects with metal wire meshes to support and contain the impacted graft and to achieve initial stability of the entire reconstruction (21).

Starting in 1981 our first femoral reconstructions were grafted without the benefit of specialized instrumentation. Trial stems were used for packing the bone chips into the localized lytic femoral lesions. In the mid-1980's this crude technology also was used in Exeter, United Kingdom, independently of our work in Nijmegen. Once again, the basic technique was aimed at closing all femoral defects, building a new medullary canal with impacted bone chips, cementing a conventional Exeter component, and manufacturing an instrumentation system. This crude technique for femoral reconstruction was modified in the 1990's in close cooperation with Ling and Gie from Exeter and with representatives from Howmedica (Staines, U.K.) for restoration of femoral bone-stock deficiencies after loosening of femoral components in total hip arthroplasty (7,8). The initial clinical experience (20) of the Exeter group with femoral reconstruction was reported in 1991. In the same year, one of us (B. W. S.) showed in animal experiments (19) the increased stability of femoral components when impacted graft and cement were combined. In similar experiments one of our colleagues (18) evaluated histologically the process of the incorporation of the chip allograft. Because the surgical technique of these studies on goats was comparable with the one used in operations on humans, it became clear that the reconstruction method resulted in rapid union of the graft with the host bone. From 24 weeks onward, little of the original bone graft remained, and a new immature trabecular bony structure formed (Fig. 1). In the course of time no signs of resorption or collapse of

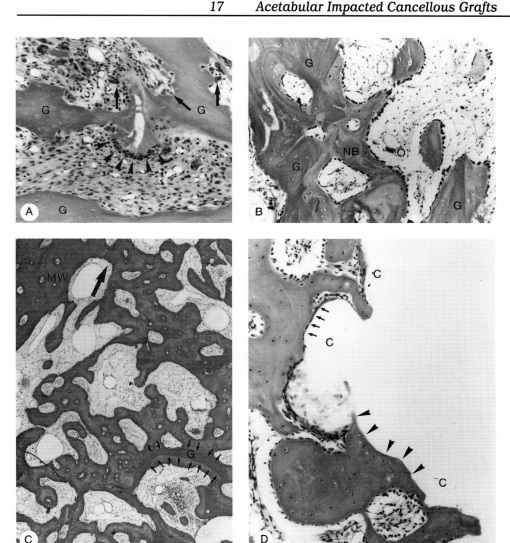

Figure 1. A and **B:** Six weeks postoperatively. **A:** The graft is invaded by vessels and a loose connective tissue with many osteoclasts (*arrows*). Locally at the transition of individual pieces of graft, microcallous phenomena were found with many active osteoblasts (*arrowheads*). Original magnification ×150. **B:** Formation of new bone (*NB*) on the remnants of the graft (*G*). Original magnification ×150. **C:** Twelve weeks postoperatively reorganized spongiosa is present in the anterior superior acetabulum. Only scarce remnants of the graft (*G, arrows*) were found in the bone. Consolidation with the medial wall (*MW, thick arrow*) was good. Original magnification ×55. **D:** Direct bone cement (*C,* removed during tissue processing) contact sites (*arrowheads*) and areas with a very thin soft-tissue interface (*arrows*). Original magnification ×160.

the reconstruction were seen. The results of these studies encouraged more extensive use of this biologic reconstruction method in clinical practice.

INDICATIONS AND PATIENT SELECTION

Progressive periprosthetic bone loss caused by aseptic loosening is considered the main indication for revision arthroplasty with bone impaction and cement. Other indications for revision arthroplasty include infection, recurrent dislocation, severe functional disability, and continuous or progressive pain. In general, the treatment strategy is focused on the degree of bone-stock loss. It must be clear that in the case of chronic infection, a delayed, two-stage exchange is recommended. Since the 1970's, regular radiographic follow-up examinations have been included in our standard postoperative protocol after primary total hip arthroplasty to detect any progressive loss of bone. In our patient series radiographic signs of loosening often preceded the clinical symptoms of failure. In all cases, the patients were in good condition and healthy without vital contraindications to revision arthroplasty. The method of reconstruction was discussed with the patients before the operation. They were sufficiently familiar with the extensive procedure and the use of allografts from our hospital bone bank.

PREOPERATIVE PLANNING

All patients undergoing total hip replacement underwent periodic follow-up examinations according to a standard protocol to monitor well-being, function, and postoperative symptoms and to prevent the occurrence of loss of bone stock in the event of loosening. A thorough physical examination was followed by laboratory tests, including erythrocyte sedimentation rate, blood cell count, and C-reactive protein determination. Very essential was the assessment of a possible diagnosis of "loosening" and to establish the cause of a failing total hip. Good-quality plain radiographs were obtained in three views, anteroposterior, axial, and abduction-exorotational, to visualize both components carefully. These formed an essential part of the routine evaluation of primary total hip arthroplasty. The radiographs were used to evaluate eventual anatomic distortions, the location and the extent of the bone lysis, the distribution of the cement, and cavitary or segmental defects. All serial radiographs were compared to monitor any progressive changes in the position of the components, the cement, and bone-stock loss over time. If loosening was suspected, preoperative planning for revision included subtraction arthrography and nuclear arthrography combined with intraarticular needle biopsy to exclude septic loosening.

HISTORY

We have no experience with cementless implants in acetabular reconstruction and therefore cannot report on this subject. From the 1970's we started to revise the first hip arthroplasties using more cement, as was recommended by Charnley. In cases of serious segmental acetabular defects, we tried metal reinforcements such as rigid Eichler and Müller rings. However, in all those reconstructions, defects remained and interdigitation of cement was absent because of a dense sclerotic and polished surface of the host bone. Cancellous bone was mainly or totally absent in all revision arthroplasties. The use of modern cementing techniques, including cement pressurization, and careful preparation of the bone bed have not improved, particularly on the acetabular side, the clinical and radiographic results of these types of revision arthroplasties performed without bone-grafting procedures.

The acetabulum is a very complex anatomic structure. This structure has not received the scientific attention that the femur has. From experiments we know that the acetabular structure is flexible and that rigid metal reinforcement does not guarantee long-lasting fixation to the bone. The combination of bone grafts in direct contact with polymethyl methacrylate (PMMA) cement was chosen to achieve stability, which is a *sine qua non* for the incorporation of bone grafts. This was proved in animal experiments in our laboratory (18). Morselized grafts derived from fresh-frozen femoral heads were used in all our operations. These grafts adapted easily and closely to the irregularities of the host bone bed without gap formation. However, when freeze-dried chip allografts were used instead of fresh-frozen allografts, gap formation often occurred. Impaction of these brittle chips was impossible because of the rigidity of the dried bone. Fresh-frozen chips are more elastic and allow tight impaction to enhance incorporation of the graft.

Studies by Roffman et al. (16) showed that new bone formation is possible in direct contact with cement. This finding was confirmed by the results of histologic studies with our animal models (3,18,19). We also have had published our data on nine core biopsies

on eight patients who underwent acetabular reconstruction with chip allograft combined
with a cemented socket. The core biopsy findings (2) represented a follow-up period of 1
to 72 months. Except for the biopsy specimen taken after 1 month, the grafts showed
different stages of incorporation. In the specimens taken at 4 months, revascularization of
the graft was found. Osteoclasts had removed parts of the graft, and woven bone had
formed on the remnants of the graft and within the stroma invading the graft (Fig. 2).
Subsequent specimens showed that this mixture of graft and new bone was in due time
remodeled into a normal trabecular bony structure with viable bone marrow that contained
little or no remnants of the original graft (Fig. 3).

The graft–cement interface was present in four biopsy specimens taken 1, 22, 28, and
72 months after revision. The specimen obtained 28 months after revision showed local
vital bone in direct contact with the cement layer; however, a local soft-tissue interface
was present. It is our experience that the size of the morselized chips should be 0.5 to 1.0
cc. Reduction of the size of chips may result in less initial stability and in early migration
of the acetabular cup.

With our reconstruction method, serious acetabular defects, segmental or cavitary, even
in combination with compromised acetabular columns, were restored successfully. The

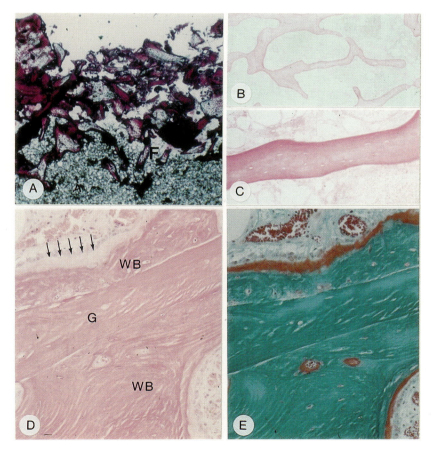

Figure 2. A through **C:** One month postoperatively. **A:** The graft–cement
interface in fuchsine-stained thick section. Cement has penetrated into the
graft. **B** and **C:** No incorporation of graft in section stained with hematoxylin
and eosin. Acellular medullary tissue is present in **C. D** and **E:** Four months
postoperatively. New woven bone (*WB*) is formed on the remnants of the
graft (*G*) by active osteoblasts (*arrows*). **D:** Section stained with hematoxylin
and eosin. **E:** Goldner-stained adjacent section. Red-stained osteoid
indicates active bone formation. Original magnification ×20 in **A** and **B,**
×90 in **C,** and ×225 in **D** and **E.**

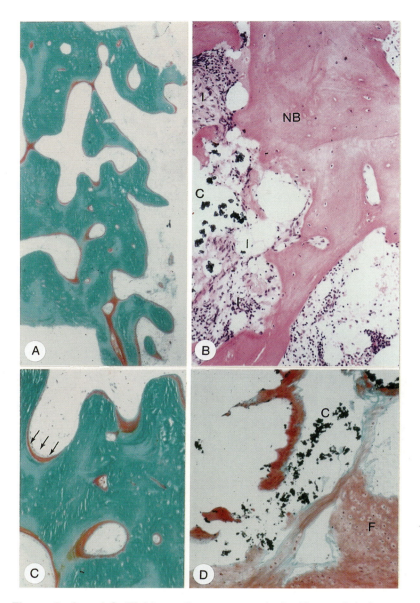

Figure 3. A and **C:** Eight months postoperatively. The graft is incorporated into a new trabecular structure. If inspected with polarized light, the structure consists mainly of woven bone with many active bone-remodeling sites indicated by the red osteoid staining. Goldner-stain, original magnification ×30. **C:** Magnification of **A.** Active osteoblasts are indicated by *arrows.* (Original magnification ×55). **B** and **D:** 28 months postoperatively. At the graft–cement (C) interface new bone (*NB*) is locally present, graft remnants are absent and a local soft-tissue interface (*I*) or fibrocartilage (*F*) is present. Hematoxylin and eosin and Goldner stain; original magnification ×140).

principles of our biologic reconstruction method are to restore normal hip mechanics, to repair acetabular integrity, and to restore the stability of reconstruction. These principles are achieved by use of the following surgical measures. Medial and peripheral segmental defects are closed with flexible metal wire mesh and fixed with screws to the iliac bone (Fig. 4). A cavitary defect remains and is filled with impacted chips, and the graft is well contained and supported. Care is taken to reconstruct the acetabulum at the anatomic location against the transverse ligament. Bone cement is used to stabilize the reconstruc-

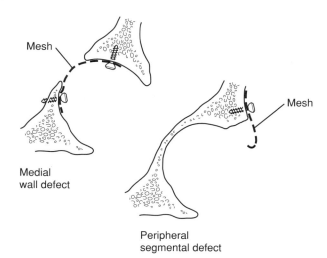

Figure 4. Diagrams of reconstruction of a medial acetabular wall defect and a peripheral segmental defect with metal wire mesh fixed with small screws. A cavitary defect remains.

tion. The impacted graft provides an ideal rough surface for interdigitation and anchorage of the pressurized cement. Since 1978 this surgical technique for acetabular reconstruction has been standardized and is uniformly used today.

STANDARD SURGICAL APPROACH

The patients are positioned on the contralateral side and stabilized on the operating table with a pubic and lumbar support. This allows free movement of the extremity and clear visualization of the posterior, lateral, and anterior aspects of the hip region. The posterolateral approach introduced by Gibson and modified by Kocher is used to expose the hip joint. A very wide exposure is used; in only three instances in our series was a trochanteric osteotomy needed. The proximal part of the femur is extensively exposed and mobilized carefully before the hip is dislocated. The entire socket of the acetabulum is visualized from the transverse ligament to the superior margin and from posterior wall to the anterior wall. Identifying important landmarks is helpful for orientation purposes when the anatomy is disturbed by scarring, distortion, and bone loss. These landmarks are the tip of the greater trochanter, the tendinous part of the gluteus maximus muscle, the lower border of the gluteus medius muscle, and the sciatic nerve. Aspiration of the hip is performed at this stage to obtain fluid for Gram staining and frozen section analysis to exclude infection. After being tested for major loosening, both components are extracted from the cement mantle. After removal of the socket and all of the cement, the fibrous interface is separated from the thin, irregular acetabular wall with sharp spoons. Removal of this interface layer leads to oozing of blood from the often sclerotic bone. At least three specimens are taken from the interfacial fibrous membrane for frozen section and bacterial culture.

A preoperative prophylactic antibiotic regimen is started. The wall and the floor of the cavity are examined to establish the integrity and bone quality and to detect any hidden defects. With a pair of scissors a flexible stainless steel mesh is trimmed and adapted to close the segmental defects. At least three screws are used to fix the wire mesh to the iliac wall. Any medial wall defects are closed in a similar manner with a metal mesh. In this way the acetabulum is contained and becomes a cavitary defect (see Fig. 4).

Drilling of multiple small holes into the sclerotic acetabular wall is performed to enhance surface contact and promote vascular invasion into the graft. A fresh-frozen femoral head from the hospital bone bank is divided into four equal parts. Substantial

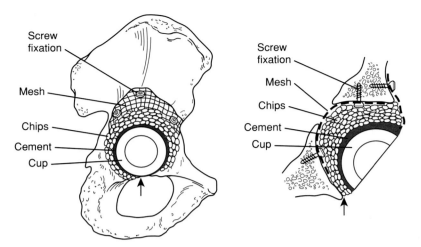

Figure 5. Diagram of reconstruction of a combined medial and peripheral segmental defect with wire mesh, impacted chip graft, and cemented cup. The cup is placed against the transverse ligament (*arrow*).

chips of 0.5 to 1 cc are cut with a rongeur from the cancellous part of the femoral head. After the acetabulum is cleaned, any small existing cavities are packed tightly with chips, and the entire socket is filled layer by layer. Impactors are used to hammer the chips *in situ,* starting with the largest possible impactor size and ending with the size suitable for a 50-mm diameter cup. Care is taken to reconstruct the socket at the level of the transverse ligament. The whole acetabular cup is surrounded by a layer of impacted allograft chips. It may become evident after impaction that the chip layer is not of an uniform thickness. Thickness depends on the local depth of the acetabular defect. After impaction, the preexisting enlarged acetabular cavity is reduced to a normal-sized acetabulum with a continuous wall of impacted chip graft. Antibiotic-loaded cement is prepared and pressure on the graft is maintained with a trial socket. After the cement is inserted and pressurized, the cup is placed and held in position with a pusher until the cement polymerizes completely (Fig. 5).

Postoperative management includes anticoagulation therapy for 3 months and systemic antibiotics for at least 24 hours. Indomethacin is administered for 5 days to prevent heterotopic ossification. Mobilization of the patient is individualized according to the different circumstances of the revision arthroplasty. A period of 3 to 6 weeks bed rest is needed after extensive acetabular reconstruction. Since the 1990's we have considered this reconstruction method out of the experimental phase. Nowadays if stable reconstruction is achieved, mobilization of the patient is similar to that after primary arthroplasty.

PATIENTS AND METHODS

In March 1996 we reviewed the cases of patients who underwent cemented acetabular reconstruction with impacted morselized bone grafts between 1979 and 1986. All had a follow-up period of at least 10 years. A total of 62 acetabular reconstructions were performed. At the time of the study, two patients were not available, leaving 60 hips in 56 patients for evaluation. The indication for revision was a loose resurfacing prosthesis in 8 instances and a loose total hip acetabular component in 52 instances. In 56 instances there was aseptic and in 4 instances septic failure. The average age at the time of the operation was 59.1 years (23 to 82 years). Thirteen patients were men and 43 were women. Ten patients (10 hips) died within 10 years of the operation, but none had undergone re-revision. All 46 of the other patients (50 hips) had a follow-up period of 10 years or more (10 to 15 years, average 12.0 years).

The defects were classified as described by D'Antonio et al. (5) on the basis of preoperative radiographs and the operative report. Thirty-seven defects were classified as cavitary and 23 as combined cavitary and segmental defects. Femoral head allografts were used in 35 cases, iliac crest autografts in 9, and combined allografts/autografts in 16. In this study the number of acetabular re-revisions was used as the sole indicator of success according to the principles of the Swedish National Hip Arthroplasty Registry.

RESULTS

None of the patients in the study had severe pain. The range of motion and all day mobility among this group of old patients was slightly diminished by age-dependent factors. The postoperative Harris hip score was good, an average of 80 points, but no preoperative Harris hip score was available for comparison of the clinical results. At the time of the follow-up study (average follow-up period 12.0 years) 5 acetabular re-revisions had been performed—2 because of septic loosening (3 and 6 years postoperatively) and 3 because of aseptic loosening (6, 9, and 12 years postoperatively). Excluding the 2 instances of septic loosening, the re-revision rate for aseptic loosening was 6%. The overall success rate of our revision procedure was therefore 94%.

PREVENTION AND MANAGEMENT OF COMPLICATIONS

Revision arthroplasty generally has a higher rate of complications than primary total hip arthroplasty. This is because the operation is more time consuming, more complex, and has greater blood loss. The patients are of old age, and many have age-related diseases. When a surgeon considers revision or a re-revision arthroplasty, selection of the patients is a very important factor for prevention of complications. Besides age-related diseases, other factors necessitate thorough preoperative investigation. These factors are preexisting infection, preoperative assessment of existing defects and bone loss, the availability of sufficient bone of good quality, the necessary instruments and implants, and the qualifications, training, and preparation of the staff.

In our study, five patients had undergone re-revision. Two procedures were performed because of recurrence of infection. Although antibiotic-impregnated bone cement and systemic antibiotic treatment had been used, the infection recurred. Three patients underwent re-revision because of aseptic mechanical loosening. Radiographic evaluation of the acetabular reconstructions revealed a too-thin layer of chip allograft. From clinical experience we know that a continuous thin graft layer, less than 0.5 cm thick, is pushed out of the acetabulum during pressurization of the cement onto the graft. The remaining graft becomes unstable and resorbs. The graft layer must be at least 5 mm thick to be stable. This is an essential part of the surgical technique. It is therefore essential to have enough graft available during the operation. Our patients also experienced migration and loosening of the component in the grafted acetabulum. When the chips are not large enough, risk for instability of the reconstruction increases. This same mechanism of failure was seen when freeze-dried bone chips were used. Because of the brittleness of these chips impaction is difficult to achieve, and the graft becomes unstable. Fresh-frozen bone grafts are recommended.

Of all the factors that determine the success or failure of a revision procedure, the surgeon and other surgical factors are probably the most important. Achieving direct stability of the reconstruction is essential to guarantee incorporation of the chip allograft and to prevent resorption of the graft and mechanical loosening of the component. Surgeons must learn the technique of approaching a serious acetabular defect with a very wide exposure and the reconstruction technique for a medial wall or segmental acetabular rim defect. They must know the basic events in graft incorporation, the advantages of host bone preparations, and the use of medium viscosity PMMA cement. From sound clinical experience and scientific data, the surgeon selects the standard components that fit in this uniform surgical procedure. It is evident that bone grafting facilities must be available.

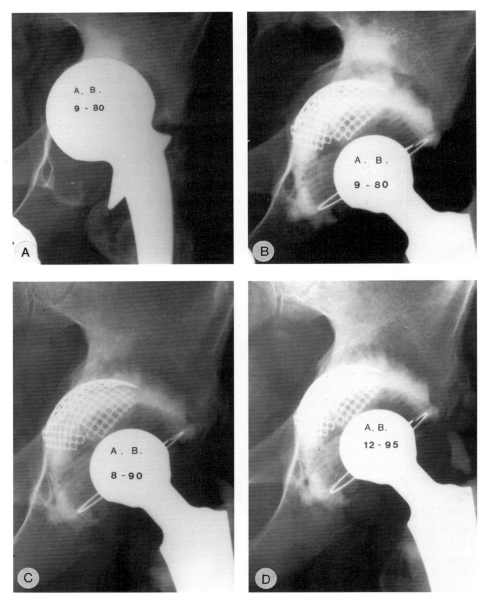

Figure 6. Radiographs of a 36-year old patient with a hemiprosthesis of the right hip that was implanted 6 years earlier after failed osteosynthesis of a femoral neck fracture. **A:** The metal head of the prosthesis is protruding through the acetabulum and has caused a central segmental defect of the acetabulum. Serial radiographs directly after (**B**), 10 years after (**C**), and 15 years after reconstruction with impacted allograft bone chips (**D**).

Dislocation of the components of a total hip replacement is frequently seen in revision arthroplasty. This is mostly caused by increased muscular laxity, malposition of the components, heterotopic ossification, and neurologic deficit. In all revisions there is atrophy of the gluteal muscles caused by a deterioration in range of motion due to the painful and invalidating loosening process. If during reconstruction hip mechanics are not anatomically restored, the risk for dislocation increases. Our reconstruction technique is aimed at this restoration of the acetabular component to the anatomic location and of the femoral component with its head center at the level of the tip of the greater trochanter. Restoration of muscular tension is mandatory. Placement of the acetabular component with an inclination of 40 degrees and a positive anteversion of 10 to 15 degrees is important. Only the surgeon is responsible for stable position of the new prosthetic components.

We are careful in exposing and incising the capsule during the revision procedure. We make a tendinous flap of the remnants of the rotators and the capsule that stabilize the joint after reattachment to the femur during closure of the wound. This is an adequate measure to prevent dislocation of the components of the total hip.

Another complication that may influence the outcome of revision arthroplasty is the occurrence of heterotopic ossification. From our research and clinical experience we know that indomethacin successfully prevents the occurrence and recurrence of heterotopic ossification. Immediately after the operation, prophylactic treatment with indomethacin is started and continued for 5 days postoperatively. The effective dosage of 50 mg three times a day had no detrimental effect on incorporation of the chip allograft.

Since the introduction of our reconstruction technique, the patients have undergone regular follow-up examinations, including critical evaluation of serial radiographs (Figs. 6 and 7). It is recognized that clinical success does not necessarily reflect the fate of the bone graft. Radiographic imaging also does not give unequivocal evidence of the long-term integrity and strength of the reconstructed acetabulum. Radiographs are at best difficult to interpret. Our clinical research is now directed at introduction of *in vivo* roentgen stereophotogramatic analysis or a similar digital technique to enable precise

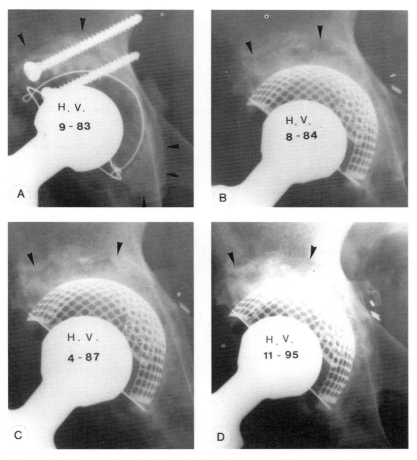

Figure 7. Status after right total hip arthroplasty (**A**) revised because of a peripheral segmental and cavitary defect (**B**). Postoperative serial radiographs show reconstruction with impacted bone chips and cement. **C:** The graft–host interface is clearly visible (*arrow*). **D:** After 11 years, the allograft has a homogeneous structure and is no longer distinguishable from host bone. No signs of migration are visible.

assessment of relative motion of the components in revision arthroplasty. With all these measures we try to prevent and manage the complications of revision total hip arthroplasty.

SUMMARY

Biologic reconstruction with bone impaction grafting and cement has gained wide clinical application in acetabular and femoral reconstruction after failed hip arthroplasty. Extensive acetabular deficiency, peripheral and medial defects, column defects, and large cavitary defects can be adequately restored with metal wire meshes to contain the graft and the cemented cup. This surgical method includes restoration of the center of rotation of the hip and correction of leg-length discrepancies. After evaluating the results of animal experiments and human core biopsies we can state that the impacted graft incorporates completely. From the third month new bone formation is evident in close contact with bone cement. *In vitro* and *in vivo* mechanical testing of reconstruction in animal experiments has shown initial and continuing stability of the acetabular and femoral components. Clinical and radiographic examination of patients treated with this technique showed, after an average follow-up period of 12 years, a success rate of 94% when re-revision rate was used as the indicator of success. We conclude that the success rate of this reconstruction is comparable with the good results of primary cemented total hip arthroplasty and exceeds the results of various other revision techniques.

REFERENCES

1. Berry DJ, Müller M. Revision arthroplasty using an antiprotrusio cage for massive acetabular bone deficiency. *J Bone Joint Surg Br* 1992;74:711–716.
2. Buma P, Lamerigts N, Schreurs BW, Gardeniers JWM, Versleyen B, Slooff TJJH. Graft incorporation after cemented acetabular revision with impaction grafting: a histological evaluation in 8 patients. *Acta Orthop Scand* 1996;67:536–540.
3. Buma P, Schreurs BW, Versleyen D, Huiskes R, Slooff TJ. Histologic evaluation of allograft incorporation after cemented and noncemented hip arthroplasty in the goat. In: Older J, ed. *Bone implant grafting.* London: Springer-Verlag 1992:12–15.
4. Bush LF. The use of homogenous bone grafts: a preliminary report on the bone bank. *J Bone Joint Surg Am* 1847;29:620–628.
5. D'Antonio JA, Capello WN, Borden LS. Classification and management of acetabular abnormalities in total hip arthroplasty. *Clin Orthop Rel Res* 1989;243:126–137.
6. Enneking WF, Mindell ER. Observations on massive retrieved human allografts. *J Bone Joint Surg Am* 1991;73:1123–1142.
7. Gie GA, Linder L, Ling RSM, Simon JP, Slooff TJ, Timperley AJ. Impacted cancellous allograft and cement for revision total hip arthroplasty. *Orthop Clin North Am* 1993;24:717–725.
8. Gie GA, Linder L, Ling RSM, Simon JP, Slooff TJ, Timperley AJ. Contained morsellized allograft in revision total hip arthroplasty: surgical technique. *Orthop Clin North Am* 1993;24:717–727.
9. Gross AE, Lavoie MV, McDermat P. The use of allograft bone in revision of total hip arthroplasty. *Clin Orthop* 1985;197:115–123.
10. Harris WH. Allografts in total hip arthroplasty in adults with severe acetabular deficiency including a surgical technique for bolting the graft to the ilium. *Clin Orthop* 1982;162:150–159.
11. Kwong LM, Jasty M, Harris WH. High failure rate of bulk femoral head allografts in total hip acetabular reconstructions at 10 years. *J Arthroplasty* 1993;8:341–347.
12. McCollum DE, Nunley JA, Harrelson JM. Bone grafting in total hip replacement for acetabular protrusion. *J Bone Joint Surg Am* 1980;72:248–252.
13. Mulroy RD, Harris WH. Failure of acetabular autogenous grafts in total hip arthroplasty. *J Bone Joint Surg Am* 1990;72:1536–1543.
14. Hastings DE, Parker SM. Protrusio acetabuli in rheumatoid arthritis. *Clin Orthop* 1975;108:76–84.
15. Parrish FF. Treatment of bone tumours by total excision and replacement with massive autologous and homologous grafts. *J Bone Joint Surg Am* 1966;64:1188–1197.
16. Roffman M, Silbermann M, Mendes D. Viability and osteogenity of bone coated with methyl-methacrylate cement. *Acta Orthop Scand* 1982;53:513–519.
17. Scales JT, Wright KWJ. Major bone and joint replacement using custom implants. In: Chao EY, Irin IC, eds. *Tumor prothesis for bone and joint reconstruction.* Stuttgart: Thieme Verlag, 1983;149–168.
18. Schimmel JW. *Acetabular reconstruction with impacted morsellized cancellous bone grafts in cemented revision hip arthroplasty* [thesis]. University of Nijmegen, 1995.
19. Schreurs BW. *Reconstructive options in revision surgery of failed total hip arthroplasties* [thesis]. University of Nijmegen, 1994.

20. Simon JP, Fowler JL, Gie GA, Ling RSM, Timperley AJ. Impaction cancellous grafting of the femur in cemented total hip revision arthroplasty. *J Bone Joint Surg Br* 1991;73:S73.
21. Slooff TJ, Huiskes R, van Horn J, Lemmens A. Bone grafting for total hip replacement in acetabular protrusion. *Acta Orthop Scand* 1984;55:593–597.
22. Sotelo-Garza A, Charnley J. The results of Charnley arthroplasty of the hip performed for protrusio acetabuli. *Clin Orthop* 1978;132:22–24.
23. Stevenson S, Xino Qing Li, Martin B. The fate of cancellous and cortical bone after transplantation of fresh and frozen tissue antigen matched and mismatched osteo chondral allografts in dogs. *J Bone Joint Surg Am* 1991;73:1143–1157.
24. Wilson PD. Experience with the use of refrigerated homogenous bone. *J Bone Joint Surg Br* 1951;33: 301–315.

Revision Total Hip Arthroplasty,
edited by Marvin E. Steinberg and Jonathan P. Garino,
Lippincott Williams & Wilkins, Philadelphia © 1999.

18

Femoral Bone Grafting: Structural Grafts

Carol R. Hutchison and Allan E. Gross

Revision of both loose and stable femoral components has become an increasing clinical problem for orthopedic surgeons. Multiple hip revisions lead to loss of bone with each operation. Loose femoral components often are associated with loss of bone stock caused by wear particles. Osteolysis caused by wear particles also may be present with a stable femoral component (18). Well-fixed femoral implants can have loss of bone stock prior to revision from stress shielding. Removal of a femoral component that is well-fixed distally usually results in further loss of bone. Full circumferential segmental bone defects or large contained defects with a thin cortical shell on the femoral side can be managed using structural proximal femoral allografts (13).

Restoration of bone stock should be one of the primary goals in planning the long-term care of patients who need revision hip arthroplasty. When it is necessary to restore bone stock, the amount and type of bone required usually preclude use of autograft bone. Allograft bone may be used in one of two forms—morselized graft or structural graft. The form in which allograft is used is determined by the type of bone defect present. The advantages of using structural allograft for reconstruction of the proximal femur include minimal invasion of distal host bone, normal transfer of forces from implant to host bone, an ideal surface for cementation of a conventional implant, and possible reattachment of soft tissues. Allograft used for structural purposes must be of strong quality with a thick cortex. A proximal femoral allograft is most appropriate for restoring normal anatomy and strength to the femoral side.

C. R. Hutchison and A. E. Gross: Division of Orthopaedic Surgery, Mount Sinai Hospital, Toronto, Ontario, Canada M5G 1X5.

CLASSIFICATION OF BONE DEFECTS

The type of bone defect can be classified with plain radiographs. More extensive radiologic imaging rarely is necessary. In classifying the bone defect, the surgeon must envision the defect as it would appear intraoperatively after the implant has been removed (Fig. 1). Bone loss may appear to be minor, contained, or noncircumferential on preoperative radiographs. However, compounding the loss of bone that occurs with removal of the implant may result in a large uncontained defect (Fig. 2). Gustilo and Pasternak (14) classified bone loss on the basis of 57 clinical cases. The classification system was based on the degree and location of cortical bone loss. D'Antonio et al. (5) produced a classification system for femoral bone loss that defined deficiencies as segmental, cavitary, or combined (segmental and cavitary). This classification also included alignment of the femur, rotational or angular deformity, femoral stenosis, and discontinuity.

We have found that the most useful classification of femoral bone defects for planning restoration of bone stock is as follows. A *contained defect* is widening of the femoral canal with an intact cortex that is substantive enough to support a femoral component. These can be managed with intramedullary impaction grafting (8). However, extremely large intramedullary defects with a thin cortical shell should be given the same consideration as uncontained circumferential defects (Fig. 3).

Uncontained defects can be cortical noncircumferential, provided the remaining cortex can support a femoral implant. These defects can be managed with strut grafts. Uncontained defects also can be cortical circumferential and are subclassified as calcar or as affecting the proximal femur. Calcar defects are less than 5 cm long and are managed with a calcar replacing revision implant. Defects of the proximal femur are longer than 5 cm and are managed with a structural femoral allograft (Fig. 4).

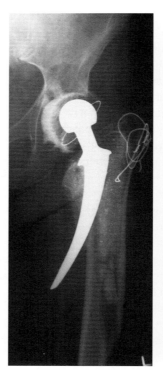 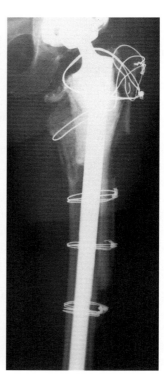

A   B

Figure 1. A: Preoperative radiograph. After removal of the implant and cement there was discontinuity and severe loss of proximal femoral bone stock. **B:** Postoperative radiograph demonstrates use of a proximal femoral allograft with a step cut and cortical strut allograft.

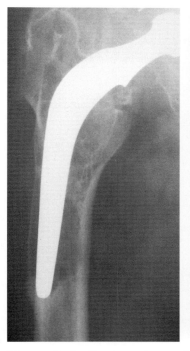
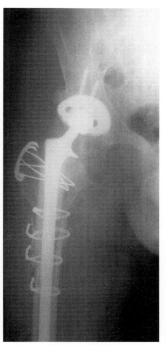

A   B

Figure 2. A: Preoperative radiograph shows a contained defect. The lateral cortical margin is thin and weak and would be unable to support an implant. **B:** Postoperative radiograph demonstrates long-stemmed femoral component cemented to allograft, uncemented in host bone distally, with host bone and cerclage wires to stabilize the junction.

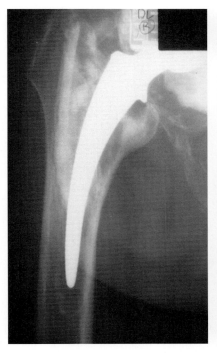
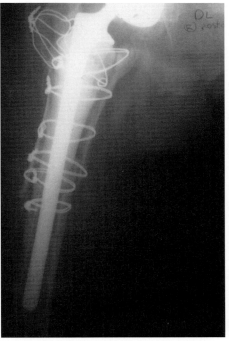

A   B

Figure 3. A: Large intramedullary defect of the right hip suitable for impaction grafting. However, this would require a large amount of morselized bone and would be a lengthy procedure. **B:** Appearance 7 years postoperatively. The defect was managed with structural support from a strong proximal femoral allograft with a thin cortical shell wrapped around the allograft.

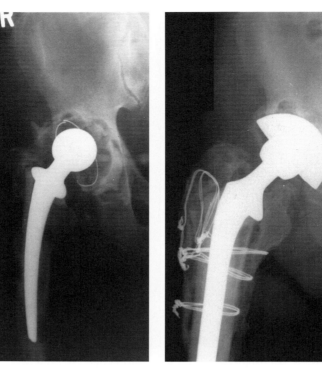

Figure 4. A: Müller cemented hip arthroplasty with cortical circumferential loss of bone stock longer than 5 cm after implant and cement removal. **B:** Transverse trochanteric osteotomy used because of loss of lateral femoral cortex. Proximal femoral allograft 2 years postoperatively. Host bone has grown into the allograft but has not replaced it.

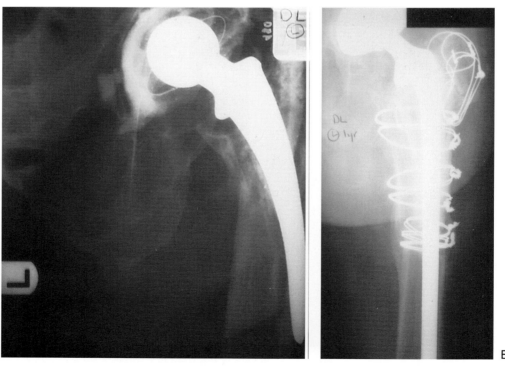

Figure 5. A: Müller arthroplasty of left hip has perforated the lateral cortex of the femur. After removal of the implant and cement there was femoral discontinuity. **B:** Proximal femoral allograft 8 years postoperatively demonstrates solid allograft–host union.

Saleh et al. (24) developed a classification system for failed total hip arthroplasty using a judgmental approach, the Delphi Group process. The resulting classification for failed femoral components is as follows:

Type I—No substantial loss of bone stock with cortical thinning less than 25%

Type II—Contained loss of bone stock with cortical thinning less than 50%

Type III—Moderate, uncontained loss of bone stock with noncircumferential bone loss or circumferential bone loss above the lower margin of the lesser trochanter

Type IV—Severe uncontained loss of bone stock with circumferential loss extending distal to the lesser trochanter

Type V—Femoral discontinuity (Fig. 5)

Interrater reliability testing produced a 0.67 ± 0.04 correlation.

SURGICAL TECHNIQUE

Revision total hip arthroplasty requiring allograft bone is performed in a laminar flow operating room at our hospital. Body exhaust systems are no longer used. There has been no increase in the rate of infection since discontinuation of the body exhaust system (4%) (17). Allograft bone is irradiated with 2.5 megarad and kept deep frozen at $-70°C$ in our bone bank. A separate sterile table is used to prepare the allograft. At the beginning of the operation the allograft is opened, cultured, and soaked in a warm povidone-iodine (Betadine; Purdue Frederick, Pickering, Ontario, Canada) and normal saline solution. Triple irrigation is used throughout the procedure with half povidone-iodine and half normal saline solution, one-third hydrogen peroxide and two-thirds normal saline solution, and 1 L normal saline solution with 50,000 units bacitracin.

SURGICAL APPROACHES

Principles for Decision Making

There are five important principles to consider when planning the surgical approach for revision hip arthroplasty. Preoperative planning of the most suitable approach is of fundamental importance to facilitate the procedure. The five key issues are as follows.

Limb-Length Discrepancy

Limb-length discrepancy up to 2 cm is managed with a standard approach or the Wagner approach (25). Discrepancies up to 4 cm are managed with the greater trochanteric slide approach or extended osteotomy (23). Discrepancies up to 6 cm are approached through a transverse greater trochanteric osteotomy. When planning to lengthen the limb more than 2 cm, the surgeon should prepare the patient and anesthetist for a wake-up test when the trial components are reduced intraoperatively. For lengthening the limb more than 3 cm, the sciatic nerve should be visualized to assess tension on the nerve.

Previous Approaches

Previous skin incisions are used as much as possible. Although compromise of the skin is a concern around the hip, this is not as much of a problem as it is in knee operations. Scarring around the sciatic nerve from a previous posterior approach may present a problem if a large limb-length discrepancy is to be corrected.

Acetabular Revision

Access to the acetabulum for extensive acetabular revision varies with the approach selected. Therefore the degree of bone loss and the surgical plan for an associated failed acetabulum must be taken into consideration. If an uncontained defect involves more than 50% of the acetabulum or there is discontinuity of the pelvis, a structural graft with a bridging roof ring is needed. The roof ring should be secured to host bone superiorly on the ilium and inferiorly in the ischium (Fig. 6). The sciatic nerve must be exposed. This cannot be achieved with the Wagner approach.

Femoral Revision

The approach selected should take into consideration whether the femoral component is loose or well fixed, cemented or uncemented (Fig. 7). Solid femoral components require a more extensive approach, such as Wagner femoral splitting or extended osteotomy.

Bone Loss

The extent and location of bone loss influence the surgical approach. If the bone loss is contained and impaction grafting is planned to restore bone stock, a Wagner approach, extended trochanteric osteotomy, or femoral split is not the preferred approach. In these cases, standard approaches or transverse trochanteric osteotomy is the favored approach.

The Approaches

Standard Approaches

The indications for use of a standard posterior or transgluteal approach are loose implants, no need for structural bone grafts, and limb-length discrepancy less than 2 cm.

Wagner

The indications for use of the Wagner approach are a solid uncemented femoral stem, such as a Lord prosthesis, and limb-length discrepancy less than 2 cm. Contraindications are acetabular major column grafts and femoral impaction grafting.

Greater Trochanteric Slide

Acetabular grafting can be performed through the greater trochanteric slide approach if there is minimal scarring and good visualization of the femoral canal. This approach is

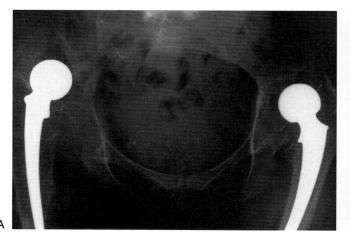
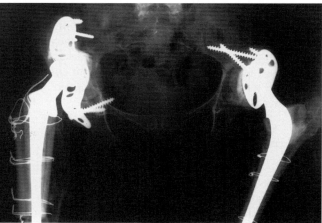

A   B

Figure 6. The patient is a woman with rheumatoid arthritis. **A:** Failed right total hip arthroplasty with large high-density polyethylene granuloma. More than 50% loss of bone stock in the acetabulum necessitates a structural allograft with a Burch-Schneider roof ring from iliac to ischial host bone. **B:** This required trochanteric osteotomy for adequate exposure.

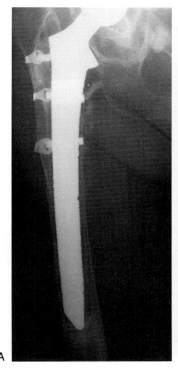
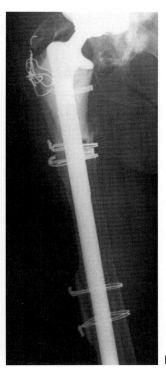

A   B

Figure 7. A: An uncemented Lord prosthesis with stress shielding. **B:** A window was made in the lateral cortex to assist in removing the loose femoral component. Appearance 7 years after loss of bone stock from stress shielding was managed with a proximal femoral allograft. The cortical window was bypassed with a long-stemmed prosthesis and a cortical strut allograft.

suitable for a well-fixed stem with proximal porous coating only. Limb-length discrepancy must be less than 4 cm. This approach is contraindicated if the femoral stem is well fixed distally.

Extended Trochanteric Osteotomy

Acetabular grafting can be performed through an extended trochanteric osteotomy if there is minimal scarring and the femoral stem is well-fixed distally. Limb-length discrepancy must be less than 4 cm. The approach is contraindicated if impaction grafting is to be performed.

The advantage of the greater trochanteric slide and extended osteotomy is that the attachment of the vastus lateralis muscle to the greater trochanter remains intact. This helps to prevent trochanteric escape and converts tensile forces on the greater trochanter to compressive forces.

Traditional Transverse Greater Trochanteric Osteotomy

Transverse greater trochanteric osteotomy provides the best access to the acetabulum for major column grafts. Limb-length discrepancy must be less than 6 cm. The approach is contraindicated if the femoral stem is well-fixed distally. Union of a transverse trochanteric osteotomy to a proximal femoral allograft is difficult to achieve. This approach has a high rate of greater trochanteric nonunion and escape (43%) (17). Because this osteotomy is superior to the origin of the vastus lateralis muscle, the pull of the gluteus medius muscle is not counteracted, resulting in tensile rather than compressive forces at the junction of the greater trochanter and proximal femoral allograft.

Details of the Greater Trochanteric Slide Approach

For failed femoral components requiring structural femoral allografts, the most frequent surgical approach we select is the greater trochanteric slide. This can be combined with a distal femoral split. The operation is performed with the patient in the lateral position. Existing scars are used as much as possible. The trochanteric osteotomy extends below the origin of the vastus lateralis muscle leaving the vastus lateralis attached to the greater trochanter. The vastus lateralis is dissected off the septum and reflected anteriorly with the trochanter and gluteus muscles to make a long, continuous sleeve. This approach decreases the risk for postoperative trochanteric escape. The transtrochanteric approach is used when there is preexisting trochanteric nonunion. The proximal femur is split to the level needed to remove the implant or to healthy host bone. At this level a step cut or oblique cut is used rather than a transverse cut. The advantages of the step cut and the oblique cut are ability to control rotation at the junction and an increase in the surface area for allograft–host bone apposition. As much soft tissue is left attached to host bone as possible. The distal femur is reamed to accommodate the femoral implant. Ideally distal press fit of the implant into host bone is achieved (Fig. 8). However, we use an implant with a smaller diameter (13 mm) to limit the amount of allograft reaming required. The allograft canal usually is smaller than the host canal, making it difficult to get a press fit in the host canal without overreaming the allograft. We prefer to sacrifice a press fit rather than weaken the allograft by overreaming. Provided the junction is adequately stabilized, a press fit of the implant into host bone is not necessary (9,12).

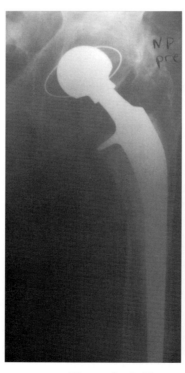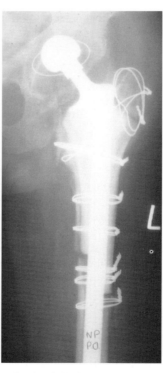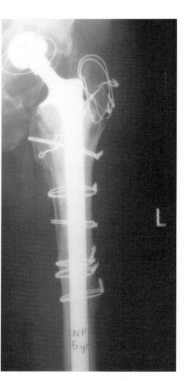

A,B   C

Figure 8. A: The patient had a failed cemented femoral component with loss of bone stock. **B:** Treatment was with trochanteric osteotomy, proximal femoral allograft, a step cut, and cerclage wires. The femoral implant is press fit into host bone distally. The junction is visible on immediate postoperative radiographs. **C:** Five years postoperatively, the allograft–host junction is solidly united, and the allograft–implant construct remains stable.

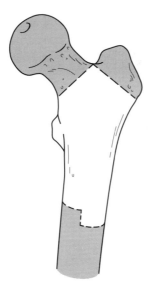

Figure 9. The proximal femoral allograft is prepared by means of removal of the femoral head and greater trochanter. The step cut is made after the orientation and length are determined. (Modified from ref. 9, with permission.)

The femoral head of the allograft and greater trochanter are removed and used for additional morselized graft (Fig. 9). The allograft is cleaned of all residual soft tissue. The intramedullary canal of the allograft is reamed to accommodate the implant. Larger allografts are preferred because they accommodate the implant and cement mantle without extensive reaming of the intramedullary cortex. Extensive reaming can weaken the

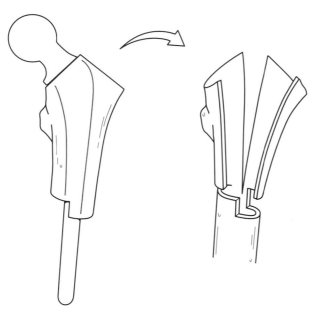

Figure 10. The implant is cemented into allograft and impacted into host bone. Cement is not used in distal host bone. Soft tissue is left attached to host bone, which is wrapped around the allograft–implant construct. (Modified from ref. 10, with permission.)

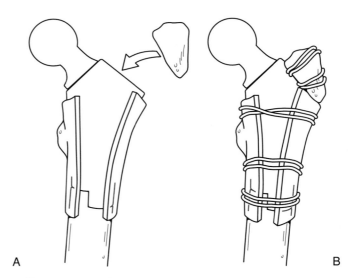

Figure 11. A: The host bone is brought down to cover the junction, and the greater trochanter is reattached. **B:** Cerclage wires are passed from posterior to anterior and tightened to stabilize the construct. (Modified from ref. 10, with permission.)

allograft. The shaft of the femoral allograft is temporarily cut to a level that allows trial reduction of the allograft–implant construct. This trial reduction confirms orientation of the implant in the allograft and the allograft–host junction. An oblique or step cut is made at the appropriate level on the allograft to correspond to the host bone cut. Oblique or step cuts help to prevent error in orientation and control rotation at the junction (22).

The allograft is irrigated with hydrogen peroxide and normal saline solution before the implant is cemented in the allograft. Cement is pressurized in the allograft canal, and the implant is inserted in the correct orientation and held in position until the cement has set. The femoral component is always cemented to the allograft. We ensure that cement is not present at the junction or on the distal aspect of the implant (Fig. 10). The allograft–implant construct is impacted into the host bone distally. In most instances we do not cement into distal host bone because this increases risk for nonunion at the allograft–host junction. The circumstance in which we would consider cementing the implant into distal host bone is if we consider this to be the last revision for the patient and the junction is in the area of the distal metaphyseal flare, where stabilization of the junction with step cuts, strut grafts, and cerclage wires is difficult to achieve. The remaining femoral allograft is cut into strut grafts and used for further structural support at the junction. Residual host proximal femur with soft tissue attached is wrapped around the junction and stabilized with cerclage wires (Fig. 11). This provides a stable construct. Any autograft available from reaming is used at the junction to promote union. Autograft may be combined with morselized allograft from the femoral head if this is not required for revision of the acetabulum.

IMPLANT DESIGN

In our view, bone ingrowth is very difficult to achieve in multiply revised total hip arthroplasties. For this reason, porous coated implants are not ideal. We aim to achieve a press fit in distal host bone. However, this is not critical to success, and we will compromise on the press fit to spare the strength of the allograft. An implant designed to be narrower at the proximal end and slightly wider (2 mm) distally is the best option. The distal width must still pass through the allograft during cementing.

MANAGEMENT OF STRUCTURAL ALLOGRAFTS

The structural allografts used are obtained from young donors with strong cortical bone. The allografts are collected and stored according to American Association of Tissue

Banks standards (6,21). The allografts are irradiated with 2.5 megarad and deep frozen at −70°C (4,22). Adhering to the explicit standards reduces the risk for transmission of the human immunodeficiency virus to less than one in one million (1,2,4). The additional irradiation decreases the risk still further (7). Immediately before use, the allograft is thawed in a warm bath of 50% normal saline solution and 50% povidone-iodine. It is important not to place drill holes in the allograft because the holes can cause graft fracture and may be a zone of revascularization that leads to local resorption of the allograft bone.

POSTOPERATIVE CARE

Our postoperative protocol for intravenous prophylactic antibiotics has been revised from 5 days to 3 days of administration of cephalosporin. The patients are usually catheterized intraoperatively, and for these patients gentamycin also is used preoperatively and for 24 hours postoperatively. The patients stay at bed rest in abduction for 3 to 5 days depending on intraoperative factors such as stability and abductor continuity. No weight bearing or touch weight bearing is performed until the allograft–host junction appears to have united on plain radiographs, usually 3 months after the operation (4). Hip spica braces are not used.

CASE STUDY

A 40-year-old male transport trailer driver was originally seen in 1986 with a failed right total hip arthroplasty. He had Legg-Calvé-Perthes disease as a child; however, he had no operations on the right hip at that time. In 1970, he was involved in a motor vehicle accident and may have suffered dislocation of the hip, which was managed with closed reduction. In 1971, the patient underwent cup resurfacing arthroplasty. In 1975, this was revised to a total hip arthroplasty. The patient was discharged in a body cast, suggesting problems during the operative procedure. The hip replacement became infected, and the patient was hospitalized for treatment with an irrigation system and intravenous antibiotics for 2 months. The implant was not removed at that time. The patient's condition remained stable until 1982, when revision of the total hip arthroplasty was performed for loosening of the femoral component.

When we first met the patient, in 1986, he reported pain and progressive shortening (limb-length discrepancy 2 cm). Radiographs revealed a loose femoral component with subsidence and lateral loss of bone stock (Fig. 12A). The acetabular component also appeared loose. Bone and gallium scan findings were consistent with aseptic loosening.

Transverse trochanteric osteotomy was the surgical approach used at the time combined with a distal femoral split. A proximal femoral allograft was used to restore the bone loss and provide a stable femoral construct. The patient continued to use one cane postoperatively. He returned to full-time work driving, loading, and unloading his transport trailer for the next 10 years. In 1996, when the patient was 50 years of age, symptoms recurred. Radiographs revealed an intact allograft, but the femoral component had loosened within the allograft (Fig. 12B and 12C).

At revision, a trochanteric slide was used. The allograft was intact. Host bone had grown into the perimeter of the allograft but had not replaced it (Fig. 12D). The thickness of the allograft cortex was well preserved. The allograft–host junction was solidly healed. Because the previous allograft had served the patient well in a high-demand lifestyle for 10 years, a second proximal femoral allograft was used for reconstruction. The bone loss and reconstruction did not have to be extended distally because the distal host bone had not been violated with the previous operation.

PREVENTION AND MANAGEMENT OF COMPLICATIONS

Infection

The incidence of infection after revision hip arthroplasty with structural femoral allografts is 4% (12). Two of our patients have required excision arthroplasty for sepsis.

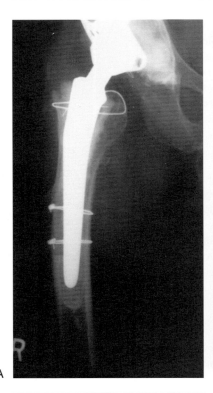

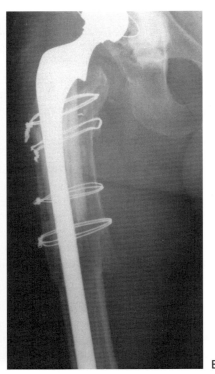

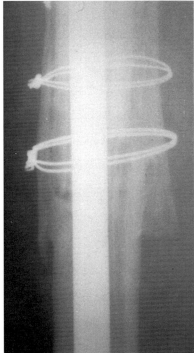

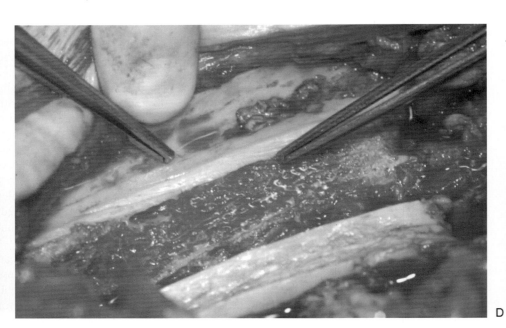

Figure 12. A: A 40-year-old transport trailer driver has a symptomatic subsiding femoral component and loss of bone stock laterally. **B:** The proximal femoral allograft 10 years after insertion. Lateral resorption has occurred. The femoral component has loosened in the cement mantle. **C:** The allograft–host junction is solidly united. Host bone has grown into the allograft medially but has not replaced it. **D:** At 50 years of age the patient underwent re-revision. Host bone has healed to allograft, but the allograft has maintained its strength and thickness.

Three patients have been treated successfully with two-stage revisions including revision of the allograft. A sixth patient had an early local wound infection, which was treated successfully with immediate irrigation and débridement and did not require re-revision. The allograft was not implicated as the cause of infection in any of these cases. Patients are treated with intravenous cephalosporin for 72 hours and intravenous gentamycin for 24 hours. The cement used for fixation of the implant to structural allograft is mixed with 1 g of cefamandole nafate. During the procedure, the surgical field is irrigated with three different irrigation solutions, including 50% normal saline solution and 50% povidone-iodine, 33% hydrogen peroxide and 67% normal saline solution, and 50,000 units bacitracin in 1 L normal saline solution.

Dislocation

The prevalence of dislocation is related to the components revised. There is a decreased prevalence of dislocation if both the femoral and acetabular components are revised during the same procedure (1.5%) (10). There is a higher incidence of dislocation when only the femoral component is revised (5.4%) (12). One of our patients has needed excision arthroplasty for management of recurrent dislocation. Patients are treated postoperatively with an abduction pillow and wedge cushion. We do not routinely use hip orthotic devices postoperatively. However, patients who have had the femoral side revised only or have a history of recurrent dislocation may be candidates for use of an abduction orthotic device. Mallory et al. (19) reported on the use of a cast brace in the postoperative management of primary and revision hip replacements. Patients who underwent revision hip arthroplasty were treated for an average of 23 postoperative days with a cast brace. There were three dislocations in the series of 37 hip revisions (8%). One hip dislocated with the cast brace in place. The advantages of a cast brace in the postoperative care after all revision hip operations is questionable. The cast brace cannot always be relied on to prevent dislocation.

Nerve Injury

The prevalence of nerve injury in revision hip arthroplasty with allograft is 1.3% (12). Five nerve injuries occurred in a series of 384 hip revisions. Three resolved spontaneously, one necessitated surgical repair, and one was followed nonoperatively.

Nonunion

Nonunion of the allograft–host junction occurs in 4% of operations (12). Nonunion is related to a femoral component that is cemented to distal host bone. The femoral stem should be cemented only to the structural allograft (3). The host–graft junction should be stabilized by use of a step cut, strut grafts (host or allograft bone), and cerclage wires. Solid distal fixation of the femoral stem with cement can cause distraction at the host–graft junction, which increases risk for nonunion. Martin and Sutherland (20) reported on four revision arthroplasties complicated by two nonunions. In all four cases, the allograft was secured to host bone with two large fragment dynamic compression (DCP) plates perpendicular to each other. Step cuts and strut grafts were not used at the allograft–host junction. Hodge (15) described seven cases of nonunion at the allograft–host junction when a transverse cut was used and the implant was cemented to distal host bone. The allograft–host junction should be secured with a step or oblique cut to control rotation, cortical strut autologous or homologous graft, cerclage wires, and morselized bone graft. We have seen five nonunions at the host–graft junction among 65 patients with proximal femoral allografts (7.7%). Three of these patients were in an early series, and the graft had been cemented to distal host bone. Nonunion should be managed by means of reinforcing the junction with strut grafts and autogenous bone graft obtained from the iliac crest for its bone induction qualities. It may be appropriate to use a biologic compound such as recombinant human bone morphogenic protein, which is being investigated for bone graft use in fracture care.

Nonunion of the greater trochanter has a much higher prevalence than nonunion at the allograft–host junction. The trochanter does not unite well to the structural allograft because this junction is under distraction rather than compression (22). In a review of 34 proximal femoral allografts followed for more than 5 years, the prevalence of trochanteric nonunion or escape was 43% (17). The incidence was not altered by the various wiring or cable techniques. The surgical approach used was transverse trochanteric osteotomy. It is anticipated that use of a trochanteric slide that leaves the vastus lateralis attached to the trochanter will decrease the prevalence of trochanteric escape and nonunion. Correlation between trochanteric escape and health status measures (including Short Form-36 physical functioning and Western Ontario and McMaster Osteoarthritis Index) ranged from Kendall Tau-B −0.196 to +0.011. The correlations between trochanteric escape and clinical measures (including 50-foot walk, up and go, limp) ranged from Kendall Tau-B +0.044 to +0.196. These correlations suggest that despite the high prevalence of trochanteric escape, health status and clinical measures are not greatly affected. Therefore, nonunion of the greater trochanter is managed nonoperatively.

Allograft Fracture

The structural femoral allografts used to restore deficient bone stock in the proximal femur are thick cortical bone. In a series of 65 proximal femoral allografts followed for more than 5 years, there was one case of noncatastrophic graft fracture in zone 7. The remaining allograft–femoral stem construct was stable, therefore it was managed nonoperatively. Martin and Sutherland (20) reported on four revision arthroplasties

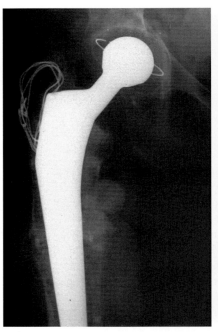
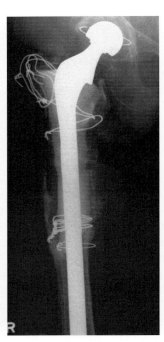
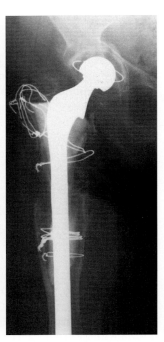

A,B   C

Figure 13. A: Preoperative radiograph of a failed total hip arthroplasty. **B:** The proximal femoral allograft at 3 years showing early signs of periosteal resorption, particularly around cerclage wires. The implant and allograft remain stable, the junction has united, and the patient has no symptoms. **C:** Seven years after the operation the allograft continues to resorb gradually. Host bone is remodeling, and there is lucency at the junction. The patient has no symptoms. Distal host bone has not been compromised and has been spared for future revisions.

complicated by three graft fractures. In all four cases, the allograft was secured to host bone with two large fragment DCP plates perpendicular to each other. Multiple screw holes were placed in the allograft, and no step cuts or strut grafts were used to stabilize the allograft–host junction. These cases emphasize the importance of avoiding drill holes in the allograft bone (3,11,12).

Allograft Resorption

Endosteal resorption was not apparent among our patients with the exception of one patient in whom the trochanter had resorbed completely from the periosteal to the endosteal surface. This suggests that the allograft is an excellent surface for cementation and high density polyethylene granuloma is not a problem. In contrast, focal periosteal resorption was present in 18 of 30 instances (17). Periosteal resorption was focal, generally measured less than 1 cm, and usually was not full thickness (Fig. 13). The most common sites of periosteal resorption were at zone 7 and around the cerclage wires. No grafts needed repeat revision for resorption. There were 4 instances of femoral component migration with subsidence up to 1 cm. These stabilized without intervention.

RESULTS

In a review of 168 proximal femoral allografts followed for an average of 5 years, 17 (10%) reoperations were related to the allografts (12). The reasons for reoperation were infection (3 instances), dislocation (8 instances), nonunion (5 instances), and amputation for chronic pain (1 instance). Success was defined as an increase in Harris hip score of at least 20 points, a stable implant, and no further surgical intervention related to the femoral side. Given this definition, the success rate was 85%. A subset of allografts in this group were followed for more than 5 years. A clinical and radiographic review of these structural

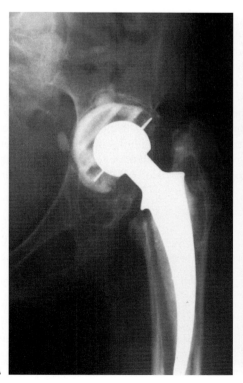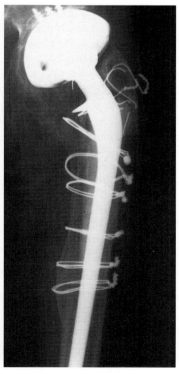

A   B

Figure 14. A: Failed cemented total hip arthroplasty with intact but weak cortical shell. **B:** The proximal femoral allograft has united to host bone but shows evidence of periosteal resorption 7 years after the operation.

femoral allografts demonstrated an 84.6% (55 of 65) success rate (17). Twenty-five of 29 additional patients who had died or were not available for the follow-up study all had successful results at the time of last follow-up examination, which was more than 5 years from reconstruction. Further surgical intervention was needed in 10 patients. Four surgical procedures were performed because of infection. Three patients were successfully treated with staged revisions. One needed débridement only. The infection was eradicated, and the allograft–prosthesis construct was left intact. The other three patients who needed further surgical intervention underwent excision arthroplasty (one patient had recurrent dislocation and two had infections).

Radiologic allograft–host union was obtained in 92.3% of cases. In all cases the allograft–prosthesis construct was structurally intact. Three nonunions were successfully managed with open reduction, internal fixation, and autogenous bone grafting. Two nonunions were stable and did not require further surgical therapy. The high rate of allograft–host union at the distal end of the allograft was not found at the greater trochanter. Trochanteric nonunion was frequent when a transtrochanteric approach was used. However, trochanteric nonunion or escape did not correlate with health status measures or functional outcome; therefore no further surgical intervention was performed for this isolated problem. The trochanteric slide approach may decrease the incidence of trochanteric escape and nonunion.

The most common radiologic feature to be detected on review of our cases was periosteal resorption (Fig. 14). This was most frequently seen around cerclage wires. Periosteal resorption was not full thickness in most instances. It is suspected that resorption occurred in areas where localized revascularization of the graft could occur. Endosteal resorption of the allograft was rare. This suggests that the allograft provides an ideal lattice for cementation. High-density polyethylene granuloma was not seen within the allograft–prosthesis construct, which is consistent with the report of Howie et al. (16).

SUMMARY

The use of structural femoral allografts is most appropriate for restoring bone stock in cases of uncontained circumferential bone defects. Bone defects should be classified on the basis of the degree of bone loss present after the implant has been removed. The most frequent and versatile surgical approach is a trochanteric slide or an extended trochanteric osteotomy. These approaches decrease risk for trochanteric escape. A step cut or oblique cut should be used at the allograft–host junction to control rotation and maintain correct orientation. The implant should be cemented to the allograft proximally and not to distal host bone. This decreases the rate of nonunion at the allograft–host junction. The strength of the allograft should be preserved during reaming. Drill holes in the allograft should be kept to a minimum to limit risk for allograft fracture. With these techniques, the long-term success rate of structural femoral allografts in revision total hip arthroplasty for the restoration of bone stock is 85%.

REFERENCES

1. Buck BE, Malinin TL, Brown MD. Transplantation and human immunodeficiency virus: an estimate of risk of acquired human immunodeficiency syndrome. *Clin Orthop* 1990;240:129–137.
2. Buck BE, Resnick L, Shah SM, Malinin TL. Human immunodeficiency virus cultured from bone: implications for transplantation. *Clin Orthop* 1990;251:249–253.
3. Chandler H, Clark J, Murphy S, et al. Reconstruction of major segmental loss of the proximal femur in revision total hip arthroplasty. *Clin Orthop* 1994;298:67–74.
4. Czitrom A, Gross AE, eds. *Allografts in orthopaedic practice.* Baltimore: Williams & Wilkins, 1992.
5. D'Antonio JA, McCarthy JC, Barger WL, et al. Classification of femoral abnormalities in total hip arthroplasty. *Clin Orthop* 1993;296:133–139.
6. Fawcett KJ, Barr HR, eds. *Tissue banking.* Arlington Va.: American Association of Blood Banks, 1987.
7. Fideler BM, Vangsness CT, Moore T, et al. Effects of gamma irradiation of the human immunodeficiency virus: a study in frozen human bone-patellar ligament-bone grafts obtained from an infected cadavera. *J Bone Joint Surg Am* 1994;76:1032–1035.
8. Gie GA, Linder L, Ling RSM, Simon JP, Slooff TJJH, Timperley AJ. Impacted cancellous allografts and cement for revision total hip arthroplasty. *J Bone Joint Surg Br* 1993;75:14–21.

9. Gross AE. Revision arthroplasty of the hip with restoration of bone stock. *Adv Operative Orthop* 1995;3:35–59.

10. Gross AE, Allen G, Lavoie G. Revision arthroplasty using allograft bone. *Instr Course Lect* 1993;42:363–380.

11. Gross AE, Allen DG, Lavoie GJ, Oakeshott RD. Revision arthroplasty of the proximal femur using allograft bone. *Orthop Clin North Am* 1993;24:705–715.

12. Gross AE, Hutchison CR, Alexeeff M, et al. Proximal femoral allografts for reconstruction of bone stock in revision arthroplasty of the hip. *Clin Orthop* 1995;319:151–158.

13. Gross AE, Lavoie MV, McDermott AGP, Marks P. The use of allograft bone in revision of total hip arthroplasty. *Clin Orthop* 1985;197:115–122.

14. Gustilo RB, Pasternak HS. Revision total hip arthroplasty with titanium ingrowth prosthesis and bone grafting for failed cemented femoral component loosening. *Clin Orthop* 1988;235:111–119.

15. Hodge WA. Cemented proximal femoral allograft in revision of total hip replacement: a report of incomplete union in seven cases. *Orthop Int Ed* 1994;2:259–266.

16. Howie D, Oakeshott R, Manthy B, Vernon-Roberts B. Bone resorption in the presence of polyethylene wear particles. *J Bone Joint Surg Br* 1987;69:165.

17. Hutchison CR, Gross AE, Leitch KK, et al. Proximal femoral allografts for revision arthroplasty of the hip. Presented at the 62nd Annual Meeting of the American Academy of Orthopaedic Surgeons; Feb. 22–26, 1995; Orlando.

18. Jasty MJ, Floyd WE, Schiller AL, et al. Localized osteolysis in stable, non-septic total hip replacement. *J Bone Joint Surg Am* 1986;68:912–919.

19. Mallory TH, Vaughn BK, Lombardi AV Jr, Kraus TJ. Prophylactic use of a hip cast-brace following primary and revision total hip arthroplasty. *Orthop Rev* 1988;37:178–183.

20. Martin WR, Sutherland CJ. Complications of proximal femoral allografts in revision total hip arthroplasty. *Clin Orthop* 1993;295:161–167.

21. Mowe JC, ed. *Standards for tissue banking*. Arlington, Va.: American Association of Tissue Banks, 1984.

22. Oakeshott RD, Morgan DAF, Zukor DJ, et al. Revision total hip arthroplasty with osseous allograft reconstruction. *Clin Orthop* 1987;225:37–61.

23. Paprosky WG, Jablonsky W, Magnus RE. Cementless femoral revision in the presence of severe proximal bone loss using diaphyseal fixation. *Orthop Trans* 1993;17:965–966.

24. Saleh KJ, Gafni A, Wong P, Hutchison CR, Gross AE. Radiographic classification for failed hip arthroplasty. *Submitted for publication.*

25. Wagner H. Revisionsprostehese fur das Huftgelenk. *Orthopade* 1989;18:438–453.

Revision Total Hip Arthroplasty,
edited by Marvin E. Steinberg and Jonathan P. Garino,
Lippincott Williams & Wilkins, Philadelphia © 1998.

19

Femoral Bone Grafting: Intramedullary Impaction Grafting

Graham A. Gie and Robin S. M. Ling

Substantial bone-stock loss in the femur after failures of total hip arthroplasty constitutes a formidable challenge to the revision surgeon. In the past few years, impaction grafting with cementing has emerged as a method that can meet this challenge in most of these difficult operations. The concept of the use of impaction of morselized allograft and cement in dealing with primary protrusio acetabuli and bone-stock loss in the acetabulum after socket loosening was introduced by Slooff et al. (28) in 1978. They built on the work of Parker and Hastings (23), McCollum and Nunley (16), Marti and Besselaar (15), and Roffman et al. (25). In 1985, at the Princess Elizabeth Orthopaedic Hospital in Exeter, United Kingdom, impaction grafting was used without cement to manage one case of femoral loosening associated with bone-stock compromise. The clinical result was satisfactory, though radiographs showed marked subsidence of the stem within the graft. As a consequence of this operation and with the experience of Slooff et al. (28) with the acetabulum in mind, the concept of impaction grafting and cement was adapted to femoral revisions and introduced into clinical practice in Exeter in the Spring of 1987 (9).

BACKGROUND

The principle that underlies impaction grafting, wherever it is used, is the achievement of implant stability by means of a combination of containment and impaction of the graft with the use of cement to immobilize the interface between cement and graft. This in

---

G. A. Gie and R. S. M. Ling: Princess Elizabeth Orthopaedic Hospital, Exeter EX2 4UE, United Kingdom.

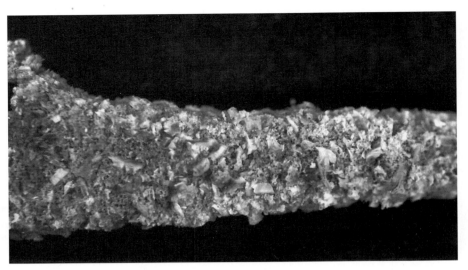

Figure 1. Specimen produced by impaction grafting in a cadaveric femur, splitting of the femur, and removal of the cortical halves. Photograph shows the grafts firmly adherent to the surface of the polymerized bone cement around the femoral component. (From ref. 9, with permission.)

effect produces a bone-coated implant (Fig. 1). Containment and impaction require full exposure of all defective areas of the femur. An effective operation *cannot* be performed through a limited exposure. Experimentally Schreurs et al. (26,27) demonstrated *in vivo* that the addition of cement made an important contribution to the stability that could be obtained by means of impaction grafting alone. The same finding emerged from an *in vitro* study by Smith et al. (29). In another *in vitro* study, Malkani et al. (14) showed that the stability of the femoral component that can be achieved by means of impaction grafting and cementing is only marginally less than that obtainable at a primary intervention with cement. What the operating surgeon must remember is that the achievement of stability in this operation is a technical matter that requires exposure, time, trouble, and familiarity with the technique.

In the initial series from Exeter (9), only milled bone from fresh-frozen femoral heads was used. Distal impaction of the bone chips on top of the intramedullary plug was performed with plug-sizing instruments. Lateral impaction of the graft against the side walls of the canal and formation of the neomedullary canal lined with impacted allograft chips were achieved by means of driving into the graft a femoral component that was one size larger than the component to be used. A problem with this early technique was difficulty achieving a neutral position for the neomedullary canal in the center of the true femoral canal. Dedicated instrumentation was developed by a number of surgeons (7,10,18,33) and made graft packing and component alignment more predictable and reproducible. These instrumentation systems are all based on use of a polished, double-tapered, collarless stem that is cemented in to a neomedullary canal formed by tight impaction of morselized allograft in the proximal femur.

The results presented in this chapter are those obtained with use of this type of stem. Because of the high compressive element of load induced by this stem design (31), these results may not apply to the use of other designs of femoral component used with impaction grafting, particularly in the longer term. Time alone will tell.

BIOLOGIC FUNDAMENTALS OF IMPACTION GRAFTING FOR THE FEMORAL COMPONENT

Much remains to be learned about the biologic fundamentals of this operation. Experimental work done with animals in Nijmegen, The Netherlands, (26,27) suggested that under appropriate mechanical conditions, substantial replacement of the graft with living bone regularly takes place. The Nijmegen group (12) also demonstrated with goats the importance of compressive loading on replacement and remodeling of the graft and the dangers of overload during the remodeling phase. Present knowledge suggests that three factors are needed for graft replacement with remodeled living bone—adequate stability, adequate blood supply, and appropriate load, the amount of which should be neither too much nor too little.

Only one report has been published on the histologic features of femoral impaction grafting found at postmortem examination. This report showed appearances that were very encouraging (13). The layer closest to the implant contained necrotic bone entombed in cement. The intermediate zone showed direct contact between methyl methacrylate and osteoid with scattered foreign-body type giant cells, an appearance similar to that described by Charnley (3) in the femur after primary cemented hip arthroplasty. No direct contact between viable mineralized bone and cement was visualized. The outer zone contained histologically normal cortex and fatty bone marrow with a few islands of dead bone. More than 90% of the total surface area of the sections of new cortical bone contained filled osteocyte lacunae. There was no continuous fibrous membrane between cement and new bone. Nelissen et al. (20) reported results on biopsy specimens from the proximal femurs of four patients 11 to 27 months after revision with impaction grafting. Since then another biopsy specimen, consisting of a circumferential section of the femur at the level of the tip of the femoral stem, has been obtained. These cases show features similar to those reported by Ling et al. (13). Three zones were noted. The inner zone contained trabeculae of partially necrotic bone, fibrosis, occasionally lymphocytes, and bone cement consistent with cemented bone graft undergoing remodeling. Several areas of viable mineralized bone were found directly adjacent to bone cement, though the importance of this is uncertain. The middle layer contained occasional particles of bone cement and viable trabecular bone in all instances.

Review of radiographs obtained at the time of revision arthroplasty suggests that some if not all of this bone is the result of incorporated and remodeled allograft. In two cases, trabecular condensation was found at the inner aspect of this zone, suggesting formation of a neocortex similar to the circumferential rim of new bone surrounding stable, conventionally cemented implants described by Jasty et al. (11). Although the neocortex is not specifically described in the histologic specimen, radiographs included in the autopsy-retrieval report by Ling et al. (13) showed a similar if incomplete neocortex around the bone cement.

Linder (personal communication, 1997) studied postmortem appearances in five cases. In each case extensive fibrous tissue was present in which were fragments of dead graft. These appearances were a good deal less optimistic than those reported by Ling et al. (13) and Nelissen et al. (20). These differences may represent in part differences in the stability of the various implants studied. The biopsy specimens obtained by Nelissen et al. all were from stable implants. The findings reported by Ling et al. were from a patient who during life had a "forgotten hip." Clinical results of this standard were regarded by Charnley as an essential prerequisite for clarifying the histologic findings between cement and bone in the femur. This level of clinical function implied excellent stability of the device, and the histologic picture would not be clouded by the effects of instability. Thus the histologic findings published so far on persons who have undergone impaction grafting are likely to represent the most optimistic end of a histologic spectrum that will almost certainly be less favourable when stability is compromised. Under those circumstances, substantially more fibrous tissue and dead graft are to be expected, as in the cases reported by Linder (personal communication, 1997).

There can be little doubt that when radiographs show substantial areas of trabecular remodeling, as in Fig. 2, living bone must have replaced substantial areas of graft. On the other hand, where there are areas of no radiologic change or areas showing what Gie et al. (9) described as trabecular incorporation, the extent of replacement of graft by living

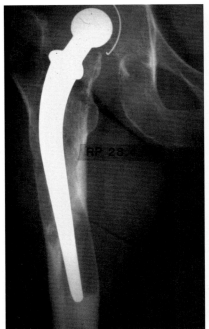
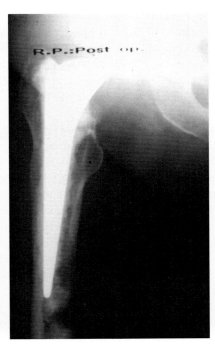
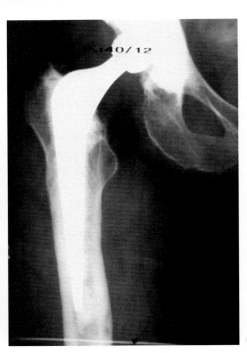

A,B   C

Figure 2. A: Preoperative radiograph shows lysis with gross thinning of the cortices in zones 2 and 5. **B:** Radiograph after revision with impaction grafting. The femoral cortex was penetrated in zone 2. **C:** Radiograph 40 months after operation shows cortical healing in zones 2 and 5 with trabecular remodeling in zone 6. Patient has no symptoms.

bone may be very much less. However, even in such cases, the clinical result may be perfectly satisfactory, and it is not certain that replacement of graft by viable bone is essential for a good, lasting clinical result.

INDICATIONS AND PATIENT SELECTION

This revision method is to be regarded as a technique in evolution. In Exeter at least, it is gradually being applied in more and more difficult situations (Fig. 3), and the longer term outcomes in these cases are not yet established. Although the results in less complicated situations are well known and no sign of deterioration with time have occurred so far (L. L. Linder, personal communication, 1997), the limitations of the method are not clear. Therefore the indications and contraindications remain to be clarified. With these points in mind, and with a follow-up period extending to almost 10 years, it can be said that in the present state of knowledge, the procedure is definitely indicated in the following circumstances.

1. The patient has mechanical failure of cemented and cementless femoral stems, regardless of the length of the latter. In the presence of infection, the procedure is performed in two stages.
2. The patient has bone loss of the proximal femur with cortical defects and thinning from stress shielding and wear-induced osteolysis.

Time may show that the procedure is indicated in situations in which there is substantial bone loss, including circumferential segmental loss more distally in the femur. Such cases are being managed now with this method in Exeter. In these cases, however, reinforcement of the femur with cortical strut allograft or a plate with a long-stemmed option to bypass the lytic or defective areas is usually advisable.

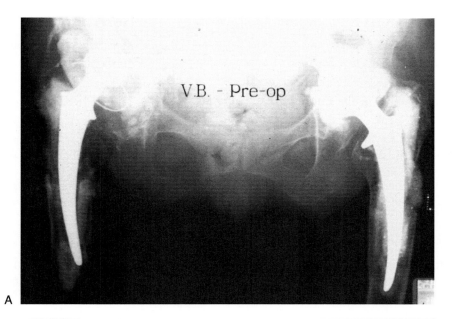

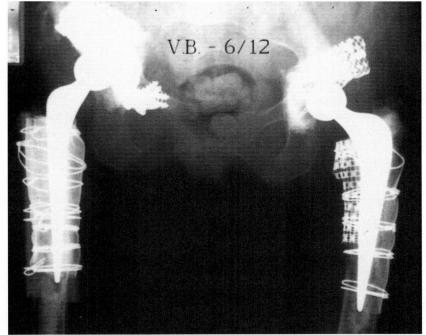

Figure 3. A: Preoperative radiograph shows severe bone loss in the proximal femur on the right with discontinuity in the proximal third of the femur and severe destruction in the acetabulum with socket migration. Similar but less severe changes are present on the left. **B:** Radiograph 6 months after revision and impaction grafting on both sides in both socket and femur. The longer-term outcome in situations of this type is not known.

The prerequisite for the procedure is that an intact femoral tube can be reconstructed and the defects covered with strut grafts or wire mesh to provide containment and allow tight packing of the bone graft and stable fixation of the cement and the femoral component in the impacted graft. The lytic lesions usually heal with time, and the femur may revert to an appearance that is virtually normal. For patients with an infected, loose total hip arthroplasty, a two-stage exchange is recommended. The infected total hip arthroplasty is removed, and the infection is treated. When the infection has been overcome, a prosthesis can be implanted with the impaction grafting technique.

PREOPERATIVE PLANNING

Preoperative planning involves establishment of the cause of the patient's symptoms, exclusion of infection, analysis of bone deficiencies, and templating.

Establishment of the Cause of the Symptoms

The clinical history and careful study of serial radiographs generally make the cause of the patient's symptoms clear. When there is doubt, observing the effect of intraarticular injection of 10 mL of 2% lignocaine (marcaine) (4) has proved to be reliable in clarifying the cause of the pain and gives the patient (and the surgeon) a good idea of the symptomatic relief that is likely to follow an effective revision procedure. It helps both surgeon and patient to come to a decision about the advisability of a revision operation.

Exclusion of Infection

Infection should be excluded along conventional lines. Every effort should be made to exclude the presence of infection preoperatively, though this is not always possible. If the surgeon embarks on a revision procedure and finds evidence of infection during or after the hip has been exposed, the procedure should be abandoned until the bacteriologic findings and antibiotic sensitivities have been clarified.

Analysis of Bone Deficiencies

Careful study of preoperative radiographs is required to give the surgeon as much information as possible about the sites and extent of bone deficiencies in the femur. These matters affect the exposure needed to provide adequate containment for the graft and generally allow the surgeon to decide preoperatively whether strut grafting or other supplementary fixation is needed. Many classifications of bone-stock loss exist. Assessment of bone-stock loss on a four-grade scale according to the Endo-Klinik classification has worked well in our unit (8).

Templating

Anteroposterior (AP) and lateral radiographs extending distally to normal diaphysis beyond the most distal lytic area are essential. These radiographs allow the surgeon to decide on the position in which the distal plug should be placed, 2 cm distal to the most distal lytic area. The radiographs should enable the surgeon to determine the distance of the planned position of the plug from the tip of the greater trochanter. This allows accurate placement of the plug during the operation with an appropriately graduated plug introducer. The surgeon should be able to estimate the size of femoral component and thus the size of the proximal femoral impactor to be used to form the neomedullary canal. A final decision on component size is not made until the operation is in progress.

SURGICAL TECHNIQUE

The technique described is based on use of the Exeter X-change instrument system (Howmedica International) (10), but whatever instrumentation is used, the general principles of the operation are the same. Prophylactic antibiotics are always given intravenously but not until specimens for bacteriologic culture have been obtained from the operative site.

Exposure

Exposure of the hip is performed according to the surgeon's preference. It is absolutely essential for the surgeon to recognize that this operation cannot be performed properly through an inadequate exposure. Free soft-tissue release is needed so that the upper end of the femur can be delivered into the wound to allow the proximal end of the canal to be opened into the greater trochanter at least 1 cm lateral to the midline axis of the canal. Only then can the new medullary canal be correctly orientated, adequately impacted, and properly cemented. Our preference is for a posterior approach that always includes a psoas tenotomy and section of the gluteus maximus tendon close to its femoral attachment. Classic trochanteric osteotomy is not favored because of possible loss of containment for the proximal and lateral part of the graft, but this objection is not valid when an extended trochanteric osteotomy is used, as described by Peters et al. (24) and Younger et al. (34). Rosenberg (personal communication, 1996) showed with *in vitro* experiments that the stability of impaction grafting after fixation of an extended trochanteric osteotomy is virtually identical to impaction grafting in intact femurs.

Removal of Old Femoral Component and Preparation of Femoral Canal

Prophylactic wiring of the femur before removal of the old implant is recommended when cortical integrity is tenuous. The old femoral component is removed, with cement if the latter has been used. All traces of cement, fibrous membrane, particulate debris, and granulomatous material are cleaned from the femoral canal, which is then thoroughly lavaged.

The next step is making good defects in the femoral canal with wire mesh (Fig. 4) secured by means of cerclage. Wire mesh used for complete, circumferential, segmental deficits of the diaphysis must be fixed with cables, and not wire; otherwise there is a danger that the distal femoral segment will be driven out of the mesh during packing and impaction of the graft. Distal lytic defects may need reinforcement with strut grafts or a plate. The deep surface of the strut should be separated from the cortex by a layer of cancellous chips before the cerclage is tightened to hold the strut. The decision whether proximal build-up of mesh in the region of the calcar is necessary should be postponed until the trial reduction is performed.

Placement of Plug

The guide wire is threaded in to a stiff medullary plug. The plug then is driven down the medullary canal to the predetermined depth with the plug introducer. The plug *must* be a tight fit in the canal. If there is a soundly fixed and noninfected plug of cement distally, the guide wire may be drilled into the cement or the plug placed on top of the cement (Fig. 5).

Graft Packing

The grafts used in the original series reported from Exeter all were milled from fresh-frozen femoral heads, though now treated bone often is used, and many surgeons use irradiated bone. All remnants of cartilage and soft tissue are removed from the femoral heads, and the entire head is placed in the bone mill. This means that the graft used does contain some small cortical fragments. There is, however, certainly no objection (and it may be advantageous) to using purely cancellous bone, though this means that more femoral heads may be needed. When bone is obtained from commercial bone banks, there are economic advantages to using distal femoral condyles (and a higher proportion of purely cancellous bone than with femoral heads).

It is becoming recognized that there are important disadvantages, from the standpoint of stability, to the use of very small chips. Results of two *in vitro* studies (5,32) supported this view. Marked reductions in stability occurred when chips smaller than 5 mm in diameter were used. These findings mean that bone mills should be driven at very low revolutions (preferably by hand only), and the cutting blades with the largest apertures should be used. Brewster et al. (2), conducted *in vitro* studies based on the principles used

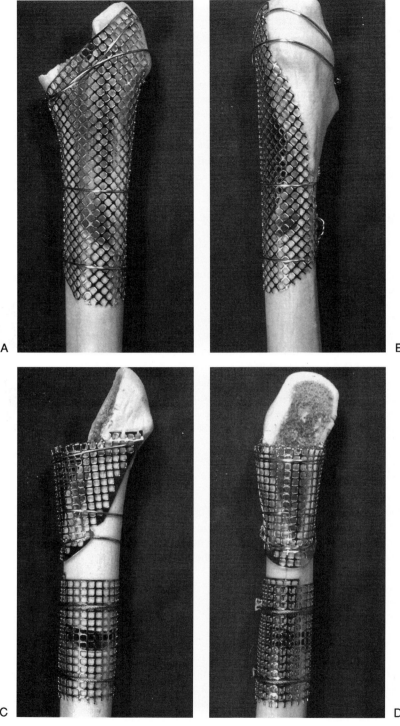

Figure 4. A and **B:** Models show method of constraining the graft with pieces of wire mesh held with cerclage wires in the presence of extensive anterior diaphyseal bone deficiency. **C** and **D:** Models show methods of constraining the graft with pieces of wire mesh held with cerclage wires in the presence of considerable deficiency of the calcar (the acetabular rim mesh is used in this situation) and of complete segmental diaphyseal deficiency of the femur. In the latter case, cables (not wires) *must* be used; otherwise inpaction of the graft may separate the mesh from the diaphyseal fragments.

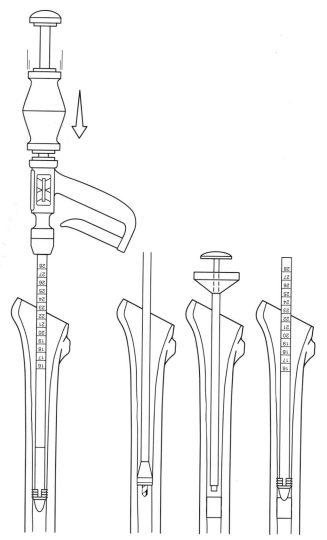

Figure 5. Diagrams show methods of plug positioning in a canal from which all cement has been removed and in a canal in which there is a satisfactorily fixed, noninfected distal cement plug.

in soil mechanics. They showed that the strongest impacted construct is achieved by use of chips of variable size. The investigators furthermore produced convincing evidence of strain hardening within the impacted graft.

Addition of antibiotic to the graft is now standard practice for impaction grafting as a second stage in a two-stage exchange performed because of infection. It also is used when there is no infection but the patient is immunocompromised or when very large amounts of graft or metal are being used. The antibiotic is added in powdered form. If no antibiotic sensitivities are available, vancomycin is used.

Trying each size of distal impactor down the canal over the guide is the best way for the surgeon to establish how far down the canal each diameter of distal impactor can be used safely without compromising the wall of the femoral canal. This is an essential step before packing starts; otherwise risk for splitting the femur increases.

The allograft chips are packed into the barrels of 20 mL syringes that have had their distal ends amputated. The chips are then ejected from the syringe barrel into the open proximal end of the femoral canal. This method prevents the loss of chips that usually occurs when the chips are inserted manually. The chips are driven into the upper part of the canal with a large-diameter, handheld, distal impactor and impacted down onto the upper surface of the plug with the largest size of impactor that will pass down over the guide wire to the plug without catching on the bony canal wall. Impaction of chips immediately above the plug should not be too vigorous; otherwise there is danger of driving the plug distally. Any tendency for this to occur can be controlled by driving a Kirschner wire across the femur and either through the plug or just below it (21). This step should always be taken when the plug is below the isthmus. The wire is removed once impaction has been completed.

Once the initial centimeter or so of canal immediately above the plug has been filled, impaction should become vigorous with firm blows of the sliding hammer. More graft is progressively inserted and impacted with increasing sizes of the distal impactors until the

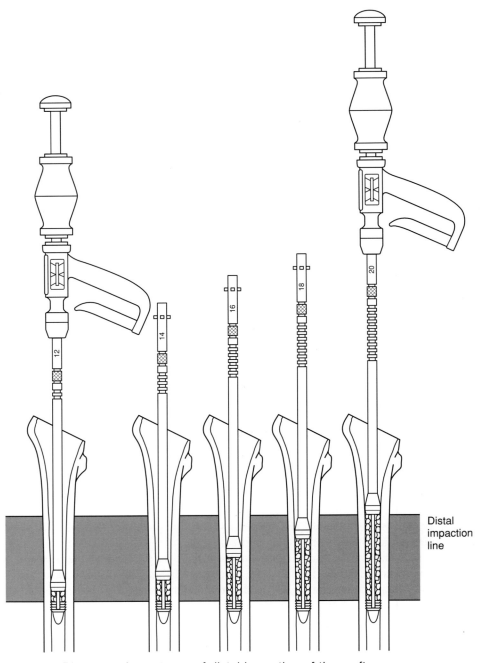

Figure 6. Diagrams show stages of distal impaction of the graft.

canal has been filled to 10 cm from its upper end (Fig. 6). Packing *must* be vigorous. The proximal impactors are then used. Some surgeons prefer to start with a proximal impactor one size smaller than the size that has been selected and subsequently change to the selected size. The proximal impactors are driven over the guide wire vigorously into the impacted graft, again with firm blows from the sliding hammer (Fig. 7). It is important for the surgeon to realize that the orientation of the proximal impactors as they are driven into the graft controls the position of the neomedullary canal that is formed. The surgeon must control the orientation of the impactors to provide the desired amount of anteversion.

More graft material is gradually introduced after each pass of the proximal impactor and impacted into the upper end of the canal with the larger distal impactors held in the hand. If the distal impactors are used with the sliding hammer at this stage, it will be impossible later to drive in the proximal impactor. The proximal impactor should be driven in so tightly that it cannot be withdrawn by hand. With these steps repeated as necessary, the femur is gradually filled and the neomedullary canal formed.

Trial reduction is appropriate just before the canal has been finally filled. The guide wire may have to be removed for this maneuver, though not always. The surgeon can then judge whether the proximal end of the femoral canal requires any build-up to support the proximal end of the graft. If it does, the acetabular rim mesh (see Fig. 4) usually is

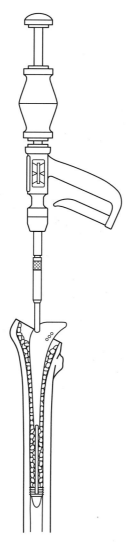

Figure 7. Diagram shows proximal impaction with proximal impactor.

appropriate. This mesh should be wired into position before the final impaction has taken place. Stability is improved if the very top of the canal is impacted with larger chips. These chips should be vigorously hammered down around the trial stem or proximal impactor with small hand impactors or the Thor spring-loaded impactor (Finsbury Instruments, Surrey, U.K.), a remarkably effective instrument.

The proximal impactor should be absolutely stable at the conclusion of impaction (Fig. 8). If it is not, it is best to extract the impactor and repack the canal more tightly. Any sudden reduction in the forces needed to drive in the proximal impactors may mean that the femur has been fractured. Under such circumstances, the fracture should be stabilized by whatever means appropriate and the packing redone.

Cementing and Introduction of Femoral Component

After removal of the guide wire, pooled blood at the distal end of the neomedullary canal stem is extracted through a suction catheter passed down the guide wire cannula of the proximal impactor or trial stem. The catheter is left in place until immediately before cement insertion.

Antibiotic-loaded cement is always used, and the surgeon should be sure that a double mix of cement is available and loaded into the cement gun approximately $1\frac{1}{2}$ minutes after the beginning of mixing at an operating theater temperature of 20°C. We have not used vacuum mixing or centrifuging. Our preference is for the use of Simplex cement. The cement gun should be fitted with a tapered gun spout to facilitate delivery of the cement into the distal part of the neomedullary canal without compromising the graft on the canal wall. Retrograde injection of cement under direct vision should begin approximately 2 minutes after the beginning of mixing. It is important that the cement dough introduced in to the canal be in a relatively low viscosity state; otherwise adequate penetration of the graft by cement cannot be achieved (1) (Fig. 9). When the canal has been completely filled, the gun spout is amputated level with the distal end of the femoral revision seal, and the seal is impacted into the upper end of the neomedullary canal. A better fit of the seal may be obtained if the surgeon uses finger pressure to flatten slightly the margins of the graft at the upper end of the canal. This should be done before cement injection starts. The femoral pressurizer seal and plate are impacted into the opening at the upper end of the neomedullary canal, and continued injection of cement allows the canal to be pressurized. Pressurization continues until the viscosity of the cement dough rises to a level judged appropriate for stem insertion. This rarely occurs before 5 minutes after the beginning of mixing. The surgeon must realize that with impaction grafting, he or she is inserting the stem into a canal that has been tailor made for the stem being used. Therefore stem insertion must take place a little earlier than in primary intervention.

The hollow centralizer is applied to the distal end of the implant, and the wings of the centralizer are cut off before insertion. The appropriate-sized, tapered, polished, collarless stem is mounted on the stem introducer and inserted to the appropriate level, as judged by the leg-length setting jig (Fig. 10). Insertion should require application of substantial force. If it does not, either the insertion is being performed too early, or the femur has been fractured. During stem insertion, the surgeon should place his or her thumb over the opening of the proximal end of the neomedullary canal medial to the stem to prevent egress of cement and maintain pressure in the canal. Oversizing the stem is a serious error that occurs at the expense of the thickness of both the graft and the cement mantle. Once the stem has reached its final position, the introducer is removed, and the horse-collar seal is applied to the upper end of the canal around the stem (Fig. 11). Digital pressure is maintained until the cement has polymerized.

POSTOPERATIVE CARE

Our practice is to mobilize the patient on the second postoperative day touch weight bearing with two elbow crutches. The patient is asked to continue this regimen for 12 weeks and then change to one crutch for 6 weeks, then two canes for 6 weeks, and

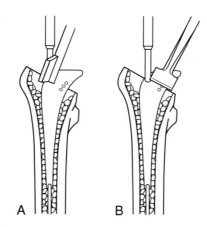

Figure 8. Diagram shows use of hand-held impactors to impact the upper end of the graft vigorously around the proximal end of the proximal impactor.

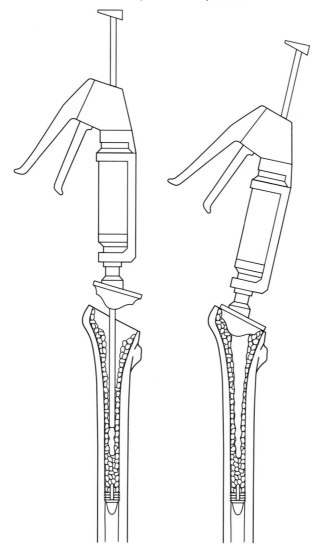

Figure 9. Diagrams show retrograde filling of the neomedullary canal with cement dough followed by cement pressurization with the half-moon proximal femoral seal and continued cement injection.

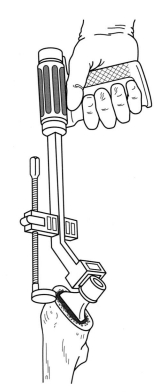

Figure 10. Diagram shows use of leg-length setting jig during stem insertion.

subsequently one cane for the ensuing 12 weeks. It is unusual, however, for patients to comply fully with this regimen. Many patients actually start full weight bearing much earlier than this. However, experiments have shown there are disadvantages to overload in the early stages after impaction grafting (12). We still believe that a relatively conservative regimen is appropriate with graduated weight bearing over time, though there is no hard evidence to support this view.

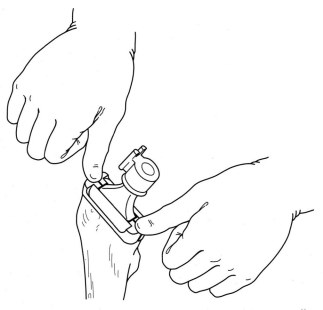

Figure 11. Diagram shows application of horse-collar proximal seal after stem positioning.

COMPLICATIONS

Apart from the general complications that may follow revision total hip arthroplasty, the specific complications of femoral impaction grafting that have emerged to date are as follows:

Femoral Fracture

Intraoperative femoral fracture is most likely to occur when inadequate soft-tissue releases have been performed during mobilization of the femur, during removal of the previous implant when the femur is structurally impaired, or during overvigorous packing of the graft. Prophylactic cerclage wiring may prevent some of these fractures. Once a fracture has occurred, it should be stabilized in the most appropriate way, and impaction grafting continued. Postoperative femoral fractures are most likely to occur when there are large lytic areas in relation to the tip of the femoral component, especially if the patient is elderly and cannot cooperate fully with a limited weight-bearing regimen. Prevention of postoperative femoral fractures involves use of a combination of strut grafts, plates, and longer stems. With these measures, fractures should become much less common. Management of femoral fractures generally involves open reduction, internal fixation, usually with a plate, and refixation of the component, when appropriate, with further impaction grafting.

Excessive Subsidence

With use of the polished, tapered, collarless type of stem, there have been reports of excessive subsidence (6,17), but equal numbers of authors have rarely seen this complication (19,22). In our experience (9) excessive subsidence is unusual and has generally been associated with defective graft packing or cementing. The probability is that excessive subsidence is generally a consequence of technical imperfections in the operation or the use of chips that are too small. In other words, it tends to occur when the primary stability produced by the surgeon at the impaction grafting procedure is inadequate (6). This reinforces the view that primary implant stability with this technique depends on the adequacy of containment and impaction of the graft and on effective cementing. These matters are under the direct control of the surgeon.

RESULTS

In our initial series of 68 cases a large proportion of cases showed trabecular remodeling and cortical healing. Radiolucent lines at the graft–host and cement–graft interfaces were uncommon and complications few. This group of patients has been under annual review since the original report. To date there is no evidence of radiologic deterioration (L. L. Linder, personal communication, 1997). Since the initial report, surgeons at our hospital have performed more than 400 operations, and the main complication is late femoral fracture. Three other series (7,18,33) had satisfactory results in the medium term with the same stem geometric configuration as in the cases reported by us. In the series treated by Elting et al. (7), there were three late femoral fractures. Appropriate prophylactic measures, as discussed earlier, should reduce the incidence of this complication. Ullmark et al. (30) reported satisfactory short-term results with the Charnley and Lubinus SPII implants.

CONCLUSIONS

The results reported from a number of centers led to guarded optimism about the long-term outcome with this procedure. It is reasonable at this stage to conclude that the technique does have a definite place in the skills of the revision surgeon. The two main problems with the procedure are the cost and availability of grafts and the fact that it is strongly technique dependent. With regard to the former, the situation may change with the introduction of bone-graft extenders and substitutes. With respect to the latter, it cannot be emphasized enough that though the operation is not usually technically difficult, the exposure, vital to an adequate operation, may sometimes be challenging. Thereafter a successful result demands attention to operative details and a commitment to take the trouble to achieve adequate and vigorous packing of the femur with graft followed by careful cementing and accurate insertion of the femoral component. On the effectiveness of these operative details depends the stability of the revision implant and its entire in-service life.

REFERENCES

1. Botha PJ, Snowdowne RB, Van Zyl AA. Allograft bone impaction grafting: what cement should be used and why? *South Afr Bone Joint Surg* 1995;5:25–28.
2. Brewster N, Madabhusi SPG, Howie CR. The material properties of morselised bone graft. In: Abstracts of Posters and Videos of the Third Congress of The European Federation of National Associations of Orthopaedics and Traumatology. Barcelona; Apr 24–27, 1997:385.
3. Charnley J. The reaction of bone to self-curing acrylic cement: a long-term histological study in man. *J Bone Joint Surg Br* 1970;52:340–353.
4. Crawford RW, Ellis AM, Gie GA, Ling RSM. Intra-articular local anaesthesia for pain after hip arthroplasty. *J Bone Joint Surg Br* 1997;79:796–800.
5. Eldridge JDJ, Hubble MJW, Nelson K, Smith EJ, le Blond R, Learmonth ID. The effect of bone chip size on initial stability following femoral impaction grafting. *J Bone Joint Surg* 1997;79[Suppl 3]:1997;79:364 [abstract].
6. Eldridge JDJ, Smith EJ, Hubble MJW, Whitehouse SL, Learmonth ID. Massive subsidence following femoral impaction grafting. *J Arthroplasty* 1997;12:535–540.
7. Elting JJ, Mikhail WEM, Zicat BA, Hubbell JC, Lane LE, House B. Preliminary report of impaction grafting for exchange femoral arthroplasty. *Clin Orthop* 1995;319:159–167.
8. Engelbrecht E, Heinert K. Klassifikation und Behandlungsrichtlinien von knockensubstansverlusten bei Revisionsoperationen am huftgelenk-mittelfristige Ergebnisse: Primare und revisionsalloartroplastik Hrgs-Endoklinik, Hamburg. Berlin: Springer-Verlag, 1987:189–201.
9. Gie GA, Linder L, Ling RSM, Simon JP, Slooff TJJH, Timperley AJ. Impacted cancellous allografts and cement for revision total hip arthroplasty. *J Bone Joint Surg Br* 1993;75:14–21.
10. Gie GA, Linder L, Ling RSM, Simon JP, Slooff TJJH, Timperley AJ. Contained morsellized allograft in revision total hip arthroplasty: surgical technique. *Orthop Clin North Am* 1993;24:717–725.
11. Jasty M, Maloney WJ, Bragdon CR, Haire T, Harris WH. Histomorphological studies of the long-term skeletal responses to well fixed cemented femoral components. *J Bone Joint Surg Am* 1990;72:1220–1229.
12. Lamerights N, Buma P, Huiskes R, Gardeniers J, Schreurs WM, Slooff TJJH. Incorporation of morsellised bone graft under controlled loading conditions. *Acta Orthop Scand* 1997; 68 Supp 277:8–9.
13. Ling RSM, Timperley AJ, Linder L. Histology of cancellous impaction grafting in the femur. *J Bone Joint Surg Br* 1993;75:693–696.
14. Malkani AL, Voor MJ, Fee KA, Bates CS. Femoral component revision using impacted morsellised cancellous allograft. *J Bone Joint Surg Br* 1996;78:973–978.
15. Marti R, Besselaar PP. Reconstruction of the acetabular roof and other bone grafts in total hip replacement and total hip revision. *J Bone Joint Surg Br* 1981;63:283 [abstract].
16. McCollum DE, Nunley JA, Harelson JM. Bone grafting in total hip replacement for acetabular protrusion. *J Bone Joint Surg Am* 1980;62:1065–1073.
17. Meding JB, Ritter MA, Keatinge EM, Faris PM. Impaction bone grafting with cemented stem in revision total hip arthroplasty: minimum two-year follow-up. *JBJS* 1997;79A:1827–1841.
18. Mikhail WEM, Timperley AJ. Tight packing of morcellized allograft: new method for managing bone lysis. *Orthop Special Ed* 1994;3:21–22.
19. Mikkelsen SS, Horlyck E. Evaluation of femoral hip arthroplasty revisions using impaction cancellous bone grafting. *Acta Orthop Scand* 1997;68[Suppl 274]:39 [abstract].
20. Nelissen RGGH, Bauer TW, Weidenhielm LRA, LeGolvan DP, Mikhail WEM. Revision hip arthroplasty with the use of cement and impaction grafting. *J Bone Joint Surg Am* 1995;77:412–422.
21. Northmore-Ball MD, Narang ON, Vergroesen D. Distal femoral plug migration with cement pressurisation in revision surgery and a simple technique for its prevention. *J Arthroplasty* 1991;6:199–201.
22. Ornstein E, Sandqvist P, Sundberg M, Franzen H, Johnsson R. 1.5 year prosthetic migration after hip revision with impacted morselised allograft: an RSA study. *Acta Orthop Scand* 1997;68[Suppl 274]:9 [abstract].
23. Parker SM, Hastings DC. Protrusio acetabuli in rheumatoid arthritis. *J Bone Joint Surg Br* 1974;74:587–596.
24. Peters PC, Head WC, Emerson RH. An extended trochanteric osteotomy for total hip replacement. *J Bone Joint Surg Br* 1993;75:158–159.
25. Roffman M, Silberman M, Mendes DG. Incorporation of bone graft covered with methylmethacrylate cement onto acetabular wall. *Acta Orthop Scand* 1983;54:580–583.
26. Schreurs BW, Buma P, Huiskes R, Slagter JL, Slooff TJ. Morsellized allografts for fixation of the hip prosthesis femoral component: a mechanical and histological study in the goat. *Acta Orthop Scand* 1994;65:267–275.
27. Schreurs BW, Huiskes R, Slooff TJJH. The initial stability of cemented and non-cemented stems fixated with a bone grafting technique. *Orthop Trans* 1991;15:439–440.

28. Slooff TJ, Huiskes R, van Horn J, Lemmens A. Bone grafting in total hip replacement for acetabular protrusion. *Acta Orthop Scand* 1984;55:593–596.
29. Smith EJ, Richardson JB, Learmonth ID, et al. The initial stability of femoral impaction grafting. *Hip Int* 1996;6:166–172.
30. Ullmark G, Lundberg B, Josefsson G, Hallin G. Impacted cortico-cancellous allografts and cement for revision total hip arthroplasty using Lubinus and Charnley prostheses. *Acta Orthop Scand* 1997;68[Suppl] 274:8 [abstract].
31. Verdonschot N, Huiskes R. Can polished stems reduce mechanical failures of the cement-bone interface in man? *Trans Eur Orthop Res Soc* 1995;5:42 [abstract].
32. Wallace IW, Ammon PR, Day R, Lee DA, Beaver RJ. Does size matter? An investigation into the effects of particle size on impaction grafting in vitro. *J Bone Joint Surg Br* 1997;79[Suppl 3]:366 [abstract].
33. Weidenhielm LRA, Nelissen RGHH, Mikhail WEM, Bauer TW. Surgical technique and early results in revision THA with a cemented, tapered, collarless, polished stem and contained morselized allograft. *J Orthop Tech* 1994;2:113–122.
34. Younger TI, Bradford MS, Magnus RE, Paprosky WG. Extended proximal femoral osteotomy: a new technique for femoral revision arthroplasty. *J Arthroplasty* 1995;10:329–338.

Revision Total Hip Arthroplasty,
edited by Marvin E. Steinberg and Jonathan P. Garino,
Lippincott Williams & Wilkins, Philadelphia © 1999.

20

Acetabular Revision: Cemented

Donald B. Longjohn, Lawrence D. Dorr, and Ye-Yeon Won

The 1960's saw the introduction by Sir John Charnley of polymethyl methacrylate cement for fixation of total hip arthroplasty components and polyethylene as a bearing surface for the acetabular component. Although initially viewed with some skepticism, the technique and materials received widespread acceptance in the early 1970's after publication of Charnley's good early results with his technique and materials.

Charnley's original indication for total hip arthroplasty was disabling arthritis of the hip of older patients that was unresponsive to all medical therapy and for which the surgical alternative was a Girdlestone operation. Heavier patients were not offered the procedure. With the increase in popularity of total hip arthroplasty and encouragement based on good early results, the technique has become one of the most common reconstructive procedures performed on adults. The indications have been expanded to include nearly all forms of arthritic conditions, including avascular necrosis, and the procedure has been increasingly performed on younger, more active, and heavier patients. Advances in technique, biomaterials, and prosthetic design, including development of bone ingrowth fixation have resulted in an overall increase in the longevity of total hip arthroplasties. However, on the basis of the sheer increase in the number of total hip arthroplasties performed and the fact that the procedure is being performed more frequently on younger, active patients, the need for revision total hip arthroplasty has risen dramatically.

Early experience with cemented revision total hip arthroplasty has been disappointing. Several reports of these early revisions demonstrated sobering results with a high

D. B. Longjohn and L. D. Dorr: University of Southern California Center for Arthritis and Joint Implant Surgery, Los Angeles, California 90033.

Y. Y. Won: Ajou University, Department of Orthopaedic Surgery, Suwon, South Korea.

incidence of radiographic loosening and re-revision rates of both components compared with the situation for primary arthroplasty (1,3,6,8,12,13,19,22). The problems related to cemented revision of the acetabulum are for the most part related to the quality of the remaining acetabular bone stock. After removal of a loose component, the acetabular bone often is sclerotic and without trabecular bone for cement interdigitation. Bone erosion due to osteolysis and mechanical damage from motion of a loose component often leaves cavitary, segmental, and combined defects in the acetabulum. These changes in the acetabular bone stock can make it difficult to obtain adequate fixation of a cemented component in revision operations and negatively affect the ability of the host bone to support a cemented or cementless component.

At present, most authors agree that uncemented fixation of the acetabulum in revision operations has better results than cemented acetabular revision. Porous coated acetabular cups have demonstrated less radiographic loosening and a lower re-revision rate (4,5,10,11,15,23). Despite these facts, there remains a role for the use of cement in revision of the acetabular component. Cemented fixation is used for fixation of a polyethylene component with a metal acetabular reinforcement ring or cage and particulate graft material, for fixation of a polyethylene component in conjunction with a large structural allograft, such as an acetabular allograft, and in selected cases for use with impaction grafting (see Chapter 17).

BACKGROUND

Early efforts at acetabular revision primarily involved recementing a new polyethylene socket into the acetabulum. Osteolysis or motion from a loose prosthesis often had resulted in large acetabular defects and loss of trabecular bone for interdigitation of cement at revision. Variable amounts of bone destruction in the acetabulum led to variable results of revision arthroplasty. Callaghan et al. (3) in 1985 reported on 139 cemented revisions. Nine percent of sockets had migrated and another 19.4% demonstrated progressive radiolucent lines. If cups with a continuous radiolucent line are included, 34.2% of revised cups were radiographically loose. Kavanagh et al. (13) in 1985 reported a 20.1% rate of probable loosening for 166 cemented acetabular revisions after a 4.5-year mean follow-up period. This statistic was based on radiographic evidence of migration or a radiolucent line greater than 1 mm. Including cups with a complete radiolucent line regardless of size increases the rate of radiographic loosening to 53%. It was interesting that only 2% of patients needed re-revision for acetabular loosening.

Amstutz et al. (1) in 1982 reviewed 66 cemented acetabular revisions performed at the University of California Los Angeles. They reported that 10% of the cups demonstrated a complete radiolucent line immediately postoperatively. This percentage increased to 71% after an average follow-up period of 2.5 years. Three percent of patients already needed a second revision by this early follow-up time. In roentgen stereophotogrammetric studies, Snorrason and Kärrholm (22) found that 11 of 15 cemented acetabular revisions had migrated within the first year and another 3 of 15 had migrated in the second year. Franzén et al. (6) found that 15 of 17 sockets revised with cement had migrated, 13 of 17 migrating within the first 4 months. More migration was seen among patients with more bone loss, and a complete radiolucent line was associated with migration. Garcia-Cimbrelo et al. (8) reported that 13% of cemented Charnley revision sockets required re-revision by 16 years of follow-up study. An additional 24% were radiographically loose after 16 years according to survivorship analysis. Raut et al. (19) found 32% acetabular loosening after 6 years of follow-up with patients 55 years or younger. In patients regarded as having good bone stock, 14% of acetabula were loose as opposed to 51% of the sockets in patients with poor acetabular bone stock, a correlation found to be statistically significant ($p = .0002$).

Of even greater concern are the results of multiple revisions. Kavanagh et al. (12) reported that 19 of 45 (42.2%) cemented acetabular revisions migrated or demonstrated radiolucent lines greater than 1 mm or progressive after a second revision. Sixty-nine percent may be considered loose radiographically if cups with a complete radiolucent line are included. After a third revision 100% of cups demonstrated radiographic signs of loosening.

Some of the best results in the literature for cemented acetabular revision were reported by Marti et al. (14). They reported a 17% rate of radiographic loosening on the basis of migration or the presence of a complete radiolucent line in 60 revisions after 5 to 14 years of follow-up study. Four sockets needed re-revision. The authors believed their rate of radiographic loosening even after a longer follow-up period is related to the older age of the patients, restoration of lost bone stock in the acetabulum with meticulous grafting technique, and use of a reinforcement ring when necessary.

Uncemented acetabular revision with bone-ingrowth components has produced better results. The most successful operations have been with hemispheric components with or without supplemental fixation such as fins, spikes, or screws. The literature reports rates of loosening from 0% to 15.2% and re-revision rates of 0% to 1.6% after an average of 17 to 52.8 months follow-up study (4,5,10,11,15,23). These results are at a shorter follow-up period than the results for cemented acetabular revision; however, with cemented acetabular revisions, complete radiolucent lines and migration often were seen early (1,6,22).

As can be seen from the aforementioned reports, the results of cemented acetabular revision are not good, especially among patients with substantial bone loss. Despite the relatively poor results of cemented acetabular revision and the encouraging early and intermediate results of uncemented acetabular revision, there is still a role for cemented fixation of the acetabular component in the revision setting. In cases of substantial acetabular bone loss, a rim fit with an uncemented cup may not be achieved, and the implant may be deemed unstable even with supplemental screw fixation. In these situations it is necessary to use another method of fixation. A solid structural allograft can be used with an uncemented or cemented cup, or an acetabular reinforcement ring or cage can be used in combination with particulate graft and possibly structural graft. With use of a large allograft and or an acetabular reinforcement ring or cage, it is necessary to use cemented fixation of a polyethylene component.

INDICATIONS AND PATIENT SELECTION

In most cases of acetabular revision, the best option is an uncemented cup with or without supplemental screw fixation. The results in the literature indicate that this technique has optimal results. However, there are situations in which cement fixation of the acetabulum is necessary. These situations include revision of the acetabulum in the face of bone loss so extensive that adequate fixation of an uncemented cup cannot be achieved.

Many acetabula in revision situations have defects that prevent reaming of the bone into a hemisphere. The more severe the osteolysis, the more difficult it is to prepare the bone for a press-fit or a rim-fit cup. If a hemisphere cannot be made, fit of the cup is severely compromised. A poorly fitted cup needs adjunctive fixation with several screws. Our experience is that if more than four screws are needed to secure the cup, there is a greater chance of the cup having failure of bony fixation. Furthermore, a poor fit increases the chance for particulate invasion at the edges of the socket. When a rim-fit socket cannot be achieved, there are three choices for fit and fixation. First is use of bulk allograft to fill the defect and allow fit of the cup. Results with bone graft have been mixed, but a failure rate of 30% or more after 6 to 10 years seems probable (16,18,21,25). Second is cancellous bone packing with a cemented socket (see Chapter 17). Little has been published on this technique, but our experience has shown it to be difficult and unpredictable. The third technique, use of a metal ring support for the osteolytic weakened bone and the bone graft, is our preferred technique. The published results have revealed an average failure rate of 20% to 25% after 5 years (9,17,18,20,24). This failure rate is similar to that of bone grafts. However, the technique that entails ring support is more predictable than that of allograft, and it is easier for less experienced revision surgeons. This technique is our primary focus in the techniques section of this chapter.

PREOPERATIVE PLANNING

Importance of Preoperative Planning

Careful preoperative planning is essential before revision total joint arthroplasty especially among patients with extensive acetabular bone loss. The surgeon must have an accurate estimation of the pattern of bone loss in the acetabulum. This is necessary to determine the inventory of materials needed to complete the operation. In centers for hip joint replacement, a large inventory of prostheses, instruments, and bone graft is available on site. At such centers, nearly any defect can be defined and dealt with at the time of the operation by an experienced revision surgeon, who has all resources needed at his or her disposal. At hospitals where complex hip revisions are not performed on a routine basis, this inventory of supplies and instruments may not be available. Special implants, instruments, and supplies have to be ordered in advance to have them available for the operation. This is a considerable cost to the hospital, particularly when large structural allografts are contemplated or custom implants may be required. Therefore it is important that the appropriate types and sizes be obtained. Even more unfortunate for surgeon and patient is to encounter unexpectedly a problem at the operation that requires a structural allograft or a different type of implant that is not available. Thorough preoperative planning in revision hip surgery benefits the patient and can help control costs.

History and Physical Examination

A careful history and physical examination are important for a patient considering revision surgery. The most common symptom of a loose acetabular component is groin pain; however, buttock pain also may occur. On occasion the presenting symptom may be thigh pain from irritation of the psoas muscle as it crosses the anterior acetabulum. Any signs or symptoms of infection, such as a history of fever or chills or vague pain in the hip with no pain-free interval since the index arthroplasty, may indicate chronic infection of the hip. Accurate assessment of the patient's preoperative activity level and an estimate of the patient's anticipated postoperative level of activity should be made because it may influence the type of acetabular reconstruction performed.

At the physical examination particular attention should be paid to the patient's gait pattern and neurologic findings. A patient with a marked abductor lurch or lateral lean indicating weakness of the hip abductors is at high risk for postoperative dislocation and loosening of the prosthesis. The same is true of patients unable to perform a side-lying straight-leg raise, also indicating weakness of the hip abductors, and of patients with a history or physical findings of neuromuscular disease.

Radiographs

The anteroposterior (AP) radiograph of the pelvis is the most valuable imaging modality in the radiologic evaluation of an acetabulum to be revised. Migration of the acetabular component can be measured with serial radiographs. An idea of pelvic bone quality can be obtained and an estimation of the extent of acetabular bone loss can be made. At our institution this is the only preoperative imaging study we obtain in most cases. Especially important is the ilioischial or Kohler's line (Fig. 1). Violation of Kohler's line on the AP pelvic radiograph indicates a substantial loss of bone from the anterior column and medial wall. In this instance, it is unlikely that 50% of an uncemented cup would be in contact with host bone and would have a higher failure rate (16). In these instances, cemented fixation of the acetabulum in conjunction with one of the techniques described later has to be used.

Other imaging studies may be useful. Judet views of the pelvis can be particularly helpful in defining deformities in the anterior and posterior columns. Computed tomography can provide information about the structure of the remaining acetabular bone. These studies are more important to surgeons at hospitals that do not have a variety of implants and graft material on site. In such situations it is especially critical to accurately define the

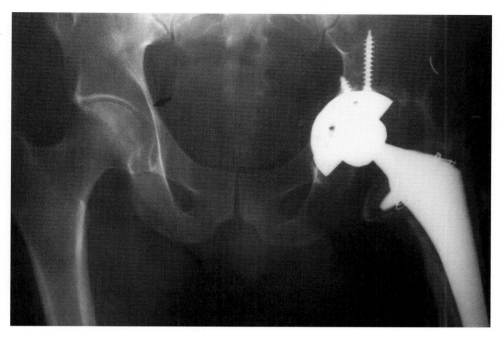

Figure 1. Anteroposterior radiograph of a pelvis. Kohler's line on the right side of the pelvis is indicated by an *arrow*. On the left side of the pelvis the apex of the acetabular cup crosses Kohler's line.

bone loss from the acetabulum to be able to order materials that may be needed at revision. Unfortunately, the ultimate decisions regarding the specific techniques needed to reconstruct an acetabulum cannot be made until the operation when the acetabulum has been exposed, the existing implant has been removed, and the defects have been defined.

SPECIFIC SURGICAL TECHNIQUES

Cementing into Acetabular Support Ring or Cage with Graft Material

Several devices have been used to reinforce the acetabular bone in arthroplasty. Many acetabular ring or cage supports are available. We describe three representative devices to provide the reader with a basic understanding of the indications and technique for implantation of acetabular support rings and cages.

Müller Roof Reinforcement Ring (Müller Ring)

The primary purpose of a Müller ring is to increase the weight-bearing area, transfer the load to the periphery, allow more lateral positioning of the socket, and protect the bone graft in the early postoperative period. This device has been of considerable value, especially in the presence of acetabular dysplasia, subchondral cysts in the acetabular roof, osteoporosis of the hip, posttraumatic acetabular wall deficiency, and loosened acetabular cups with osteolysis. The surgeon must be aware that the outer diameter of the last reamer should be 2 mm greater than the diameter of the ring to be inserted; thus a 52-mm reamer is needed to allow press fit of a 50-mm Müller ring. Commercially available sizes are 36 to 58 mm in 2-mm increments (Fig. 2–4).

Acetabular Roof Reinforcement Ring with a Hook (Ganz Ring)

The acetabular roof reinforcement ring with a hook, or Ganz ring, was developed to enable the acetabular roof to be reinforced in cases of superior acetabular rim defect and

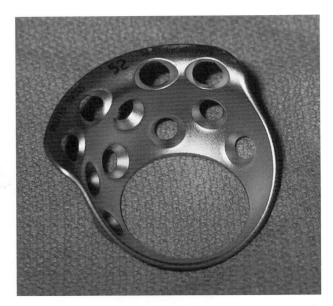

Figure 2. Photograph of a Müller ring. The ring is made of titanium and is available in diameters from 36 mm to 58 mm. The large central hole allows graft material to be packed into the acetabulum even after the ring has been implanted. It also allows cement to interdigitate with the graft material.

restore the correct center of rotation of the hip. The Ganz ring hooks onto the cortical bone of the cotyloid notch and limits superior displacement (Fig. 5). When the acetabulum has substantial superior erosion, the Ganz ring should be positioned against the bone graft at the level allowed by the hook placement on the cotyloid cortical bone. As with the Müller ring, the Ganz ring should be 2 mm smaller than the last acetabular reamer. Commercially available sizes are 36 to 64 mm in 2-mm increments.

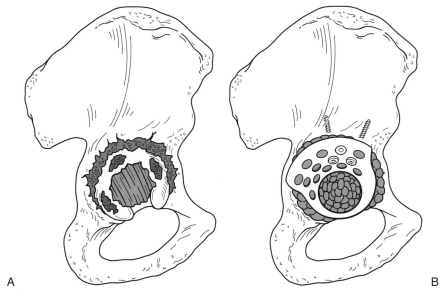

A   B

Figure 3. A: Acetabulum with segmental bone loss from the medial wall and from around the rim. Cavitary defects are present. **B:** Acetabulum reconstructed with particulate graft material and a Müller ring. At least two screws are used to fix the ring to the pelvis.

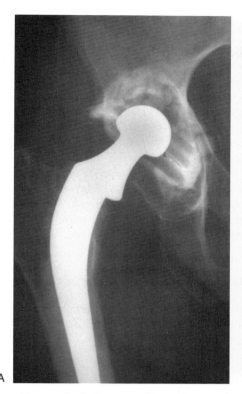
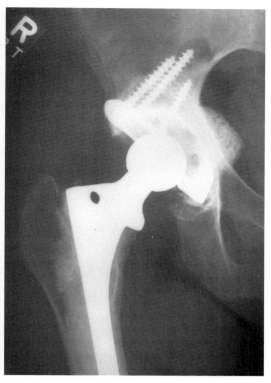

A   B

Figure 4. A: Preoperative anteroposterior (AP) radiograph of the right hip of a patient
with juvenile rheumatoid arthritis with a loose polyethylene cup. Substantial bone loss
is mostly cavitary in nature with superior migration of the cup. **B:** Postoperative AP
radiograph of the same patient as in **A.** At the operation it was not possible to revise
the socket with a press-fit porous acetabular component. The acetabulum was
therefore reconstructed with a Müller ring and corraline hydroxyapatite granules.

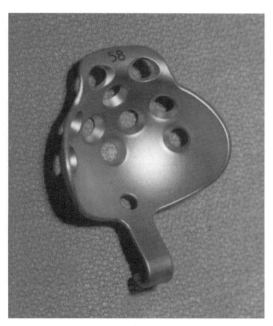

Figure 5. Photograph shows Ganz ring. The
distinguishing feature of the Ganz ring is the
inferior hook, which is designed to be inserted at the cotyloid notch and serves to
limit superior displacement. The Ganz ring
is available up to a diameter of 64 mm to
allow reconstruction of larger defects and
acetabula.

Antiprotrusio Cage (Burch-Schneider Cage)

The antiprotrusio cage has been used at the Müller Center (Berne, Switzerland) in cases of massive pelvic bone loss since 1975. The antiprotrusio cage or Burch-Schneider cage (Sulzer, Winterthur, Switzerland) was designed by Burch in 1974 and modified by Schneider (Figs. 6 and 7). It is made of rough blasted titanium with a superior flange that rests against the ilium and an inferior flange designed to be driven into the ischium or attached to its surface. The device can bridge areas of acetabular bone loss, provide support for the acetabular socket, and allow pelvic bone grafting in an environment protected from excessive stress. Biomechanically the Burch-Schneider cage provides a large contact area between the implant and remaining pelvic bone, distributing joint forces over a large area, and theoretically decreasing the likelihood of implant migration. It also allows the management of bone deficiency with morselized or bulk bone grafts placed deep to it and thus protected from forces that might contribute to graft failure. The Burch-Schneider cage is commercially available in two sizes, 44 and 50 mm.

Technique for Acetabular Revision with Ring or Cage Support

The technical use of metal ring supports involves specific technical maneuvers to perform the operation successfully. The technique is described in steps. The technique for removal of the previous implant and removal of previous cement is not detailed herein.

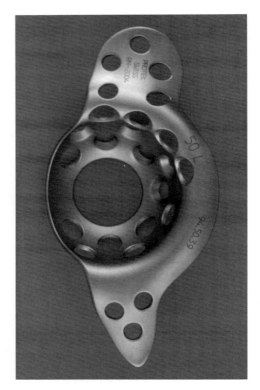

Figure 6. Photograph shows Burch-Schneider antiprotrusio cage, which has a large superior flange, triangular inferior flange, and reinforced posterior rim. This device also is made of titanium and comes in two sizes, 44 mm and 50 mm. As with the Müller ring, a larger central hole is used to pack graft material and to allow cement interdigitation with the graft.

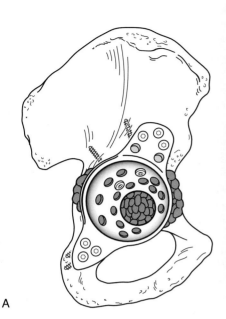 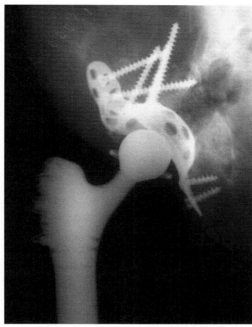

A   B

Figure 7. A: Acetabulum with pelvic discontinuity has been reconstructed with a Burch-Schneider cage with screw fixation into the ischium through the inferior flange. In this way the Burch-Schneider cage functions as a posterior plate and an acetabular support cage. This links the superior pelvis to the inferior pelvis through the ischium and ilium. Careful contouring of the cage is needed to prevent retroverting the cage or placing it in a vertical position. **B:** Postoperative radiograph of an acetabulum with pelvic discontinuity reconstructed with a Burch-Schneider cage. The inferior flange has been applied to the outside of the ischium and fixed with screws. The defects have been filled with cancellous allograft chips and demineralized bone putty. Because of abductor weakness and the use of an oncologic-type endoprosthesis with the resultant loss of proximal soft-tissue attachment, the patient is at increased risk for dislocation; therefore constrained polyethylene has been used.

Step 1: Removal of All Fibrous Tissue

After removal of the previous implant and fixation surface, the remaining acetabular bone is cleaned of all fibrous tissue. This can be done with a curette or a high-speed burr. The fibrous tissue has to be removed from all cavitary defects and from the acetabular surface.

Step 2: Determining Pelvic Continuity

Once the bone is cleaned, it must be determined whether there is discontinuity of the acetabular columns. This is first done by means of inspection. To confirm that the acetabulum is intact, force is applied on the columns to determine that they move jointly. If discontinuity of the acetabulum is present, use of a posterior plate is recommended in combination with the acetabular ring. In such situations, we have used a Burch-Schneider cage (antiprotrusio cage) without a posterior plate. When this is done the inferior flange of the cage is carefully contoured to rest on the ischium instead of being driven into the ischial bone. Screws are then placed into the ischium through holes in the inferior flange of the cage. In this way the Burch-Schneider cage acts as both an acetabular support device and as a posterior plate (see Fig. 7).

Step 3: Reaming of the Acetabulum

Reaming of the acetabulum is performed. Reaming does not have to produce a hemisphere. Often with thin, osteolytic acetabular bone, development of a hemisphere destroys too much bone of the acetabulum. This is why a rim-fit cup cannot be used in these acetabula. If it is possible to ream the acetabulum to a hemisphere with adequate bony support, a rim-fit cup should be used. Therefore in these instances the reaming is done simply to shape the acetabular bone to allow the ring to be press fit adequately between the level of the anterior inferior spine and the ischium. Reaming also helps to provide a bleeding bony bed for incorporation of the bone graft.

Step 4: Identifying the Defects, Choosing a Ring or Cage, Grafting

The defects are identified. Often there is a central medial defect and superior cavitary defects. Most often the anterior wall also is missing. A missing anterior wall differs from absence of the anterior column. If the acetabular bone has a half-moon shape, so that there is no medial wall or anterior column (and therefore no link between the pelvis at the level of the anterior inferior spine and the pubis), a Burch-Schneider cage (antiprotrusio cage) should be used (see Fig. 6). If only the anterior wall is absent, a Müller ring (see Fig. 3) or a Ganz ring (see Fig. 5) can be used.

The defects present have to be bone grafted to allow bone healing for improved support of the acetabular cup. We have used two types of graft. The first is corticocancellous demineralized bone. The second is hydroxyapatite granules. In most instances, we have not used solid bulk allograft to treat these patients and believe that it is seldom required. If a solid bulk allograft is used it should be used only as a plug that prevents cement from being pressurized into the pelvis. Corticocancellous bone chips or hydroxyapatite granules are preferred, because they heal much more quickly and completely than does a bulk allograft. We pack the bone graft or hydroxyapatite granules into position with a reamer used in reverse. We also use sufficient graft material to fill the defects completely, so that the ring chosen fits snugly against graft.

The choice of ring used depends on the defect present. If there is discontinuity or absence of an anterior column, a Burch-Schneider cage (antiprotrusio cage) is preferred. If the posterior column is absent, we may use a plate and solid bone graft to reconstitute the posterior column and use a Burch-Schneider cage. We may alternatively use the Burch-Schneider cage contoured to serve as a posterior plate with screws placed through the inferior flange into the ischium. If a defect of the superior acetabular rim raises the center of rotation of the hip more than 2.5 cm, we do not use a Müller ring. For successful use, the Müller ring must be placed onto the superior rim of the remaining acetabulum (see Fig. 3). If the rim is severely deficient or is so high that reconstruction of the hip is compromised, we use a Ganz ring (see Fig. 5). The Ganz ring hooks onto the cortical bone of the cotyloid notch. Superior displacement is limited by this hook. When the acetabulum has extensive superior erosion, we prefer to pack the superior cavity with bone graft and place the Ganz ring against the bone graft at the level allowed by the hook placement on the cotyloid cortical bone. In these instances it may be necessary to use solid graft material. The ring and screws protect the graft from excess stress, decreasing risk for collapse of the graft.

Step 5: Press Fit of the Ring or Cage

Either a Müller ring or a Ganz ring should have an anterior posterior press fit into the remaining bone of the acetabulum. The Burch-Schneider cage ideally should be press fit, but it is linked superiorly and inferiorly to bone. If a Müller ring or Ganz ring is sized incorrectly so that it floats within the acetabulum or bone graft, the stability of the construct is reduced considerably. With the Müller ring, the press fit is enhanced by the superior support of the acetabular bone. The Müller ring or Ganz ring is inserted into the acetabulum by means of tapping it in with a large bone tamp. The need to tap in the ring assures a good press fit. The press fit of the Müller ring or the Ganz ring is augmented by at least two screws into the ilium. With the Ganz ring, these screws may pass through bone graft before they engage the ilium.

The Burch-Schneider cage can be difficult to insert because of the superior and inferior flanges. The flanges usually have to be bent to conform to the shape of the acetabulum. The inferior flange is driven into the ischium from within the acetabulum into a slot previously made with an osteotome. When the flange is driven into the ischium, a vertical orientation of the cage can be avoided. When pelvic discontinuity exists, a Burch-Schneider cage can be used to bridge the defect by use of the cage as a combination cage–posterior plate. In this situation the inferior flange can be contoured and fixed to the outside of the ischium with screws (see Fig. 7). Care must be taken to bend the inferior flange correctly. If the flange is undercontoured, the cage will be placed in a vertical position and will not be able to provide good superior coverage for the polyethylene cup, which may result in lateralizing the hip center.

Step 6: Orienting the Ring or Cage

With either the Müller ring, the Ganz ring, or the Burch-Schneider cage, the posterior cup must be covered. If the posterior wall or posterior column is too deficient to allow adequate posterior coverage of the cup by bone, the metal ring must be tilted within the acetabular cavity so that it maintains an anterior posterior press fit but at the same time has posterior coverage for the cup. Use of a cup one size smaller than might otherwise be used is recommended in this situation so that the posterior cup is entirely covered by the metal ring support. When this is done, only the hood should protrude above the posterior metal support for the posterior wall of the cup. The orientation between the polyethylene cup and ring should be optimal. Increased shearing load between differently oriented components may cause early loosening at the polyethylene–cement interface. We have had one cup loosen and dislocate out of a Burch-Schneider cage. This occurred in a hip in which we did not have good coverage of the posterior polyethylene by the metal support. We now always tilt the posterior rim of whichever metal support we choose so that the posterior polyethylene is completely supported (except for the hood). Tilting of the metal support for posterior cup coverage should not be done at the expense of firm anterior posterior press fit of the ring. Use of the size metal support necessary to accomplish both an anterior posterior press fit and posterior wall support is recommended.

Step 7: Inserting Screws

The screws should be placed in the areas of the acetabulum that provide the best bone stock, thus allowing introduction of the largest possible screws while minimizing risk for damage to vital intrapelvic structures or posterior structures. The screws must be as long as possible and fully threaded to provide the largest possible contact area between implant and bone, thus decreasing local stress and strain. Fully threaded titanium 6.5-mm cancellous bone screws should be used. The posterosuperior acetabular quadrant offers the best bone stock and is relatively safe for placement of the screws. The first screw should not be introduced through the outer holes of the ring if it can be avoided, because this screw can tilt the ring outward and displace the inferior ring from the acetabular floor. Inserting the first screw into the ilium through the acetabular portion of the ring or cage prevents outward tilting of the ring and secures firm seating of the ring into the dome. During insertion of screws, the assistant pushes the ring or cage against the acetabular inner wall with a large bone tamp or similar instrument. Whenever possible, screws are not inserted into the pubis or ischium, because it is difficult to achieve adequate purchase of the screws in these areas. With Burch-Schneider cages, additional screws may be placed if necessary transversely into the ilium through the superior flange. Again, the first screws should be placed through the rim oriented upward into the ilium if such fixation can be achieved. If the transverse screws are placed into the ilium first, the inferior portion of the cage may pull away from the socket. This is especially true if the superior flange is not contoured to fit snugly against the ilium. Screws can be placed into the ischium through the inferior flange if that method is selected. Care must be taken to avoid damage to the sciatic nerve by a drill or a retractor while placing ischial screws.

Step 8: Orientation of the Polyethylene Cup

The cup inclination must be correct for stability of the hip. We recommend an abduction or theta angle of no more than 45 degrees and approximately 20 degrees of anteversion. This almost always means that the superior cup is not covered by the metal ring and must be covered with cement. As much as one third of the superior cup may be left uncovered by the metal ring support. The anteversion of the cup must be such that the posterior wall of the cup is covered (see Step 6). We prefer to use a hood to provide additional coverage for the femoral head. We may also use a protrusio plastic, which extends the lateral walls of the cup by 5 mm. The protrusio plastic is used if necessary to prevent the cup from being buried below the metal walls of the ring, which can lead to impingement of the femoral neck on the edge of the ring or cage and result in dislocation of the hip.

Step 9: Cementing the Polyethylene Cup

After irrigation of the acetabulum to clear blood and debris (with care not to dislodge the bone graft), the acetabulum including the ring or cage device and bone graft is packed with dry gauze. When the polymethyl methacrylate cement has reached a doughy consistency, the gauze is removed (again, with care not to disrupt the bone graft). A bolus of cement is dropped into the acetabulum and pressurized into the ring and bone graft with the bulb portion of a large irrigation syringe or commercial pressurizing device. This forces the cement through the holes of the ring and into the bone graft and spreads it evenly inside the ring. After the cement is pressurized for approximately 1 minute, a second small bolus of cement is dropped into the socket, and the cup is introduced and correctly positioned as described in Step 8. The cup is seated into the cement with an acetabular impactor maintaining the proper cup orientation. Excess extruded cement is cleared from around the acetabular cup with a curette. Pressure is maintained on the cup until the cement has hardened.

In summary, the four most important factors to achieve success with use of an acetabular ring or cage support are as follows: (a) The ring must achieve press fit within the acetabulum. (b) The defects must be bone grafted. (c) The posterior wall of the cup must be covered to prevent the cup from spinning out of its fixation. (d) The cup must have correct orientation to prevent hip dislocation.

Cementing with Solid Graft

We reconstruct nearly all bone-deficient acetabula with a ring support and particulate graft. In the past we used bulk allograft to reconstruct the acetabulum and have used femoral heads, distal femurs, and whole acetabular allografts. In the Results section we report our results and the results of others with this technique. Paprosky and Magnus (16) recommend use of a distal femoral allograft contoured in the shape of the number 7 and fixed to the ilium with screws oriented obliquely. If Kohler's line is intact they believe they have 30% to 60% contact between cup and graft, and they recommend uncemented fixation in such cases. If Kohler's line were not intact, a larger portion of the cup would be in contact with graft and not host bone. In these situations, Paprosky and Magnus recommend use of a whole acetabular allograft and cemented fixation. We believe that if we cannot reconstruct an acetabular defect with particulate graft and an acetabular support ring or cage, we need a whole acetabular allograft. We use this graft in conjunction with a Burch-Schneider cage. Our studies have shown that in most instances the bulk of the allograft remains necrotic even when there is union at the graft–host junction. When whole acetabular allografts are used, it is necessary to cement the cup, because ingrowth cannot be expected from the allograft. Garbuz et al. (7) reported improved results of structural allograft reconstruction when a reinforcement ring was used and recommend use of a ring or cage whenever a massive allograft is used on the acetabular side.

There may be times when it may be advantageous to use solid graft in addition to particulate graft and a reinforcement ring. Solid allograft such as femoral heads or condyles or bone graft substitute material such as coralline hydroxyapatite blocks may be useful to fill large superior defects in conjunction with a reinforcement ring. The ring support ideally should be stable against host bone, but in cases of substantial superior defect, solid or impacted particulate graft material can help provide additional support to the ring. In such situations, weight bearing should be protected for an extended period of time until the graft shows radiographic signs of incorporation.

Technique of Reconstruction with Acetabular Allograft

The technique for reconstruction of the acetabulum with bulk allograft is described in detail in Chapter 16. We describe our technique for reconstruction with an acetabular allograft.

The acetabulum is exposed and cleared of all fibrous tissue. This step is performed with curettes and a high-speed burr. The acetabulum is reamed to help shape it for the allograft and to make a bed of bleeding bone for incorporation of the graft. Reaming does not have to produce a hemisphere as in reaming for placement of an uncemented cup. The acetabular defects are then identified. If it is determined that the acetabulum cannot be reconstructed with either an uncemented cup or a reinforcement ring with particulate graft material, the decision is made to use a large allograft.

Massive superior defects combined with complete loss of the medial wall and one or both columns may necessitate use of solid allograft. A hemipelvis allograft is our preferred graft material. Portions of the ilium, pubis, and ischium are removed from the graft as necessary to allow it to be placed in the defect. The hemipelvis should be

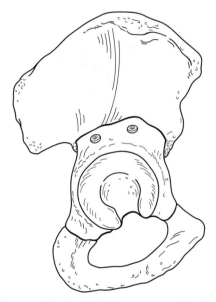

Figure 8. Acetabulum reconstructed with an entire acetabular allograft. A hemipelvis allograft has been prepared by making beveled cuts in the pubis, ischium, and ilium to allow the graft to be press fit into the host pelvis and to maximize contact of the allograft with host bone. The allograft has been fixed to the ilium with lag screws. The acetabulum now can be reamed and a Burch-Schneider cage applied for additional fixation and to protect the allograft. A polyethylene cup then is cemented into the cage.

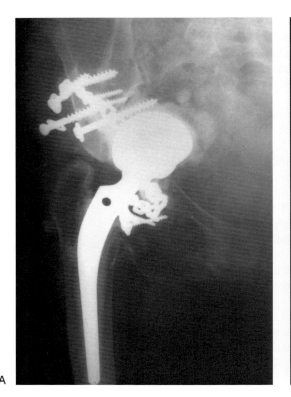

A

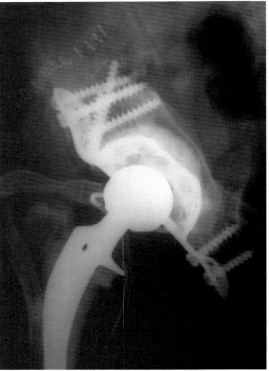

C

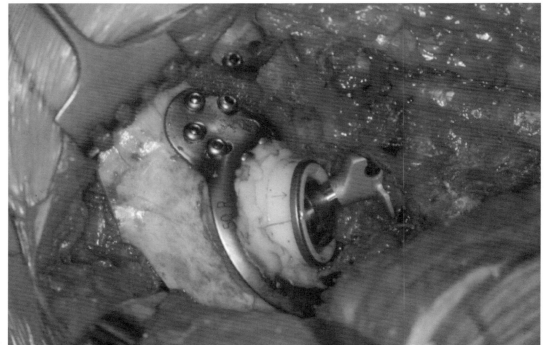

B

Figure 9. A: Preoperative radiograph of a failed right acetabulum of a patient with rheumatoid arthritis. The acetabulum had been reconstructed 3 years previously with a distal femoral allograft, pelvic reconstruction plates, and a cemented metal-backed cup. At that time there was documented pelvic discontinuity at the posterior column and between the ischium and the pubis. The acetabular cup has now migrated through the pelvis, indicating a severe medial defect. Much of the superior graft has resorbed, and bone loss appears substantial. **B:** Intraoperative photograph of the acetabulum reconstructed with an entire acetabular allograft formed from a hemipelvis and fixed to the host bone with screws and a Burch-Schneider antiprotrusio cage. The entire posterior column was missing from the ischium to the level of the greater sciatic notch. (Continued)

shaped in such a way as to maximize contact of the graft with the host bone. Beveled cuts should be made to enable the graft to be press fit into the defects with maximum contact with host bone. (Fig. 8) This is necessary to provide the best chance for the graft to unite to the pelvis. Particulate graft material may be used to fill small voids or defects between the graft and host bone. The graft should be fixed to the host pelvis with 6.5-mm cancellous lag screws. Screws directed obliquely into the ilium generally provide the best fixation. Lag screws into the pubis are difficult to place and may risk damage to vessels or the femoral nerve. Lag screws into the ischium may be placed but may not achieve good purchase in osteoporotic bone. If lag screws alone cannot provide adequate stability, additional fixation with pelvic reconstruction plates along the posterior and possibly anterior column may be needed. This requires a fairly extensive exposure. We have not found this necessary for most patients who have needed a hemipelvis allograft for reconstruction of a failed arthroplasty. The allograft socket is now reamed appropriately to prepare it for placement of a cage and cemented fixation of a polyethylene cup. Care is taken not to remove too much bone and weaken the graft. Several holes are drilled in the socket with a one-fourth-inch drill bit approximately 5 mm deep to help provide additional cement interdigitation. With the advent of acetabular reinforcement rings and cages, we now recommend that a Burch-Schneider cage be carefully contoured and placed within the acetabular allograft. The cage is fixed to the allograft and host bone with lag screws that ideally will pass through the cage and allograft and into the host bone. The superior flange may be in direct contact with host ilium and allow screw placement directly into host bone superiorly. Inferiorly, the lower flange may be driven into the host ischium but usually should be fixed with screws into host bone if possible, because often in defects requiring a large bulk allograft there is pelvic discontinuity. The cage now provides additional fixation for the graft and also helps protect the graft from uneven compressive forces (Fig. 9).

Once the allograft and cage have been securely fixed to the host bone, the graft is prepared to accept a cemented cup. The socket is then irrigated by means of pulsatile lavage and packed with dry gauze. A polyethylene cup of the appropriate size to fit within the allograft and cage in the correct orientation is selected. It should be large enough to avoid sinking into the cage and socket such that impingement of the femur may result. Trial sockets if available or reamer shells can help determine the correct size. The cup is then cemented into the allograft in the same manner described for cementing a cup into a ring support (Fig. 9B,C).

Figure 9. (*Continued*) There was a thin rim of remaining anterior column, but a fracture with fibrous union only in this area left a discontinuity between the ilium and the pubis. There was a large medial defect, which was continuous with the sciatic notch. Superiorly only iliac wing remained. The bone loss was too severe for reconstruction with particulate graft and a cage alone. The acetabular graft was formed from an entire hemipelvic allograft segment. This was made with a high-speed burr into a 7-shaped configuration, and beveled cuts were made in the ischium and pubis. This allowed the graft to be press fit into the remaining host pelvis and maximized contact of the graft with the host bone. The acetabular allograft was reamed and prepared for cemented fixation, and the Burch-Schneider cage was contoured and fit to the graft and host pelvis. The screws in the superior flange of the cage pass through the cage and the outer table of the graft and into host bone. Two oblique screws pass though holes on the inside rim of the cage, though the graft, and into host ilium. Inferiorly two screws are placed through the cage directly into host ischium. A constrained polyethylene liner has been cemented into the cage–allograft construct because of marked hip abductor weakness with high risk for postoperative dislocation. **C:** Postoperative radiograph shows acetabulum reconstructed with an entire-acetabulum allograft and a Burch-Schneider cage. Screws pass through the cage and allograft and then into the host ilium. In the inferior aspect screws were placed directly into the host ischium. A constrained polyethylene liner has been cemented into the construct. Cement protrudes through the center hole and the smaller holes of the cage and into the allograft. The locking ring is seen around the elevated rim of the constrained liner.

POSTOPERATIVE CARE

Weight-bearing Restrictions and Precautions

After extensive acetabular reconstruction, weight bearing is limited as long as necessary until it is felt that the reconstruction can support the patient's weight. With use of a Müller ring that achieves a firm press fit with host bone and is supplementally fixed with screws with no structural supporting graft material (excluding filler graft material in cavitary defects), the decision can be made to allow the patient weight bearing as tolerated, provided that the femoral reconstruction does not warrant limited weight bearing. In acetabular reconstructions requiring more extensive use of particulate graft and with weak supporting host bone, weight bearing is limited to toe touch until radiologic evidence of incorporation of the graft is seen. With cavitary defects alone weight bearing usually can be started more quickly than with defects that involve segmental bone loss. When a ring support is used, weight bearing generally is limited for 6 weeks to 3 months. For reconstructions of hips with loss of an acetabular column, pelvic discontinuity or hips requiring reconstruction with a large, solid allograft, weight bearing may be limited to toe touch for several months until radiologic evidence of healing is seen.

Often in large acetabular reconstructions substantial work has been done on the femoral side or a trochanteric osteotomy has been performed. Patients are instructed in postoperative dislocation precautions depending on the approach used, that is, posterior, anterolateral, or anterior. If a trochanteric osteotomy has been performed (which we recommend in the form of an extended slide and reattach with at least two cerclage cables), the patient should wear a short pantaloon spica cast to protect the fixation. These patients should follow trochanteric slide precautions, which limit weight bearing to toe touch and restrict active straight leg raising and hip abduction to help prevent displacement of the trochanter until the cast has been placed.

Patients who have had loss of an acetabular column with extensive use of particulate graft and a Burch-Schneider cage, use of a large structural allograft, or otherwise have thin, weak supporting host bone also wear a pantaloon spica cast postoperatively and perform only toe-touch weight bearing until radiographic evidence of healing has occurred. Our patients do not receive casts until surgical drains are removed and the wound is clean and dry.

PREVENTION AND MANAGEMENT OF COMPLICATIONS

Dislocation

The rate of postoperative dislocation in revision hip surgery is much higher than that in primary arthroplasty. As can be seen from our early results with ring supports, dislocations were frequent. Dislocations can be prevented with careful attention to the correct orientation of the acetabular cup within the ring. Patients at high risk for dislocation also should wear a pantaloon spica cast or brace postoperatively for 6 to 8 weeks to allow the soft tissues to heal.

Patients who have weak abductors from neuromuscular disease, disuse atrophy, scar tissue, or loss of the greater trochanter are at particular risk for dislocation. For these patients, especially those with loss of the greater trochanter, strong consideration should be given to use of a constrained acetabular cup. We have cemented a constrained acetabular polyethylene cup into acetabular reinforcement rings for patients at high risk for dislocation for the past 2 years and have seen only one dislocation of a head out of the constrained liner. So far no cups have dissociated from the rings.

Nerve Damage

Care must be taken when using the Burch-Schneider cage to avoid dennervation of the gluteus medius muscle with resulting abductor weakness and increased risk for dislocation. The Burch-Schneider cage has an extended superior flange that rests on the ilium and allows placement of transverse screws. This superior flange requires elevation of the gluteal muscles off the lateral ilium. Often the superior rim of the acetabulum has been eroded and the superior edge is displaced superiorly. This means that the superior flange of the Burch-Schneider cage is placed high on the ilium, where innervation of the gluteus medius occurs. Because of the threat of dennervation, we recommend use of a Burch-Schneider cage only when discontinuity or a ''half moon'' acetabulum exists. In other acetabular deficiencies, a Müller or Ganz ring can be used.

Care must be taken to avoid damage to the sciatic nerve when driving the inferior flange of the Burch-Schneider cage into the ischium or especially when exposing the lateral ischium for placement of screws through the inferior flange should this method of fixation to the ischium be chosen. The sciatic nerve also may suffer stretch injury. This is more likely when there has been long-standing superior displacement of the femoral head as in developmental dysplasia of the hip. In any case, if the hip center is restored to a near anatomic position, the leg is lengthened and the potential for stretch injury to the sciatic nerve exists. The sciatic nerve can be palpated where it crosses over the ischium. This can be done without completely dissecting out the nerve and potentially compromising its vascularity. Sometimes the nerve can be difficult to palpate because of an overlying layer of scar tissue. In this case, this layer can be incised longitudinally with an electrocautery while an assistant monitors the foot for any ''jump''. With incision of the scar-tissue layer, the surgeon's fingers are allowed access into the fatty tissue layer that surrounds the nerve.

The tension on the sciatic nerve can be estimated by means of palpation. If the nerve is tethered across the ischium and palpated to be ''tight like a banjo string,'' risk for injury is high. Patients whose hip center has been markedly lowered but whose sciatic nerve is not felt to have excessive tension are treated in the same manner as patients with developmental dysplasia of the hip. They are positioned postoperatively with the knee in flexion to help keep tension off of the sciatic nerve. The patients are gradually allowed to straighten the knee by themselves. With this technique, the incidence of postoperative nerve palsy can be lessened.

RESULTS

Acetabular Reinforcement Rings

Berry and Müller (2) performed the first comprehensive study of the midterm performance of the Burch-Schneider antiprotrusio cage to manage massive acetabular bone deficiency in revision total hip arthroplasty. Thirty-two of 42 (76%) of the reconstructions showed no evidence of acetabular failure or loosening after a mean follow-up period of 5 years (2 to 11 years). Berry and Müller defined loosening as breakage, bending, or loosening of the screws that secure the cage to the pelvis, a change in position, or development of a continuous cement–bone radiolucent line wider than 2 mm. Before 1982, they used cement only to fill defects. Since then, morselized bone graft has been used. The graft appeared to be incorporating, as shown by radiographic remodeling in 12 hips that could be assessed, and there was no graft resorption.

In 1994, Zehntner et al. (24) reported the results of acetabular reconstructions with frozen femoral head allografts and the Müller acetabular reinforcement after an average follow-up period of 7.2 years (range 5.5 to 10 years) in 27 patients and hips. The deficiencies, according to the American Academy of Orthopaedic Surgeons (AAOS) classification, were 1 segmental, 14 cavitary, and 12 combined cavity and segmental. Twenty-two (82%) of the reconstructions were classified as adequate and 5 (18%) as inadequate. Reconstructions were considered adequate if an appropriately sized ring had been used in accordance with the recommendations of the authors (contact on host pelvic bone cranially, posteriorly, and inferomedially). Radiographic evaluation revealed acetabular component migration of more than 2 mm in 12 reconstructions (44%). Of these, cranial migration averaged 4 mm (range 2 to 9 mm) in inadequate reconstructions, whereas it averaged only 2 mm (range 1 to 4 mm) in adequate reconstructions. The incidence of migration in adequate reconstructions for segmental only and combined cavitary and segmental defects was 6 of 12 (50%), whereas it was 1 of 10 among reconstructions of cavitary deficiencies. Kaplan-Meier survivorship analysis revealed a 79.6% probability of survival at 10 years with revision as the end point for failure. It was concluded that durability of the reconstruction can be expected if support of the metallic reinforcement device is provided by host bone.

Peters et al. (17) reported on a retrospective review of 28 acetabular revisions with the Burch-Schneider antiprotrusio cage and cancellous allograft bone with a 33-month average follow-up period. Twenty-two hips had AAOS type III (combined segmental and cavitary bone loss) acetabular deficiency, 5 hips had type II (cavitary bone loss), and 1 hip had type I (segmental bone loss). After the operation, 80% of the patients had mild or no pain and 80% functioned as at least a community ambulator. Marked component migration was documented in 14% of the acetabular reconstructions. The hip center was improved from a preoperative side-to-side difference of 12.5 mm to 4.9 mm at final evaluation. Average medial wall bone stock improved from 1.9 mm before the operation to 10.1 mm after revision. No patients needed revision of the antiprotrusio cage for problems related to the acetabular reconstruction.

Haentjens et al. (9) reported the 5-year results of cemented acetabular reconstruction with a Müller ring for 43 patients. The same group's results had been previously reported after a 40-months follow-up period. At 5 years they reported excellent, very good, or good results for 82% of patients compared with 87% at 40 months. They found a high incidence of nonprogressive radiolucent lines at the cement–bone interface that did not correlate with the clinical results. Progressive radiolucencies or radiolucencies around screws were, however, predictive of failure.

Rosson and Schatzker (20) reviewed the 5-year results of 66 acetabular reconstructions with either the Müller ring or Burch-Schneider cage. Five Müller rings needed re-revision. The authors found that the practice of grafting the defects reduced the incidence of failure from 13% to 6% and the incidence of circumferential radiolucent lines from 39% to 2%. They concluded that the Burch-Schneider cage should be used for medial segmental defects and extensive cavitary and combined defects and that bone defects should be filled with graft instead of cement.

From September 1992 to July 1994, 111 acetabular reconstructions were performed by one of us (L. D. D.) on 109 patients. Acetabular ring supports were used in 23 hips in 22 patients (20.7% of the cases). Acetabular reinforcement rings used included 12 Burch-Schneider, 5 Müller, and 4 Ganz. All but one were fixed with a minimum of two screws (range one to five screws). Twenty of 21 acetabula were bone grafted before ring insertion and then polyethylene cups were cemented into the ring supports.

The preoperative Harris hip scores averaged 46.7 points (range 20 to 83 points). The Harris hip scores at the time of most recent follow-up examination or revision operation averaged 73.4 points (range 50 to 92 points) and were similar among the three types of ring supports used. Five patients needed further revision hip operations. Two patients with Burch-Schneider rings had vertical cup positions and needed exchange and repositioning of the polyethylene cup. One patient sustained dissociation of the polyethylene cup from the acetabular reinforcement ring and needed cemented fixation of a new cup. A patient who sustained a femur fracture 6 months postoperatively underwent open reduction and internal fixation. These four patients retained their original acetabular reinforcement ring. One patient had an infection 10 months postoperatively and underwent two-stage exchange. This hip demonstrated progressive radiolucent lines before exchange. Evidence of radiolucent lines (2 to 4 mm) was seen in seven other cases, and all were seen initially on the postoperative radiograph. Four of these seven hips showed no progression or change in the lines at last follow-up examination. Two demonstrated graft incorporation and disappearance of lines after an average of 17 months; one showed progression of radiolucent lines. Among the rest of the hips, incorporation of bone graft was demonstrated after an average of 15 months. Medial ring support migration more than 3 mm was not seen in any hip. Vertical cup migration more than 3 mm was seen in two hips: one with a Burch-Schneider and one with a Müller ring. Patients with Burch-Schneider rings had the highest incidence of dislocation and largest opening ring angle. The postoperative dislocation rate was 33% (7 of 21). Two of the first three hips with ring support dislocated. Five of seven dislocations occurred among patients with Burch-Schneider cages. The hips that dislocated had absent or severely weak gluteus medius function, sometimes in combination with a vertical cup position (18).

We have improved the orientation of the ring and cage support and the orientation of the cup within the support. We also have begun using constrained polyethylene cups to treat patients with severely weakened abductors. It is important to remember that these are the results of our early experience with acetabular ring supports. Our complication rate was high because we were learning the technique of this method of reconstruction without the benefit of instruction. Our purpose is to make the reader aware of these complications and teach methods to help avoid the complications we experienced in our early endeavors.

We have used various types of particulate graft material, including demineralized allograft bone chips and coralline-derived hydroxyapatite granules, in acetabular reconstruction. We performed a randomized study that at the time of this chapter had not yet been published, comparing these two types of graft material in acetabular revision. Thirty-seven consecutive cases of complex acetabular reconstruction were randomized with 15 in the hydroxyapatite granule group and 22 in the demineralized bone allograft chip group and followed for a minimum of 2 years (2 to 4 years). Cementless cups were used in 16 hips. Twenty-one acetabular reinforcement rings were used, which included 5 Ganz rings, 5 Müller rings, and 11 Burch-Schneider cages. Fifty-seven percent of acetabular defects were type III according to the AAOS classification. Computerized graphic analysis was used for quantitative determination of radiologic incorporation. There was no statistical difference in demographic data, acetabular defect, or type of ring support between the two groups. Radiologic incorporation was demonstrated in 12 of 15 hips (80.0%) in the hydroxyapatite group and 18 of 22 hips (81.8%) in the demineralized bone allograft chip group, and there was no statistical difference ($p = .89$). One autopsy retrieval of hydroxyapatite granules confirmed healing. On the basis of this data we support the use of either bone graft material with ring reinforcement for acetabular reconstruction.

Bulk Solid Allograft

A study was performed by one of us (L. D. D.) to evaluate the use of solid intact allograft in revision total hip arthroplasty reconstruction among 22 patients with marked insufficiency of acetabular or proximal femoral bone stock. Entire cadaveric acetabular allografts were used to augment severe bone loss of the acetabulum among 8 of 22 patients who underwent revision total hip arthroplasty with noncemented implants. The average follow-up period was 4 years. The average time to radiographic union of the acetabular allografts was 11 months. Superior migration of the allograft occurred in 4 patients (50%) and ranged from 10 to 20 mm. Varus tilt of the acetabular component within the allograft was found in 3 patients. Reoperation on 2 patients revealed nonunion of 90% of the graft. Union did not occur in areas where there was no direct contact of the allograft with the host bone. On the basis of this study, we determined that the successful use of acetabular allografts requires that most of the allograft be contiguous to host bone and not to soft tissue. When large solid allografts are used, such as entire-acetabulum allografts, the *component should be cemented into the graft,* because bone ingrowth cannot be expected to occur with allograft bone (25).

Shinar and Harris (21) reported that despite good early results (5 year follow-up period) at their institution, acetabular reconstruction with bulk structural autogenous grafts and allografts from the femoral head in complex total hip arthroplasty was much less successful in the long term. At an average of 16.5 years postoperatively, 9 of the 15 acetabular components supported by allograft and 16 (29%) of the 55 supported by autogenous graft were revised ($p = .03$). However, the total rate of loosening of acetabular components was 10 of 15 (67%), and the rate of revision was 33 of 55 (60%). All of the sockets had been inserted with cement and all of the grafts united. Regression analysis revealed that a younger age at the time of the operation and the extent of coverage of the acetabular component by the graft were associated with the need for revision. Twenty-one (78%) of the 27 acetabular components that remained rigidly fixed were supported by graft over less than 50% of the contact area, whereas only 9 (36%) of the 25 that were revised were so supported ($p < .05$). None of the 9 acetabular components with 30% of the contact area or less covered by graft were revised.

Garbuz et al., (7) reported the results of the placement of a massive structural acetabular allograft in conjunction with a revision total hip arthroplasty in 32 patients (33 hips) were evaluated at a minimum of 5 years. The graft supported more than 50% of the cup in all patients. Eight hips were reconstructed with a cup cemented into an acetabular allograft and roof reinforcement ring. Fourteen cups were cemented into an allograft without a ring, 7 were uncemented, and 4 were bipolar cups. After an average follow-up period of 7 years, 7 hips needed another revision, but the structural allograft was intact and had been used to support the cup at the repeat revision. Eight hips had loosening of the prosthesis and failure of the allograft. The result was considered a clinical and radiographic success when the hip score had increased at least 20 points, the cup was stable, the allograft had united, and no additional operation was necessary. According to these criteria, the rate of success was 55% (18 of 33 hips). The only factor that was found to be clinically important with respect to outcome was the method of reconstruction. Seven of the 8 hips that had been reconstructed with use of a roof-reinforcement ring and a structural allograft had a successful result after an average of 7.5 years (range 5 to 11 years). Two of 14 cemented cups without a ring failed, 3 of 7 uncemented cups failed, and 2 of 4 bipolar cups failed. Because of the high rate of success with cemented fixation into acetabular reinforcement rings, the authors advocate this method of reconstruction whenever a massive allograft is used on the acetabular side.

Paprosky and Magnus (16) reported the results of 69 acetabular revisions that required allograft reconstruction. Distal femoral allografts united to host bone, and there was no migration of uncemented cups after 5 years of follow-up study if Kohler's line was intact on the preoperative radiographs. When Kohler's line was not intact, 70% of the uncemented cups had migrated more than 4 mm. In cases in which Kohler's line was violated and whole acetabular allografts with cemented cups were used, all 14 of these demonstrated union at the graft–host junction and no change in the cement graft interface at a minimum follow-up period of 2 years. Overall, the authors reported 76% good to excellent results. This study emphasized the limitations of uncemented fixation with allograft when there is severe loss of bone stock and an insufficient area of contact between cup and host bone. In these situations cemented fixation and a larger graft performed better.

On the basis of these results from the literature, it can be seen that the results of complex reconstruction of the acetabulum in revision arthroplasty are not as good as in those hips with good bone stock. It appears that early efforts at reconstruction with particulate graft and acetabular support rings and cages have produced results comparable to fairly recent results of reconstruction with large bulk allograft. Bulk allograft demonstrates inconsistent incorporation and a high incidence of resorption and collapse. On the other hand it appears that hydroxyapatite granules and demineralized bone allograft bone chips both have a high rate of radiologic incorporation with no significant difference found between the two. When large bulk allografts are used, better results are obtained with the additional use of a support cage.

SUMMARY AND CONCLUSIONS

The results in the literature for cemented revision of the acetabulum are inferior to those for uncemented revision. Cemented fixation is less effective in cases of bone loss and cannot be expected to achieve adequate interdigitation in the remaining sclerotic host bone. There are, however, cases in which the defects present preclude use of an uncemented cup. In such situations other methods of reconstruction have to be employed. Reconstruction with acetabular reinforcement rings or cages, depending on the shape and severity of the defects present, is recommended in most cases. Particulate graft material is recommended to reconstitute bone defects because it is more reliably and readily incorporated. The use of a support ring or cage protects and contains the graft. The results of reconstruction with support rings and cages compares favorably with those of reconstruction with bulk solid allograft, yet the technique is easier for most surgeons to perform. When this method is used, the acetabular polyethylene is cemented into the ring or cage and the graft. Proper surgical technique and adherence to the principles described are necessary for a successful outcome.

There are cases in which the defects are so large that a stable construct cannot be obtained with use of a cage and particulate graft. Fortunately, these cases are infrequent. In these circumstances, use of a large bulk allograft is required and an entire acetabular allograft usually is the best choice. Use of an acetabular reinforcement ring or cage is recommended in conjunction with use of a large bulk allograft to provide additional fixation and to help dissipate weight-bearing forces to protect the graft. Cemented fixation of the cup is required because bone ingrowth cannot be expected to occur from the allograft.

REFERENCES

1. Amstutz HC, Ma SM, Jinnah RH, et al. Revision of aseptic loose total hip arthroplasties. *Clin Orthop* 1982;170:21–33.
2. Berry DJ, Müller ME. Revision arthroplasty using an anti-protrusio cage for massive acetabular bone deficiency. *J Bone Joint Surg Br* 1992;74:711–715.
3. Callaghan JJ, Salvati EA, Pellici PM, et al. Results of revision for mechanical failure after cemented total hip replacement, 1979 to 1982: a two to five-year follow-up. *J Bone Joint Surg Am* 1985;67:1074–1085.
4. Dorr LD, Wan Z. Ten years of experience with porous acetabular components for revision surgery. *Clin Orthop* 1995;319:191–200.
5. Engh CA, Glassman AH, Griffin WL, et al. Results of cementless revision for failed cemented total hip arthroplasty. *Clin Orthop* 1988;235:91–110.
6. Franzén H, Mjöberg B, Önnerfält R. Early migration of acetabular components revised with cement: a roentgen stereophotogrammetric study. *Clin Orthop* 1993;287:131–134.
7. Garbuz D, Morsi E, Gross AE. Revision of the acetabular component of a total hip arthroplasty with a massive structural allograft: study with a minimum five-year follow-up. *J Bone Joint Surg Am* 1996;78: 693–697.
8. Garcia-Cimbrelo E, Munuera L, Diez-Vazquez V. Long-term results of aseptic cemented Charnley revisions. *J Arthroplasty* 1995;10:121–131.
9. Haentjens P, De Boeck H, Handelberg F, Casteleyn PP, Opdecam P. Cemented acetabular reconstruction with the Müller support ring: a minimum five-year clinical and roentgenographic follow-up study. *Clin Orthop* 1993;290:225–235.
10. Harris WH, Krushell RJ, Galante JO. Results of cementless revisions of total hip arthroplasties using the Harris-Galante prosthesis. *Clin Orthop* 1988;235:120–126.
11. Hedley AK, Gruen TA, Ruoff DP. Revision of failed total hip arthroplasties with uncemented porous-coated anatomic components. *Clin Orthop* 1988;235:75–90.
12. Kavanagh BF, Fitzgerald RH Jr. Multiple revisions for failed total hip arthroplasty not associated with infection. *J Bone Joint Surg Am* 1987;69-A:1144–1149.
13. Kavanagh BF, Ilstrup DM, Fitzgerald RH Jr. Revision total hip arthroplasty. *J Bone Joint Surg Am* 1985;67:517–526.
14. Marti RK, Schüller HM, Besselaar PP, et al. Results of revision of hip arthroplasty with cement: a five to fourteen-year follow-up study. *J Bone Joint Surg Am* 1990;72:346–354.
15. Padgett DE, Kull L, Rosenberg A, et al. Revision of the acetabular component with out cement after total hip arthroplasty: three to six year follow-up. *J Bone Joint Surg Am* 1993;75:663–673.
16. Paprosky WG, Magnus RE. Principles of bone grafting in revision total hip arthroplasty: acetabular technique. *Clin Orthop* 1994;298:147–155.
17. Peters CL, Curtain M, Samuelson KM. Acetabular revision with the Burch-Schneider anti-protrusio cage and cancellous allograft bone. *J Arthroplasty* 1995;10:307–312.
18. Possai KW, Dorr LD, McPherson EJ. Metal ring supports for deficient acetabular bone in total hip replacement. *Instr Course Lect* 1996;45:161–169.
19. Raut VV, Wroblewski BM. Revision of the acetabular component of a total hip arthroplasty with cement in young patients with out rheumatoid arthritis. *J Bone Joint Surg Am* 1996;78:1853–1856.
20. Rosson J, Schatzker J. The use of reinforcement rings to reconstruct deficient acetabulae. *J Bone Joint Surg Br* 1992;74:716–720.
21. Shinar AA, Harris WH. Bulk structural autogenous grafts and allografts for reconstruction of the acetabulum in total hip arthroplasty: sixteen-year-average follow-up. *J Bone Joint Surg Am* 1997;79:159–168.
22. Snorrason F, Kärrholm J. Early loosening of revision hip arthroplasty: a roentgen stereophotogrammetric analysis. *J Arthroplasty* 1990;5:217–229.
23. Tanzer M, Drucker D, Jasty M, et al. Revision of the acetabular component with an uncemented Harris-Galante porous-coated prosthesis. *J Bone Joint Surg Am* 1992;74:987–994.
24. Zehntner MK, Ganz R. Midterm results (5.5–10 years) of acetabular allograft reconstruction with the acetabular reinforcement ring during total hip revision. *J Arthroplasty* 1994;9:469–479.
25. Zmolek JC, Dorr LD. Revision total hip arthroplasty: the use of solid allograft. *J Arthroplasty* 1993;8:361–370.

Revision Total Hip Arthroplasty,
edited by Marvin E. Steinberg and Jonathan P. Garino,
Lippincott Williams & Wilkins, Philadelphia © 1999.

21

Acetabular Revision: Uncemented

Andrew H. Glassman

Acetabular reconstruction remains a challenge in revision total hip arthroplasty. Technical difficulties derive in large part from the varying degrees of bone-stock damage that exist after acetabular failure and implant removal. In contrast to the femur, there is little bone-stock reserve in the acetabulum. Acetabular component position plays a pivotal role in determining hip biomechanics and stability against dislocation, yet the bone available to contain and secure an acetabular component in the anatomic position is extremely limited.

The state of the art in complex revision is in flux. The reported results of acetabular revision with cemented components have been less than ideal (11–14,17,18,22). On the other hand, the early and intermediate-term results of cementless revision have been very encouraging (11,12,19,22). Debate continues regarding the utility of structural allografting (3,4,6–8,13,14,18,20), the importance of restoring the hip center to anatomic position (8,18), and the use of special components, including reinforcement rings or cups (1,3,4,6,7,17), bilobed or elliptical cups (20), constrained liners, and custom components. Given the spectrum of conditions a revision surgeon may encounter, it is clear that no single technique is optimum in all cases. One must be familiar with a variety of techniques and implants. Furthermore, today's health care environment demands that the costs associated with various constructs be weighed against the physical demands and life expectancy of the patient.

A. H. Glassman: The Anderson Clinic, and Joint Replacement Service, Pentagon City Hospital, Arlington, Virginia 22206.

INDICATIONS

The most common indication for acetabular revision is aseptic loosening (12,14,19,22). The clinical and radiographic features are well known and covered in Chapter 3. Another indication is recurrent dislocation caused by component malposition. Radiographic findings may include vertical cup orientation on the anteroposterior (AP) view with or without retroversion (in cases of recurrent posterior dislocation) or excessive anteversion (in cases of anterior dislocation) on the true acetabular lateral view. It must not be assumed that suboptimal acetabular component orientation alone is responsible for recurrent dislocation. Careful analysis of femoral component version, leg length, and the status of the greater trochanter and abductors is essential. One occasionally may encounter a case of recurrent dislocation in which femoral and acetabular component position and leg length are ideal. This appears to be more common with late dislocation. Revision of the acetabular component to a constrained design is one effective solution in such situations (Fig. 1).

During the past 15 years, cementless acetabular fixation has become the preference of most surgeons. At present, revision for aseptic loosening of these components appears to be less common than for cemented cups at similar follow-up times. Unfortunately, polyethylene wear and osteolysis around cementless cups have supplanted aseptic loosening as a leading reason for reoperation. Whether and when surgical intervention for wear-related problems is indicated and whether acetabular component revision versus polyethylene exchange with bone grafting should be performed depend on a variety of considerations. Important determinants are the patient's age, sex, body habitus, and activity level, the location and extent of any osteolytic lesions, the presence of associated soft-tissue masses or cysts, acetabular component design, femoral component design, and the need for revision of the femoral component. For example, reoperation would be strongly indicated for a young, active, heavy man with eccentric wear. Factors favoring polyethylene exchange alone include minimal osteolysis, accessibility of lytic lesions to bone grafting, and acceptable acetabular component design. Alternatively, revision of the entire component is preferred if osteolysis is extensive or the lesions are inaccessible without removal of the acetabular shell.

Formal revision also is indicated, even in the absence of marked osteolysis, if the existing acetabular component is known to be of poor design. Multiple screw holes, an inadequate locking mechanism for the liner, poor shell–liner congruence or support, and areas of excessively thin polyethylene all have been identified in various early designs of cementless acetabular components. In such cases, polyethylene exchange alone, particularly in the case of a young and active patient is unlikely to provide a satisfactory long-term result. In fact, replacement liners are no longer available for certain of these cups. For an elderly, low-demand person with eccentric wear and minimal osteolysis, observation with regular radiographic examination is reasonable. For patients who need femoral revision, we regularly exchange the polyethylene liner. A particularly difficult problem commonly encountered at my institution is the presence of a well-functioning, bone-ingrown, cementless femoral component (often extensively porous coated), with a fixed, 32-mm millimeter femoral head, eccentric polyethylene wear, and osteolysis. For a young person, unless the revision acetabular component can accommodate a liner with 8 to 10 mm of polyethylene thickness, the femoral component is exchanged to one that will accommodate a smaller prosthetic head. For an elderly person, the patient's general health, activity level, and life expectancy must be carefully considered, particularly if the femoral component is extensively coated. For such a person we would be more willing to perform isolated acetabular revision and accept a polyethylene thickness of 6 to 8 mm.

It is now known that osteolysis may manifest itself in unexpected ways. The process extends to contiguous areas, including the abdomen, pelvic cavity, and inguinal canal. Such problems, discussed in detail later, may not be initially recognized as hip-related problems. Most often they are a strong indication for acetabular revision.

The indications for revision with a cementless acetabular component versus a cemented one are controversial and largely a matter of surgeon preference. The prerequisites for

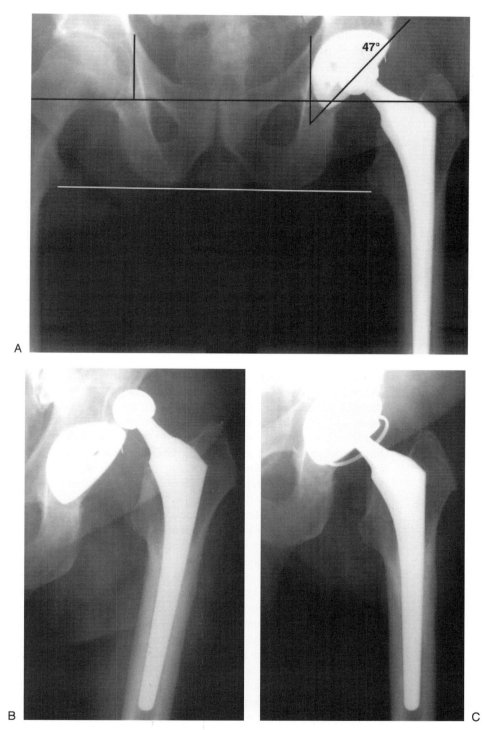

Figure 1. A 59-year-old man underwent cementless primary left total hip replacement 5 years previously for a diagnosis of avascular necrosis, probably related to ethanol use. **A:** Leg lengths were equal and component position appears satisfactory. **B:** The patient then sustained five posterior dislocations. **C:** Revision with a constrained polyethylene insert was performed.

biologic fixation, namely, the ability to achieve initial mechanical implant stability and apposition of the ingrowth surface to an adequate area of well vascularized host bone, must be met if cementless technique is chosen.

PREOPERATIVE PLANNING

Careful preoperative planning is the cornerstone of successful acetabular revision. Its importance increases in proportion to the complexity of the case. Preoperative planning takes place at a variety of levels, including the clinical evaluation, assessment of bone-stock damage, templating, and implant selection.

Clinical Evaluation

The general clinical evaluation is covered elsewhere in Chapters 8 through 10. Certain aspects pertinent to acetabular revision merit emphasis. As always, infection must be ruled out. The primary disease must be appreciated and understood. Certain conditions, most noteworthy rheumatoid arthritis, metabolic bone disease, and Paget's disease, compromise the quality of remaining acetabular bone stock and the ability to achieve primary mechanical stability with cementless components. Under these circumstances it may be necessary to use a cemented acetabulum, often in conjunction with support rings or cages and bone graft (Fig. 2). Osteoporosis, whether generalized or from disuse, has a similar effect. Other conditions, such as arthrokatadysis and developmental dysplasia are associated with focal bony deficiencies that may not have been adequately addressed at primary arthroplasty.

The status of the soft tissues, including skin, fascia, and muscle, is critical. The presence and location of prior incisions (sometimes multiple) is recorded. Narrow islands of skin between previous incisions may be markedly attenuated and the underlying subcutaneous tissue atrophic. In select instances, consultation with a plastic surgeon should be considered. Preliminary scar revision or flap closure after the revision can then be planned. Fascial defects also should be documented. The status of the abductor muscles is assessed critically. A careful neurologic examination of the entire lower extremity is undertaken and if necessary supplemented with electrodiagnostic studies. Any preexisting nerve deficit should be carefully documented, both for preoperative planning and medical-legal purposes. When no deficit is clinically evident, any history of transient nerve palsy is carefully sought. For example, a patient with a primary diagnosis of fracture dislocation, prior internal fixation, and transient sciatic palsy would be expected to have scarring of the sciatic nerve, which may be tethered to the posterior column. Formal sciatic neurolysis, possibly in collaboration with a neurosurgeon, should be considered.

A careful review of systems is conducted with particular attention to the gastrointestinal, genitourinary, and circulatory systems, especially if intrapelvic protrusion of the existing acetabular component or internal fixation devices is found or if substantial polyethylene wear or osteolysis is present. If indicated, a barium enema examination, intravenous pyelography and cystography, arteriography, or arthrography is performed in search for fistulas or to assess the proximity of implants to the ureters, intestine, or major blood vessels (2). Osteolysis is now known to manifest itself in varied and sometimes unusual ways. A case in point is that of a 60-year-old woman who found a painful mass in her groin $2\frac{1}{2}$ years after ipsilateral primary cementless total hip replacement. With a presumptive diagnosis of inguinal hernia, the area was explored and the inguinal canal was found to contain several hundred milliliters of jet-black fluid. An intraoperative contrast study revealed communication with the hip joint. Radiographs performed after referral to our service demonstrated marked eccentricity of the femoral head (Fig. 3). At acetabular revision, the polyethylene liner was found to be fractured peripherally, and the prosthetic femoral head was articulating against the titanium acetabular shell as the source of dramatic metallosis, cyst formation, and dissection into the inguinal area.

The reports from all previous operations should be obtained and examined for comments regarding abnormalities encountered and implants used. The manufacturer, design, and size of each existing implant must be obtained.

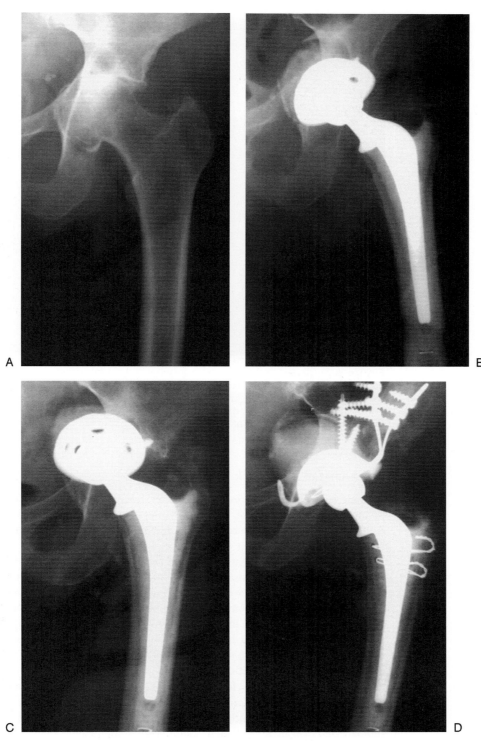

Figure 2. A 75-year-old woman with severe, steroid-dependent rheumatoid arthritis. **A:** Preoperative radiograph shows marked protrusio. **B:** Immediately postoperative radiograph after hybrid total hip replacement and morselized femoral head autograft of medial wall defect. **C:** Radiograph 6 weeks postoperatively shows loss of acetabular fixation. **D:** After revision with allografting, acetabular support cage, and cemented polyethylene cup.

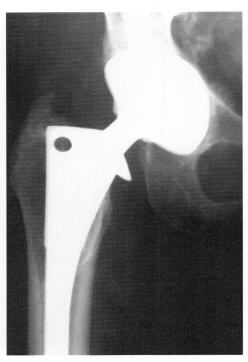

Figure 3. A 60-year-old woman underwent right primary total hip replacement $2\frac{1}{2}$ years earlier for osteoarthritis. **A:** Radiograph performed after exploration of the inguinal canal returned jet-black fluid. Eccentricity of the femoral head is present within the acetabular shell. **B:** After cup revision, bone grafting, and débridement of metallosis dissecting into the inguinal canal.

Assessment of Bone-Stock Damage

The goals of acetabular revision are to reestablish component fixation, restore the center of hip rotation to optimize joint mechanics and stability, and reconstitute bone stock. Achieving these goals requires an assessment of the bone available for component fixation and the location and extent of any defects.

For most patients, conventional AP pelvic and cross-table acetabular lateral radiographs (2,21) are sufficient for assessing bone-stock damage. Judet internal and external pelvic oblique views are useful for evaluating the integrity of the anterior and posterior columns. Special studies such as computerized tomographic scans with or without three-dimensional reconstructions and models can provide further anatomic detail. However, scatter and artifacts from existing hardware combined with the cost of these studies limits the utility of such techniques to selected cases (7,20). Full assessment of the existing anatomy and bone-stock damage ultimately is made at the operation.

A variety of systems for classifying bone-stock damage have been developed (2,3,4,6,7,13,14). From a practical standpoint, most such systems are acceptable for the individual surgeon, assuming they are used appropriately. However, adaptation of a standardized classification system facilitates communication regarding the specifics of an individual case and provides for the more rapid accumulation of data regarding recognized types of defects and the outcomes of their management with different techniques. As such, the American Academy of Orthopaedic Surgeons (AAOS) Committee on the Hip has developed a classification system for deficiencies of the acetabulum. This system (Table 1) is used in this chapter, and the reader is encouraged to consider its use in his or her practice.

The system includes two basic categories of deficiencies: segmental and cavitary. The first represents a loss in the supporting wall of the acetabulum and the second a volumetric loss of bone stock. The two types can and usually do occur in combination. Pelvic

Table 1. *American Academy of Orthopaedic Surgeons classification of acetabular deficiencies*

Type	Deficiency
I	Segmental deficiency
	Peripheral
	Superior
	Anterior
	Posterior
	Central (medial wall absent)
II	Cavitary deficiencies
	Peripheral
	Superior
	Anterior
	Posterior
	Central (medial wall intact)
III	Combined deficiencies
IV	Pelvic discontinuity
V	Arthrodesis

discontinuity indicates disruption of both the anterior and posterior columns with separation of the acetabular cavity into superior and inferior segments. Arthrodesis is not considered herein. Each category of deficit and the technical requirements for its revision are discussed in the section on surgical technique.

The status of several key landmarks is helpful in assessing bone-stock damage. Violation of Kohler's line or of the radiographic teardrop is indicative of severe damage to the medial wall and anterior column (13,14). Lysis of the ischium denotes posterior wall involvement (13). The normal head center is 14 to 15 mm above the interteardrop line (18,20). Cephalic migration more than 2 cm is indicative of a moderate or severe (major columnar) type III deficit (3,20).

Templating

The purpose of templating is to assist in selecting the design, size, and location of the revision components. It is also an appropriate time to review the status of the existing acetabular and femoral implants. The manufacturer and design of these implants should be known from operative records. This is essential when exchange of polyethylene with retention of the shell is contemplated. When a femoral component with a modular head is to be retained, the length of the existing head must be determined. The availability and size range of replacement heads must be established, because acetabular revision commonly alters the center of hip rotation, and leg length must then be adjusted. Identification of an existing cementless cup is especially important when the revision is performed for reasons other than loosening, e.g., when the component is well fixed. Fixation screws from different manufacturers may require specific screwdrivers for removal. Many companies also provide implant-specific tools for removal of polyethylene liners and extraction devices for the metallic shell. The presence of lugs or spikes is recorded, because one must navigate around them during division of the bone–implant interface. Dedicated instruments must be available for the removal of cementless components.

The templating procedure begins with establishment of a coordinate system on an AP pelvic radiograph (23). Except in the most severe cases of acetabular damage, the teardrops can be located and a horizontal line drawn across their inferior borders. Vertical lines that pass through the medial aspects of the teardrops are drawn perpendicular to the first line. When the teardrop on one or both sides is obliterated, the superior medial aspects of the obturator foramina (4) or the inferior borders of the ischia can be used for the horizontal axis and the center of the symphysis pubis for the vertical axis. The center of the normal hip is located with a concentric circle template.

The coordinates of this point are measured in millimeters and transcribed to the side to be revised. If the contralateral hip is abnormal, the method of Ranawat et al. (15) can be used to estimate the position of the hip center. The magnification is determined by means of measuring the femoral head, the true diameter of which is known, and templates of corresponding magnification are used.

Templates for porous hemispheric cups are used first. The inferior medial corner of the cup ideally, should fall just below the inferior border of the teardrop, and the most medial projection of the cup should approximate the lateral aspect of the teardrop. I prefer an opening angle (abduction) of 45 degrees (18). The cup should be adequately contained superiorly and laterally. These ideals are not always met in the revision setting; rather the surgeon optimizes the fit possible and compromises the position (usually more superior or medial than ideal) and orientation (generally more vertical). When the template size and position have been optimized, the center of the cup is marked through the hole on the template, and the contours of the cup traced onto the radiograph.

Acceptable deviations from ideal positioning vary with surgeon preference, bone quality, and patient factors such as activity level, life expectancy, and ability to tolerate a more lengthy and complicated reconstruction and rehabilitation, as might be involved with structural allografting. Also important is the compatibility of the new acetabular position with the existing femoral component if it is to be retained, particularly if it is of monoblock design. Certain departures from the ideal are unsatisfactory for use of a standard component without structural grafting. The limits used in my practice include an opening angle that exceeds 55 degrees, lack of superior lateral coverage, and cephalic translation of the hip center in excess of 2 cm. Even if the proposed construct appears acceptable at this point, it is important to assess the template on the true acetabular lateral view. A jumbo cup large enough to fill a superior lateral segmental defect on the AP radiograph may exceed the AP dimension of the acetabular cavity on the lateral view.

At this point, it is generally possible to classify the patient into one of three categories. In the first category are patients who can, with confidence, be treated with a standard porous hemispheric cup, perhaps with adjunctive screw fixation and possibly addition of morselized graft for small, contained defects. A second category includes patients who clearly cannot be treated in this way. Examples are patients with massive segmental and combined segmental/cavitary losses, which preclude adequate containment of a hemispheric cup without structural allografting or a special implant such as an oblong or custom cup or reinforcement ring or cage. Patients with pelvic discontinuity also fall into this category, although a standard porous hemispheric cup may be suitable after the anterior and posterior columns are reconstructed.

The third category falls between the first two. It includes patients who may or may not be amenable to the use of a standard cup without structural grafting or internal fixation techniques. Within this category are those patients for whom such a construct is possible but probably not optimal. An example is a young and active person in whom a hemispheric cup could be placed in the "high" position but for whom it is desirable to restore normal hip mechanics and augment bone stock for future reconstructions. Also included are patients for whom the acetabular reconstruction being contemplated may not be compatible with an existing femoral component the surgeon prefers to retain. Placement of a standard acetabular component in the high position may provide for adequate containment and fixation but lead to unacceptable shortening, impingement, and abductor insufficiency, even with trochanteric advancement. This is clearly a concern for monoblock femoral components but also may be a problem with modular designs. The longest neck length may still be inadequate, and most likely will have a skirt that further potentates impingement and dislocation with a high cup position. Such patients can sometimes be treated with a cup that will accept a lateralized polyethylene liner, which must be special-ordered in advance. A related situation is that in which the socket has always been in the high position, as in severe developmental dysplasia. Among such patients, the abductors, entire femur, and sciatic nerve are all shortened. If the acetabulum is reconstructed in the anatomic position, it may be impossible to reduce the hip without releasing the abductors and shortening the femur. Even then, there is risk for stretch injury to the sciatic nerve. The most important point is that when patients fall into the third or questionable category, the final determination as to the best method of reconstruction is made intraoperatively. As such, several different operative plans must be formulated during templating, and appropriate implants, graft materials, and instruments must be available to implement each.

SURGICAL TECHNIQUE

Exposure

Because the technical aspects of various exposures are presented in Chapter 12, discussion herein is limited to the selection of exposure for acetabular revision. Considerations include whether the stem also is to be revised and if so the exposure required for that procedure, the location and extent of acetabular bone-stock damage, and the techniques (bone grafting, plating) necessary to reconstruct those deficits, the status of the greater trochanter, leg-length discrepancy, and the anticipated need to shorten or lengthen the limb substantially, and finally the patient's body habitus. In my practice, four approaches have proved effective for acetabular revision with or without concomitant femoral revision—the posterior lateral approach, the standard transtrochanteric approach, sliding trochanteric osteotomy (5) and its variant the extended trochanteric osteotomy, and the extensile approach of Reinert et al. (16). General guidelines for selection of each are presented in Table 2. In the presence of osteolysis of the trochanter or its bed, trochanteric osteotomy should be undertaken only if absolutely necessary and then with great caution, because the risk for nonunion or fragmentation is increased. Isolated cup revision in the presence of a well-fixed, smooth, cemented stem can sometimes be facilitated with the tap in–tap out procedure, in which the stem is removed from its intact mantle during exposure and reinserted after cup revision (10). Whereas standard trochanteric osteotomy, sliding trochanteric osteotomy, and extended trochanteric osteotomy can provide equivalent acetabular exposure, the latter two are preferred when complex femoral component revision is needed.

Regardless of the operative approach, the entirety of the remaining acetabular rim and the origins of the ilium, the ischium, and the pubis must be fully exposed. My preference is to orient the new acetabular component according to these internal landmarks, as opposed to relying on an external aiming guide. In certain situations, access must be gained to the entire anterior or posterior column or even the pelvic aspect of the acetabulum.

Acetabular Reconstruction

After exposure is obtained, all existing implant materials, including cement, screws, and plates, are removed. If loosening has occurred a membrane of variable thickness covers

Table 2. *Selection of surgical approaches for acetabular revision*

Posterior lateral approach
  Isolated cup revision without structural grafting
  Polyethylene exchange
  Cup and simple stem revisions (unstable, short stem)
  Osteolysis of the greater trochanter
  No substantial change in leg length required
Standard trochanteric osteotomy
  Trochanteric nonunion
  Isolated cup revision necessitating structural grafting
  Segmental or combined segmental/cavitary defect necessitating structural grafting
  Obese or large patient
Sliding trochanteric osteotomy or extended trochanteric osteotomy
  Segmental or combined segmental/cavitary defect necessitating structural grafting
  Complex femoral revision or substantial leg lengthening needed
Extensile approach (16)
  Massive acetabular damage necessitating total allograft
  Pelvic dissociation necessitating anterior and posterior column plating
  Intrapelvic protrusion of components, especially if vascular compromise is involved

the acetabular floor and must be removed. This is undertaken cautiously when the medial wall is deficient, because the membrane may be adherent to vital intrapelvic structures, which can be avulsed.

At this point, true assessment of bone-stock damage and the requirements for reconstruction is made. The rim is examined for segmental defects. Cavitary defects within the acetabulum are documented. The integrity of the anterior and posterior columns is assessed. An overall impression is gained regarding the ability of the rim to provide mechanical support for the new cup and of the bed to provide for bone ingrowth.

In many situations, such as early loosening of either a cemented or cementless component, the acetabular cavity retains its hemispheric shape and remains centered in the anatomic position. Segmental (type I) defects are minimum and often symmetric. Cavitary defects are limited to cement anchoring holes or perhaps focal areas of osteolysis. The remaining rim is mechanically supportive, and the cavity retains sufficient bone that after reaming is capable of providing for bone ingrowth. The sphericity of the cup is confirmed with acetabular trials or sizers with multiple perforations through which contact with the acetabular cavity is assessed. In such cases, a standard porous hemispheric cup can be used. The socket is serially reamed with cheese grater–type reamers in 1-mm increments. With judicious reaming, most minor surface irregularities are removed until a uniform, bleeding, hemispheric surface and firm peripheral rim purchase are achieved. This yields a situation similar to that found in primary acetabular arthroplasty. I prefer to press fit the new cementless component by underreaming by 1 to 2 mm relative to the cup diameter. Others favor line-to-line preparation followed by adjunctive screw fixation and have shown excellent results in terms of fixation and no adverse effects from the use of screws (19).

Isolated segmental (type I) defects are usually minor, herein defined as involving less than 30% of the acetabular rim. More severe segmental defects are most often accompanied by cavitary damage to the underlying bone, that is, they comprise combined defects. In my practice, patients with minor defects of the posterior or superior rim are treated with a standard porous hemispheric cup as long as 70% to 75% of the rim is intact and supportive (18). Adjunctive screw fixation is frequently added. Isolated segmental defects of the anterior rim usually are ignored or packed with morselized allograft (12). Large segmental defects of the posterior or superior rim, as might be encountered in developmental dysplasia and fracture dislocation, are managed according to their extent and the principles outlined later for combined (type III) defects.

Contained cavitary (type II) defects left by cement, osteolysis, or component migration are filled with cancellous bone. I prefer fresh-frozen femoral head allograft. Although this can be prepared by hand with rongeurs or with a bone mill, I prefer to fix the head in a vise and ream it with acetabular reamers beginning with a 36-mm reamer and progressively increasing the size until all cancellous bone is evacuated. This produces uniform particles of optimum size for packing that are neatly retained within the reamer. The graft is tightly packed into the defects by hand or with a small tamp. I do not routinely use reverse reaming because it spreads the graft over the healthy areas of host bone and interposes dead bone between the porous cup surface and viable host bone. If reverse reaming is used, these surfaces should be wiped clean of graft before the socket is impacted. Isolated cavitary (type II) or combined segmental/cavitary (type III) defects of the medial wall are treated in a similar way as long as the remaining rim is intact and mechanically supportive (Fig. 4). Morselized graft is packed centrally, and a porous cup is fixed on the acetabular rim (6,12). The cup used must be sufficiently large to ensure rim support.

The AAOS classification of acetabular bone stock damage is qualitative (20). In recognition of this fact, several investigators have subdivided the more severe, that is, type III, defects on a quantitative basis to better define how various situations are best managed (3,4,6,7,9,13,14,20). Although terms and treatment philosophies differ, there is general agreement regarding the recognized patterns of type III defects. I divide type III defects into mild, moderate, and severe on the basis of the extent of acetabular damage. Mild

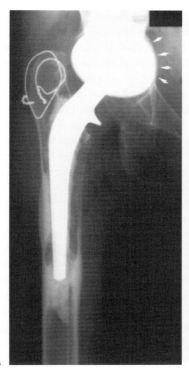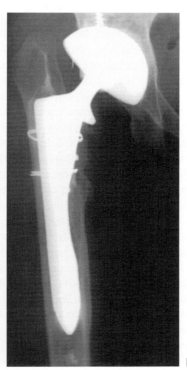

A   B

Figure 4. A 57-year-old woman with an original diagnosis of severe developmental dysplasia. She underwent right primary cemented total hip replacement at the age of 41 years. The acetabular component loosened and was revised to a cement-less component 7 years later. She sought treatment at 53 years of age with severe groin and buttock pain. **A:** Prerevision antero-posterior radiograph demonstrates acetabular loosening and a severe combined cavitary and segmental defect of the medial wall. There was dramatic osteolysis around the cemented femoral component. **B:** Four years after revision of both components and massive morselized allograft of the central wall and femur with insertion of a jumbo cup and extensively porous coated stem. Reconstitution of the medial wall is shown.

defects are defined as those involving less than 25% of the acetabulum; moderate defects, 25% to 50%; and severe defects, more than 50%. This division has practical importance in that each category warrants distinctly different treatment. Mild type III defects have already been discussed; management with a porous hemispheric cup without support graft works well as long as 70% to 75% of the porous surface of the acetabular component is in contact with viable host bone (18).

Management of moderate and severe defects presents greater challenges, choices, and controversies. Defects of more than 25% most commonly involve the posterior or superior rims or both in combination with the subjacent acetabular cavity. The cavitary defect may exceed the segmental defect with excavation of the superior or posterior bone beneath a partially intact, overhanging rim. A key feature of moderate defects is that the posterior column remains intact and supportive. Whether the anterior column is intact does not affect reconstruction. Some moderate segmental or combined defects can be reduced in size by centralizing the cup, as in instances of developmental dysplasia, by means of deliberately reaming more cephalad and placing the cup slightly high or by means of concentric reaming and expansion of the socket and the use of a larger cup (12).

I manage most moderate type III defects with cementless cups in one of two ways—bulk allografting (3,4,6,7,9,13,14), or high cup placement (8,18). Each technique has its advocates and critics. Acetabular revision ideally returns the hip center to its anatomic position to restore leg length, proper hip mechanics, and stability against dislocation; restores bone stock should future reconstruction be needed; and provides reliable long-term fixation. Most moderate type III defects involve cephalad translation of the hip center. Returning the hip center to anatomic position can be accomplished with a solid allograft, which also restores bone stock. Unfortunately, in some series this technique has been associated with late graft collapse and cup migration (8). Other authors (13,14) report much lower incidences of graft failure and contend that when failure does occur, the remaining bone graft is viable and sufficient for fixation of another cup without further grafting. Advocates of a high hip center (8,18) report excellent fixation with cementless cups and contend that leg length and hip mechanics can be compensated for by use of a long neck length or calcar replacement femoral prosthesis. Proponents of allografting concede that within certain limits, high hip placement is more reliable and provides acceptable hip mechanics. Advocates of a high hip center concede that some severe defects can only be managed with grafting.

My recommendations are as follows. For moderate type III defects in which a cup can be adequately contained no higher than 2 cm above the anatomic position, a cementless cup and high hip center are used. Above this level, the bone stock available for containment and fixation dwindles rapidly. Although fixation can be achieved with a small or miniature cup, I avoid this because it necessitates use of a small head and long neck length, usually requiring a skirt. This reduces the ratio of head-to-neck diameters, which when combined with a high hip center increases the likelihood of impingement and dislocation. When this technique is used, 70% to 75% of the porous surface of the cup should be contained by the remaining host bone (18). Adjunctive screw fixation is recommended. When there is a compelling reason to leave a monoblock (fixed head) femoral component *in situ* and the head center will be moved cephalad, a cup that will accommodate a lateralized polyethylene liner should be considered, and the trochanter may have to be advanced. Patients must be counseled that their leg may be shorter after the operation.

When the foregoing technique would result in a head center greater than 2 cm above anatomic position, I recommend use of solid allograft. Such defects correspond closely with the type 2 defects described by Paprosky et al. (13,14) and the minor column defects described by Gross, Garbuz, and Morsi et al. (3,4,6,7,9) managed with so-called bulk allografts and shelf allografts, respectively. The details of these techniques are presented in Chapter 18. The important principle of such grafts, emphasized by both groups mentioned, is that although the graft may augment component fixation, host bone remains the principal means of support. I prefer use of fresh-frozen distal femoral allograft fixed with large screws and washers (Fig. 5), although proximal tibia and portions of whole acetabular grafts also have been recommended. Large grafts are supplemented with plate fixation. Another critical point is that after reaming of the composite acetabulum, at least 50% of the porous surface of the revision cup must be in contact with viable, bleeding, host bone. If not, a cemented cup should be used (6).

Using the above criteria, there are cases that on preoperative templating fall into a gray zone and are amenable to treatment with either of the aforementioned techniques. In such cases, various other patient factors must be considered, including age, weight, demand level, life expectancy, and ability to comply with the prolonged period of protected weight bearing required after allograft reconstruction. It is also important to remember that for certain patients, return of the head center to the anatomic position may cause serious technical difficulties in terms of relocating the femoral component and avoiding neurovascular stretch injury.

On rare occasions an oblong porous coated component is used. These have the theoretic advantage of providing bone ingrowth fixation to host bone and restoring the hip center without reliance on bone graft. A disadvantage is that bone stock is not restored. Also, it remains to be shown that stable biologic fixation can be obtained as reliably as for conventional porous hemispheric cups. Fixation failure of these devices has been attributed to the lack of instruments available when they were first introduced and to the limited porous coating on some designs, particularly custom-made implants (20). They are

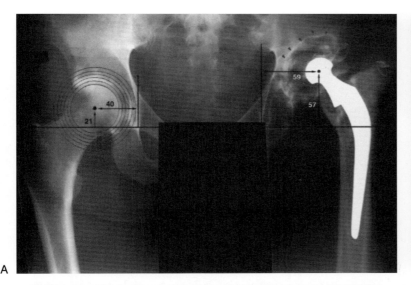

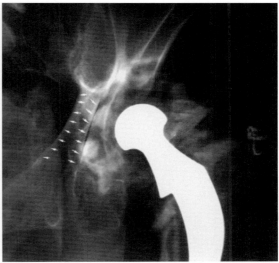

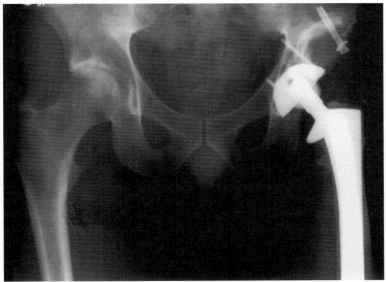

Figure 5. A 40-year-old man sustained a posterior fracture-dislocation at 21 years of age. A cemented Charnley total hip replacement was performed 1 year later. Prerevision radiographs showed aseptic loosening of both components and a moderate type III deficit with posterior and superior cavitary and segmental defects. **A:** Anteroposterior pelvic radiograph. The hip center is translated 36 mm cephalad and 19 mm laterally. **B:** Internal oblique Judet view shows an intact anterior column and deficient posterior rim. **C:** Five years after revision with a distal femoral allograft and cementless cup. The graft has healed and the cup appears stable. The hip center now is 7 mm cephalad and 12 mm medial to that of the right hip.

of particular value to patients averse to the use of allograft bone (Fig. 6). When using an oblong cup, it is important to use a component large enough to to be fixed on the cortical rim of the remaining ilium. In my experience, the likelihood of subsidence and loosening is far greater if the superior aspect of the cup falls entirely inside a combined segmental/cavitary defect.

Severe type III defects involve more than 50% of the acetabulum. These defects correlate with the major columnar defects described by Gross, Garbuz, and Morsi et al. (3,4,6,7,9) and with the type 3 defects described by Paprosky et al. (13,14). This degree of damage has important mechanical and biologic consequences. Mechanically, the anterior and posterior columns are no longer supportive. The bone graft necessary to reconstruct such defects is truly structural in that it must bear most of the load transmitted across the hip joint. Moreover, there is now clinical and radiographic evidence that such grafts fare better if supplemented with a roof-reinforcement ring or cage (3). The biologic consequences are that after reconstruction, the composite acetabular bed comprises less than 50% host bone, and the use of a cementless acetabular component is contraindicated. A cemented polyethylene socket must be used. This also is true if a roof-reinforcement cage is used.

Pelvic discontinuity occurs when there is disruption of both the anterior and posterior columns. In the classic form, there is a transverse fracture of the acetabular cavity and

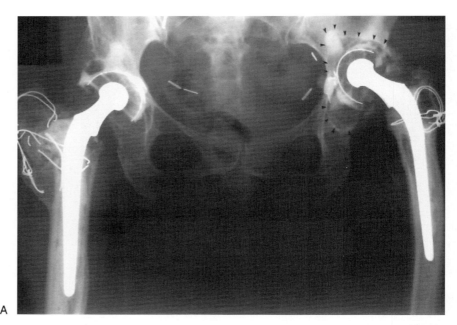

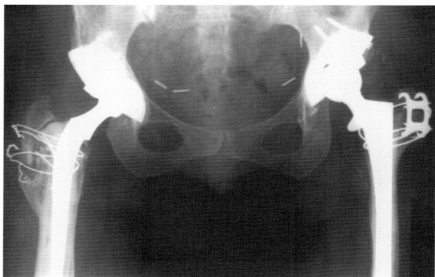

Figure 6. A 62-year-old woman with an original diagnosis of severe bilateral developmental dysplasia had undergone pelvic and femoral osteotomy of both hips as a child and bilateral cemented total hip replacement at 43 years of age. She sought treatment because of left hip pain. **A:** Anteroposterior pelvic radiograph shows superior, medial, and posterior combined cavitary and segmental (type III) defects on the left. The femoral component is fractured and there is apex lateral bowing of the femur. The patient was adverse to the use of an allograft. The right socket also appears loose. **B:** On the left she underwent acetabular revision with an oblong cup, corrective femoral osteotomy, and femoral revision with a long, extensively porous coated stem. On the right she underwent only acetabular revision. Six and four years after left and right revision, respectively, she has no symptoms, and both acetabular components appear stable.

medial wall with separation of the acetabulum into superior and inferior portions. In practice, there may be little visible separation on preoperative radiographs, and the diagnosis requires critical inspection of the internal and external oblique Judet views. The first step in reconstruction is internal fixation with anterior and posterior pelvic reconstruction plates. Solid interfragmentary compression of the posterior column is

Table 3. *Management of acetabular deficits*

Defect	Management
Type 1 (segmental)	
Minor (>70% of rim intact)	Porous hemispheric cup
Major (<70% of rim intact)	Manage as a type III defect (shelf allograft or high hip center)
Type II (cavitary)	
Cement anchoring holes or lytic defects	Morselized allograft and porous hemispheric cup
Protrusio	Morselized allograft and porous hemispheric cup
Type III (combined)	
Minor (<25% of acetabulum involved)	Porous hemispheric cup with or without screws Morselized graft of cavitary defects
Moderate (25%–50% of acetabulum involved)	
Hip center <2 cm above normal	Porous hemispheric cup, high hip center Morselized graft of cavitary defects
Hip center >2 cm above normal	Porous hemispheric cup Bulk allograft Morselized graft of cavitary defects or Oblong porous cup with screw fixation
Severe (>50% of acetabulum involved)	Cemented polyethylene cup Structural allograft Roof ring or cage
Type IV (pelvic discontinuity)	Anterior and posterior column plating Address remaining defects as above

critical to success. After restoration of pelvic continuity, the acetabular cavity may be remarkably normal in appearance, and in such cases a cementless cup is used. Although adjunctive screw fixation may be used, I prefer column plates as the primary internal fixation device. In other cases, substantial bony deficits remain after internal fixation. These must be classified intraoperatively and treated accordingly. When both pelvic discontinuity and a substantial acetabular defect are present, use of a ring or cage, such as the Burch-Schneider, combined with a bone graft and a cemented socket may be indicated. My recommendations for acetabular revision are summarized in Table 3.

POSTOPERATIVE CARE

The nature of the acetabular revision is but one factor to be considered in the postoperative care of these patients. The following guidelines are based on the assumption that the femoral component has not been revised and that the patient is otherwise healthy. For type I and most type II defects managed with porous hemispheric cups without shelf allografts, I use a standard protocol for routine primary cementless or hybrid total hip replacement. This includes an initial 6-week period of touch-down weight bearing with crutches or a walker followed by 4 to 6 weeks with a single crutch, and then use of a cane for as long as the patient feels is necessary for comfort and safety. For shelf allografts (moderate type III defects) and severe protrusio, touch-down weight bearing is continued for 3 months or until graft union is visible on radiographs. Progression to full weight bearing takes place between 3 and 6 months postoperatively (3,14). For severe type III reconstructions in which a structural allograft has been used, and most cases of pelvic discontinuity, touch-down weight bearing is continued for 6 months. In addition, I prefer that the patient use a hip abduction orthosis for the first 3 postoperative months.

RESULTS

As might be expected, the reported results of acetabular revision with cementless components vary with the degree of bone stock present, and this is not always clearly defined in published results. The results in series in which most defects were type I or type II and were managed with standard cementless components have been extremely favorable. Padgett et al. (12) and Silverton et al. (19) reported on 138 such consecutive cases 3 to 6 years and 7 to 11 years postoperatively. Although many operations included use of morselized allograft, only two involved bulk allografts. In no case did any cup require revision for aseptic loosening at either period of follow-up study.

The results of more severe defects are more difficult to decipher, depending on the cases included and the method of treatment. Morsi et al. (9) reported results of management of a series of 29 type II defects with shelf allografts with a minimum follow-up period of 5 years. Eighty-six percent of operations were considered successful, both clinically and radiographically, and only three cups (10.3%) loosened. In two cases, the graft survived and facilitated successful repeat revision. However, 12 of the cups were cemented, and the fixation mode of the failed cups was not specified. The authors emphasized the predictability of this technique provided that at least 50% of the cup is supported by host bone. Citing a 47% failure rate of bulk allografts (50% among revision operations) at a minimum follow-up period of 8 years, Kwong et al. (8) and Schutzer and Harris (18) condemned this practice and recommended use of a porous cup and high hip center. At relatively short follow-up periods (2 to 5 years), the latter group reported no re-revisions for aseptic loosening among 49 patients treated in this manner.

Paprosky et al. (13,14) reported a 19% failure rate of major bulk allografts and cementless cups at mean follow-up period of 5.7 years. Their only failures were in cases in which the graft supported more than 50% of the cup (severe type III defects). Similarly, Garbuz et al. (4) reported a 24% failure rate at a minimum follow-up period of 5 years for 33 cases in which graft supported more than 50% of the cup, although only seven of the components used were cementless. In the same study they reported a 100% success rate when the same defects were treated with a roof support ring and cemented cup.

SUMMARY

Acetabular revision encompasses a broad range of situations, the elements of which include bone-stock damage, the primary disease process, the status of the femoral component, and patient factors, including age, health, demand level, and life expectancy. The goals are to reestablish stable implant fixation, to optimize the location of the hip center, and to replace bone stock. These goals must be prioritized on a case-by-case basis. The keys to successful revision are thorough knowledge of the various patterns of bone-stock damage and the ability to recognize them, careful preoperative planning, familiarity with various methods of reconstruction, and meticulous surgical technique. Porous hemispheric acetabular components are extremely versatile and can be used successfully to manage most failed sockets. In certain circumstances they must be supplemented with solid or morselized graft. When properly used, cementless acetabular revision can be expected to yield a high rate of success.

REFERENCES

1. Berry DJ, Müller ME. Revision arthroplasty using an anti-protrusion cage for massive acetabular bone deficiency. *J Bone Joint Surg Br* 1992;74:711–715.
2. D'Antonio JA, Capello WN, Borden LS, Bargar WL, Bierbaum BF, Boettcher WG, Steinberg ME. Classification and management of acetabular abnormalities in total hip arthroplasty. *Clin Orthop* 1989;243: 126–137.
3. Garbuz D, Morsi E, Gross AE. Revision of the acetabular component of a total hip arthroplasty with a massive structural allograft. *J Bone Joint Surg Am* 1996;78:693–697.
4. Garbuz D, Morsi E, Mohamed N, Gross AE. Classification and reconstruction in revision acetabular arthroplasty with bone stock deficiency. *Clin Orthop* 1996;323:98–107.
5. Glassman AH, Engh CA, Bobyn JD. A technique of extensile exposure for total hip arthroplasty. *J Arthroplasty* 1987;2:11–21.
6. Gross AE, Allan G, Catre M, Garbuz DS, Stockley I. Bone grafts in hip replacement surgery: the pelvic side. *Orthop Clin North Am* 1993;24:679–695.
7. Gross AE, Garbuz D, Morsi ES. Acetabular allografts for restoration of bone stock in revision arthroplasty of the hip. *Instr Course Lect* 1995;45:135–142.

8. Kwong LM, Jasty M, Harris WH. High failure rate of bulk femoral head allografts in total hip acetabular reconstructions at 10 years. *J Arthroplasty* 1993;8:341–346.
9. Morsi E, Garbuz D, Gross AE. Revision total hip arthroplasty with shelf bulk allografts: a long-term follow-up study. *J Arthroplasty* 1996;11:86–90.
10. Nabors ED, Liebelt R, Mattingly DA, Bierbaum BE. Removal and reinsertion of cemented femoral components during acetabular revision. *J Arthroplasty* 1996;11:146–152.
11. Nivbrant B, Karrholm J, Onsten I, Carlsson A, Snorrason F. Migration of porous press-fit cups in hip revision arthroplasty: a radiostereometric 2-year follow-up study of 60 hips. *J Arthroplasty* 1996;11:390–396.
12. Padgett DE, Kull L, Rosenberg A, Sumner DR, Galante JO. Revision of the acetabular component without cement after total hip arthroplasty: three to six year follow-up. *J Bone Joint Surg Am* 1993;75:663–673.
13. Paprosky WG, Magnus RE. Principles of bone grafting in revision total hip arthroplasty: acetabular technique. *Clin Orthop* 1994;298:147–155.
14. Paprosky WG, Perona PG, Lawrence JM. Acetabular defect classification and surgical reconstruction in revision arthroplasty. *J Arthroplasty* 1994;9:33–44.
15. Ranawat CS, Dorr LD, Inglis AE. Total hip arthroplasty in protrusio acetabulae of rheumatoid arthritis. *J Bone Joint Surg Am* 1980;62:1059–1064.
16. Reinert CM, Bosse MI, Poka A, Schacherer T, Brumback RJ, Burgess AR. A modified extensile exposure for the treatment of complex or malunited acetabular fractures. *J Bone Joint Surg Am* 1988;70:329–337.
17. Rosson J, Schatzker J. The use of reinforcement rings to reconstitute deficient acetabulae. *J Bone Joint Surg Br* 1992;74:716–720.
18. Schutzer SF, Harris WH. High placement of porous-coated acetabular components in complex total hip arthroplasty. *J Arthroplasty* 1994;9:359–367.
19. Silverton CD, Rosenberg AG, Sheinkop MB, Kull LR, Galante JO. Revision of the acetabular component without cement after total hip arthroplasty: a follow-up note regarding results at seven to eleven years. *J Bone Joint Surg Am* 1996;78:1366–1370.
20. Sutherland CJ. Treatment of type III acetabular deficiencies in revision total hip arthroplasty without structural bone-graft. *J Arthroplasty* 1996;11:91–98.
21. Sutherland CJ. Radiographic evaluation of acetabular bone stock in failed total hip arthroplasty. *J Arthroplasty* 1988;3:73–79.
22. Weber KL, Callaghan JJ, Goetz DD, Johnston RC. Revision of a failed cemented total hip prosthesis with insertion of an acetabular component without cement and a femoral component with cement. *J Bone Joint Surg Am* 1996;78:982–994.
23. Yoder SA, Brand RA, Pedersen DR, O'Gorman TW. Total hip acetabular component position affects component loosening rates. *Clin Orthop* 1988;228:79–87.

Revision Total Hip Arthroplasty,
edited by Marvin E. Steinberg and Jonathan P. Garino,
Lippincott Williams & Wilkins, Philadelphia © 1999.

22

Femoral Revision: Cemented

Craig G. Mohler and Dennis K. Collis

Cemented revision on the femoral side is a complex procedure. Many surgeons have stopped using cement when revising the femoral component because of their own results and negative reports in the literature (1,2,16,18,19,25,27). However, excellent results can be obtained if proper indications and appropriate surgical techniques are used (3,9,11,13,15,20,22,31).

BACKGROUND

Many techniques are used for revision of the femoral component. All involve the basic techniques of either cemented or uncemented revision. Uncemented revision has two basic techniques—fully porous coated and partially porous coated femoral components. Both cemented and uncemented revisions may involve some form of associated bone grafting, either intramedullary or extracortical, or may depend only on the patient's existing bone stock. This chapter focuses on the latter situation. Structural and morselized allografting types of cemented revision are discussed elsewhere.

INDICATIONS AND PATIENT SELECTION

The two basic primary indications for revision hip surgery are intolerable pain and progressive bone loss. Femoral components can be revised with cement for most patients who have a loose femoral component. If bone stock loss is massive, structural allografting has to be accomplished; those indications are discussed in Chapter 18. If intramedullary endosteal bone loss is substantial, morselized internal grafting may be indicated as

---

C. G. Mohler and D. K. Collis: Department of Orthopaedics, University of Oregon, Portland, and Sacred Heart Medical Center, Eugene, Oregon 97401.

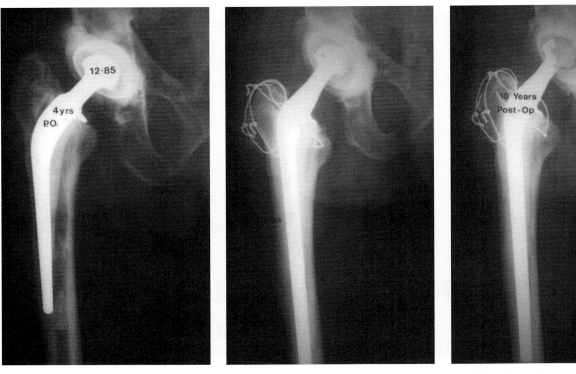

A,B   C

Figure 1. Images of a 68-year-old man 4 years postoperatively with a loose femoral prosthesis and substantial bone loss. **A:** Before revision. **B:** After revision. **C:** Ten years after revision.

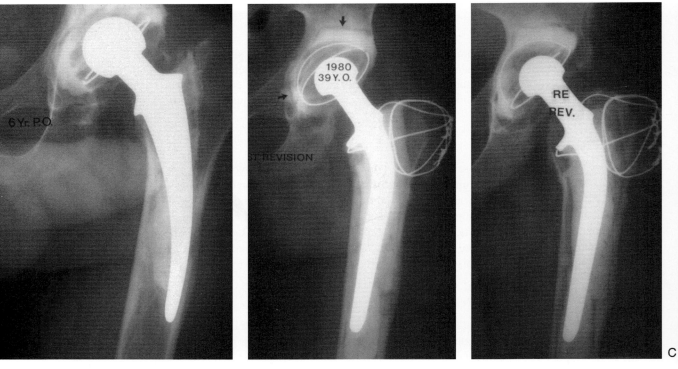

A,B   C

Figure 2. Images of a 38-year-old man who needed revision of a loose, subsided femoral component that had been implanted 6 years earlier. Because of the wide femoral canal, uncemented revision would have been difficult. **A:** Before revision, there is a wide femoral canal and thin femoral cortical bone. **B:** After revision with cement. **C:** Sixteen years postoperatively the patient has pain and needs another revision, but the femoral cortex is no less than at the time of the first revision (**A**) (This revision was done with impaction grafting).

discussed in Chapter 19. A patient older than 60 years of age with adequate residual bone stock is the ideal candidate for revision with a cemented stem with no associated bone grafting. If it is believed that the previous components and cement can be removed and still leave reasonable bone stock for cement–surface interdigitation, this clearly is the method of choice.

The older the patient, the more likely it is that a greater amount of bone loss may be accepted. That is, no grafting and purely standard cementing techniques are used (Fig. 1). A guideline is that if a patient is younger than 60 years, has a normal life expectancy, and has substantial bone loss, plans must be made for bone grafting, because the expectation for long-term successful revision diminish for younger patients. For patients younger than 50 years, the surgeon might best plan to use uncemented devices if they appear to be applicable and bone graft as necessary. However, there are situations in which patients in their forties and fifties are clearly candidates for a cemented stem (Fig. 2). These situations are when remaining bone stock allows adequate cement technique and yet the bone stock is deficient or deformed enough that standard uncemented techniques are not likely to produce a good result.

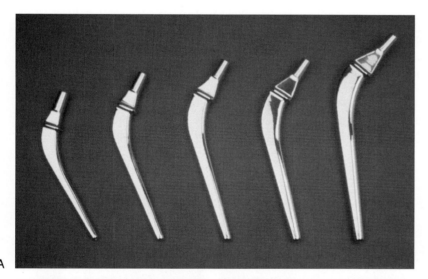

A

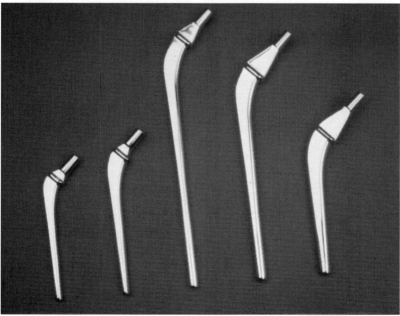

B

Figure 3. A versatile hip system applicable to all situations in which cement is used on the femoral side. (Hermitage System, Zimmer, Warsaw, Indiana) **A:** Proportional stem and neck lengths for different-sized femurs in primary and revision total hip arthroplasty. Seven different modular heads are available that adjust in length. **B:** Five specialty stems for revision THR are, from left to right, *(1)* Developmentally Dysplastic Hip stem for small femurs, *(2)* straight stem for valgus femurs, *(3)* extra long stem for diaphyseal fracture treatment, *(4)* long neck, long stem, *(5)* long neck, large stem.

PREOPERATIVE PLANNING

As is necessary with any revision operation, careful preoperative planning is imperative. First the patient must be carefully examined to rule out infection (1,32). The bony anatomy has to be assessed with radiographs, which expose the entire existing component and surrounding bone in two planes (4,6). If bone lysis is apparent, oblique radiographs sometimes are helpful. Computed tomographic scans are of occasional benefit, although radiographic scatter caused by the implant may markedly diminish the value of these studies. Appropriate laboratory assessment, including complete blood cell count, erythrocyte sedimentation rate, C-reactive protein, and possibly hip aspiration to rule out infection, is warranted. The surgeon must have a complete cemented system to replace the absent bone. Usually a versatile system that has multiple stem and neck lengths and modular heads is adequate (Fig. 3). We prefer the Heritage system prosthesis (Zimmer, Warsaw, Ind.). There is occasional need for a calcar or proximal femoral replacement prosthesis (Fig. 4) (8), but most standard revision cemented systems allow adequate replacement of proximal femoral bone loss. Canal dimensions of the intramedullary area have to be templated so that an adequate-sized prosthesis is available for the bone loss. Prostheses of adequate stem length must be available so that at least the distal part of the stem can be cemented into bone of adequate quality (32). A stem should be made of one of the superalloys such as forged cobalt chrome or titanium with a high fatigue strength. Our strong preference is that the stem have a smooth surface. The prosthesis should have no sharp corners. Although the stem may have to be longer than primary cemented stems, lengths of more than 200 mm are used only in unusual circumstances, even if the upper half of the femur does have substantial bone deficiency (see Fig. 4). Adequate blood must be available. Usually in revisions, homologous blood should be available in addition to any autologous blood that the patient is able to donate. The basic preoperative planning outlined in Chapter 11 is clearly valuable in cemented total hip revision.

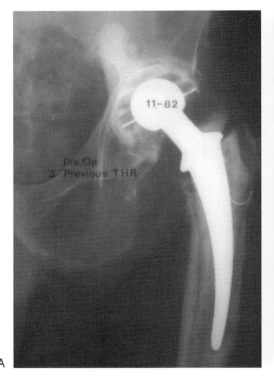
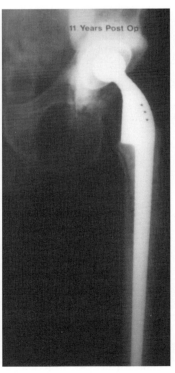

Figure 4. Images of a 56-year-old man with ten previous hip operations and marked bone loss (type III). **A:** Before third revision total hip arthroplasty with deficient proximal femur. **B:** Proximal femoral replacement.

SPECIFIC SURGICAL TECHNIQUES

Approach

When the surgeon is planning to cement a femoral component in a revision operation, it is important that the appropriate surgical approach be anticipated. We recommend that a transtrochanteric approach be used in most instances. This almost always allows access to the intramedullary canal for prosthesis and cement removal and careful cementing of the new prosthetic device. The recently popularized extended trochanteric approach should be avoided if possible; that approach makes it much more difficult to accomplish good cementing technique for the new prosthesis. Efforts to approach the femur either anteriorly or posteriorly with only soft-tissue dissection while avoiding trochanteric osteotomy in most instances do not offer adequate exposure.

Technique

Preoperative insertion of a Foley catheter under sterile conditions is useful to measure intraoperative urine output and should be strongly recommended for expected long operations. After induction of anesthesia, the procedure begins with positioning of the patient. The patient is placed in a lateral decubitus position with a vacuum-pack bean bag or appropriate pelvic positioners to secure the torso. The down leg must be carefully padded to prevent contralateral limb problems such as compartment syndrome, which has been reported in hip revision surgery. After a povidone-iodine (Betadine) scrub of the entire lower extremity from midabdomen to the knee, the skin is cleaned with alcohol, which defats the skin and enhances adherence of iodoform-impregnated drapes. The unprepared leg and foot are wrapped in sterile towels and covered with impervious stockinette.

Before the incision is made, the location of previous incisions should be verified. Although not as critical as in revision knee surgery, previous incisions should be used if properly located, rather than making a narrow skin bridge between the old and the new incision, which may invite skin necrosis. For most revision hip operations, a long, direct, lateral skin incision is performed.

The greater trochanter is exposed and osteotomized with a curved gouge just below the vastus lateralis ridge (12). Care is taken to pass this gouge in a superior medial direction and then reflect the trochanter proximally. This often requires release of portions of the pseudocapsule to allow the trochanter to be retracted proximally. The trochanter is then secured proximally to the hip capsule with an abductor retractor, which has holes that allow fixation with two smooth Steinman pins in the ilium. Another pin is placed in the proximal femur just distal to the trochanteric osteotomy. With the proximal and distal pins parallel to each other, a measurement is made for future leg-length determination. It is very important to excise an adequate amount of hip capsule and surrounding soft tissue. Once this is accomplished the hip can be easily dislocated and the femoral component and any surrounding cement can be removed, usually, in our experience, with hand tools. The techniques for removal of the prosthesis are described in Chapter 13. Care must be taken to avoid perforation of the femoral canal so that good pressurization can be accomplished when the prosthetic component is being cemented. Final preparation is carefully done with a high-speed burr to roughen possibly sclerotic, smooth cortical bone. This preparation of the canal for recementing is greatly facilitated with a lighted canal irrigator, which simultaneously illuminates and irrigates the canal. If no infection is present and portions of previous cement seem well interdigitated, these certainly can be left, but usually all cement is extracted.

On occasion, a solid distal cement plug need not be removed and can be used for plugging the canal for reinsertion of the new prosthetic device. Once the canal is ready for recementing, trial reductions should be accomplished. If the bone stock has been perforated, it is usually best to select a stem of adequate length to bypass the defect by at least two cortical diameters (Fig. 5). If an extensive perforation of the cortex exists, cortical onlay grafting may be used. We prefer temporarily to occlude moderate

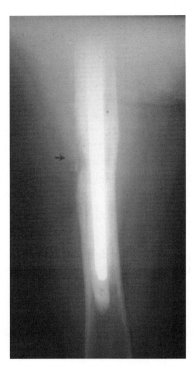

Figure 5. Revision bypasses femoral defects by several centimeters.

perforations during cementing with the fingers of the surgical assistant. This allows removal of any extruded cement, which could possibly interfere with contact between cortical graft and the cortex of the femur. Some surgeons have tried to occlude perforations with removable rubber dams and tight-fitting hose-type clamps, but we have not used these devices. Trial reductions are accomplished so the appropriate head and neck lengths can be selected. The trial position of the prosthesis must be carefully marked on the femoral neck region so that the level of the new prosthesis is well delineated. In addition to leg length, stability must be verified so that with appropriate leg length determined, the surgeon is sure that the head is stable in the acetabulum throughout at least 90 degrees of flexion, some adduction and internal rotation, and 40 or 50 degrees of external rotation. At this time, anteversion and retroversion must be identified and the position of the prosthesis clearly determined so that during cementing of the prosthesis this position is achieved. With trochanteric osteotomy, it is quite simple to allow the femur to be in a position parallel to the floor and the tibia in a position perpendicular to the floor. This allows determination of appropriate anteversion-retroversion.

After removal of the trial prosthesis, the proximal femur is again exposed. Pulsatile lavage is carried out with a canal irrigator and brush to clean vigorously the cancellous surfaces. The canal then is plugged distally (10). This can often be done with a standard polyethylene cement restrictor, which should be placed approximately 2 cm distal to the tip of the new prosthesis. If the stem to be cemented passes beyond the diaphysis and the polyethylene restrictor cannot be secured, a separate batch of cement may be mixed to form an actual cement plug distal to the tip of the stem (28). After this has been appropriately placed, a long, thin sponge soaked in 1:100,000 epinephrine solution is packed into the canal while cement mixing begins. One must be prepared to have plenty of cement available, particularly if stems of 200 mm or more in length are going to be used. Up to four packs and on occasion five packs of cement must be available. A powdered antibiotic (1.2 g tobramycin) can be added to every 80 grams of cement mixed if an antibiotic is desired. For routine revisions in which little chance of infection exists, no antibiotics have to be mixed with the cement. Some form of porosity reduction of the cement should be used, either a vacuum mixture or centrifugation (5).

After complete preparation of the femoral canal, the trochanteric wires are placed. Two are placed through the lesser trochanter and brought circumferentially around the femur. The two others are placed in a vertical direction through drill holes through the lateral aspect of the femur, at least 1 to 2 cm distal to the osteotomy cut.

An important technique of cement insertion is that the cement be allowed to reach a fairly doughy stage before insertion into the canal. This prevents blood from intermixing with a liquid and allows better cement to be interdigitated into the interstices of the bone. Just before insertion of the cement, the epinephrine sponges are removed, suction is used carefully to remove any distal fluid that has collected, and a dry sponge is used further to dry the canal.

Cement insertion is performed in a retrograde direction using a long-tipped introducer and cement gun. Pressurization is performed with a proximal femoral pressurizer (24). The cement is inserted into the canal 5 to 6 minutes after mixing the monomer with the polymer, when it no longer sticks to the surgeon's gloves. The prosthesis is then placed in the proximal cement bed 6 to 7 minutes after mixing and gradually and progressively inserted more fully over a 2-minute period. This allows progressive injection of the cement into the bony trabeculae. It is essential that cementing be completed before the cement becomes so viscid as to prevent complete insertion of the prosthesis. It is inserted to the appropriate depth. Care is taken to replicate the stem position selected during trial reduction. Excess cement is cleaned from around the proximal femur while the stem is held in place by the surgeon. Strict attention must be paid at this time to avoid any stem movement while the cement cures. After total cement curing, the chrome cobalt femoral head selected may be inserted, or a second trial reduction may be performed with a variety of trial heads to determine final leg length. The actual prosthetic modular head then is impacted onto the trunnion.

After cementing of the prosthesis, the leg is abducted and placed on a Mayo stand, and the trochanter is reattached with the four wires previously placed (30). The two proximal ends of the vertical wires are passed up over the greater trochanter and with a large-bore needle are passed through the tendinous portion of the abductor insertion. The two circumferential wires are placed through the anterior aspect of the trochanter and abductor muscle mass approximately 1 cm apart. The trochanter is grasped with a bone clamp and reduced to its trochanteric bed. The wires are tightened sequentially, the vertical wires being tightened first with a wire tightener and partially twisted. After all four wires are initially tightened, the surgeon returns to the first wire to be sure that they are snug before final twisting and cutting of the wires. The wires then are bent and impacted into the side of the greater trochanter to diminish their prominence. At this point, the vastus lateralis fascia should be repaired over the trochanteric wires to further cover them. The wound is closed in the standard manner with interrupted sutures in the fascia lata. Thin wires are placed through the superficial surface of the tensor fascia lata and are brought outside the subcutaneous tissue to allow application of a compression bolster to the lateral aspect of the hip. The subcutaneous tissue and skin are closed in the standard manner.

POSTOPERATIVE CARE

The patient is taken to the recovery room and placed in balanced suspension, which allows the patient to move but have the hip protected from excessive motion. The balanced suspension is removed on the first postoperative day, and gait training is begun with weight bearing restricted to 25% to 30% with use of a walker or crutches. The drains are removed on the first postoperative day, and the bolster dressing is changed on the second or third postoperative day. If trochanteric repair is not as secure as desired or soft-tissue deficiency has been found during the operation, the patient can be placed in a brace or single-hip spica cast before discharge. This is not usually necessary. The patient also can be treated with an abduction brace. Throughout the postoperative stay some form of anticoagulation is used. Patients use crutches to walk with 25% to 50% weight bearing for the first 6 weeks after the operation. The patient then uses a cane for another 6 to 8 weeks. Radiographs are taken 6 weeks, 3 months, 6 months, one year, and then every two years, thereafter.

PREVENTION AND MANAGEMENT OF COMPLICATIONS

The four most common complications after revision total hip replacement are dislocation, infection, neurovascular injury, and femoral fracture.

Dislocation

Dislocations have been reported to occur among as many as 20% of patients after revision total hip replacement (35). Early dislocation is treated by means of expedient reduction, usually in the operating room, and application of external immobilization and a spica cast or commercially available brace for 6 weeks. Trochanteric displacement nonunion may lead to postoperative dislocation and, if so, should be rectified by appropriate repair. Component malposition, particularly acetabular retroversion, may lead to early dislocation after the operation and may necessitate re-revision if repeated dislocations occur.

Infection

The risk for sepsis after revision total hip arthroplasty has been reported to be at least double that encountered in primary total hip replacement (23,32). Draining wound hematomas must be aggressively managed by means of débridement in the operating room to prevent infection. Early deep sepsis within 2 weeks of an operation may be managed successfully by means of débridement and retention of the components combined with administration of culture-specific intravenous antibiotics for 4 to 6 weeks. The expected cure rate approaches 70%. Proper, careful surgical technique and meticulous wound hemostasis combined with prophylactic administration of antibiotics may help decrease the rate of this complication. The role of antibiotic-loaded cement in preventing infections in total hip revision performed for aseptic loosening is not clear. Use of Antibiotic-loaded cement usually is indicated to provide a safety factor in revision total hip arthroplasty.

Neurovascular Injury

Neurovascular injury in revision total hip replacement is more common than in primary total hip replacement, chiefly due to scaring, making exposure more difficult, and aberrant retractor placement (29). Care must be taken when placing retractors, particularly anterior and posterior acetabular retractors, to avoid injury to the iliac and femoral vessels and sciatic nerve, respectively. Sciatic and peroneal nerve palsies following revision total hip replacement can occur from lengthening, retractor placement, and excessive postoperative bleeding. The prognosis for recovery of function in patients with nerve palsies following revision total hip replacement, as would be expected, is directly related to the degree of neural injury. Nerve palsies in patients who recover some motor function immediately following have a better prognosis than those with severe dysesthesia or those who continue to have a complete nerve palsy by the time of discharge (34). In most cases, postoperative nerve palsies should be observed and recovery documented using electroconductive studies. Immediate intervention is rarely necessary except for stretch-induced nerve palsies caused by obvious overlengthening of a limb, in which case shortening of the modular femoral neck may be beneficial.

Femoral Fracture

Postoperative femoral shaft fractures can occur when the canal is violated during cement removal (21). If femoral canal perforation is identified during cement removal, it is best to proceed with insertion of a longer-stemmed component to bypass the defect in the femoral canal by two cortical diameters to prevent postoperative fractures. A defect in the femoral canal can be identified on postoperative radiographs when a bolus of cement is seen in the soft tissue surrounding the proximal femur. Canal perforation often is not recognized until the initial postoperative radiographs are examined. If it can be clearly documented that the perforation is well above the tip of the stem, no intervention is necessary. If a defect clearly extends distally past the tip of the stem, casting or bracing is appropriate. If the defect is large enough, application of strut allografts may be necessary to prevent late fracture.

RESULTS

The initial results with the cemented techniques of the early 1970s were not particularly impressive (1,26). A Mayo clinic study of 166 hips followed 4.5 years after revision in which cement was used a second time revealed only 52% good or excellent results (16). Fifteen of the 166 hips had already needed revision. Another report from New York of 99 revisions followed 8.1 years found 63% good and excellent results and 29% failures, failure defined as the need for revision (26). A study of 139 revisions performed in the same institution (The Hospital for Special Surgery, New York) with improved surgical techniques from 1979 to February 1982 still found only a 59% rate of excellent results, a 29% rate of progressive radiolucency, and an 8.6% rate of second revision after an average of only 3.6 years (2).

In a more encouraging report from Boston of 43 hips revised with cementing techniques developed after 1976, only one hip needed revision by 74 months (9). The same group of patients was observed an average of 15 years (22). Four of 36 for whom the index procedure had been a first femoral revision, later experienced failure of the hip, and 3 of 7 for whom the revision was a second or third revision experienced failure. Thus the overall revision rate for the 35 surviving hips was 20% at 15 years. This group of patients was relatively young, having the index revision at an average of 51 years of age. In this same group of patients, 2 had radiographic loosening of the femoral component. The combined loosening and femoral revision rate was 26%. Marti et al. (20) in 1990 reported 85% survivorship at 14 years for 80 revisions. Seventy-five of the operations had been performed on patients for whom the initial revision was performed after the patient was 60 years of age. Kershaw et al. (18) reported reasonable results of 276 cemented revisions performed between 1977 and 1986 with an average follow-up period of 75 months. Only ten femoral components required re-revision because of recurrent loosening.

The personal results of one of us (DRC.) with revision of the femoral component using cement a second time have been reasonably good (3). Between 1974 and 1990 he performed 205 revisions of loose cemented total hip replacements. In 140 of these, the revision was done with cement. Because 30 of these were revisions of surface arthroplasties they were excluded from analysis, leaving 110 hips in which a stem was cemented into a femur a second time. The average age of the patients was 66.9 years and 90 of the hips were older than 60 years. All patients were operated on with the trochanteric osteotomy approach. We believe this approach allows proper positioning of the components and tensioning of the hip. Only two dislocations occurred in the postoperative period. One femoral shaft fracture occurred interoperatively; this was in the very first revision performed in 1974. Other postoperative complications included 12 recognized femoral perforations. Two postoperative femoral fractures occurred and were associated with considerable trauma but did appear to be related to perforation that had occurred at the operation. Among the four patients with nerve palsies, three recovered completely, and the fourth had only partial residual weakness in ankle dorsiflexion. Two deep wound infections necessitated Girdlestone resection, but another prosthesis was reimplanted. The clinical results among these patients were excellent. The average Iowa hip rating was 89.5, and 89% of the patients reported little, if any, pain. Ninety-three percent of the patients had mild or no limp. The average arc of flexion was 110 degrees, 87% of the patients could flex past 90 degrees.

Eighteen of the revisions were done with techniques of the 1970s. In 1996 we evaluated the results for hips implanted between 1980 and 1991 and followed at least 5 years after

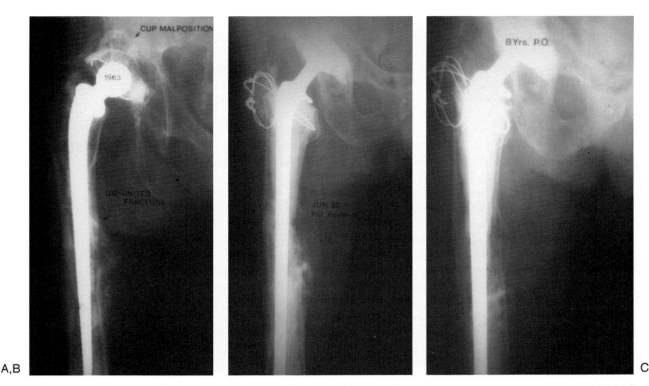

Figure 6. Images of a 75-year-old man with loose cemented long stem and midshaft femoral nonunion. **A:** Before revision. **B:** After cemented rerevision. **C:** Eight years postoperatively and doing well.

the operation. Ninety-two hips were replaced in patients with an average age of 69.3 years. Twelve of these revisions were done for patients younger than 60 years. Stem length of the revision component was 140 mm or less in 45 hips, between 140 and 200 mm in 37 hips, and more than 200 mm in only 10 hips (Fig. 6) (33). In all prostheses, second- and third-generation cementing techniques were used. Antibiotics were used in the cement in 36% of the operations. Bone stock of the revised component was believed to be type II or III bone loss among 52% of patients (see Figs. 2, 3, and 5). Clinical results showed an average Iowa hip rating of 90.6 at last follow-up examination, 89% of patients having mild or no pain. Thirty-three percent of patients did use some support. Eight stems (11%) had the required re-revision an average of 6 years after the initial operation. Among the patients older than 65 years at the time of revision, only two needed re-revision, and one had radiologic loosening.

SUMMARY

A revision operation on the femoral side with a cemented component is an excellent procedure for many hips. Previously failed uncemented stems usually can be revised with a cemented femoral component. If cement has been used previously on the femoral side and reasonable bone stock remains, excellent results with cement the second time can be expected. If extensive bone loss has occurred, femoral allografting may be necessary. In most cases, however, moderate osteolysis or bone deficiencies can be made up with a cemented femoral component technique, often without supplemental grafting.

It is very important that second- and third-generation cementing techniques be used. The canal must be cleaned of all debris, dried thoroughly, and prepared so that a rough surface is available for cement interdigitation. The cement itself must be prepared with a porosity-reduction technique and placed in the canal of the femur at the proper stage. A modern prosthetic design should be used, and the stem must bypass defects or extensive perforations for an adequate distance. These techniques usually result in a painless and stable hip. Good to excellent results can be anticipated among a high percentage of patients for 5 to 10 years. Longer follow-up data on these techniques are only now becoming available. We prefer cemented revision on the femoral side for patients older than 60 years with adequate bone stock and for selected patients younger than 50 years who are not considered good candidates for uncemented techniques.

REFERENCES

1. Amstutz HC, Ma SM, Jinnah RH, Mai L. Revision of aseptic loose total hip arthroplasties. *Clin Orthop* 1982;170:21–33.
2. Callaghan JJ, Salvati EA, Pellicci PM, Wilson PD, Ranawat CS. Results of a revision for mechanical failure after cemented total hip replacement. 1979–1982. *J Bone Joint Surg Am* 1985;67:1074–1085.
3. Collis DK. Revision total hip arthroplasty with cement. *Semin Arthroplasty* 1993;4:38–49.
4. D'Antonio JA, Bargar WL, Borden LS, et al. Classification of femoral abnormalities in total hip arthroplasty. *Clin Orthop* 1993;296:133–139.
5. Davies JP, Jasty M, O'Connor DO, Burke DW, Harrigan TP, Harris WH. The effect of centrifuging bone cement. *J Bone Joint Surg Br* 1989;71:39–42.
6. Estok DM, Harris WH. Long-term results of cemented femoral revision surgery using second generation techniques: an average 11.7-year follow-up evaluation. *Clin Orthop* 1994;299:190–202.
7. [Deleted in proof.]
8. Harris WH, Allen JR. The calcar replacement femoral component for total hip arthroplasty: design, uses and surgical technique. *Clin Orthop* 1981;157:215–224.
9. Harris WH, McCarthy JC, Jr, O'Neill DA. Femoral component loosening using contemporary techniques of femoral cement fixation. *J Bone Joint Surg Am* 1982;64:1063–1067.
10. Harris WH, McGann WA. Loosening of the femoral component after use of the medullary plug cementing technique: follow-up note with a minimum 5-year follow-up. *Bone Joint Surg Am* 1986;68:1064–1066.
11. Herberts P, Ahnfelt L, Malchau H, Strömberg C, Andersson GBJ. Multicenter clinical trials and their value in assessing total joint arthroplasty. *Clin Orthop* 1989;249:48–55.
12. Jensen NF, Harris WH. A system for trochanteric osteotomy and reattachment for total hip arthroplasty with a ninety-nine percent union rate. *Clin Orthop* 1986;208:174–181.
13. Katz RP, Callaghan JJ, Solomon PM, Johnston RC. Cemented revision total hip arthroplasty using contemporary techniques: a minimum 10-year follow-up study. *J Arthroplasty* 1994;9:103 (abstract).
14. [Deleted in proof.]
15. Kavanagh BF, Fitzgerald RH. Multiple revisions for failed total hip arthroplasty not associated with infection. *J Bone Joint Surg Am* 1987;89:1144–1149.
16. Kavanagh BF, Ilstrup DM, Fitzgerald RH. Revision total hip arthroplasty. *J Bone Joint Surg Am* 1985;67:517–526.
17. [Deleted in proof.]
18. Kershaw CJ, Adkins RM, Dodd CAF, et al. Revision total hip arthroplasty for aseptic failure: a review of 276 cases. *J Bone Joint Surg Br* 1991;73:564–568.
19. Lawrence JM, Engh CA, Macalino GE. Revision total hip arthroplasty: long-term results without cement. *Orthop Clin North Am* 1993;24:635–644.
20. Marti RK, Schüller HM, Cesselarr PP, et al. Results of revision of hip arthroplasty with cement: a five to 14 year follow-up. *J Bone Joint Surg Am* 1990;72:346–354.
21. Morrey BF, Kavanagh BF. Complications with the revision of the femoral component of total hip arthroplasty: comparison between cemented and uncemented techniques. *J Arthroplasty* 1992;7:71–79.
22. Mulroy WF, Harris WH. Revision total hip arthroplasty with use of so-called second generation cementing techniques for aseptic loosening of the femoral component: a 15-year average follow-up study. *J Bone Joint Surg Am* 1996;78:325–330.
23. Nassar SA. Prevention and treatment of sepsis in total hip replacement surgery. *Orthop Clin North Am* 1992;23:265–277.
24. Oh I, Bourne RB, Harris WH. The femoral cement compactor: an improvement in cementing technique in total hip replacement. *J Bone Joint Surg Am* 1983;65A:1335–1338.
25. Pellicci PM, Wilson PD, Sledge CB, et al. Revision total hip arthroplasty. *Clin Orthop* 1982;170:34–41.
26. Pellicci PM, Wilson PD, Sledge CB, et al. Long-term results of revision total hip replacement: a follow-up report. *J Bone Joint Surg Am* 1985;67:513–516.
27. Retpen JB, Jensen JS. Risk factors for recurrent aseptic loosening of the femoral component after cemented revision. *J Arthroplasty* 1993;8:471–479.
28. Rubash HE, Harris WH. Revision of nonseptic loose, cemented femoral components using modern cementing techniques. *J Arthroplasty* 1988;3:241–248.
29. Schmalzreid TP, Amstutz HC, Dorey FJ. Nerve palsy associated with total hip replacement. *J Bone Joint Surg Am* 1991;73:1074–1080.
30. Schutzer SF, Harris WH. Trochanteric osteotomy for revision total hip arthroplasty: 97% union rate using a comprehensive approach. *Clin Orthop* 1988;227:172–183.

31. Stromberg CN, Herberts P, Ahnfelt L. Revision total hip arthroplasty in patients younger than 55 years old: clinical and radiologic results after 4 years. *J Arthroplasty* 1988;3:47–59.
32. Tsukyama DT, Estrada R, Gustilo RB. Infection after total hip arthroplasty: a study of the treatment of 106 infections. *J Bone Joint Surg Am* 1996;78:512–523.
33. Turner RH, Mattingly DA, Scheller A. Femoral revision total hip arthroplasty using a long-stem femoral component: clinical and radiographic analysis. *J Arthroplasty* 1987;2:247–258.
34. Wasielewski RC, Crossett LS, Rubash HE. Neural and vascular injury in total hip arthroplasty. *Orthop Clin North Am* 1992;23:219–235.
35. Williams JF, Gottesman MJ, Mallory TH. Dislocation after total hip arthroplasty: treatment with an above-knee hip spica cast. *Clin Orthop* 1982;171:53–58.

Revision Total Hip Arthroplasty,
edited by Marvin E. Steinberg and Jonathan P. Garino,
Lippincott Williams & Wilkins, Philadelphia © 1999.

23

Femoral Revision: Uncemented

C. Anderson Engh, Jr. and Charles A. Engh, Sr.

For the past two decades most revision hip operations involved removal of the femoral prosthesis for aseptic loosening. In the series of Schulte et al. (23) with cemented Charnley components, 50% of revisions involved a femoral component. In a report by Kavanagh et al. (13), 57% of revisions involved a cemented femoral component. In our experience, less than 25% of total hip revisions involve the femoral component. Moreland (18) reported that 14% of the revisions in his primary cementless series involved the femoral component. In our series of cementless anatomic medullary locking (AML; DePuy, Warsaw, Ind.) hips, 22% of the revisions involved a femoral component (7). This change in pattern of revision surgery is attributed to the following four factors: development of durable cementless femoral components (7,10); Improvement in techniques used for cementing femoral prostheses (20); availability of modular femoral components; and increased incidence of acetabular revision for polyethylene wear problems encountered with some uncemented acetabular components (2,7,16). Although symptomatic loosening of a femoral stem is less common now than previously, it still represents a difficult problem for the revision surgeon. Patients with a loose stem are older and have more disability than patients are at the time of the primary operation. If the femur has been damaged by osteolysis or if removal of the failed femoral component is difficult, the femur available for reconstruction will be damaged, making reconstruction more difficult.

The goals of revision surgery are clear cut for patients. Patients hope to gain relief from thigh pain, a return of leg length lost to subsidence of the loose prosthesis, and improved hip function with the strength necessary to climb stairs or walk distances without crutches.

C. A. Engh, Jr., and C. A. Engh, Sr.: Anderson Orthopaedic Research Institute, Alexandria, Virginia 22030.

However, having already had one failure, patients are not as optimistic as they were the first time. As a result, they often are satisfied with a less than normal hip, provided they can have some assurance that the new prosthesis will not loosen.

The surgeon's task in revision surgery is well defined. The surgeon must satisfy the patient's expectations by producing durable femoral fixation and appropriate hip biomechanics in a femur that is deformed and has deficient proximal bone stock. These factors have an effect on both the design of the femoral prosthesis and on the method by which it will become connected to the femoral cortices. We prefer to bypass the proximally damaged bone and fix a porous surfaced implant to the most proximal portion of the femoral diaphysis that is strong enough to support body loads. The bone must be viable enough to grow into the porous surface of the implant and adapt to the changing concentration of body loads that will be applied to this area.

BACKGROUND

Many revision surgeons now agree that in most cases the initial stability of a revision stem must be achieved within the femoral diaphysis distal to proximally damaged bone. Even proponents of cemented femoral revision routinely use a component longer than the primary component. The longer stem allows initial cement fixation to both distal cortical bone and proximal distorted bone while re-establishing hip biomechanics. However, cemented femoral revision implants do not always provide a durable cement–bone interface. The initial results of cemented revision demonstrated a re revision plus impending failure rate of approximately 40% (1,4,6,12,14,25). Second-generation revision techniques improved the results but the re revision plus impending failure rate remained greater than 10% (9,17,21,22).

Although many experienced hip surgeons prefer certain proximally coated stems, the authors elected to perform revision operations with fully porous coated stems to lessen the incidence of failure due to stem loosening. Two femoral revision techniques are used. These include stems with porous coating on only the upper half of the stem and those with coating on the entire stem surface. For primary operations we have used implants with porous coating on only the upper part of the stem. However, for revision procedures when

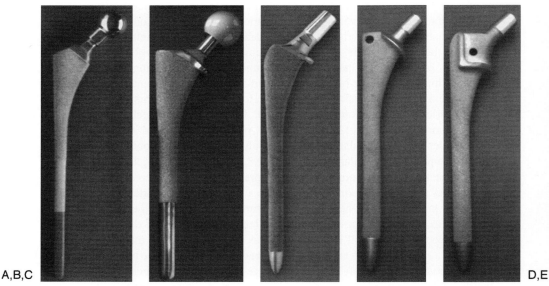

A,B,C   D,E

Figure 1. Current porous coated stems designed for predominantly diaphyseal fixation. **A:** Mallory-Head revision stem (Biomet, Warsaw, Ind.). **B:** Universal (Biomet). **C:** Versys (Zimmer, Warsaw, Ind.). **D:** AML Solution (DePuy, Warsaw, Ind.). **E:** AML Solution calcar replacement stem (De Puy).

the bone is weak, has a poor blood supply, and has a distorted proximal shape, we favor coating on the entire stem so that the coating can be placed in contact with a greater amount of normal-appearing bone (8). Figure 1 shows examples of this kind of implant.

We accept the fact that it is not possible in femoral revision surgery to fit an implant as well proximally as distally and believe it is easier to obtain fixation in healthy diaphyseal bone. We prefer to bypass the proximally damaged bone and fix a fully porous surfaced implant to the most proximal 5 cm of the femoral diaphysis that appears radiographically normal. This bone is both strong enough to support weight bearing and viable enough to rapidly osseointegrate with the implant.

INDICATIONS AND PATIENT SELECTION

Many revision surgeons believe that there are specific indications for or contraindications to the different femoral revision techniques. Therefore, different techniques are used by the same surgeon in different situations. The predominant reason for different techniques is variance in bone stock. We believe the technique of distal porous fixation in revision femoral surgery can be used reproducibly in most situations. This versatility is particularly important because bone stock is difficult to evaluate on preoperative radiographs. It is even more difficult to judge the amount of bone stock that will remain after removal of the failed implants and cement. We acknowledge that other techniques that allow more proximal stress transfer may spare bone stock from stress shielding or even increase bone stock in the case of proximal allografting, but these techniques are not suited to all cases. Because the technique of distal femoral porous fixation works for simple femoral revision as well as complex revisions and can address complications that arise during revision, every revision hip surgeon should be familiar with the technique.

The indications for choosing this technique are the same as those outlined in Chapters 15 and 20. The most frequent indication is patient dissatisfaction caused by aseptic loosening. The most important symptom is thigh pain on weight bearing. There are also indications when well-fixed stems have to be removed, but these are much less frequent. These indications include recurrent dislocation that cannot be handled with acetabular revision, thigh pain with a well-fixed stem, and distal femoral osteolysis. The only contraindication to this technique is active infection.

Although the technique is potentially applicable to all femoral revisions, there are some patient-selection considerations. The surgeon must ensure that the patient's goals of pain relief and function can be achieved and that unrealistic patient goals are discussed before revision. Surgeons should be especially cautious about revising what appears to be a well-fixed cemented or cementless femoral component because of unexplained pain. The surgeon must also be sure the patient understands and will abide by the perioperative physical restrictions. In particular, this means that the patient must follow dislocation precautions. Even more specific to this technique is recognition that the patient must follow the weight-bearing restrictions required to provide an appropriate mechanical and biologic environment for bone ingrowth. These weight-bearing precautions can range from immediate full weight bearing to no weight bearing for 3 months. Patients who cannot follow instructions should not undergo revision surgery.

PREOPERATIVE PLANNING

The goals of femoral revision surgery are to obtain durable fixation, restore the anatomical integrity of the hip, and ensure that the patient has the best available articular bearing surface. These goals can be addressed with radiographs, a physical examination, and operative notes describing the existing implants.

In addition to defining the indication for surgical treatment, radiographs are used for determining the 5 to 10 cm section of healthy diaphyseal bone where initial and subsequent durable fixation will occur. The physical examination, specifically leg lengths, are combined with the anteroposterior (AP) radiograph to plan surgical therapy in such a way that hip biomechanics are reestablished. The previous operative note is needed to

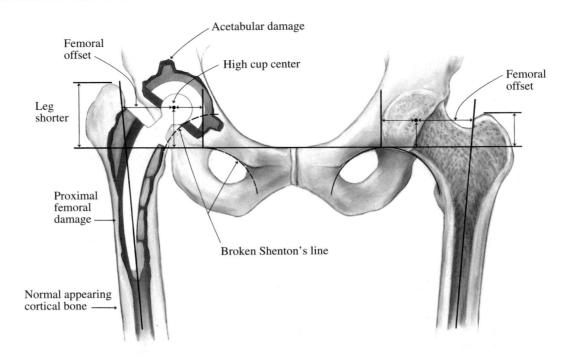

Figure 2. Example of a failed hip arthroplasty.

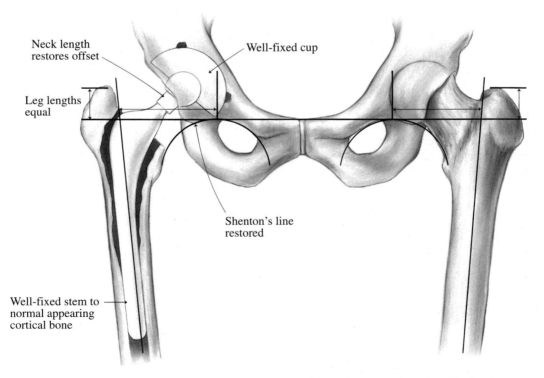

Figure 3. The ideal reconstruction includes normal hip biomechanics, durable fixation to host bone, and the best possible articular surface.

determine the size and modularity of the existing implants so that implant-specific extraction tools and modular replacement parts are available. Many early metal-backed components were nonmodular. In some cases, the surgeon may decide not to exchange the polyethylene liner. However, in cases with a damaged liner, the surgeon may not have a choice. In these situations, the surgeon must have a custom replacement liner, be prepared to remove a well-fixed acetabular component, or cement a smaller polyethylene liner into the existing metal shell. Without documentation of the existing implants, the surgeon cannot be sure that the best available articular bearing surface will be implanted.

A failed hip typically has damaged acetabular bone with an elevated head center, a disruption of Shenton's line, femoral bone damage, and leg-length discrepancy (Fig. 2). An ideal reconstruction reestablishes hip biomechanics by means of matching a stable acetabular component with a femoral component that has an acceptable neck geometry. When seated in the femur, the stem corrects leg-length discrepancy and reestablishes acceptable hip-joint mechanics (Fig. 3).

The actual templating process to plan the ideal reconstruction (Fig. 4) is done in five steps. Step 1 determines the diaphyseal fixation point on the AP radiograph (Fig. 5). Using this diaphyseal segment of bone, the surgeon is able to judge the diameter of the stem and the centerline of the femur. Step 2 determines the acetabular center (Fig. 6). If the acetabular component is not to be revised, it is the existing acetabular center. If an acetabular revision is necessary, the position of the new acetabular center has to be estimated. Step 3 focuses on a head–neck segment and the seating level of the prosthesis. Using the center line of the femur, the surgeon selects a component with an appropriate combination of neck shaft angle, base neck length, and varying lengths of modular heads.

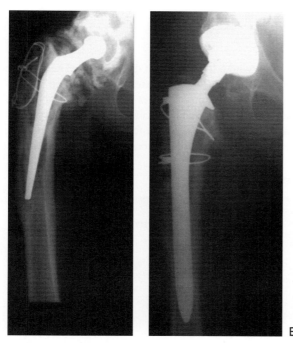

Figure 4. A: Radiograph shows a failed arthroplasty. The fixation has failed and the hip biomechanics are poor. **B:** The same hip reconstructed. Diaphyseal fixation is obtained with an extensively porous coated femoral component. The porous coated acetabular component is fixed to host bone. Trochanteric osteotomy was needed for exposure and to accommodate the new femoral component. A long neck ball was used to improve offset.

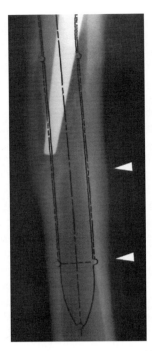

Figure 5. Step 1. The first 5 to 10 cm of healthy diaphyseal bone is chosen. The appropriate diameter template is used. Varus-valgus positioning of the component is determined with the diaphyseal fixation point.

Choosing a component with adequate offset directly correlates with the stability of the hip joint. The component-seating level is determined in Step 3. If 1 cm of leg-length correction is necessary, the seating level or vertical position of the stem in the femur should be one that places the femoral head center 1 cm directly above the acetabular center (Fig. 7). At this point, the relation between femoral bony landmarks, especially the tip of the greater trochanter, and component landmarks such as the lateral edge of the component

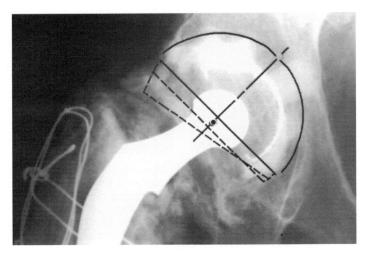

Figure 6. Step 2. The position of the new acetabular component is estimated, and the center of the bearing surface is marked.

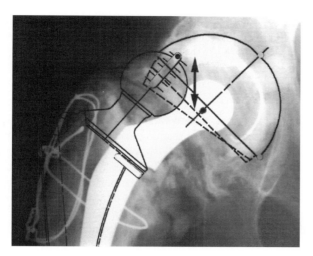

Figure 7. Step 3. The femoral component is raised and lowered while the appropriate neck length is chosen to correct offset and leg length. In this case, leg length is corrected but offset is decreased.

are marked as references to be used in the operation. The length of the stem is one that allows a minimum of 5 to 10 cm of porous contact with diaphyseal bone at the fixation point at this seating level. In most instances, this is done with an off-the-shelf prosthesis. In the occasional severely deformed or destroyed femur, a longer stem has to be cut off. Step 4 confirms that the medial to lateral dimensions of the proximal portion of the stem are not too large to fit within the femoral metaphysis at the planned seating level (Fig. 8).

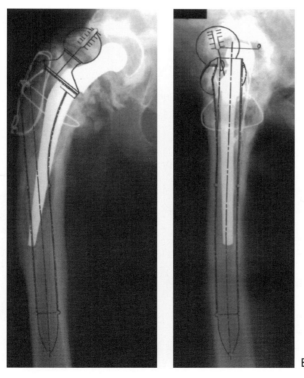

Figure 8. A: Step 4. Anteroposterior sizing is good medially and poor laterally. A trochanteric osteotomy is needed to place this femoral component. **B:** Step 5. A bowed component is needed to obtain distal fixation on the lateral radiograph.

The fifth and final step is to make certain on the lateral radiograph that with the planned length stem seated to the appropriate depth, the prosthesis fits the bow of the femur. If it does not, a bowed femoral prosthesis is necessary (see Fig. 8).

SURGICAL TECHNIQUE

The surgical technique closely follows the preoperative planning. Successful surgical technique involves precise cylindrical reaming and impacting of the appropriate cylindrical stem into the femur. Our routine revision approach is the posterior approach. We perform a trochanteric osteotomy 40% of the time. The osteotomy can be for acetabular or femoral exposure. In cases with minimal bone destruction in which a 6-inch (15 cm) stem is used, a trochanteric osteotomy is usually not necessary. However, in cases that require an 8-inch (20 cm) or longer stem, a trochanteric osteotomy greatly facilitates removal of the existing implant, removal of a canal plug, and reaming of the diaphyseal bone (Fig. 9).

The surgical technique often requires removal of bone or cement plugs. Direct visualization of canal plugs with or without a trochanteric osteotomy facilitates removal. The usual technique involves drilling through the plug with a one-fourth-inch (0.6 cm) drill and removing either the bone or the cement with specially designed femoral curettes. To prevent eccentric reaming, complete removal of the canal plug is critical.

Precise reaming over 5 to 10 cm at the diaphyseal fixation point is the critical surgical step. The only way to ensure precise reaming is to be certain that the diaphysis directs the reamer. In other words, the reamer cannot impinge on a distal bone plug or retained cement. The reamer must be free proximally and cannot impinge on the greater trochanter or overhanging proximal soft tissue. If there is any doubt about reamer direction, reamer impingement, retained cement, or bone plugs, an AP and a lateral radiograph are obtained.

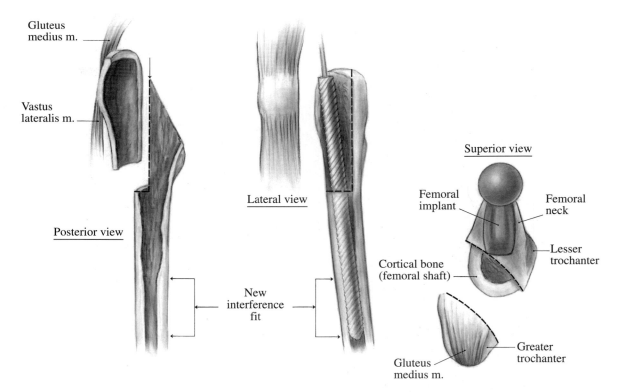

Figure 9. A trochanteric osteotomy facilitates acetabular and femoral exposure. The osteotomy allows unobstructed access to the femoral diaphysis for precise reaming.

A trochanteric osteotomy allows accurate machining of the diaphysis with straight reamers in cases that necessitate use of a long stem or have excessive anterior femoral bow. Without the osteotomy, the straight reamers would penetrate the anterior femoral cortex.

In most instances, we advocate use of straight, rigid reamers. Occasionally we use thin-shafted, rigid reamers and never use flexible reamers over a guide wire. The more rigid the reamer, the more precise is the reaming. Precise reaming is critical to preventing femoral fractures during impaction and ensuring maximum contact between bone and porous coating.

Reaming is done in 0.5-mm increments. Appropriate reamer tightness requires both irrigation to prevent bone necrosis and frequent cleaning of cortical bone from the reamer tip. However, the reamer should not require excessive force to advance. Reamers of increasing size typically advance easily down the femur. The last two reamers need a gentle push. The last reamer may have to be removed and the tip cleaned multiple times to remove caked-on cortical bone. Reaming is stopped at a size 0.5 mm smaller than the actual size of the implant.

After reaming, sizing of the diaphysis is confirmed. In straightforward operations, the appropriate diaphyseal diameter and length of cortical contact are inferred from the feel of the reamer. We strongly advocate use of intraoperative radiographs in operations that require stems longer than 8 inches (20 cm) and greater than 16.5 mm in diameter, in operations on patients with osteoporotic femurs, or operations on femurs that have an abnormal reamer feel. Radiographs with the reamer in place confirm that the stem diameter is appropriate and that the length of contact with diaphyseal bone is 5 to 10 cm.

We always use trial components to confirm that the combination of femoral and acetabular component position results in appropriate leg lengths and a stable hip joint. We do not use radiographs to confirm leg length. Our primary technique involves securing the foot of the leg not being operated on to the table with the knee in 70 to 90 degrees of flexion before preparation. No pillows are placed between the legs. Before hip dislocation, the heels and soles of the feet are placed side by side and the femurs are measured at the tibial tubercle. This distance is recorded and compared with the same measurement with the trial components in place. An additional technique for patients who do not have a trochanteric osteotomy is to place a Steinmann pin in the ilium, bend it twice so that it touches the greater trochanter, and use this point as a reference for both length and femoral offset. Using these two intraoperative measuring techniques makes it possible to adjust the trial components to obtain the planned leg-length correction. If hip joint stability, leg length, and offset are not appropriate at trial reduction, additional measures such as changing the stem version, neck length, prosthesis-seating level, and polyethylene insert are explored.

The final step is impaction of the femoral component. When the porous coated prosthesis is inserted, it should be impossible to push it manually the last 7 to 10 cm into the femur. Insertion requires consistent blows with a hammer. With each impaction, the stem should drop 2 to 5 mm. For the last 2 cm, it should drop only 1 mm with each impaction. If more than this amount of force is required, the stem should be removed and the intramedullary canal prepared with a drill the same size as the stem. In every case, surgeons must have an instrument that creates a metal to metal, motion-free connection to the implant to allow removal of partially impacted stems. The potential for a partially impacted stem is another reason we advocate use of a straight cylindrical stem. A straight stem can be knocked out without danger of femoral fracture, whereas a curved or anatomic stem partially impacted must be removed with great care to prevent femoral or trochanteric fracture.

COMPLICATIONS

The most common technical complications of revision surgery with a distally fixed stem are: failure of bone ingrowth, recurrent dislocations, femoral perforation, and distal femoral fractures caused by using a stem that is either too long or too large in diameter

(5). The incidence of each of these complications can be decreased with modification of the surgical technique (24). Failure of bone ingrowth is related to surgical technique, bone stock, and patient compliance. Stems that are not inserted tightly need a more prolonged period of protected weight bearing for success.

Dislocations and leg-length inequality problems can be decreased by use of trial components to check leg length and hip stability. When only the femoral component needs to be revised, the rasp that corresponds to the size of the porous coated implant is seated. Different head and neck possibilities are tried until correct leg length and added hip stability are obtained. If the hip is unstable because the orientation of the well-fixed cup is not compatible with rotation of the stem, it may be necessary to remove the well-fixed cup and change its orientation to achieve stability. When the cup and the stem are well aligned but the hip still dislocates, the surgeon must be prepared to advance the trochanter.

Femoral perforations can be prevented by means of obtaining intraoperative radiographs with a drill in place. Anterior perforations are usually caused by drilling too far down a curved femur with a straight drill. Lateral perforations usually are caused by incomplete cement or bone pedestal removal. We routinely obtain radiographs for patients who need more than an 8-inch (20 cm) stem, have had removal of a bone pedestal or cement plug, or who have a canal larger than 16.5 mm. These are the cases in which the feel of the drill may not be adequate. The radiographs ensure that all retained cement or bone pedestals are removed and that reamer alignment and cortical contact are appropriate.

Femoral fractures occur when the stem is inserted too tightly. Precise technique, use of intraoperative radiographs, and surgical experience can prevent this complication. The most common type of fracture is one that occurs during impaction. The stem, which has been advancing 1 mm with every blow of the hammer, suddenly advances 3 to 5 mm. When this happens, we check the stability of the femur with a dislocation and reduction maneuver and obtain radiographs. If a nondisplaced fracture is seen and the femoral component is stable, no additional operative fixation is used. However, the weight-bearing status of the patient is kept at 0% to 25% for 6 weeks. All displaced fractures are treated with cables, strut allografts, and 3 months of protected weight bearing.

POSTOPERATIVE CARE

The postoperative rehabilitation plan is based on three factors and on the patient's ability to comply with the rehabilitation plan. The three factors are the quality of acetabular and femoral component fixation, hip joint stability, and abductor function. Component fixation determines weight-bearing status; hip joint stability determines the range of motion; and abductor function determines the ability to do repetitive strengthening exercises. The patient's ability to comply with a rehabilitation plan is a combination of the person's cognitive function and physical ability. The rehabilitation timetable is arbitrarily divided into the hospital stay and 6-week intervals that correspond to the timing of follow-up visits.

The initial rehabilitation plan is defined immediately after the operation. Weight-bearing status depends on component fixation. The categories of weight bearing are none, 25%, 50%, and full weight bearing. Acetabular components that are not revised or are revised with an intact rim and cavity can bear weight as tolerated. Acetabular components that have some rim or cavity defects treated with or without particulate graft are allowed 50% weight bearing for 6 weeks, then full weight bearing. Acetabular components that require extensive grafting or supplemental screw fixation are 25% or no weight bearing for 6 weeks to 3 months. In the case of the femoral component, all femoral revisions are placed on protected weight-bearing status. The quality of femoral fixation is based on the tightness of impaction and the fit seen on the recovery room radiograph. If both metaphyseal and diaphyseal fixation are good, the patient is allowed 50% weight bearing for 6 weeks. This amount is followed by advancement to weight bearing as tolerated over the second 6 weeks. Patients with good diaphyseal fixation but minimal or no metaphyseal fixation perform 25% weight bearing for 6 weeks, then 50% weight bearing for the next

6 weeks, and weight bearing as tolerated after 3 months. Patients with suboptimal diaphyseal fixation, femoral perforation, or femoral fracture perform no weight bearing for 6 weeks and advance after 6 weeks on the basis of the radiographic findings and clinical judgment. These patients also wear an above-knee brace or single leg spica cast, depending on the adequacy of femoral fixation. Because both the acetabular and femoral fixation determine the weight-bearing status differently, the weight-bearing plan that is the most restrictive is the one followed.

The range of motion for all patients who undergo revision is 0 to 70 degrees. Hip joints without a tendency to dislocate follow this range of motion for 6 weeks. Hips that have a tendency to dislocate on the table are braced for 6 weeks. At the operation, the hip must flex 90 degrees and internally rotate 60 degrees, or a brace is ordered. It is preferable to improve the operative range of motion by adjusting component orientation, component selection, or trochanteric advancement. When these options do not work or are not a viable alternative, a brace is used.

Abductor muscle function is the third determinant or contributor to the rehabilitation plan. Patients with intact abductors and no trochanteric osteotomy are allowed to do active repetitive strengthening exercises from day one. Patients who need a trochanteric osteotomy are allowed active exercises based on the quality of trochanteric fixation. Patients with suboptimum osteotomy fixation, who do not have functioning abductors to start with, or who are not expected to regain abductor function, wear a brace, perform 25% weight bearing, and do not perform repetitive flexion or abduction exercises for 6 weeks.

Often these fairly straightforward plans are altered if the patient cannot follow instructions. The reasons for inability to follow instructions usually are related to physical handicaps such as obesity, rheumatologic involvement of other joints, and a long list of chronic medical conditions, cognitive disorders, or straightforward noncompliance. We do not hesitate to place revision patients in a cast or brace, with their consent, if they do not seem capable of protecting the reconstruction. In these cases, the rehabilitation plan is often more restrictive and prolonged.

In terms of hospital care, all patients sit and dangle their legs within 12 hours of the operation and are in a chair or walking with supervision in the first 24 to 36 hours. This activity requires experienced nurses and therapists who can monitor vital signs when they initially mobilize the patients. By 48 hours after the operation, the patients are seen in the gymnasium. Before discharge, patients are able to transfer with minimal assistance, follow weight-bearing and dislocation precautions, climb stairs, and walk 100 feet (30 meters). At discharge, the summary of the specifics of the rehabilitation plan is dictated, given to the patient, and faxed or electronically transmitted to all caregivers to ensure continuity of care after the patient leaves the hospital.

RESULTS

A review of published results confirms the success of this technique. The first report from our institution by Lawrence et al. (15) reviewed the cases of 81 patients who underwent revision between 1980 and 1986. All had a minimum 5-year follow-up period with a mean follow-up period of 9 years (range 5 to 13 years). In this series, the femoral re-revision rate was 10% and the mechanical loosening rate was 11%. Clinical success was measured in terms of function, physician-defined success, and patient satisfaction. In terms of pain and walking, 87% of patients improved and 93% of patients were satisfied with the outcome of their revision hip arthroplasty. At final follow-up examination (including all interim procedures), only 5% had an unstable implant. However, 12% had partial success with a stable implant but without improved function. In a more recent report, Moreland and Bernstein (19) reported the results for 175 patients who underwent femoral revision between 1984 and 1991. The mean follow-up period was 5 years (range 2 to 10 years). The results were considerably better, with a femoral re revision rate of 4% and a mechanical loosening rate of 4%. For this series the authors not only reported improved pain and walking scores but also addressed thigh pain and stress shielding. Thigh pain was reported in 8% of patients, and in only one half of these patients was this pain considered severe. The pain correlated with preoperative osteoporosis and failure of bone ingrowth. Severe stress shielding was reported in 8% of hips, and no patient had failure or complications attributed to stress shielding. The stress shielding was statistically associated with preoperative osteoporosis and large stem size.

Most published results involve revision of failed cemented femoral components. We reviewed revision of failed porous coated femoral stems with extensively porous coated femoral revision components. In that series, 21 cases were followed for a mean 6.3 years (minimum 5 years). There were no femoral rerevisions or cases of mechanical loosening. The mean time to failure of the initial cementless femoral component was only 2.6 years. In every case, the failure was diagnosed when pain was associated with migration or varus tilt of the stem. The revision procedure was uncomplicated because the failed cementless stem was easily disimpacted in each case. This is contrasted to the failed cemented component that loosens late and in which the revision procedure is complicated by cement removal.

SUMMARY

Although many experienced hip surgeons prefer certain proximally coated components, we believe that use of extensively porous coated femoral components gives better results

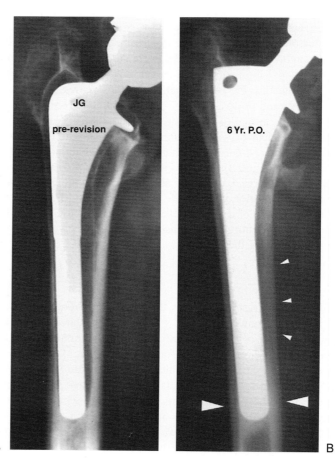

Figure 10. A: Loose femoral component with osteolysis, widening radiolucencies, and calcar hypertrophy. **B:** Bone-ingrown, fully porous coated femoral component. Cortical hypertrophy (*large arrows*) at the termination of the porous coating with proximal stress shielding (*small arrows*) confirms osseointegration.

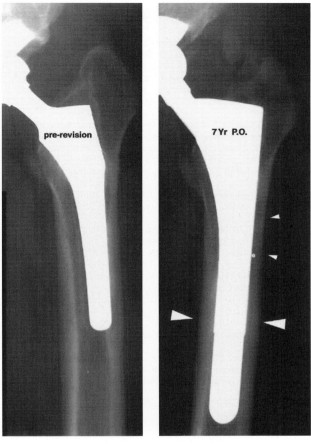

Figure 11. A: Loose femoral component with proximal radiolucencies adjacent to the porous coating and migration into varus position. **B:** The revision femoral component is osseointegrated. Cortical hypertrophy (*large arrows*) and proximal stress shielding (*small arrows*) are characteristic radiographic findings of osseointegration.

in revision femoral operations and is a reproducible technique that can be applied to many femoral revision situations. The technique, which is well documented in the literature, involves choosing 5 to 10 cm of diaphyseal bone and reaming that point cylindrically for a porous coated femoral stem (8). Surgical implantation is uncomplicated because the femoral diaphysis aligns the component and imparts a reproducible press-fit sensation during impaction. The complications are well documented and can be avoided with adequate exposure, use of intraoperative radiographs, and surgical experience. However, particular attention is needed when extensive bone damage is present, a stem longer than 6 inches (15 cm) is required, and when large diameter stems are used (5). Bone ingrowth is easy to diagnose radiographically (Fig. 10). Distal spot welds with proximal stress shielding are favorable signs that indicate osseointegration. When osseointegration is diagnosed, femoral stability is exceptionally durable (7,19) (Fig. 11). In the occasional case in which fixation fails, rerevision is uncomplicated. The only criticism that warrants concern is stress shielding and associated proximal bone loss. This complication occurs among 24% of primary operations and 8% of revision procedures. Stress shielding has not been a clinical problem and occurs only with bone-ingrown implants (3,19).

REFERENCES

1. Amstutz HC, Ma SM, Jinnah RH, Mai L. Revision of aseptic loose total hip arthroplasties. *Clin Orthop* 1982;170:21–33.

2. Bono JV, Sanford L, Toussaint JT. Severe polyethylene wear in total hip arthroplasty: observations from retrieved AML PLUS hip implants with an ACS polyethylene liner. *J Arthroplasty* 1994;9:119–125.

3. Bugbee WD, Culpepper WJ, Engh CA Jr, Engh CA. Long-term clinical consequences of stress shielding in cementless total hip arthroplasty. *J Bone Joint Surg* 1997;79-A(7):1007–1012.

4. Callaghan JJ, Salvati EA, Pellocci PM, Wilson PD, Ranawat CS. Results of revision for mechanical failure after cemented total hip replacement, 1979 to 1982. *J Bone Joint Surg Am* 1985;67:1074–1085.

5. Egan EJ, DiCesare PE. Intraoperative complications of revision hip arthroplasty using a fully porous-coated straight cobalt-chrome femoral stem. *J Arthroplasty* 1995;10[Suppl]:s45–s51.

6. Engelbrecht DJ, Weber FA, Sweet MB, Jakim I. Long-term results of revision total hip arthroplasty. *J Bone Joint Surg Br* 1990;72:41–45.

7. Engh CA Jr, Culpepper WJ, Engh CA. Long-term results of the anatomic medullary locking prosthesis in total hip arthroplasty. *J Bone Joint Surg* 1997;79-A(2):177–184.

8. Engh CA, Culpepper WJ, Kassapidis E. The revision of failed porous-coated femoral prostheses, using larger, more completely porous-coated components. *Clin Ortho* 1998;347(Feb):168–178.

9. Franzen H, Mjoberg B, Onnerfalt R. Early loosening of femoral components after cemented revision. *J Bone Joint Surg Br* 1992;74:721–724.

10. Heekin RD, Callaghan JJ, Hopkinson WJ, Savory CG, Xenos JS. The porous-coated anatomic total hip prosthesis, inserted without cement. *J Bone Joint Surg Am* 1993;75:77–91.

11. [Reserved]

12. Kavanagh BF, Fitzgerald RB Jr. Multiple revisions for failed total hip arthroplasty not associated with infection. *J Bone Joint Surg Am* 1987;69:1144–1149.

13. Kavanagh BF, Myrna DA, Ilstrup DM, Stauffer RN, Coventry MB. Charnley total hip arthroplasty with cement: fifteen-year results. *J Bone Joint Surg Am* 1989;71:1496–1503.

14. Kershaw CJ, Adkins RM, Dodd CAF et al. Revision total hip arthroplasty for aseptic failure: a review of 276 cases. *J Bone Joint Surg Br* 1991;73:564–568.

15. Lawrence JM, Engh CA, Macalino GE, Lauro GR. Outcome of revision hip arthroplasty done without cement. *J Bone Joint Surg Am* 1994;76:965–973.

16. Maloney WJ, Herzwurn P, Paprosky W, Rubash HE, Engh CA. Treatment of pelvic osteolysis associated with a stable acetabular component inserted without cement as part of a total hip replacement. *J Bone Joint Surg Am* 1997;79(11):1628–1634.

17. Marti RK, Schüller HM, Cesselarr PP, et al. Results of revision of hip arthroplasty with cement: a five to fourteen year followup study. *J Bone Joint Surg Am* 1990;72:346–354.

18. Moreland JR. AML at 5 years: young and old. 26th Annual Course, Total Hip Replacement, Harvard Medical School; 1996; Boston.

19. Moreland JR, Bernstein ML. Femoral revision hip arthroplasty with uncemented, porous coated stems. *Clin Orthop* 1995;319:141–150.

20. Mulroy Jr. RD, Harris WH. The effect of improved cementing techniques on component loosening in total hip replacement: an 11-year radiographic review. *J Bone Joint Surg Br* 1990;72:757–760.

21. Pellicci PM, Wilson PD, Sledge CB, et al. Long term results of revision total hip replacement. *J Bone Joint Surg Am* 1985;67:513–516.

22. Rubash HE, Harris WH. Revision of nonseptic, loose, cemented femoral components using modern cement techniques. *J Arthroplasty* 1988;3:241–248.

23. Schulte KR, Callaghan JJ, Kelley SS, Johnson RC. The outcome of Charnley total hip arthroplasty with cement after a minimum twenty-year follow-up: the results of one surgeon. *J Bone Joint Surg Am* 1993;75:961–975.

24. Taunton OD, Culpepper WJ, Engh CA. Treatment of complications in cementless total hip arthroplasty. Presented at the 1997 American Academy of Orthopaedic Surgeons Specialty Day Meeting of the Hip Society; February 16, 1997; Boston.

25. Turner RH, Mattingly DA, Scheller A. Femoral revision total hip arthroplasty using a long stem femoral component: clinical and radiographic analysis. *J Arthroplasty* 1987;2:247–258.

Revision Total Hip Arthroplasty,
edited by Marvin E. Steinberg and Jonathan P. Garino,
Lippincott Williams & Wilkins, Philadelphia © 1999.

24

Postoperative Management

Norman A. Johanson

The diversity of conditions and levels of severity encountered in revision total hip replacement preclude development of rigorous protocols or pathways for patient care. The surgeon determines the pathway and the important management needs on the basis of the type and severity of the failure, important technical factors encountered during the operation, joint stability, and quality of prosthetic fixation. Other factors that may influence the postoperative course, such as comorbidity, blood loss, and the patient's vitality and cognitive function, are assessed. Ultimately the care plan is individualized to match the patient's motivation and potential with the structural integrity of the implant and surrounding bone and soft tissue.

The postoperative course can be viewed from three general perspectives—medical, physical, and psychosocial. Comprehensive care would include a mixture of all three of these factors to obtain the optimal outcome. Medical issues directly influenced by or under the control of the surgeon include blood loss, salvage, and transfusion; thromboembolic prophylaxis and treatment; and perioperative antibiotic coverage. The institution and maintenance of physical mobilization and weight bearing is the surgeon's highest-profile activity. There must be a clear understanding among all hospital and outpatient staff regarding the desired level of transfer activities, walking support, and weight-bearing status. This requires a multidisciplinary approach by the physician, nurses, physical therapists, and ancillary personnel. Revision surgery is almost certain to have some feature that requires an exception to the rules that have been developed for routine primary total hip replacement. The effectiveness with which the exceptions are communicated may have an impact on the outcome of surgical treatment. The psychosocial component is no less important than either of the others, particularly in the context of managed care cost-containment strategies. The patient's social comorbidities may have as much to do with the outcome as the implant used, mode of fixation, or amount of bone graft used in

N. A. Johanson: Department of Orthopaedic Surgery, Temple University School of Medicine, Philadelphia, Pennsylvania 19140.

the reconstruction. Home discharge for an elderly patient who lives alone in the inner city may carry more risk for a bad outcome than for a patient who goes home to a supportive environment with ready resources for maximizing the comfort and safety of the home.

The volume of revision total hip replacement is rising with the increasing volume of hip replacements being performed. They are more complex, more expensive, and require more preoperative planning and surgical expertise to achieve acceptable results. Failures of revision tend to occur sooner and usually present even more complex and costly problems than primary procedures and first-time revisions. The best opportunity for achieving good results is the first. This is true for both primary and revision operations. Optimizing postoperative medical, physical, and psychosocial care is an integral part of cutting the losses that are inherent in revision total hip replacement.

MEDICAL MANAGEMENT

Blood Loss, Salvage, and Transfusion

Because of the increase in operative time and extent of surgical exposure in revision total hip replacement the average blood loss is considerably greater than in a primary operation (2). Therefore strategies that minimize blood loss, enhance the salvage of blood, and involve autologous blood transfusion have been formulated with the goal of accelerating normalization of the patient's sense of vitality and functional status. The patterns of use of transfusion, however, are changing in the face of cost constraints placed on hospitals and blood banks. Clinical judgment regarding the suitability of transfusion continues to be the most important factor in the decision (4). The pressure has been to raise the threshold of transfusion to keep blood use to a minimum. One institution reported the charge for one unit of autologous blood to be $114, whereas the charge for a unit of homologous packed red blood cells was $78 (15). Intraoperative salvage of blood by use of the Cell-Saver system (Haemonetics, Braintree, Md.) resulted in charges of $839 for up to 4 hours of use. It was concluded that more than ten units of blood would have to be salvaged for use of the Cell-Saver system to be deemed cost effective. Analyses such as these point toward important realities and suggest trends but are clouded in their accuracy by the murky distinction between hospital costs and charges. In summary, unless more than five units of blood loss is anticipated, it seems reasonable to rely on the autologous blood program and, if necessary, banked blood for transfusion.

Use of genetically recombinant erythropoietin has been advocated for enhancement of vigor and a sense of vitality after elective operations such as hip replacement. Hemoglobin levels have been found to be maintained at higher perioperative levels (5). When combined with an autologous blood donation program, use of erythropoietin may increase the amount of blood that can be collected preoperatively (7). Although this drug is a promising ally in approaching surgical procedures with high anticipated blood loss, its efficacy and cost effectiveness in more routine conditions has yet to be demonstrated.

Antithrombotic Prophylaxis

Because of the high rate of deep venous thrombosis after total hip replacement without prophylaxis it is generally accepted that some form of anticoagulation be used (17). The most popular medical prophylaxis includes warfarin, low-molecular-weight heparin, low-dose unfractionated heparin, or aspirin (18). Mechanical means of prevention of deep venous thrombosis after total hip replacement have gained considerable popularity as either stand-alone or adjuvant agents. Sequential compression boots and foot pumps have been shown to be effective prophylactic tools (17). The rapid decline in length of hospital stay has presented the surgeon with a dilemma, especially when using warfarin, which takes 2 or more days to reach anticoagulant blood levels. The management and dosing of warfarin is critical for avoiding either nontherapeutic levels or high levels that lead to bleeding complications. Many patients discharged within 4 or 5 days have too short a period for establishing a stable warfarin dosage. It is now common for anticoagulation to be handled by a primary care physician, who may not have the same approach to managing warfarin dosing as the surgeon. An alternative to routinely discharging patients taking warfarin is early screening with either venography or venous duplex imaging. If no proximal thrombi are identified, the patient is discharged with a 6-week regimen of aspirin or low-molecular-weight heparin, both of which do not require monitoring of prothrombin time for dosage determination.

Screening and Therapy for Deep Venous Thrombosis

Venography has been considered to be the standard for diagnosis of deep venous thrombosis (14). Duplex venous imaging has been developed in many centers as the procedure of choice for diagnosing deep venous thrombosis because in skilled hands the technique is as sensitive as venography, less painful, and may be repeated as many times as appropriate. The decision to use venous duplex imaging should be based on the local success of an institution in matching the sensitivity of venography. Currently there is some controversy as to the cost effectiveness of any screening strategy compared with a routine 6-week warfarin or low-molecular-weight heparin regimen (14). If thrombosis is found while the patient is still in the hospital, a more aggressive approach to anticoagulation may be triggered, particularly if the thrombus is proximal to the knee. A 6-week to 3-month course of warfarin keeping the international normalized ratio (INR) between 2.5 and 3 is recommended for all proximal thrombi, whereas a prophylactic warfarin regimen with no screening would maintain the INR between 2 and 2.5 for 6 weeks.

Perioperative Antibiotics

Because of the frequent uncertainty regarding sepsis in failed total hip replacement administration of all antibiotics should be held until satisfactory intraoperative cultures are obtained. A broad spectrum antibiotic such as cefazolin (1 g every 8 hours) may be started and continued for 48 hours or until the definitive intraoperative culture report is obtained. Even if a preoperative positive culture result is obtained, if no clinical suspicion of infection is present (radiographic or systemic) there does not appear to be any advantage to tailoring the routine prophylactic regimen. Barrack and Harris (3) reported that among 270 preoperative aspirations, none of the 6 infections occurred in the absence of a high clinical suspicion. On the other hand Padgett et al. (12) reported a 30% rate of positivity of intraoperative cultures, only one of which was found to be an infection. Fitzgerald et al. (6) stated that positive culture results for specimens obtained intraoperatively from hips previously operated on were more likely to be significant, and they recommended appropriate antibiotic therapy for 3 to 6 weeks after the operation. Therefore, if there is no pre- or postoperative clinical suspicion of infection, and the intraoperative culture results are negative, prophylactic antibiotics may be stopped at 48 hours. If a positive culture result is obtained, appropriate antibiotics should be given postoperatively unless this is considered a false-positive result.

PHYSICAL MANAGEMENT

Wound Management

When making the incision for revision total hip replacement the surgeon often uses all or a part of the scar left from previous procedures. When a completely different approach is planned, caution is used in making parallel incisions, which should be separated by at least 5 cm. In a posterior approach when an anterior or lateral approach has been performed, the previous scar should intersect at as close to a right angle as possible. This minimizes the potential for wound necrosis. The extensive incisions that may be needed in performing revision total hip replacement are most commonly encountered during difficult femoral stem extraction or massive structural allografting. Wound necrosis in the gluteal region, where incisions may be parallel or divergent, and intramuscular or subfascial hematoma formation are the most common cause of wound problems. The use of deep and superficial drains to eliminate accumulation of blood in the resulting dead space is recommended. Meticulous multilayered surgical closure is the most important preventive strategy for minimizing the dangers associated with wound hematoma.

Diagnosis of wound hematoma requires regular inspection and palpation of the thigh and gluteal region. If more than the expected swelling is found in the thigh in association with unremitting pain; bloody drainage, and increasing localized erythema, a subfascial hematoma should be suspected. An unexpected drop in hemoglobin level may offer supporting evidence of hematoma, but blood cell counts often are difficult to interpret in light of the marked fluid shifts during the early postoperative period. A computed tomographic scan of the thigh may help locate a fluid collection, but findings of this sort often are nonspecific. Accurate and timely diagnosis depends primarily on the clinical judgment of the surgeon.

Management of postoperative wound hematoma depends on the size of the hematoma, the amount and appearance of drainage, and associated systemic signs of infection. If a draining hematoma is left without definitive therapy more than a few days there is high risk for development of infection in a retrograde direction through the evolving sinus tract. Therefore the decision to incise and drain a draining hematoma is made promptly. A nondraining but painful swollen thigh is observed for 2 weeks. In the absence of any systemic signs of infection (increasing fever, erythrocyte sedimentation rate, or white blood cell count) or local erythema, swelling and pain should begin to subside in 2 weeks as the hematoma resorbs. If it appears that the hematoma is about to drain spontaneously or if there is suspicion of infection, the conservative approach is surgical exploration, evacuation, and irrigation of the subfascial space and collection of multiple cultures of fluid and tissue. This preventive strategy helps to rule out an insidious infection and makes both patient and surgeon more comfortable. After incision and drainage, the wound is closed over suction drains, which remain until the drainage is minimal and the final culture result is negative. A broad-spectrum antibiotic such as cefazolin (1 g every 8 hours) is continued until infection is ruled out.

Bed Rest

The use of prolonged in-hospital bed rest as a distinctive treatment modality is rapidly disappearing from orthopedic practice. If a patient is not acutely ill with an illness or mechanical complication such as a fracture that necessitates surgical intervention or traction, there is little justification for bed rest in the acute care setting. A postoperative patient with substantial structural compromise of the supporting bone (either host or graft) around the implant or jeopardized soft-tissue integrity may be a candidate for a period of bed rest with or without a spica cast either in a skilled nursing facility or at home (8).

Transfer Activities

Transferring a patient in and out of bed may result in torsional stress at the hip joint unless transfer is performed with maximal assistance under ideal conditions with an experienced therapist or member of the nursing staff. If the patient is moved into the sitting position and asked to come independently to the standing position, considerable posterior torsional moment around the femoral component results. When fixation is considered compromised because of poor bone stock, the patient should receive maximum assistance in transfers until stability is achieved according to radiographic criteria. It is common during a revision procedure to encounter a widened, smooth, sclerotic femoral canal and cavitary defects in the acetabulum that may compromise bone contact and implant stability for both cemented and cementless components. Intraoperative observation and judgment are essential for deciding the appropriate restrictions in postoperative transfer activity.

Weight Bearing

There are many philosophies in the management of weight bearing status even after primary total hip replacement. It is not surprising that a uniform protocol for weight bearing after revision operations would be both impossible and dangerous. The severity of the condition that resulted in the need for revision is a primary factor in predicting optimal postoperative weight-bearing status. Preoperative bone quality is most commonly compromised by wear-induced osteolysis. Thinning of cortical bone predisposes to compromised fixation or fracture if distal load transfer to good bone is not achieved. The technical difficulty of the operation is an important factor (8). The surgeon must assess how much additional damage to bone occurred during implant removal and reinsertion. Windows placed in the femoral cortex for cement removal, especially if not bypassed by two canal diameters by the revision implant, may act as stress risers for propagation of a fracture under normal weight-bearing conditions. Partial weight bearing for up to 12 weeks may be needed to allow the femur to remodel. Longitudinal cracks in the femur may propagate during implant removal or insertion. If a crack is recognized before insertion of the revision prosthesis, cables may be placed. If the resulting fracture stability is satisfactory and the remainder of the revision proceeds uneventfully, a normal weight-bearing schedule may be implemented. If the crack occurs during revision implant insertion, it is more difficult to assess the stability of the fracture. If the crack extends below the level of the lesser trochanter, cables are applied. Postoperative weight-bearing status depends on the extent of the crack, the quality of the bone, and the quality of distal femoral fixation. If allograft is used to augment bone stock, there may be no compromise in weight-bearing status. On the other hand, structural bulk allograft used to augment deficient bone stock or to enhance the stability of fracture fixation may require an extended period of bed rest followed by 3 to 6 months of no weight bearing.

Determining the appropriate weight bearing status based on acetabular component stability may be difficult because of the variable amount of contained and uncontained bone loss (13). After reaming, the amount of rim remaining, particularly in the anterior and posterior columns, and prosthetic contact and support from the dome are the primary determinants of prosthetic stability (16). This construct may be augmented by one or more screws. In general, if the acetabular component is stable enough after impaction not to require screws, full weight bearing may be allowed. If stability is questionable and screw fixation is necessary but bony coverage is present with at least 75% of the rim and 25% of the dome, a partial weight-bearing regimen with crutches for 8 to 12 weeks is recommended. If stability, coverage, and bony contact are severely compromised, screw fixation followed by 3 months of no weight bearing is recommended. Alternatively, a bulk allograft may be used, which would require no weight bearing for 6 to 12 months.

Trochanteric Precautions

When the greater trochanter has been removed during a revision operation, it is reattached to the proximal femur with wire, cables, adjuvant mesh, specialized gripping devices fastened with wires or cables, or a broad-headed bolt inserted through a hole in the femoral prosthesis. No single method has been proved definitively to be superior to another, and each has its own particular advantages and pitfalls (9–11). The technique used should be familiar to the surgeon and appropriate for the quality of trochanteric bone, abductor mechanism, and bony bed of the proximal femur to which the trochanter is attached. The bone quality of the trochanteric fragment is determined by the location of the osteotomy and the amount of bone destroyed by osteolysis or the effects of previous surgical intervention. In general postoperative management after trochanteric osteotomy and reattachment is determined by the surgeon's confidence in the bone quality and the security of fixation. Normal trochanteric bone with a flexible abductor mechanism attached to a healthy bed of proximal femoral bone may result in virtually no deviation from routine postoperative weight bearing and exercise. A small wafer of trochanter brought down to the proximal femur only after extensive abductor release may be treated with extensive protective measures such as abduction bracing or casting, limited weight bearing with crutches for 6 to 8 weeks, and graduated adduction to stretch the gluteus medius.

The complications of trochanteric fixation failure include acute dislocation, limp, painful nonunion, and painful broken hardware (1). Reoperation to establish secure fixation is indicated unless the patient's medical condition does not allow or the condition is chronic and in the surgeon's judgment the abductor mechanism is irreversibly contracted. In many cases a stable, fibrous union is established with little resulting pain or impairment. The key to proper patient care when there is tenuous trochanteric fixation is careful radiographic follow-up evaluation and assessment of the patient's symptoms combined with measures to minimize stress on the abductor mechanism until sufficient healing has occurred.

Prevention of Dislocation

The incidence of dislocation after revision operations is much higher than after primary total hip arthroplasty. The usual postoperative hip precautions are used after revision operations with modifications according to the degree of bone-stock compromise, prosthetic fixation, trochanteric fixation, and overall stability of the joint. Compromised acetabular fixation may result in tilting to a more vertical or retroverted position. Compromised torsional stability of the femoral component may result in retroversion during activities such as stair climbing or rising from a sitting position. Migration of this sort may lead to dislocation. Acute loss of trochanteric fixation may result in prosthetic dislocation, which necessitates open reduction and reattachment. If no prosthetic migration has occurred and the greater trochanter is well fixed, dislocation usually can be treated with closed reduction followed by abduction bracing with a flexion stop. In more complex situations in which muscle strength, spasticity, or patient compliance is in doubt, a spica cast or rigid brace may be used. Otherwise surgical correction of the underlying cause of joint instability may be necessary.

Exercise and Activity

Exercise after revision total hip replacement must be tailored to the abilities and goals of the patient and the mechanical stability of the implants, bone, and soft tissue. In general, walking with or without support is the safest and most effective exercise for restoration of strength and overall conditioning, and it may be used to supplement the standard regimen. After 4 to 6 weeks water walking may be instituted. After 6 to 8 weeks the patient may begin to use an exercise bike without resistance but with care to avoid excessive flexion. Radiographic confirmation of prosthetic position and fixation precedes each substantial change in exercise regimen. The use of aggressive weight-training programs provides no improvement in the overall symptomatic and functional outcome of surgical treatment and may actually increase risk for mechanical failure of the implants, particularly in cementless procedures.

Six to 12 weeks after stable total hip revision, the patient may return to activities of daily living and light duties at work. After a complicated operation with some degree of inherent instability, these activities should be postponed for 3 to 6 months or longer.

PSYCHOSOCIAL MANAGEMENT

Expectations of Revision Surgery

Loosening, implant breakage, and infection are associated with considerable pain before revision surgery. Successful revision surgery for these conditions most likely results in satisfactory pain relief and functional gain—outcomes that are readily understood and appreciated by the patient. When discussing revision total hip replacement, it is important to emphasize the limitations, risks, and potential for inferior durability compared with primary total hip replacement.

Conditions such as polyethylene or other particulate wear and painless osteolysis demand in-depth explanation in terms that help the patient understand the potentially disastrous effects of the problem if left unmanaged and the preventive benefits of revision surgery. On the other hand, these factors must be weighed against the actual risks of revision. Removal of a well-fixed stem or socket alone may result in morbidity and bone loss, possibly in excess of the short-term effects of the condition being treated. As with the primary operation, the decision to operate is shared by patient and surgeon to promote acceptance and satisfaction with the outcome. The least invasive procedure is performed (exchange of a modular head or socket to arrest generation of wear debris). The operation is tailored to the patient's current medical condition and activity level. If the patient thoroughly understands the rationale and treatment alternatives before undergoing a revision operation, the postoperative course is more tolerable.

Cognitive Function

A patient's understanding of the rationale and expected outcomes of revision total hip replacement has an important effect on the speed and ease of surgical recovery. Cognitive impairment naturally obfuscates a timely progression of inpatient mobilization, physical therapy, and instruction in activities of daily living and ultimately delays hospital discharge or transfer to alternative levels of care. If there are limitations and precautions that have to be observed, such as protected weight bearing or limited active abduction, the patient's cognitive function may influence the outcome. Causes of cognitive impairment include hypersensitivity to or overuse of certain medications such as narcotic analgesics and sedatives, heightened anxiety, cerebral vascular compromise due to hypotension, hypoventilation, atherosclerosis, metabolic encephalopathy, or a combination of two or more of these factors. Elderly patients are particularly prone to postoperative cognitive impairment, even in the absence of important preoperative signs and symptoms. Depression may complicate patients' recovery, sapping them of the motivation necessary to complete rigorous physical therapy.

In the setting of a postoperative cognitive impairment, a thorough neurologic evaluation is performed to rule out treatable or reversible conditions. The carotid arteries are checked for the presence of bruits, and cardiopulmonary status is evaluated and optimized. A minimum amount of narcotic analgesics and sedatives is administered. The patient is encouraged to remain active during the day to avoid reversal of normal sleep patterns. Frequent checks of vital signs, serum blood chemistry, hemoglobin and hematocrit, and arterial blood gases and chest radiography should be routine in the care of patients with cognitive impairment. Magnetic resonance imaging or computed tomography of the head is considered, especially in the setting of new focal neurologic signs. If at all possible, physical therapy and mobilization are continued to prevent pulmonary and thromboembolic complications. If metabolic and neurologic causes of cognitive impairment have been ruled out, a psychiatric examination should be performed. Temporary medical management of acute psychiatric disorders related to surgical intervention and hospitalization may be particularly helpful in facilitating postoperative recovery.

Family Support and Public Resources

A supportive family with resources to assist the patient's recovery is a most important determining feature of the rate and quality of postoperative recovery. This is true for primary operations but is particularly applicable in revision, in which there may be special needs and treatment options that necessitate close, continuous monitoring. As the managed care model begins to affect the elderly and lower socioeconomic strata of our society there will be a much more restrictive approach to the services that people need in lieu of the support of a healthy and financially secure family (3). Most typical managed care organizations do not highly regard social comorbidity as a determinant of covered services, simply because up to this point they have focused their efforts on recruiting a healthy and employed population. This will not be possible when entire populations of low-income people are moved precipitously into a managed care environment. Surgeons who practice revision surgery need to be mindful that 3 or 4 days after an operation, they might lose control of the patient's care, and worse yet, the patient may be transferred into a setting in which the caregivers have little or no knowledge of appropriate patient care.

As a result there will be pressure either to limit the extent of surgical intervention that alters the routine postoperative course or to stop performing revision operations altogether. These pressures must be resisted and quality medical care must be maintained.

As in all areas of medicine, the social and economic impact of decisions and policy are at center stage. Revision total hip replacement will be discussed more and more in terms of cost and benefit. It is especially important for surgeons who perform revision to be active participants in the debate and solidify their role as patient advocates. The postoperative care of patients who undergo revision operations can be complex and fraught with risk. The protection that has been available in the form of additional services, including length of hospital stay and home care, is jeopardized. It is still unclear how deep the reductions in care can be before quality suffers. In this sense patients who need revision procedures are highly vulnerable and are likely to suffer first.

REFERENCES

1. Amstutz HC, Maki S. Complications of trochanteric osteotomy in total hip replacement. *J Bone Joint Surg Am* 1978;60:214–216.
2. Barrack RL. Economics of revision total hip arthroplasty. *Clin Orthop* 1995;319:209–214.
3. Barrack RL, Harris WH. The Value of aspiration of the hip joint before revision total hip arthroplasty. *J Bone Joint Surg Am* 1993;75:66–76.
4. Consensus Conference. Perioperative red cell transfusion. *JAMA* 1988;260:2700–2703.
5. deAndrade JR, Jove M, Landon G, Frei D, Guilfoyle M, Young DC. Baseline hemoglobin as a predictor of risk of transfusion and response to epoetin alfa in orthopedic surgery patients. *Am J Orthop* 1996;25:533–542.
6. Fitzgerald RH Jr, Peterson FA, Washington JA II, Van Scoy RE, Coventry MB. Bacterial colonization of wounds and sepsis in total hip arthroplasty. *J Bone Joint Surg Am* 1973;55:1242–1250.
7. Goodnough LT, Rudnick S, Price TH, et al. Increased preoperative collection of autologous blood with recombinant human erythropoietin therapy. *N Engl J Med* 1989;321:1163–1168.
8. Gross ARE, Hutchison CR, Alexeeff M, Mahomed N, Leitch K, Morsi E. Proximal femoral allografts for reconstruction of bone stock in revision arthroplasty of the hip. *Clin Orthop* 1995;319:151–158.
9. Krengel WG, Turner RH. Trochanteric revision. In: Turner RH, Scheller AD, eds. *Revision total hip arthroplasty.* New York: Grune & Stratton, 1982:249–263.
10. McGrory BJ, Bal BS, Harris WH. Trochanteric osteotomy for total hip arthroplasty: six variations and indications for their use. *J Am Acad Orthop Surg* 1996;4:258–267.
11. Nercessian OA, Newton PM, Joshi RP, Sheikh B, Eftekhar NS. Trochanteric osteotomy and wire fixation: a comparison of 2 techniques. *Clin Orthop* 1996;333:208–216.
12. Padgett DE, Silverman A, Sachjowicz F, Simpson RB, Rosenberg AG, Galante JO. Efficacy of intraoperative cultures obtained during revision total hip arthroplasty. *J Arthroplasty* 1995;10:420–426.
13. Paprosky WG, Magnus RE. Principles of bone grafting in revision total hip arthroplasty: acetabular technique. *Clin Orthop* 1994;298:147–155.
14. Pellegrini VD Jr, Clement D, Lush-Ehmann C, Keller GS, Evarts CM. Natural history of thromboembolic disease after total hip arthroplasty. *Clin Orthop* 1996;333:27–40.
15. Rollo VJ, Hozack WJ, Rothman RH, Chao W, Eng KO. Prospective randomized evaluation of blood salvage techniques for primary total hip arthroplasty. *J Arthroplasty* 1995;10:532–539.
16. Silverton CD, Rosenberg AG, Sheinkop MB, Kull LR, Galante JO. Revision total hip arthroplasty using a cementless acetabular component: technique and results. *Clin Orthop* 1995;319:201–208.
17. Wilson MG. Orthopedic surgery. In: Goldhaber SZ, ed. *Prevention of venous thromboembolism.* New York: Marcel Dekker, 1993:373–404.
18. Zimlich RH, Fulbright BM, Friedman RJ. Current status of anticoagulation therapy after total hip and total knee arthroplasty. *J Am Acad Orthop Surg* 1996;4:54–62.

Revision Total Hip Arthroplasty,
edited by Marvin E. Steinberg and Jonathan P. Garino,
Lippincott Williams & Wilkins, Philadelphia © 1999.

25

Results

Robert B. Bourne and H. A. Crawford

Low-friction arthroplasty has evolved as one of the most successful medical interventions of the twentieth century (3,52). To date, more than six million total hip replacements have been performed worldwide, dramatically improving quality of life and providing outstanding durability for 10 or more years. The success of total hip replacement has led to a broadening of the indications for this procedure, particularly to younger and younger, more active patients. As such, aseptic loosening, wear-induced osteolysis, infection, and dislocation have prompted an ever increasing need for revision total hip replacement (Fig. 1).

In many countries, revision total hip arthroplasty represents as many as 10% to 20% of all total hip replacements performed. In the United States, 1995 figures revealed that 169,803 primary and 28,129 (11%) revision total hip replacements were performed, increases of 3% and 2.5% from 1994 data. Revision total hip replacement presents its own challenges in terms of determining the failure mechanism, exposure, extracting the implants, selecting the proper revision implants, dealing with bone defects, optimizing results, and cost containment.

In this chapter, acetabular and femoral revisions are dealt with separately, so that the reader may deal with one issue at a time. Whenever possible, 10-year follow-up data are relied on, but the evolutionary nature of revision total hip arthroplasty makes this impossible in all instances.

RESULTS OF ACETABULAR REVISION

The success or failure of revision acetabular reconstruction is largely proportional to the presence or absence of substantial acetabular bone loss (25,29). Every acetabular revision has

R. B. Bourne and H. A. Crawford: Department of Surgery, Division of Orthopaedic Surgery, The University of Western Ontario and London Health Sciences Center, London, Ontario, Canada N6A 5A5.

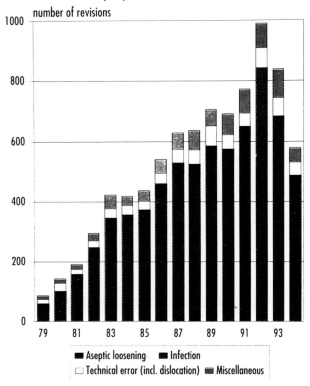

Figure 1. Reasons for revision total hip arthroplasty as determined from the Swedish Hip Registry.

some degree of bone deficiency, ranging from relatively minor to severe. In simplest terms, most acetabular bone defects are contained, uncontained, or combinations of both. Several studies have suggested that structural allografts are needed in approximately one fourth of acetabular revisions (58). The clinical outcomes of acetabular revision requiring structural allografts have been demonstrated to be inferior to those that do not require such reconstruction

Table 1. *American Academy of Orthopaedic Surgeons classification of acetabular bone deficiency*

Type	Deficiency
I	Segmental
	Peripheral
	Superior
	Anterior
	Posterior
	Central (medial wall absent)
II	Cavitary
	Peripheral
	Superior
	Anterior
	Posterior
	Central (medial wall intact)
III	Combined
IV	Pelvic discontinuity
V	Arthrodesis or ankylosis

Table 2. *Garbuz-Gross classification of acetabular bone defects*

Type	Defect
1	Contained cavitary
2A	Segmental >50% host support
2B	Segmental <50% host support

(34). Without a universally accepted classification system, it is difficult to compare the clinical results of one series with those of another. Many classification systems exist, but unfortunately one is not universally accepted. The American Academy of Orthopaedic Surgeons (AAOS) study group proposed the useful classification system outlined in Table 1 (9).

Several authors have found the AAOS classification to be not specific enough, particularly with issues such as host bone support for the acetabular reconstruction, elevation of the joint line, or a description of rim support of the implant. Garbuz, Gross, and Morsi et al. (17,19,21,50) proposed a simple classification system, which has proved useful in our hands (Table 2). Garbuz et al. found that type 1 contained defects were treated with morselized allograft/autograft with 90% success among 54 patients after 7 years of follow-up study (17). Type 2A segmental defects were treated with structural allografts with 90% success after 7 years of follow-up study among 29 patients. Only one allograft did not unite with the host. Patients with Type 2B segmental defects and less than 50% host support presented the main problems in this series. Among 33 patients with Type 2B defects observed 7 years, 45% of those treated with segmental allografts alone needed re-revision. Conversely, among 8 patients with type 2B defects treated with segmental allografts and reinforcement rings, a 100% success rate was achieved. The importance of host bone support cannot be emphasized enough. The efficacy of reinforcement rings in complex acetabular revision procedures is now recognized (19). The value of such a classification system in analyzing like clinical problems and directing proper interventional strategies is clear.

Debate also exist as to the advantages of accepting a high hip center as opposed to use of a structural allograft (39,47,67,70). Proponents of a high hip center suggest that as long as the acetabular socket is not lateralized, forces through the hip are not increased. Several clinical studies have demonstrated the effectiveness of a high hip center. Most authors

Table 3. *Results of acetabular revision arthroplasty*

Authors	No. of hips	Follow-up period (yr)	Rate of good to excellent results	Re-revision rate	Radiographic loosening rate
Cemented					
Izquierdo and Northmore-Ball (33)	148	5.5	95%	—	10%
Kavanagh et al. (37)	166	4.5 (2–10.5)	62%	2%	20%
Pellicci et al. (59)	99	8.1 (5–12.5)	63%	3%	—
Mulroy and Harris (53)	29	15.1 (14.2–17.5)	55%	38%	62%
Raut et al. (63–65)	87	6 (1.9–18.1)	91%	10%	30%
Kershaw et al. (38)	60	6.3 (2.5–12)	44%	3%	8%
Weber et al. (72)	56	6.4 (5–8)	92%	0%	21%
Impaction grafting–cemented					
Azuma et al. (2)	24	5.8	—	0%	8%
Levai and Boisgard (42)	39	3	—	7%	—
Sloof et al. (68)	88	5.8	89%	5%	—
Cementless					
Lawrence et al. (40,41)	43	9 (5–13)	83%	7%	11%
Paprosky and Magnus (58)	316	5.1	76%	—	—
Silverton et al. (67)	138	8.3 (6.5–11.3)	58%	5%	5%
Lachiewicz and Hussamy (39)	60	5 (2.9.8)	80%	0%	0%
Dorr and Wan (11)	139	4.3 (2–9.8)	77%	4.3%	1%
Weber et al. (72)	61	6.4 (5–8)	92%	0%	2%

Values in parentheses are ranges.

accept elevation of the hip center by 1.5 to 2 cm. If the hip center is elevated more than 2 cm, various studies have suggested higher failure rates, increased risk for instability, leg-length problems, and altered hip kinematics. As a consequence, if the hip center is elevated more than 2 cm, most authors prefer to restore the center of rotation of the hip.

The choice of acetabular component is controversial. Reports in the literature do not advocate use of bipolar devices (6). Debate exists about whether the revision acetabular component should be cemented or cementless. Much of the controversy arises from the lack of a universally accepted classification system and hence an inability to compare

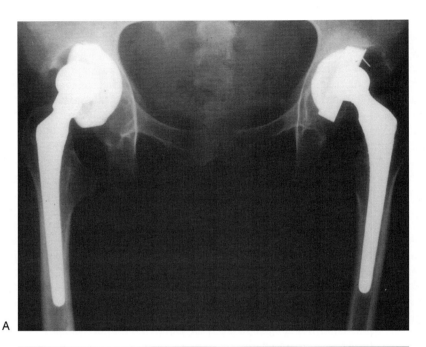

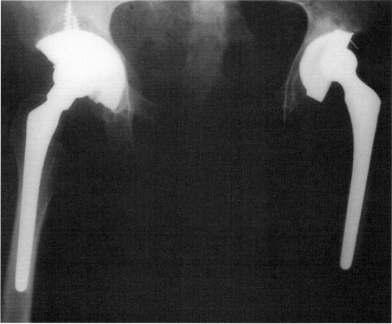

Figure 2. Contemporary cementless acetabular revision total hip arthroplasty of right hip. **A:** Failed cementless acetabular component with a contained defect. **B:** Revision acetabular arthroplasty with morselized allograft, screw fixation, and cementless Reflection socket (Smith and Nephew, Memphis, Tenn.).

cemented with cementless devices in like clinical situations. Although good results have been quoted for both cemented and cementless acetabular revisions, the trend in 1997 is toward cementless revision, provided there is at least 60% viable host bone contact and a stable acetabular reconstruction. Table 3 summarizes the most recent results with cemented (with or without impaction grafting) and cementless revision acetabular reconstruction. Our current approach to various acetabular reconstructions is summarized as follows.

Contained Defects

A contained acetabular defect implies an enlarged acetabular socket with retained structural support and usually sclerotic bone. Initially only ultrahigh-molecular-weight polyethylene (UHMWPE) acetabular components were available. Historically, most surgeons simply removed the loose acetabular component and pseudomembrane, made multiple cement-seating holes, and recemented a larger UHMWPE acetabular component in place. The results of such an approach were somewhat disappointing and are summarized in Table 3.

The less than stellar results of use of cemented acetabular components in the management of contained defects led surgeons to seek new solutions. Cementless fixation supplemented with screw and occasionally fin fixation has gained considerable support (39). With this approach, the opening of the acetabulum is enlarged with reamers so that at least anterior and posterior rim support can be achieved for the cementless implant. Morselized, cancellous autograft/allograft is used to fill small bony defects. Dome or rim screw fixation usually is used to enhance cementless acetabular cup fixation. The results of this approach have been encouraging and are summarized in Table 3. Lessons learned have been the need for thicker polyethylene (at least 6 mm, preferably 8 to 10 mm), conforming polyethylene, and a secure polyethylene locking mechanism. Advances have been made in the proper placement of acetabular component fixation screws, polishing of the metal backing, and design and number of screws used. An example of such a revision acetabular arthroplasty is shown in Fig. 2.

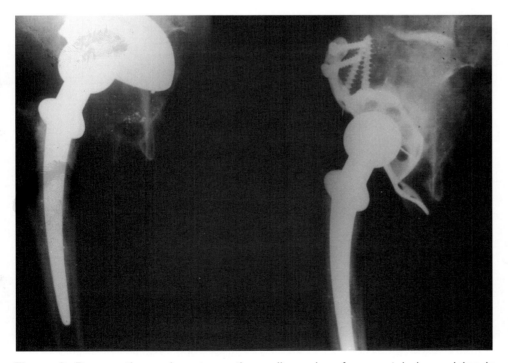

Figure 3. Preoperative and postoperative radiographs of an acetabular revision in which structural and morselized allograft reconstruction was supported by a Burch-Schneider ring (Sulzer, Winterthur, Switzerland).

Noncontained Acetabular Defects

Noncontained acetabular defects include an absent acetabular rim, column, or medial wall. Each is dealt with separately.

Acetabular Rim Defects

The most common sites for a rim defect are posterosuperior, superior, and anterior. Cement fixation of an all-polyethylene acetabular socket has not met with stellar results because unsupported cement performs poorly (see Table 3). Structural allografts with femoral head or distal femur have been proposed for these defects. Debate exists with regard to the efficacy of femoral head allografts (29,30,34,71). Paprosky and Magnus (58) has popularized a figure seven, distal femoral allograft construct with encouraging results. Cementless acetabular socket fixation has been advocated when there is at least 60% living bone against the cementless socket. Cemented fixation is advocated otherwise. Allograft has been used with less frequency in rim defects. Instead, jumbo cementless acetabular components have been used with supplemental dome and rim screw fixation. Morselized autograft/allograft has been used to fill in any defects (39,55).

Column Defects

Anterior and posterior column defects are less commonly encountered. Many anterior rim and column defects can be ignored. Posterior and posterolateral column defects usually necessitate reconstruction. Femoral head allografts often are too small to reconstruct a posterosuperior column defect. The use of a figure seven, distal femoral allograft has proved useful in these unusual situations (58). Cement fixation of an all polyethylene acetabular component usually is advisable in these situations because more

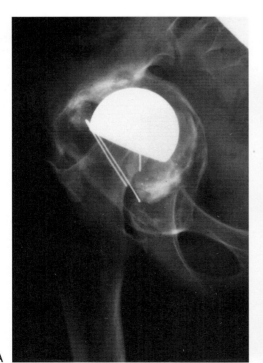
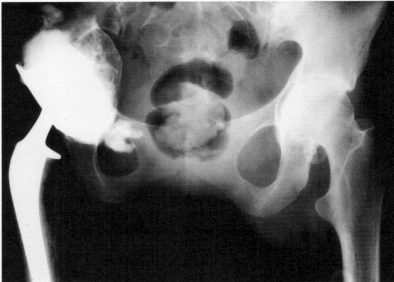

A   B

Figure 4. Fourteen-year follow-up status of a failed surface replacement salvaged with cemented femoral and acetabular components, morselized bone graft and an antiprotrusio ring (Howmedica, East Rutherford, N.J.). **A:** Preoperative appearance. **B:** Postoperative appearance at 14 years.

than 60% of the acetabular socket is made up of allograft. If there is less than 50% host support, the use of a reinforcement ring is advised in conjunction with a structural allograft (Fig. 3) (60).

Medial Wall Defects

Noncontained, medial-wall defects are relatively common. Most are less than 1 to 2 cm in diameter. Hastings demonstrated the efficacy of particulate allograft, wire mesh, and cementing an all-polyethylene socket in this instance (24a). Sloof et al. (68) developed an impaction grafting technique in which the noncontained defect is made a contained defect and an all-polyethylene socket is cemented into the densely compacted cancellous allograft. Others have advocated the use of protrusio rings in association with particulate graft. With large, noncontained medial-wall defects, use of protrusio cages such as Burch-Schneider rings and allograft are gaining support. An example of 14-year follow-up status after the use of particulate graft, wire mesh, and a protrusio ring is shown in Fig. 4.

RESULTS OF FEMORAL REVISION

As with acetabular revision arthroplasty, femoral revision total hip replacement is influenced greatly by the bone defect present (10,28,66,69). This is an important consideration in assessment of the results of revision operations, because the bone defect can determine implant selection, surgical technique, and outcome. Numerous classifications of bone defects exist. The AAOS classification of femoral bone defects is outlined in Table 4. Our preference is to use a classification based on the cancellous bone remaining and the intactness of the cortical tube (Table 5). We use this classification to discuss the results of revision of femoral components.

Other factors also affect the clinical outcome of femoral revision operations. The mechanism of failure of the primary component may contribute to failure of the revision component. For example, revision for sepsis results in a higher infection rate in revision operations than revision for aseptic loosening (73). Revision for instability has a higher incidence of recurrent instability than other revisions (74). Patients with osteolysis may be predisposed to further osteolysis after revision.

When interpreting results one has to be aware of the different methods of analysis. It is important to know whether the patients were in a consecutive series or whether they were selected for a particular technique. Different authors use different hip scores in their assessments. For example, the Harris hip score may not be as rigorous as the d'Aubigne score (23). The hip scores also are used to assess the acetabular side of the total hip revision, so when one looks at the results of femoral revision in isolation, this must be taken into account.

Survivorship analysis is another method of looking at total hip revision outcome. Survivorship can be affected by patients' being "lost to follow-up" skewing the results and by the choice of "end point" for survivorship analysis. For example, some authors use re-revision as the end point whereas others combine this point with definite radiologic

Table 4. *American Academy of Orthopaedic Surgeons classification of femoral bone deficiency*

Defect type	Description
I	Segmental
II	Cavitary
III	Combined (segmental and cavitary)
IV	Malalignment
V	Femoral stenosis
VI	Femoral discontinuity

Table 5. *Bourne-Rorabeck classification of femoral bone deficiency*

Defect type	Description
1	Intact cancellous bone, intact cortical tube
2	Deficient cancellous bone, intact cortical tube
3	Deficient cancellous bone and cortical tube
4	Absent cancellous bone and cortical tube

loosening for survivorship analysis. This raises the problem of interpretation of radiographs for loosening and the definitions of "definitely" or "probably" loose.

Clinical results can be satisfactory despite evidence of loosening. This often makes the decision to revise an arthroplasty more difficult. The length of follow-up period also affects the results of revision hip operations. It has been found in primary hip replacement that follow-up evaluation has to be long term (more than 10 years) to have any meaningful result. Pellicci et al. (59) showed this deterioration in time when they reviewed 110 revision hip replacements at an average of 3.4 years and then at an average of 8.1 years; they found 29% of replacements had failed in the intervening period. This length of follow-up period is more difficult to attain in revision hip surgery because fewer revisions are performed, so to accumulate a large series, many years elapse. It is important to know whether the results are minimum 5-year results or an average, for example, 2- to 14-year results with a mean 5-year follow-up period. Early surveillance is extremely important in assessing a new implant or surgical technique, because early failure can alert the surgeon to a design problem that can result in implant modification or implant withdrawal. An example of this was the early failure of the proximally coated uncemented revision prostheses that subsided soon after insertion. Finally, patients who undergo hip revision often have undergone multiple operations since the index procedure, making them a very heterogeneous group. Using the classification outlined in Table 5, we examine the published results of femoral revision (Tables 6 and 7) under each category to attempt to compartmentalize this heterogeneous group.

Type 1: Intact Cancellous Bone, Intact Cortical Tube

Examples of a revision total hip replacement with intact cancellous bone and cortical tube include revision of a surface replacement arthroplasty or press-fit endoprosthesis

Table 6. *Results of uncemented femoral revision*

Authors	Component	No. of hips	Follow-up period (yr)	Femoral re-revision or loosening rate
Hedley et al. (27)	PCA	61	1 minimum	9.5% femoral loosening
Gustilo and Pasternak (22)	Bias	57	2.8 mean	4% femoral loosening
Harris et al. (24)	Harris-Galante	23	2 minimum	4% femoral loosening
Engh et al. (15)	AML	127	4 mean	4% femoral loosening
Lawrence et al. (40,41)	AML		7.4 mean	5.7% re-revision
Moreland and Bernstein (48)	AML/Solution	175	5 mean	4% re-revision
Paprosky et al. (57)	Solution	311	5.8 mean	6% re-revision
McCarthy et al. (cited in 7 and 8)	S-ROM	133	5 mean	1.5% re-revision
Durkin et al. (12)	S-ROM		5 minimum	4% re-revision
Mulliken et al. (51)	Mallory-Head	52	4.6 mean	10% re-revision
Woolson and Delaney (cited in 24)	Harris-Galante	25	5.5 mean	20% re-revision

AML, anatomic medullary locking implant (Depuy, Warsaw, Ind.); Bias, Bias component (Zimmer, Warsaw, Ind.); Harris-Galante, Harris-Galante component (Zimmer); Mallory-Head, Mallory-Head stem (Biomet, Warsaw, Ind.); PCA, porous coated anatomic implant (Howmedica, Rutherford, N.J.); Solution, Solution stem (Depuy); S-ROM, S-ROM stem (Joint Medical Products, Stamford, Conn.).

Table 7. *Results of cemented femoral revision*

Authors	No. of hips	Follow-up period (yr)	Femoral rerevision rate
Pellicci et al. (59)	110	8.1 mean	19 (%)
Amstutz et al. (1)	66	2.1 mean	9 (%)
Morrey and Kavanagh (49)	94	—	15 (%)
Estok and Harris (16)	38	11.7 mean	10.5 (%)
Katz and Callaghan (35)	79	10.0 minimum	9.5 (%)
Raut et al. (63–65)	351	6.0 mean	1.6 (%)
Mulroy et al. (52)	43	15.1 mean	20 (%)
Izquierdo and Northmore-Ball (33)	112	6.5 mean	3.6 (%)
Huo and Salvati (32)	113	4.1 mean	3 (%)
Kershaw et al. (38)	220	6.3 mean	4.5 (%)
Pierson and Harris (62)	29	8.5 mean	10 (%)

(Fig. 5). The proximal femur in such cases is essentially the same as the surgeon might encounter with a primary total hip replacement. Either cemented or cementless revision total hip replacements suffice under such circumstances. The results of such revisions are usually as good as primary total hip replacement; most of the long-term problems appear on the acetabular side.

Type 2: Deficient Cancellous Bone, Intact Cortical Tube

A femoral component revision with deficient cancellous bone and an intact cortical tube represents the most common femoral revision scenario. Aseptic loosening of a cemented total hip replacement represents the most common failure mechanism leading to this bone

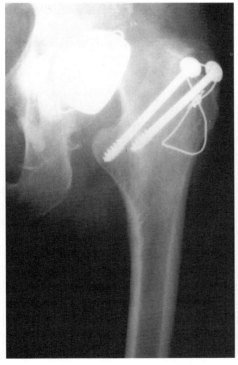
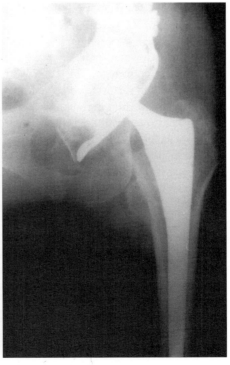

A   B

Figure 5. Type 1 femoral revision of a failed surface replacement arthroplasty (Burch-Schneider ring, Sulzer, Winterthur, Switzerland; Synergy cementless femoral component, Smith and Nephew, Memphis, Tenn.). **A:** Preoperative appearance. **B:** Postoperative appearance.

defect pattern. Simply removing the loose implant and accompanying pseudomembrane and cementing another implant in place with early cementing techniques led to disappointing results. Amstutz et al. (1) at a mean follow-up time of only 2.1 years reported a re-revision rate of 9% and radiographic evidence of femoral loosening in 29%. In another series, Morrey and Kavanagh (49) reported on 94 cemented revisions with probable loosening in 53% and a reoperation rate of 15%.

The main cause of failure of these early-generation cementing techniques was aseptic loosening at the cement–bone interface caused by difficulty obtaining good interdigitation into the sclerotic bone (5). Barrack et al. (4) showed radiographically that modern cementing techniques can give a white-out appearance at the cement–bone interface, indicating complete fill of the medullary canal (4). Dohmae et al. (10) looked at the changes in shear strength at the cement–bone interface in femurs of fresh human cadavers prepared for primary and first and second revisions. First-revision interface shear strength was reduced to 20.6% of primary strength and second revision interface strength to 6.8% of primary strength. This led to the introduction of second- and third-generation cementing techniques with better canal preparation and cement pressurization. The results of these revisions were superior. Estok and Harris (16) reviewed 38 cemented hip revisions after an average follow-up period of 11.7 years and found a re-revision rate of 10.5% for aseptic loosening of the femur and 10.5% definite loosening of the femoral component. This was a 90% survival rate of femoral stems and a 78% frequency of well-fixed femoral stems at an average follow-up time of 11.7 years. Katz and Callaghan (35) reviewed 79 consecutive hip operations in which a cement gun and plug were used. After a minimum follow-up period of 10-years, 9.5% had been re-revised; however, when radiographic "failure" (definite or probable loosening) was added to this re-revision rate, there was a 26.1% failure rate. Raut et al. (63–65) reviewed 351 cemented revision femoral stems after a mean of 6 years and found that 72.1% of patients were pain free. There was radiographic loosening of the femoral stem in 10 (2.8%), and 9 patients had undergone re-revision for mechanical loosening of the stem.

Mulroy and Harris (53) reviewed 43 consecutive operations on unselected patients after an average of 15.1 years of follow-up study. Seven (20%) patients needed revision because of aseptic loosening. Two other patients had radiographic loosening. The authors concluded that younger patients have distinctly poorer results when cemented femoral revisions are performed. This conclusion was confirmed by Retpen and Jensen (66) for a series of 160 consecutive cemented first revisions performed for aseptic loosening. They reported the risk for recurrent loosening was increased if the revision femoral stem did not "overbridge" the tip of the primary stem by one width of the femoral shaft, if the cement mantle was less than 2 mm around the femoral stem, and if the patient was young.

Distally fixed, cementless femoral components have proved useful with cancellous deficiency and an intact cortical tube (Fig. 6). Some surgeons depend entirely on distal support, some fill the ectatic proximal femur with morselized bone graft, and others remove longitudinal strips of cortical bone from the ectatic area and reduce the size of the proximal femoral canal. The results of these cementless revisions are discussed with deficient cancellous bone and cortical tube defects.

Gie et al. (18) popularized impaction grafting and cement fixation of a femoral component in the presence of an intact cortical tube and deficient cancellous bone (Fig. 7). This technique seems to hold great promise in that it adds rather than subtracts bone in the proximal femur. This technique requires an intact femoral tube; therefore any structural defects must be filled with bone graft or wire mesh. Gie et al. reported short-term results of 18 to 49 months for 56 hips revised with this technique. The results were extremely good and histologic studies on retrieved implants showed reconstitution of the proximal bone. Elting et al. (13) reported the results of femoral component revision with compressed morselized cancellous allograft 2 to 5 years after hip revision. Among 56 patients available for review, the authors found that for 93% of the revised femurs, the radiographs showed graft incorporation and bone remodeling. Three femoral implants had

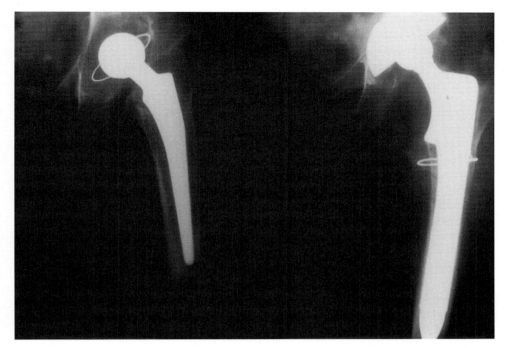

Figure 6. Type 2 femoral revision depending on distal femoral fixation with a calcar replacement Solution stem (DePuy, Warsaw, Ind.).

to be re-revised because of late fracture of the femoral shaft. These early results from two separate groups suggested this technique may be successful; however, longer-term follow-up evaluation is needed.

Lieberman et al. (43) described cement-within-cement revision hip arthroplasty. When there is a well-fixed cement–bone interface and the femoral component has loosened within the cement, when the femoral component has to be removed for access to the acetabulum, or when the femoral component has to be revised for component malposition, cementing a revision component into the old intact cement mantle was performed in 19 revision hip arthroplasties. There were two interoperative perforations of the femur, but no

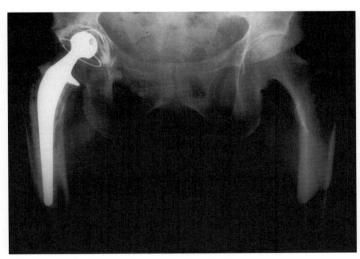
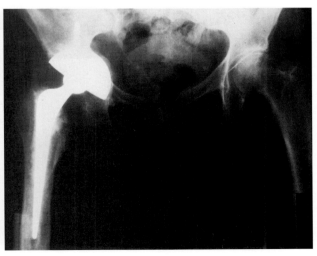

A   B

Figure 7. Type 2 femoral revision with impaction grafting and the Exeter stem (Howmedica, East Rutherford, N.J.). **A:** Preoperative appearance. **B:** Postoperative appearance.

femoral component had been revised for loosening and all the stems were radiographically stable after an average follow-up period of 59 months. This represents another method for revising a failed cemented hip joint replacement.

Type 3: Deficient Cancellous Bone and Cortical Tube

Femoral revision in the face of deficient cancellous and cortical bone presents a challenge. Cemented fixation in such circumstances has proved less than desirable. Because of the deficiency of the proximal femur, a long-stemmed cemented prosthesis has to be used. Good cement pressurization is difficult to achieve and cement often extrudes into the soft tissue. Re-revision of these long-stemmed cemented components is fraught with difficulty trying to remove all the cement. To overcome the proximal bone defect, proximal femoral replacement cemented prostheses have been used for revision operations. Malkani et al. (44) reported on 50 consecutive operations with this implant on hips that had undergone an average of 3.1 previous operations. For the 33 hips that were assessed with an average follow-up period of 11.1 years, the authors reported a high failure rate; 11 hips dislocated and 4 femoral components loosened, necessitating re-revision. This discouraging report, especially with the early cemented revisions, led to the development of cementless hip revision arthroplasty.

The principles of initial implant stability, the ability to bypass the femoral defects and the concept of distal diaphyseal fixation have led to the development of many different types of cementless implants (54,56). The bony defects can be filled with bone graft or specialized components, for example, a calcar replacement implant (26) (Fig. 8). The initial results of cementless femoral revision were not good because of implant design and patient selection. The initial cementless components relied on proximal fit and fill of the femoral canal but because of bone deficiencies did not achieve initial stability. Likewise, some of the implants were only partially porous coated and this led to poor bone ingrowth and subsequent implant subsidence and loosening. Peters et al. (61) reported on 49 cementless revisions with a noncircumferential porous coated, curved, long-stemmed

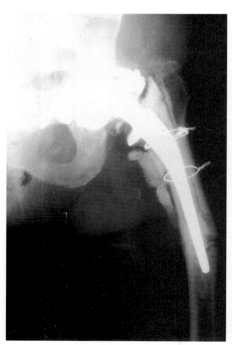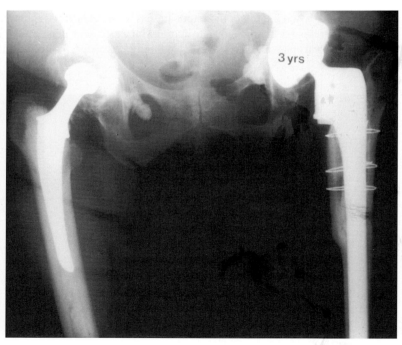

Figure 8. Type 3 femoral revision with a calcar replacement cementless femoral component and strut grafting. **A:** Preoperative appearance. **B:** Postoperative appearance with Mallory-Head stem (Biomet, Warsaw, Ind.).

prosthesis. They showed that 45% of the patients exhibited progressive subsidence and that this subsidence was proportional to the preoperative bone defects. After an average of 7.2 months, there was only a 37% chance of survival with progressive subsidence or revision as the end point.

In 1988, the early results of cementless femoral revision arthroplasty were presented at the meeting of The Hip Society. All components were proximally porous coated (51). Hedley et al. (27) reported a 9.5% femoral loosening rate after 1 year with the porous coated anatomic (PCA; Howmedica, East Rutherford, N.J.) femoral component. Gustilo and Pasternak (22) had a 4% femoral revision rate after a mean follow-up period of 2.8 years with the Bias (Zimmer, Warsaw, Ind.) component. Harris et al. (24) reported on use of the Harris-Galante component (Zimmer) with a 2-year minimum follow-up period and a 4% rate of femoral loosening. In the same year, Engh et al. (15) reported on use of the anatomic medullary locking prosthesis (AML, DePuy, Warsaw, Ind.) with a mean follow-up period of 4 years and a 4% rate of femoral loosening. These early results and other reports of high incidences of subsidence of uncemented components led to redesign of the femoral stem with more emphasis on initial stability with diaphyseal fit. This distal fit can be with a fully coated porous coating or with distal fluting. The results with these prostheses are superior to those with the earlier uncemented femoral revisions.

Lawrence et al. (40,41), using the AML prosthesis, which was extensively porous coated, conducted prospective follow-up studies with their patients for a mean of 7.4 years. The re-revision rate was only 5.7%, and the radiographic loosening rate was 1.1%. Moreland and Bernstein reported on use of 175 extensively porous coated prostheses with an average follow-up period of 5 years. Ninety-six percent of the components were still in place. Re-revision had been performed on two patients for recurrent dislocation and two patients for pain. One of the patients with pain had stable fibrous ingrowth and the other had bony ingrowth. The authors found that severe stress shielding occurred among 7.6% of their patients and that it occurred more commonly if there was preoperative osteoporosis or a large diameter prosthesis was used. Paprosky et al. (57) in a series of 311 revisions with extensively coated cementless femoral prostheses with a mean follow-up period of 5.8 years had a revision rate of 6% because of aseptic femoral loosening caused by use of an undersized stem.

Bone-stock deficiencies can be replaced with femoral strut allografts when cementless revision total hip arthroplasty is performed (14). Deficiencies within the calcar region can be replaced with a calcar-replacing prosthesis, because small calcar allografts have been shown to resorb in most instances. Large circumferential defects are probably best replaced with proximal femoral allografts, and the results of these are discussed later. Pak et al. (56) in a review of 95 cortical strut grafts used with a fully coated porous implant found that 87 of the 95 grafts showed radiographic evidence of graft incorporation an average of 4.75 years after the operation. Emerson et al. (14) found that cortical strut allografts unite by 8.4 months on average and that the overall rate of strut union is 96.6%. They showed that both the graft and the host bone remodel. Head et al. (26) found that 98% of cortical onlay grafts united with evidence of revascularization and some with complete incorporation. In a series of 174 patients, only 6 patients underwent revision because of femoral failure.

A more recent design of femoral component is the modular S-ROM prosthesis (Joint Medical Products, Stamford, Conn.), which relies on distal diaphyseal fit with a fluted stem and a proximal truncated modular cone to fit into the proximal femur (7,8). This modularity allows the component to be used in femurs with a variety of deficiencies as long as there is proximal intact femur to allow bony ingrowth. Initial concerns with fretting of the metal surfaces have not been substantiated in clinical review. McCarthy et al. (cited in 7 and 8) reported on 133 hip operations with the S-ROM prosthesis with a mean follow-up period of 5 years and a 1.5% re-revision rate and a 4% subsidence rate. In another series using the same prosthesis with a minimum 5 year follow-up period, Durkin et al. (12) had only two re-revisions of the femoral stem in 46 consecutive revision total hip joint replacements. They detected no substantial osteolysis, and there was no problem with the modular junctions of the prosthesis.

Type 4: Absent Cancellous Bone and Cortical Tube

Revision procedures on hips that have undergone multiple operations and sustained considerable proximal bone loss present the biggest challenge to surgeons. This is especially so in the care of young patients for whom further revision can be predicted. It is therefore essential to try to restore bone stock. If structural allografts are not indicated, whole proximal femoral allografts have to be used. The results with cemented proximal femoral replacement prostheses have been poor. Gross et al. (20,21) reported on 168 proximal femoral allografts with an average follow-up period of 4.8 years. They had a re-revision rate of 10.1%. Three patients underwent revision because of infection, 8 because of dislocation, 5 because of nonunion of the graft, and 1 because of pain. Radiographic results showed minor resorption in only 6 patients. Chandler et al. (7,8) reviewed 30 hips that needed proximal femoral allografts (7,8). After an average of 22 months of follow-up study, all but two grafts had united. Five revisions had dislocated, there was 1 nonunion, 1 graft resorption, and 1 infection that necessitated resection arthroplasty. Both groups cemented into the allograft proximally and relied on distal press fit for initial stability (Fig. 9). This allows early weight bearing, loading of the proximal femur, and restoration of deficient bone stock. The best results are achieved when a step cut is made in the graft–host interface, cerclage wire is used when necessary, and the host–graft site is autografted with or without strut grafting. The high complication rate with proximal femoral allografts means this technique is reserved for patients who need multiple revisions and have severe proximal femoral deficiency that precludes use of strut allografts and long-stemmed uncemented components.

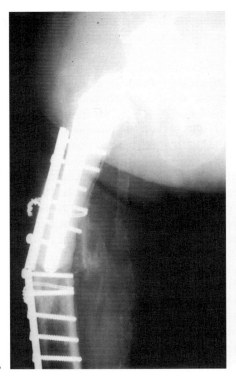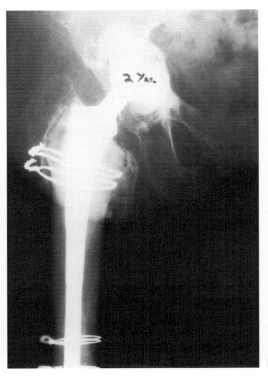

A   B

Figure 9. Type 4 femoral revision with allograft-implant composite in which the implant is cemented into the allograft and press fit distally (Biomet, Warsaw, Ind.). **A:** Preoperative appearance. **B:** Postoperative appearance.

SUMMARY

Revision total hip replacement will become more prevalent in the years ahead (31,36,45,46). Prevention is always the best treatment and will involve better patient selection, improved surgical techniques, and dedicated revision implants. This chapter provides guidelines for contemporary revision hip operations based on scientific fact. Undoubtedly, the field of revision hip surgery will continue to evolve.

REFERENCES

1. Amstutz HC, Steven ME, Ma SM, Jinnah RH, Mai L. Revision of aseptic loose total hip arthroplasties. *Clin Orthop* 1982;170:21–33.
2. Azuma T, Yasuda H, Okagaki K, Sakai K. Compressed allograft chips for acetabular reconstruction in revision hip arthroplasty. *J Bone Joint Surg Br* 1994;76:740–744.
3. Barrack RL. Economics of revision total hip arthroplasty. *Clin Orthop* 1995;319:209–214.
4. Barrack RL, Mulroy RD Jr, Harris WH. Improved cementing techniques and femoral component loosening in young patients with hip arthroplasty: a 12 year radiographic review. *J Bone Joint Surg Br* 1992;74: 383–389.
5. Callaghan JJ, Salvati EA, Pellicci PM, Wilson PD Jr, Ranawat CS. Results of revision for mechanical failure after cemented total hip replacement, 1979 to 1982. *J Bone Joint Surg Am* 1985;67:1074–1085.
6. Cameron HV, Jung YB. Acetabular revision with a bipolar prosthesis. *Clin Orthop* 1990;251:100–103.
7. Chandler HP, Ayres DK, Tan RC, Anderson LC, Varma AK. Revision total hip replacement using the S-ROM femoral component. *Clin Orthop* 1995;319:130–40.
8. Chandler HP, Clark J, Murphy S, et al. Reconstruction of major segmental loss of the proximal femur in revision total hip arthroplasty. *Clin Orthop* 1994;298:67–74.
9. D'Antonio JA, Capello WN, Borden LS, et al. Classification and management of acetabular abnormalities in total hip arthroplasty. *Clin Orthop* 1989;243:126–137.
10. Dohmae Y, Bechtold JE, Sherman RE, Puno RM, Gustilo RB. Reduction of cement–bone interface shear strength between primary and revision arthroplasty. *Clin Orthop* 1988;236:214–220.
11. Dorr LD, Wan Z. Ten years of experience with porous acetabular components for revision surgery. *Clin Orthop* 1995;319:191–200.
12. Durkin RC, Namba RS, Murray WR. Revision total hip reconstruction with a modular cementless femoral component: a 5 year minimum follow-up study. Presented at the 64th Annual Meeting of the American Academy of Orthopaedic Surgeons; 1997 Feb 13–17; San Francisco.
13. Elting JJ, Mikhail WE, Zicat BA, Hubbell JC, Lane LE, House B. Preliminary report of impaction grafting for exchange femoral arthroplasty. *Clin Orthop* 1995;319:159–167.
14. Emerson RH, Melinin TI, Cuellar PD, Head WC, Peters PC. Cortical strut allografts in the reconstruction of the femur in revision total hip arthroplasty: a basic science and clinical study. *Clin Orthop* 1992;285:35–44.
15. Engh CA, Glassman AH, Griffin WL, Mayer JG. Results of cementless revision for failed cemented total hip arthroplasty. *Clin Orthop* 1988;235:91–110.
16. Estok DM, Harris WH. Long-term results of cemented femoral revision surgery using second-generation techniques: an average 11.7-year follow-up evaluation. *Clin Orthop* 1994;299:190–202.
17. Garbuz D, Morsi E, Mohamed N, Gross AE. Classification and reconstruction in revision acetabular arthroplasty with bone stock deficiency. *Clin Orthop* 1996;324:98–107.
18. Gie GA, Linder L, Ling RSM, Simon JP, Sloof TJJH, Timperley AJ. Impacted cancellous allografts and cement for revision total hip arthroplasty. *J Bone Joint Surg Br* 1993;75B:14–21.
19. Gross AE, Allan DG, Catre M, Garbuz DS, Stockley I. Bone grafts in hip replacement surgery: the pelvic side. *Orthop Clin North Am* 1993;24:679–696.
20. Gross AE, Hutchison CR, Alexeeff M, Mohamed N, Leitch K, Morsi E. Proximal femoral allografts for reconstruction of bone stock in revision arthroplasty of the hip. *Clin Orthop* 1995;319:151–158.
21. Gross AE, Lavoie MV, McDermott P, Marks P. The use of allograft bone in revision total hip arthroplasty. *Clin Orthop* 1985;197:115–122.
22. Gustilo RB, Pasternak HS. Revision total hip arthroplasty with titanium ingrowth prosthesis and bone grafting for failed cemented femoral component loosening. *Clin Orthop* 1988;235:111–120.
23. Harris WH. Tramautic arthritis of the hip after dislocation and acetabular fractures: treatment by mold arthroplasty. *J Bone Joint Surg Am* 1969;51:737–755.
24. Harris WH, Krushell RJ, Galante JO. Results of cementless revisions of total hip arthroplasties using the Harris-Galante prosthesis. *Clin Orthop* 1988;235:120–126.
25. Havelin LI, Vollset SE, Engesaeter LB. Revision for aseptic loosening of uncemented cups in 4,352 primary total hip prostheses: a report from the Norwegian Arthroplasty Register. *Acta Orthop Scand* 1995;66: 493–500.
26. Head WC, Wagner RA, Emerson RH, Malinin TI. Revision total hip arthroplasty in the deficient femur with aproximal load-bearing prosthesis. *Clin Orthop* 1994;298:119–125.
27. Hedley AK, Gruen TA, Rueoff DP. Revision of failed total hip arthroplasties with uncemented porous coated anatomic components. *Clin Orthop* 1988;235:75–90.
28. Hoagland T, Razzano CD, Marke KE, Wilde AH. Revision of Mueller total hip arthroplasty. *Clin Orthop* 1981;161:180–185.
29. Hooten JP, Engh CA Jr, Engh CA. Failure of structural acetabular allografts in cementless revision arthroplasty. *J Bone Joint Surg Br* 1994;76:419–422.
30. Hooten JP, Engh CA, Heekin RD, Vinh TM. Structural bulk allografts in acetabular reconstruction: analysis of two grafts retrieved at post-mortem. *J Bone Joint Surg Am* 1996;78:270–275.

31. Hunter GA, Welsh RP, Cameron HV, Bailey WH. The results of revision of total hip arthroplasty. *J Bone Joint Surg Br* 1979;61:419–421.
32. Huo MH, Salvati EA. Revision of total hip replacement using cement technique. *Orthopedics* 1993;7: 58–64.
33. Izquierdo RJ, Northmore-Ball MD. Long term results of revision hip arthroplasty: survival analysis with special reference to the femoral component. *J Bone Joint Surg Br* 1994;76:34–39.
34. Jasty M, Harris WH. Salvage total hip reconstruction in patients with major acetabular bone deficiency using structural femoral head allograft. *J Bone Joint Surg Br* 1990;72:63–67.
35. Katz RP, Callaghan JJ. Cemented revision total hip arthroplasty using contemporary techniques: a minimum ten year follow-up study. *J Arthroplasty* 1994;9:103 (abstract).
36. Kavanagh BF, Fitzgerald RH. Multiple revisions for failed total hip arthroplasty not associated with infection. *J Bone Joint Surg Am* 1987;69:1144–1149.
37. Kavanagh BF, Ilstrup DM, Fitzgerald RH Jr. Revision total hip arthroplasty. *J Bone Joint Surg Am* 1985;67:519–526.
38. Kershaw CJ, Atkins RM, Dodd CAF, Bulstroke CJK. Revision total hip arthroplasty for aseptic failure: a review of 276 cases. *J Bone Joint Surg Br* 1991;73:564–568.
39. Lachiewicz PF, Hussamy OD. Revision of the acetabulum without cement with use of the Harris-Galante porous-coated implant: two to eight-year results. *J Bone Joint Surg Am* 1994;76:1834–1839.
40. Lawrence JM, Engh CA, Macalino GE. Revision total hip arthroplasty: long-term results without cement. *Orthop Clin North Am* 1993;24:635–644.
41. Lawrence JM, Engh CA, Macalino GE, Lauro GR. Outcome of revision hip arthroplasty done without cement. *J Bone Joint Surg Am* 1994;76:965–973.
42. Levai JP, Boisgard S. Acetabular reconstruction in total hip revision using a bone graft substitute: early clinical and radiographic results. *Clin Orthop* 1996;330:108–114.
43. Lieberman JR, Moeckel BH, Evans BH, Salvati EA, Ranawat CS. Cement-within-cement revision hip arthroplasty. *J Bone Joint Surg Br* 1993;75:869–871.
44. Malkani AL, Settecerri JJ, Sim FH, Chae EY, Wallrichs SL. Long term results of proximal femoral replacement for non-neoplastic disorders. *J Bone Joint Surg Br* 1995;77:351–356.
45. Mallory TH. Preparation of the proximal femur in cementless total hip revision. *Clin Orthop* 1988;235: 47–60.
46. Marti RK, Schuller HM, Besselaar PP, Haasnoot ELV. Results of revision of hip arthroplasty with cement. *J Bone Joint Surg Am* 1990;72A:346–354.
47. McGann WA, Welch RB, Picetti GD III. Acetabular preparation in cementless revision total hip arthroplasty. *Clin Orthop* 1988;235:35–46.
48. Moreland JR, Bernstein ML. Femoral revision hip arthroplasty with uncemented, porous coated stems. *Clin Orthop* 1995;319:141–150.
49. Morrey BF, Kavanagh BF. Complications with revision of the femoral component of total hip arthroplasty: comparison between cemented and uncemented techniques. *J Arthroplasty* 1992;7:71–79.
50. Morsi E, Garbuz D, Gross AE. Revision total hip arthroplasty with shelf bulk allografts: a long-term follow-up study. *J Arthroplasty* 1996;11:86–90.
51. Mulliken BD, Rorabeck CH, Bourne RB. Uncemented revision total hip arthroplasty. *Clin Orthop* 1996;325:156–162.
52. Mulroy WF, Estok DM, Harris WH. Total hip arthroplasty with use of so-called second generation cementing techniques: a fifteen year-average follow-up study. *J Bone Joint Surg Am* 1995;77:1845–1852.
53. Mulroy WF, Harris WH. Revision total hip arthroplasty with use of so-called second generation cementing techniques for aseptic loosening of the femoral component. *J Bone Joint Surg Am* 1996;78:982–994.
54. Nelson IW, Bulstrode CJ, Mowat AG. Femoral allografts in revision of hip replacement. *J Bone Joint Surg Br* 1990;72:151–152.
55. Padgett DE, Kull L, Rosenberg A, Sumner DR, Galante JO. Revision of the acetabular component without cement after total hip arthroplasty. *J Bone Joint Surg Am* 1993;75:663–673.
56. Pak JH, Paprosky WG, Jablonsky WS, Lawrence JM. Femoral strut allografts in cementless revision total hip arthroplasty. *Clin Orthop* 1993;295:172–178.
57. Paprosky WG, Jablonsky W, Magnus RE. Cementless femoral revision in the presence of severe proximal bone loss using diaphyseal fixation. *Orthop* 1993;17:965–966.
58. Paprosky WG, Magnus RE. Principles of bone grafting in revision total hip arthroplasty: acetabular technique. *Clin Orthop* 1994;298:147–155.
59. Pellicci PM, Wilson PD Jr, Sledge CB, Poss R, Callaghan JJ. Long-term results of revision total hip replacement: a follow-up report. *J Bone Joint Surg Am* 1985;67:513–516.
60. Peters CL, Curtain M, Samuelson KM. Acetabular revision with the Burch-Schneider antiprotrusio cage and cancellous allograft bone. *J Arthroplasty* 1995;10:307–312.
61. Peters CL, Rivero DP, Kull LR, Jacobs JJ, Rosenberg AG, Galante JO. Revision total hip arthroplasty without cement: subsidence of proximally porous coated femoral components. *J Bone Joint Surg Am* 1995;77:1217–1226.
62. Pierson JI, Harris WH. Cemented revision for femoral osteolysis in cemented arthroplasties: results in 19 hips after a mean 8.5 year follow-up. *J Bone Joint Surg Br* 1994;76:40–44.
63. Raut VV, Siney PD, Wroblewski BM. Cemented Charnley revision arthroplasty for severe femoral osteolysis. *J Bone Joint Surg Br* 1995;77:362–365.
64. Raut VV, Siney PD, Wroblewski BM. Cemented Charnley revision arthroplasty in patients with rheumatoid arthritis. *J Bone Joint Surg Br* 1994;76:909–911.
65. Raut VV, Siney PD, Wroblewski BM. Cemented revision for aseptic acetabular loosening: a review of 387 hips. *J Bone Joint Surg Br* 1995;77:357–361.
66. Retpen JB, Jensen JS. Risk factors for recurrent aseptic loosening of the femoral component after cemented revision. *J Arthroplasty* 1995;8:371–378.

67. Silverton CD, Rosenberg AG, Sheinkop MB, Jull LR, Galante JO. Revision of the acetabular component without cement after total hip arthroplasty. *J Bone Joint Surg Am* 1996;78:1366–1370.
68. Sloof TH, Schimmel JW, Buma P. Cemented fixation with bone grafts. *Orthop Clin North Am* 1993;24:667–677.
69. Snorrasen F, Kaarholm J. Early loosening of revision hip arthroplasty: a roentgen stereophotogrammetric analysis. *J Arthroplasty* 1990;5:217–229.
70. Tanzer M, Drucker D, Jasty M, McDonald M, Harris WH. Revision of the acetabular component with an uncemented Harris-Galante porous-coated prosthesis. *J Bone Joint Surg Am* 1992;74:987–994.
71. Trancik TM, Stulberg BN, Wilde AH, Feiglen DH. Allograft reconstruction of the acetabulum during revision total hip arthroplasty: clinical, radiographic and scintigraphic assessment of the results. *J Bone Joint Surg Am* 1986;68:527–533.
72. Weber KL, Callaghan JJ, Goetz DD, Johnston RC. Revision of a failed cemented total hip prosthesis with insertion of an acetabular component without cement and a femoral component with cement: a five to eight-year follow-up study. *J Bone Joint Surg Am* 1996;78:982–994.
73. Went P, Krismer M, Frischut B. Recurrence of infection after revision of infected hip arthroplasties. *J Bone Joint Surg Br* 1995;77:307–309.
74. Wyssa B, Raut VV, Siney PD, Wroblewski BM. Multiple revisions for failed Charnley low friction arthroplasty. *J Bone Joint Surg Br* 1995;77:303–306.

Revising the Infected Total Hip

Revision Total Hip Arthroplasty,
edited by Marvin E. Steinberg and Jonathan P. Garino,
Lippincott Williams & Wilkins, Philadelphia © 1998.

26

Diagnosis and Evaluation

Bassam A. Masri, Eduardo A. Salvati, and Clive P. Duncan

Although excellent functional outcomes continue to be enjoyed after total hip arthroplasty, deep infection complicates about 1% of primary operations and 2% to 4% of revision procedures (8,24). Infection after total hip arthroplasty continues to be an unexpected and devastating complication for the patient and a burden on the health care system (28), because of the very large numbers of arthroplasties being performed in North America. An infected arthroplasty is expensive to treat, yet poorly remunerated by paying agencies, requiring prolonged hospitalization and at least one to two operations to achieve a cure. In United States alone, the cost per year to manage the 3,500 to 4,000 infected arthroplasties is 150 to 200 million dollars (28). The incorrect diagnosis of a chronically infected hip replacement as aseptic loosening leads to inappropriate surgical procedures that have high failure rates. Reimplantation of an arthroplasty in an infected bed without appropriate débridement is likely to result in persistent infection. The failure is disappointing to both patient and surgeon, because salvage of the joint is much more complex. The consequences of misdiagnosis are great, and efforts to improve the accuracy of the diagnosis of infection after total hip arthroplasty are paramount.

Infection after total hip arthroplasty presents a diagnostic challenge because there is no single test that is a standard. The diagnosis of infection therefore relies on the judgment and experience of the surgeon as he or she assembles the pieces of a diagnostic puzzle. The various diagnostic modalities include an accurate history, physical examination, and

B. A. Masri: Department of Orthopaedics, University of British Columbia, Vancouver, British Columbia, Canada V5Z 4E1.

E. A. Salvati: Department of Orthopaedic Surgery, Hip and Knee Service, The Hospital for Special Surgery and New York Hospital, Cornell University College of Medicine, New York, New York 10021.

C. P. Duncan: Department of Orthopaedics, University of British Columbia, Vancouver, British Columbia, Canada V5Z 4E1.

radiographic examination and simple laboratory investigations such as erythrocyte sedimentation rate (ESR) or measurement of acute-phase reactant levels. More sophisticated tests include nuclear imaging and molecular biologic techniques. In our experience, the most direct and predictable diagnostic test is hip aspiration. These various diagnostic modalities are discussed in this chapter, as is our preferred approach to the investigation of a possibly infected hip replacement.

NONINVASIVE DIAGNOSTIC TESTS

Laboratory Investigations

Erythrocyte Sedimentation Rate

The ESR is a measurement of the physiologic response of red blood cells stimulated to agglutinate by acute-phase reactant proteins. The most common use of the ESR in orthopedics is in the diagnosis and follow-up of infection. Eftekhar (5) found elevation of the ESR among more than 75% of his patients with infected total joint replacement prostheses. In a study of 79 patients undergoing revision total hip replacement with no known factors that would elevate the ESR, it was found that in the noninfected group, 27 of 28 had an ESR less than 35 mm/hour with only one more than 35 mm/hour (31). The sensitivity of an ESR greater than 35 mm/hour in differentiating septic and aseptic loosening was 98%, and the specificity was 82% (31). In our prospective study of 202 revision total hip arthroplasties (30), the sensitivity of the ESR for the diagnosis of infection was 82%, the specificity was 85%, the predictive value of a positive test result was 58%, and the predictive value of a negative test result was 95% (Table 1). In this study, an elevated ESR was defined as more than 30 mm/hour. This is similar to other reports in the literature. Other factors may cause elevation of the ESR, including concomitant infection, inflammatory arthritis, collagen vascular disease, recent surgical intervention, and some malignant diseases. Accordingly, a normal ESR can be used safely to rule out infection, whereas an elevated ESR cannot necessarily be used with confidence to confirm a diagnosis of infection, and other tests are necessary to rule out infection. In addition to its role in the diagnosis of infection after total hip arthroplasty, the ESR may be of use in determining the persistence of infection after revision. If the ESR is greater than 30 mm/hour 6 months after two-stage revision, there is a 62% chance of persistence of infection (25).

C-Reactive Protein

The C-reactive protein (CRP) is one of the acute-phase proteins that contribute to elevation in the ESR and may be a more sensitive indicator of infection (26). All diseases

Table 1. *Diagnostic value of routine investigations*

Diagnostic test	Sensitivity	Specificity	Predictive value of positive test	Predictive value of negative test
ESR	82%	85%	58%	95%
CRP	96%	92%	74%	99%
Preoperative aspiration	86%	94%	67%	98%
Repeat aspiration[a]	81%	97%	77%	97%
Frozen section	80%	94%	74%	96%
Intraoperative cultures	94%	97%	77%	99%

Information from a prospective series of 202 consecutive revision total hip replacements (30).

[a] Repeat aspiration refers to reaspiration of the hip joint when there is discordance between aspiration results and clinical and laboratory features.

ESR, erythrocyte sedimentation rate; CRP, C-reactive protein.

resulting in an increase in acute-phase reactants may result in an increase in CRP, and the results among these patients have to be interpreted with caution. As a screening test for patients with failed total hip arthroplasty, CRP is a valuable tool because it is inexpensive and readily available. The CRP level decreases sooner after infection has resolved than does ESR, and therefore it is of more use in the follow-up evaluation of infection. The ESR may take as long as 1 year after an uncomplicated procedure to return to normal levels, whereas CRP level returns to normal within 3 weeks (29). In our prospective series of 202 revision total hip arthroplasties, the sensitivity of CRP for the diagnosis of infection was 96%, the specificity was 92%, the predictive value of a positive test result was 74%, and the predictive value of a negative test result was 99% (30). A positive test result was defined as a CRP level greater than 10 mg/L.

White Blood Cell Count

An increase in neutrophil count on a manual differential, particularly when a shift to the left is found, suggests ongoing infection. However, the white blood cell (WBC) count is rarely abnormal among patients with a chronically infected joint arthroplasty. The WBC count is therefore of minimal use in the diagnosis of chronic infection after total hip arthroplasty. In our prospective review of 202 consecutive revision total hip arthroplasties, we found the sensitivity of WBC count to be 20%, the specificity to be 96%, the predictive value of a positive test result to be 50%, and the predictive value of a negative test result to be 85% (30).

Radiographic Investigations

Plain Radiographs

There are very few specific radiographic features consistent with infection, and none is pathognomonic (2). Loosening is not a necessary feature of infection, and most patients with acute infection have solidly fixed components. However, late prosthetic loosening frequently complicates protracted chronic infection. Two radiographic features, although not diagnostic of infection, may be suggestive of infection—a lacy periosteal reaction and osteolysis (Fig. 1). The rapid onset of osteolysis or endosteal scalloping (2), particularly in the absence of obvious causes, such as thin or faulty polyethylene, excessive polyethylene wear, or incorrect placement of the acetabular component with excessive lateral opening, should raise the index of suspicion for infection. The importance of comparing serial radiographs cannot be overemphasized, because some of the radiographic findings may be subtle, and only in comparison with previous good-quality radiographs can their true importance be established.

Magnetic Resonance Imaging

Magnetic resonance imaging is of occasional value in the investigation of infected total hip arthroplasty, particularly to delineate the extent of periprosthetic abscesses and their intrapelvic extension. If the femoral component is fixed with radiolucent cement, plain radiography does not demonstrate the full extent of the cement mantle, and magnetic resonance imaging does, because cement produces a signal void within the medullary canal of the femur (6) (Fig. 2). Knowledge of the extent of the cement within the medullary canal of the femur assists with preoperative planning and improves the safety of the revision procedure.

Ultrasonography

Ultrasonography may be of occasional value in the diagnosis of infected joint arthroplasty (9). We use it when the index of suspicion for infection is high, and routine hip aspiration gives normal results. In some instances, ultrasonography helps identify the

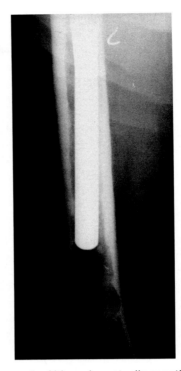

Figure 1. Although not diagnostic of infection, endosteal scalloping distal to the stem tip, as seen here, is a worrisome feature suggestive of infection, particularly when polyethylene wear is not severe and the duration of implantation has not been long.

location of abscesses, and the needle can be redirected to obtain an abnormal aspirate (Fig. 3). One report in the literature suggests that a thickened hip joint capsule suggests infection (9).

Radionuclide Scans

Technetium-99m Bone Scan

Much work has been performed on the role of nuclear imaging in the diagnosis of the infected joint replacement (see Fig. 3B). Although this field is rapidly evolving, these tests are expensive and have little more diagnostic value than ESR. Developments such as immunoglobulin G (IgG)–labeled scans, however, may improve the diagnostic accuracy in the future. However, a normal bone scan should rule out the presence of infection and mechanical complications in a total hip replacement (13), leading the surgeon to search for other factors that can cause hip pain, such as bursitis, lumbosacral disease, or other causes of referred pain.

^{99m}Tc bone scans are sensitive but not specific (22). Although most patients with infection have an abnormal bone scan, aseptic loosening of total hip replacements also causes increased radionulcide uptake on ^{99m}Tc bone scans. The test therefore cannot be used to differentiate the two main differential diagnoses of failed arthroplasty. The scan also is abnormal for as long as 1 year after uncomplicated arthroplasty (3). Heterotopic ossification, inflammatory conditions, fractures, and tumors also cause abnormal uptake in periprosthetic tissue.

Indium-111 Scan

Because of the inaccuracy of ^{99m}Tc scans, other techniques have been investigated. Indium-111–labeled WBC scans are highly sensitive in the diagnosis of conditions with

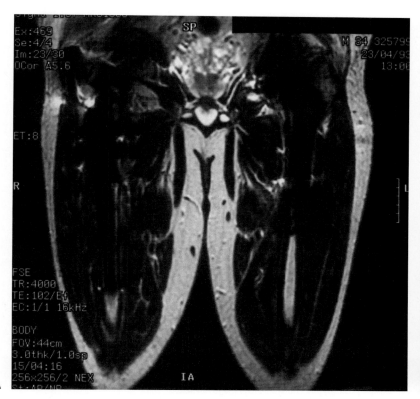
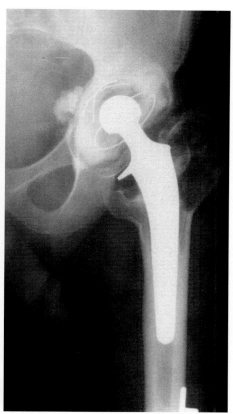

Figure 2. A: Magnetic resonance image shows the distal extent of radiolucent cement in the left femur, which cannot be seen on the plain radiograph (**B**).

increased vascularity and WBC uptake. In chronic osteomyelitis with poor vascularity, these scans often are normal. Although some studies have suggested that ^{111}In scans are useful for the diagnosis of infected total hip arthroplasty (21), others have shown that they are of little use (17). Okerlund et al. (17) showed that the predictive value of a positive ^{111}In scan is only 63%.

The two techniques therefore have been combined into a sequential bone and WBC scan protocol (11,20). The sensitivity and specificity of combined scans are higher than those of individual scans (11), particularly if the head of the prosthesis is specifically inspected (20). These techniques cannot be recommended for routine investigation of failed total hip arthroplasty. They have a limited role in difficult situations in which other tests have negative results or are inconclusive despite a high index of suspicion for infection and in the case of patients for whom hip joint culture results are confounded by inappropriate administration of antibiotics before referral.

Gallium-67 Scan

Gallium citrate accumulates in areas of infection and neoplasia, but its presence is nonspecific for the diagnosis of the infected total hip arthroplasty. In our opinion, gallium scans have no important role in the diagnosis of the infected total hip replacement.

Immunoglobulin-G scan

In an effort to improve the specificity of nuclear imaging, radioactive labeled IgG has been used as a tracer in the investigation of musculoskeletal sepsis (23). In principle, this test is not unlike ^{111}In-labeled WBC scans, in which the radionuclide targets areas of acute inflammation.

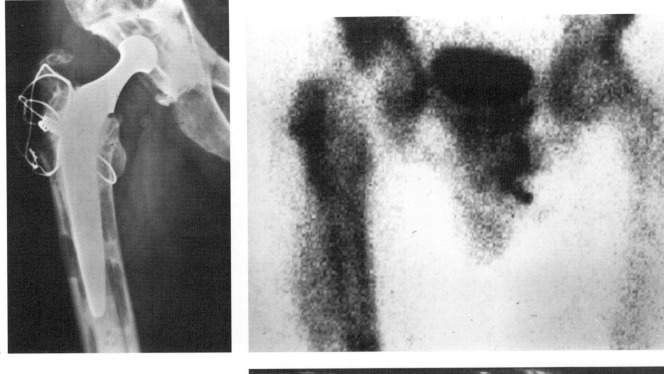

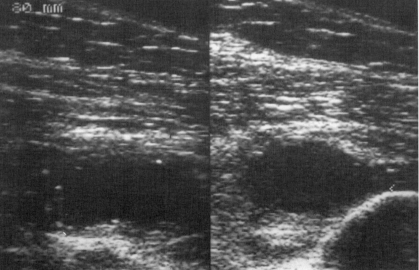

Figure 3. A: Plain radiograph shows extensive femoral lysis. **B:** Increased uptake on the bone scan is compatible with but not diagnostic of infection; however, the findings at ultrasonography (**C**) are suggestive of infection with abscess formation, which was confirmed with hip aspiration.

Because immunoglobulins may have a more specific affinity for areas of acute inflammation than the crude preparation of the WBC used in ^{111}In scanning, IgG may be a better carrier for the radioisotope (18,19). In one study of this test for the diagnosis of musculoskeletal infection (18), the sensitivity was 74% and the specificity was 100%. In another study, the sensitivity of ^{111}In-labeled IgG scans was 77.8%, and the specificity was 95.5% for the diagnosis of infection after total hip arthroplasty (19). Although no studies have compared ^{111}In-labeled IgG with ^{111}In-labeled WBC scanning in the diagnosis of infected total hip arthroplasty, animal studies comparing these two techniques have found that the latter is more sensitive in the diagnosis of infection (7). Until studies comparing these two modalities in the diagnosis of infected total hip arthroplasty clarify their value, we cannot recommend routine use of ^{111}In-labeled IgG scans. In our practice, nuclear scans play a limited role in the diagnosis of infection after total hip arthroplasty.

INVASIVE DIAGNOSTIC TESTS

Hip Joint Aspiration and Arthrography

If infection is suspected, hip joint aspiration is mandatory to confirm the presence of infection and to determine the identity and sensitivity profile of the infecting organism. It is performed preferably with fluoroscopy in the radiology suite under strict aseptic conditions and with local anesthesia. Arthrography is used to confirm intraarticular placement of the needle (Fig. 4). By itself, arthrography is rarely useful in the diagnosis of infection, although the accumulation of contrast material in pockets may suggest abscess formation. In the case of normal aspiration results, arthrography may help in redirecting the needle to an abscess to obtain a positive aspirate. A number of recent reviews have assessed the value of preoperative aspiration. Opinions vary from its being a valuable test to be performed on every revision hip replacement to its having little value (2,16).

Part of the difference in opinion may relate to the technique of aspiration. Although hip aspiration is a simple procedure, technique has to be strict and subsequent handling of the aspirate prompt and meticulous; otherwise the accuracy of the test diminishes markedly. Aspiration should be performed with strict aseptic technique and fluoroscopic control. Local anesthetic should not be injected into the joint, because some local anesthetic preparations are bacteriostatic. The samples should be sent immediately to the laboratory in a transport system with a culture medium to be incubated as soon as possible, to decrease the risk for a false-negative aspiration result, particularly when the organism is of poor vitality. We request a Gram stain "stat" to assure immediate processing of the specimen by the bacteriologist. Some authors have advocated use of a blood-culture bottle for synovial fluid aspiration; however, this practice may increase the risk for a false-positive culture result. In a study of the blood culture system (1) for analysis of prosthetic joint aspiration samples, the false-positive rate was 58%. At present, we no longer use a blood culture system for the transport of hip joint aspiration samples.

The value of the hip aspiration is not limited to whether the culture shows bacterial growth. In adjunctive tests that may be performed on the aspirate to confirm or rule out a diagnosis of infection also are important. If enough fluid is aspirated, a complete blood cell count and differential may give valuable information. If the blood cell count shows more than 25,000 leukocytes/mL, and the differential count reveals that more than 25% are polymorphonuclear leukocytes (PMNs), infection should be suspected. The higher the number of PMNs, the greater is the possibility of infection. Fluid should be analyzed for glucose and protein levels. In normal synovial fluid, protein levels are about one-third serum levels, whereas in infection, they approach serum levels. Glucose values in synovial fluid are similar to those in plasma. In the presence of infection, the synovial glucose levels are lowered, perhaps because of consumption of glucose by bacterial organisms and inflammatory cells or because of abnormalities in the cellular transport mechanisms. Thus a higher protein level and a lower glucose level suggest infection. Cultures obtained from draining sinuses are unreliable, because they often grow mixed flora and not necessarily the main pathogen causing the deep periprosthetic infection.

In our prospective series of 202 consecutive revision total hip arthroplasty procedures, routine hip joint aspiration was performed to determine the role of hip aspiration and other tests in the diagnosis of infection (30). The sensitivity of a preoperative aspiration for the diagnosis of infection was 86%, the specificity was 94%, the predictive value of a positive test result was 67%, and the predictive value of a negative test result was 98%. These figures are comparable with values reported by other authors. The aspiration of clear synovial fluid with normal cultures can reliably exclude infection for most patients. Routine preoperative aspiration cannot be recommended for routine revision total hip replacement on the basis of our data and a review of the literature. We agree with the recommendation of Lachiewicz et al. (12) that selective aspiration in suspicious circumstances is an invaluable tool for the diagnosis of infection.

In addition to routine microbiologic analysis of hip aspiration samples, more

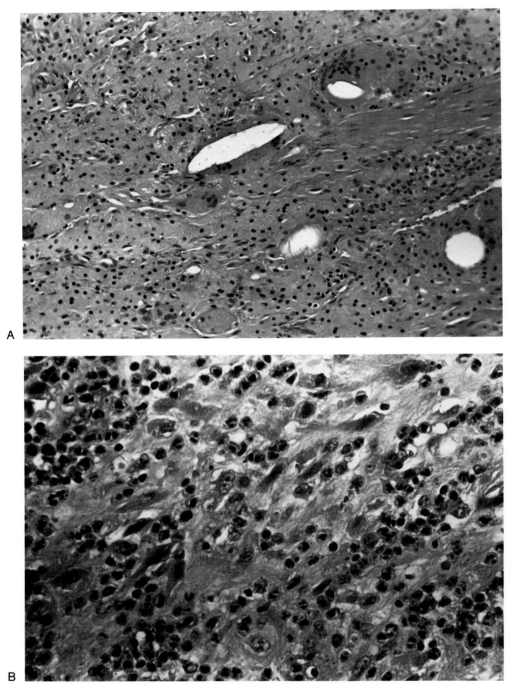

Figure 4. A: Photomicrograph shows no acute inflammatory cells, suggesting there is no infection. **B:** Section shows numerous polymorphonuclear leukocytes, suggesting infection.

modern molecular biologic techniques are being developed. The presence of bacterial deoxyribonucleic acid (DNA) or ribonucleic acid (RNA) remnants within the tissues may be determined with polymerase chain reaction techniques. Because very small quantities of DNA may be found in a specimen, the DNA can be replicated and increased in volume by means of polymerase chain reaction. The specimen is cycled in an amino acid broth to allow exposure and polymerization of the DNA chains. After 30 to 40 cycles, sufficient volumes of DNA are available for analysis. Comparing the

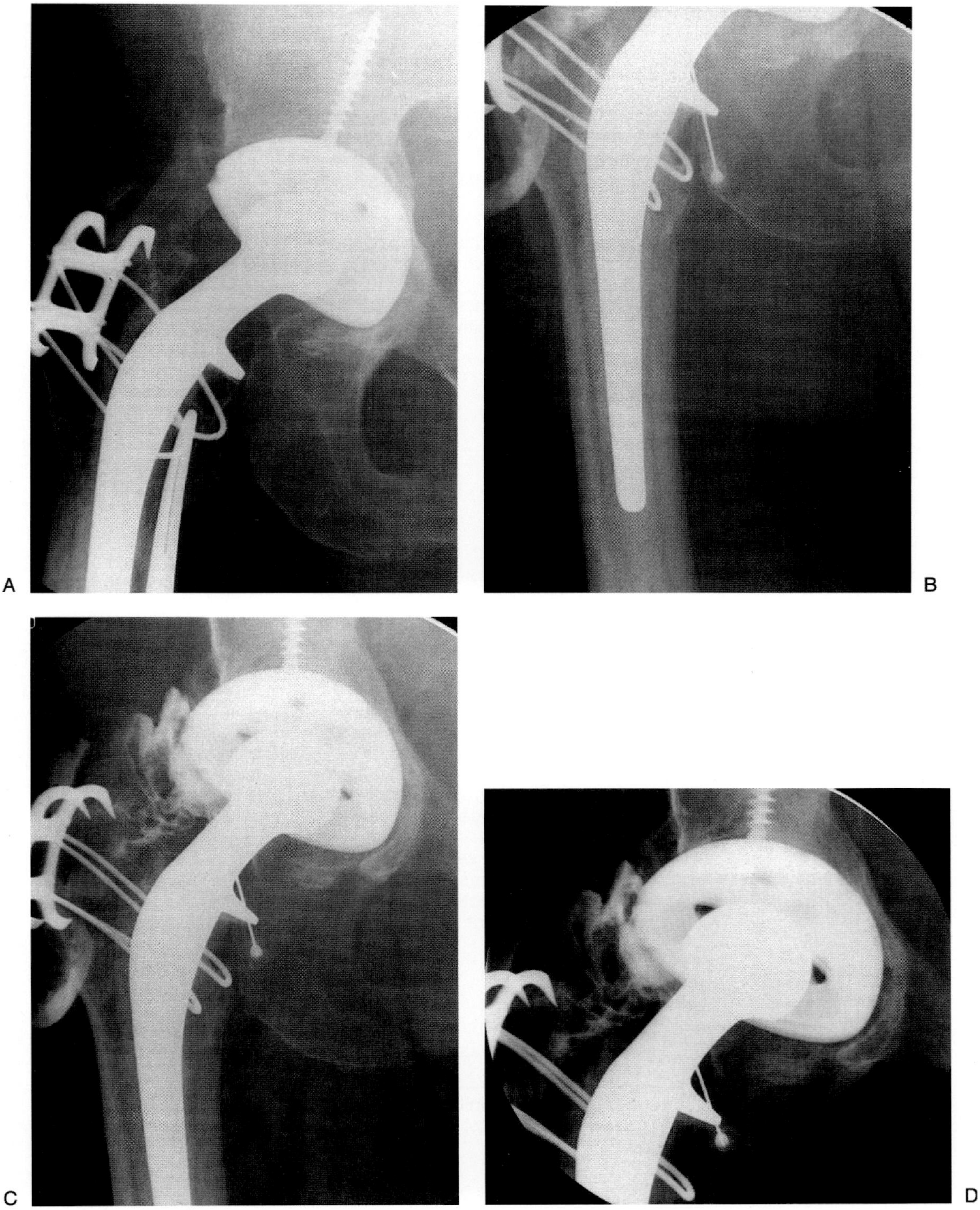

Figure 5. Hip joint aspiration is done in the fluoroscopy suite by an experienced musculoskeletal radiologist. Under sterile conditions, the hip joint is located with an instrument (**A**) to allow correct insertion of the needle into the hip joint (**B**). Contrast agent is then injected to confirm the intraarticular position of the needle (**C**). After the needle is withdrawn, the contrast agent remains in the hip joint, showing no extraarticular extravasation and no focal fluid collections in direct communication with the joint (**D**).

Table 2. *Criteria for the diagnosis of deep hip infection*

Category	Maximum points per category	Subcategory
Clinical diagnosis	2 points; 1 point for each subcategory	History of hip infection within 3 years Clinical signs and symptoms of infection
Condition of wound	3 points	Draining wound or sinus communicating with hip joint
Laboratory findings	2 points; 1 for each positive subcategory	ESR >30 mm/hr WBC >11,000 with shift to the left (> 5% bands)
Radiographic findings	3 points; 1 for each positive subcategory	Plain radiographs showing loosening, settling, wandering, or bony resorption adjacent to the hardware or prosthesis Arthrogram or sinugram showing sinus tracts or soft-tissue abscess communicating with the joint or demonstration of contrast agent between acrylic and bone, suggesting septic loosening Nuclear scan showing increased uptake compatible with infection or loosening
Bacteriologic findings	10 points; 4 points for the initially positive Gram stain, preoperative culture, or intraoperative culture with 2 additional points for each subsequent specimen positive for the same organism	Hip aspirations Gram stain Culture Intraoperative specimen Gram stain Culture
Intraoperative observations	6 points; 4 points for subcategory A and 2 points for subcategory B	A: Gross periprosthetic infection Purulent fluid in joint B: Appearance of tissue suggestive of infection Boggy edematous capsule Inflamed synovium
Histopathologic findings	3 points	Acute inflammation on surgical specimen

Fifteen or more points indicate definite infection.
ESR, erythrocyte sedimentation rate; WBC, white blood cell count. (Adapted from ref. 10, with permission.)

obtained DNA sequence with a number of standard sequences can show the fingerprint of the infecting organism. These techniques are in development and hold promise for improved diagnostic accuracy (8). Although the sensitivity of this test is high, the specificity is low. Because this test depends on the availability of minuscule amounts of genetic material, DNA from dead microorganisms can be detected. It is difficult to differentiate an infection that has been successfully treated from a clinically active infection.

Intraoperative Tests for the Diagnosis of Infection

Despite an extensive and normal preoperative investigation, the surgeon occasionally is faced with intraoperative findings that suggest infection. The gross appearance of the tissues, however, is not always diagnostic of infection. In the absence of features such as florid synovitis, pus within the joint, and abscess formation and in the absence of preoperative features that suggest infection, it is safe to assume that infection is not present. It is up to the surgeon's judgment to determine whether it is safe to proceed with the revision procedure or perform the first stage of a two-stage exchange arthroplasty while awaiting the results of the final cultures. Whenever there is doubt at the time of the operation, it is safer to proceed with a two-stage exchange arthroplasty. Feldman et al. (7) correlated intraoperative surgical opinion with the pathologic diagnosis for a sensitivity of 70% and a specificity of 87%. Because of the relatively poor sensitivity and specificity of the gross appearance of the tissues at the time of revision total hip arthroplasty, a variety of adjunctive tests can be performed to rule out infection. These include an immediate Gram stain and culture of the synovial fluid and frozen section of the inflamed tissues.

Gram Stain and Intraoperative Frozen Section

Despite the widespread use of Gram staining at the time of revision total hip arthroplasty, there has been questionable support in the literature (4). In our experience, the false-negative rate of Gram staining is so high that it cannot be relied on unless the infection is so overt that a large load of bacteria is present to allow observation of bacteria on the Gram stain. This is the exception rather than the rule.

Intraoperative frozen section (Fig. 5) of the periprosthetic tissues also has been used (7,14,15). The most inflamed appearing tissue at the time of the operation should be sampled by the surgeon, and the microscopic specimen should be examined by the pathologist under low power first to study the most inflamed portion of the sample. Mirra et al. (15) reported the criteria of more than five PMNs per high power field as suggestive of infection. With these criteria, the sensitivity was 100% and the specificity was 96% (7). In a follow-up study by the same group (14), with the more stringent criterion of at least ten PMNs per high power field overdiagnose of infection was less likely, with a sensitivity of 84% and a specificity of 99%. In our prospective series of 202 revision total hip arthroplasties (30), with more than five PMNs per high power field as the diagnostic criterion, the sensitivity was 80%, the specificity was 94%, the predictive value of a positive test result was 74%, and the predictive value of a negative test result was 96%.

Intraoperative Cultures

Intraoperative cultures often are considered the standard for the diagnosis of infected arthroplasties. The area that appears to be most inflamed should be sampled, and at least three tissue samples should be sent for culture to improve the yield and decrease the likelihood of a false-negative culture result. All cultures should be incubated for at least 5 days. Unfortunately, errors in culture technique can occur, antibiotics may have been administered preoperatively without the knowledge of the surgeon, and antibiotics may have been added to the irrigation fluid before harvesting of tissue for culture. Sampling error at the time of the operation also may occur. All these factors can contribute to a false-negative culture result. Contamination of the tissue samples at the time of transfer to the culture media or in the laboratory may contribute to false-positive results. In our prospective series of 202 revision total hip arthroplasties (30), at least three intraoperative tissue samples were obtained. With the arbitrary criterion that at least two samples had to be positive to be considered a true-positive culture result, the sensitivity of this test was 94%, the specificity was 97%, the positive predictive value was 77%, and the negative predictive value was 99%.

In 1979, we (10) proposed criteria based on a point system to determine whether the surgeon is dealing with a definite infection. These criteria assign points for different findings at history, examination of the wound, radiography, bacteriologic examination, intraoperative observations, and histopathologic examination (Table 2). A total of 29 points is possible. If the patient's numeric value totals 1 to 6 points, the joint is considered at high risk for infection; 7 to 14 points, suspected of being infected; and greater than 15 points, definitely infected.

PROTOCOL FOR THE DIAGNOSIS OF INFECTION

A high index of suspicion is essential, particularly when a patient has a persistently painful arthroplasty despite unremarkable radiographs. A careful history and physical examination should precede any tests for the diagnosis of infection. The patient should be carefully questioned regarding any wound-healing complications, early local or distant infections, or prolonged administration of antibiotics after the operation. Delays in discharge from the hospital also suggest an early complication. Questions regarding recent infections, such as skin infections or ulcerations, urinary tract infections, and dental infections or manipulations can be revealing. Radiographs should be obtained and compared with previous ones. In the early postoperative period, ectopic ossification can explain persistent pain.

The next investigation should be an ESR and C-reactive protein. If both tests are normal, no further tests are necessary. If the ESR or CRP is elevated and the suspicion for infection is high, a hip joint aspiration with the patient off all antibiotics for at least 4 weeks can be performed. If aspiration results confirm infection, the surgeon may proceed with the most appropriate treatment. If the aspiration result is negative, and the index of suspicion remains high, aspiration is repeated with the guidance of arthrography or ultrasound. If the aspirate remains negative, ancillary tests, such as a repeat hip aspiration with arthroscopic means, tissue culture, or sequential technetium-indium nuclear scanning, may be performed. If all these test results are normal, the surgeon may finally have to resort to intraoperative tests such as Gram stain, blood cell count, differential, and frozen section at the time of revision arthroplasty to differentiate aseptic loosening and infection. If the frozen section analysis has normal results, we proceed with revision total hip arthroplasty. Several intraoperative tissue cultures are obtained for all patients. If unexpected positive intraoperative cultures are obtained, a 6-week course of intravenous antibiotics is administered after the revision. A minimum postpeak serum bactericidal titer of 1:8 against the patient's own infecting organism is obtained followed perhaps by oral suppressive antibiotic therapy.

Although many tests have been recommended for the diagnosis of infected total hip arthroplasty, the rational use of these tests in a sequential manner allows the correct diagnosis of infection in most instances. This minimizes complications, morbidity, and cost of treatment of incorrectly diagnosed infected total hip arthroplasty.

REFERENCES

1. Baker S, Fraise AP. Use of Sentinel blood culture system for analysis of specimens from potentially infected prosthetic joints. *J Clin Pathol* 1994;47:475–476.
2. Barrack RL, Harris WH. The value of aspiration of the hip joint before revision total hip arthroplasty. *J Bone Joint Surg Am* 1993;75:66–76.
3. Brause BD. Infections associated with prosthetic joints. *Clin Rheum Dis* 1986;12:523–536.
4. Chimento GF, Finger S, Barrack RL. Gram stain detection of infection during revision arthroplasty. *J Bone Joint Surg Br* 1996;78:838–839.
5. Eftekhar N. Diagnosis of infection in joint replacement surgery. In: Eftekhar N, ed. *Infection in joint replacement surgery: prevention and management.* St. Louis: Mosby, 1984:115–130.
6. Fehrman DA, McBeath AA, DeSmet AA, Tuite MJ. Imaging barium-free bone cement. *Am J Orthop* 1996;25:172–174.
7. Feldman DS, Lonner JH, Desai P. The role of intraoperative frozen sections in revision total joint arthroplasty. *J Bone Joint Surg Am* 1995;77:1807–1813.
8. Garvin K, Hanssen A. Infection after total hip arthroplasty. *J Bone Joint Surg Am* 1995;77:1576–1588.
9. Graif M, Schwarts E, Strauss S, Mouallem M, Schecter M, Morag B. Occult infection of hip prosthesis: sonographic evaluation. *J Am Geriatr Soc* 1991;39:203–204.
10. Hughes PW, Salvati EA, Wilson PD, Blumenfeld EL. Treatment of subacute sepsis of the hip by antibiotics and joint replacement: criteria for diagnosis and evaluation of twenty-six cases. *Clin Orthop* 1979;141: 143–157.

11. Johnson JA, Christie MJ, Sandler MP, Parks PFJ, Homra L, Kaye JJ. Detection of occult infection following total joint arthroplasty using sequential technetium 99-m HDP bone scintigraphy and indium 111 WBC imaging. *J Nucl Med* 1988;29:1347–1353.
12. Lachiewicz PF, Rogers GD, Thomason HC. Aspiration of the hip joint before revision total hip arthroplasty. *J Bone Joint Surg Am* 1996;78:749–754.
13. Lieberman JR, Huo MH, Schneider R, Salvati EA, Rodi S. Evaluation of painful hip arthroplasties: are technetium bone scans necessary? *J Bone Joint Surg Br* 1993;75:475–478.
14. Lonner JH, Desai P, DiCesare PE, Steiner G, Zuckerman JD. The reliability of analysis of intraoperative frozen sections for identifying active infection during revision hip or knee arthroplasty. *J Bone Joint Surg Am* 1996;78:1553–1558.
15. Mirra JM, Amstutz HC, Matos M, Gold R. The pathology of the joint tissues and its clinical relevance in prosthesis failure. *Clin Orthop* 1976;117:221–240.
16. Mulcahy DM, Fenelon GC, McInerney DP. Aspiration arthrography of the hip joint: its uses and limitations in revision hip surgery. *J Arthroplasty* 1996;11:64–68.
17. Okerlund M, Chehabi H, Huberty J, Rosen-Levin E, Murray W, Hattner R. Indium-111-granulocyte studies in the evaluation of complicated post-operative hip prostheses. *J Nucl Med* 1988;29:883 (abst).
18. Oyen WJ, Claessens RA, van der Meer JW, Corstens FM. Detection of subacute infectious foci with indium 111-labeled autologous leukocytes and indium 111-labeled human nonspecific immunoglobulin G: a prospective study. *J Nucl Med* 1991;32:1854–1860.
19. Oyen WJ, van Horn JR, Claessens RA, Sloof TJ, van der Meer JW. Diagnosis of bone, joint and joint prosthesis infections with In-111-labeled nonspecific human immunoglobulin G scintigraphy. *Radiology* 1992;182:195–199.
20. Palestro CJ, Kim CK, Swyer AJ, Capozzi JD, Solomon RW, Goldsmith S. Total-hip arthroplasty: periprosthetic indium-111-labeled leukocyte activity and complementary technetium-99-m-sulfur colloid imaging in suspected infection. *J Nucl Med* 1990;31:1950–1955.
21. Pring DJ, Henderson RG, Rivett AG, Kausz T, Coombs RR, Lavender JP. Autologous granulocyte scanning of painful prosthetic joints. *J Bone Joint Surg Br* 1986;68:647–652.
22. Reing CM, Richin PF, Kenmore PI. Differential bone-scanning in the evaluation of a painful total joint replacement. *J Bone Joint Surg Am* 1979;61:933–936.
23. Rubin RH, Fishman AJ. The use of radio-labeled nonspecific immunoglobulin in the detection of focal inflammation. *Semin Nucl Med* 1994;24:169–179.
24. Salvati EA, Robinson RP, Zeno SM, Koslin BL, Brause BD, Wilson PDJ. Infection rates after 3175 total hip and total knee replacements performed with and without horizontal unidirectional filtered air-flow system. *J Bone Joint Surg Am* 1982;64:525–535.
25. Sanzen L. The erythrocyte sedimentation rate following exchange of infected total hips. *Acta Orthop Scand* 1988;59:148–150.
26. Sanzen L, Carlsson AS. The diagnostic value of C-reactive protein in infected total hip arthroplasties. *J Bone Joint Surg Br* 1989;71:638–641.
27. Schauwecker DS, Carlson KA, Miller GA, Kalasinski LA, Katz BP. Comparison of In-111 nonspecific polyclonal IgG with indium-111-leukocytes in a canine osteomyelitis model. *J Nucl Med* 1991;32:1394–1398.
28. Sculco T. The economic impact of infected total joint arthroplasty. *Inst Course Lect* 1993;42:349–351.
29. Shih LY, Wu JJ, Yang DJ. Erythrocyte sedimentation rate and C-reactive protein values in patients with total hip arthroplasty. *Clin Orthop* 1987;225:238–246.
30. Spangehl MJ, Duncan CP, O'Connoll JX, and Masri BA. Prospective analysis of preoperative and intraoperative studies for the diagnosis of infection in revision total hip arthroplasties. Presented at the 64th Annual Meeting of the American Academy of Orthopaedic Surgeons; 1997 Feb. 13–17; San Francisco.
31. Thoren B, Wigren A. Erythrocyte sedimentation rate in infection of total hip replacements. *Orthopedics* 1991;14:495–497.

Revision Total Hip Arthroplasty,
edited by Marvin E. Steinberg and Jonathan P. Garino,
Lippincott Williams & Wilkins, Philadelphia © 1999.

27

Infecting Organisms and Antibiotics

Amy L. Graziani, Janet M. Hines,
Amy S. Morgan, Rob Roy MacGregor,
and John L. Esterhai, Jr.

The purpose of this chapter is to discuss the specific organisms commonly involved in total hip arthroplasty infection and prophylactic and therapeutic antibiotic treatment regimens.

PATHOGENS THAT COMPLICATE TOTAL HIP ARTHROPLASTY

The potential number of organisms involved in infections of total hip arthroplasty is broad but for the most part predictable. Consideration of the microbial epidemiologic situation is particularly useful in the treatment of patients with clinical evidence of joint infection in whom an organism does not grow. The spectrum depends to a certain extent on the time elapsed from the original arthroplasty. Infections that arise within the first several weeks to months after arthroplasty are most often related to perioperative contamination, presumably caused by loss of the usual physical barriers. Later infections may be related to intraoperative contamination of the joint with less virulent organisms, such as coagulase-negative staphylococci. Two years after arthroplasty, infections are

A. L. Graziani: Department of Pharmacy Services, Hospital of the University of Pennsylvania, Philadelphia, Pennsylvania 19104.

A. S. Morgan: Philadelphia College of Pharmacy and Science, Philadelphia, PA 19104.

J. M. Hines and Rob Roy MacGregor: Division of Infectious Disease, Department of Internal Medicine, University of Pennsylvania School of Medicine, Philadelphia, Pennsylvania 19104.

J. L. Esterhai, Jr.: Department of Orthopaedic Surgery, Hospital of the University of Pennsylvania, University of Pennsylvania School of Medicine, Philadelphia, Pennsylvania 19104.

more likely to be related to hematogenous seeding. In such cases, microbiologic status is determined by the apparent source of bacteremia. Dental infections are associated with bacteremia caused by viridans Streptococcus and anaerobic organisms. Cellulitis or cutaneous abscesses may be associated with *Staphylococcus aureus* or streptococcal bacteremia. The Enterobacteriaciae, enterococci, and gastrointestinal anaerobes are most likely with intestinal and bladder origins.

Coagulase-negative staphylococcal and skin flora anaerobic infections such as *Proprionibacterium acnes* are frequent contaminants of surgical specimens and are common pathogens in prosthetic joint infections. This diagnostic situation may be clarified if the organism is isolated from a single specimen, in enrichment broth only, in which case the organism is viewed as a contaminant. On the other hand, if bacteria with the same antibiotic resistance profile are identified in multiple specimens, it is likely that the cultured organism is a pathogen. Often in prosthetic hip revision, multiple specimens from different sites are not obtained, or they all are subject to the same collection and processing techniques that allowed contamination of the first specimen. We advocate obtaining multiple specimens for microbiologic and pathologic examination from different sites. Each specimen is handled with instruments not used during earlier dissection.

MOLECULAR MECHANISMS OF ADHESION

The presence of a foreign body alters host–parasite interaction in favor of the parasite. Implantation elicits a characteristic host response that results in production of an encapsulating material known as *extracellular slime substance*. This substance is important in making infections of prosthetic devices difficult to treat without removal of the entire device, cement, and glycocalyx. The pathogenesis of prosthetic joint infection begins with adhesion of the organism to the biomaterial. Most pathogenetic studies are performed with coagulase-negative staphylococci. Nonspecific interactions between the bacterium and the implant include electrostatic forces, van der Waals forces, and hydrophobicity. The prosthetic material and the potential pathogen become coated by host proteins including fibronectin, vitronectin, collagen, and fibrinogen, which act as receptors and ligands to bind the foreign body and organism together. The organism further encases itself in glycocalyx, the precise composition of which has not been determined but is probably glycerol teichoic acid (9).

Extracellular slime protects bacteria from the immune system. Glycocalyx stimulates monocytes to produce prostaglandin E_2, which inhibits T-lymphocyte proliferation (17), B-lymphocyte blastogenesis, and immunoglobulin production. It inhibits chemotaxis, opsonization, and degranulation. It also blunts the effect of antimicrobial therapy. The minimum inhibitory concentration for *Staphylococcus epidermidis* in the presence of slime (either adherent to a polymer surface or grown in a medium that promotes slime production) is considerably higher than that for *Staph. epidermidis* organisms grown in conventional media.

Surgical technique can increase the potential for infection. Site preparation by means of reaming can disrupt the blood supply immediately adjacent to the prosthesis. This dysvascular interval can inhibit optimal host cell, humoral factor, and antibiotic penetration. Although neither the heat of the polymethyl methacrylate (PMMA) polymerization nor the local concentration of monomer have been found to be important in the development of the zone of necrosis, it is likely that both contribute to the potential for infection. The presence of PMMA increased markedly the likelihood of infection with *Staph.* epidermidis or *Escherichia coli*. Multiple studies have demonstrated the toxicity of PMMA monomer in vitro, specifically on bactericidal serum factors, terminal complement components, phagocytosis and intracellular killing by polymorphonuclear cells, and lymphocyte function. PMMA monomers can reach concentrations surrounding the prosthesis sufficient to cause damage.

PERIOPERATIVE USE OF ANTIBIOTICS

The presence of an infection at a distant site during an operation has been associated with subsequent prosthetic joint infection. Patients should undergo thorough preoperative screening for the presence of pulmonary, genitourinary, skin, and dental infections. Infections should be treated and eliminated before the operation.

The incidence of deep wound infections after total hip replacement decreases with the use of prophylactic antimicrobial agents. The benefit of ultraclean air systems in addition to antimicrobial prophylaxis is not clear. These systems may provide a further decrease in the incidence of wound infection. Prophylactic agents should have antimicrobial activity against *Staphylococcus* sp and *Streptococcus* sp, good tissue penetration, low toxicity, and low cost. First-generation cephalosporins meet these criteria and have been shown to be effective prophylactic agents. The administration of antimicrobial agents for a short duration (24 to 48 hours) after the operation is effective in preventing infection.

We recommend intravenous administration of cefazolin, 1 g within 2 hours of skin incision. Ideally, the infusion should be completed 30 minutes before the operation to ensure adequate cefazolin levels. An additional 1-g dose is administered if the operation lasts longer than 4 hours. Cefazolin 500 mg every 8 hours is continued for 24 hours postoperatively. In institutions with a high incidence of methicillin-resistant *Staph. aureus* or coagulase-negative staphylococcus infections, vancomycin should be considered for antimicrobial prophylaxis either alone or in combination with other agents. Patients with a history of severe allergic reaction (urticaria, angioedema, anaphylaxis) to penicillins, cephalosporins, meropenem, or imipenem should receive vancomycin 1 g 2 hours before incision and every 12 hours thereafter for 24 hours (14). Dosage adjustment for vancomycin is required for patients with impaired renal function. The incidence of postoperative infection is increased among elderly and obese persons and those who have malnutrition, diabetes, rheumatoid arthritis, or psoriasis or are undergoing corticosteroid therapy. It is particularly important that patients with these diagnoses undergo meticulous preoperative examination and preparation.

ANTIBIOTICS: LATE PROPHYLAXIS

The incidence of late hematogenous prosthetic joint infection is approximately 0.3%. Late prosthetic joint infection caused by hematogenous spread from a distant site of infection is well documented. The incidence after procedures known to induce transient bacteremia, such as dental manipulation, gastrointestinal endoscopy, and urologic procedures, is unknown. In retrospective studies of the causal relationship between dental procedures and late prosthetic joint infection, the incidence was 0.04% to 0.05%. When dental procedures were identified as the likely cause of late prosthetic joint infection, hematogenous spread was probably caused by chronic dental infection rather than transient bacteremia from dental manipulation. Case reports have implicated dental and urologic procedures as the cause of late prosthetic joint infection (6). Reports of late prosthetic joint infection from dental procedures have been challenged because organisms have not been isolated from both the infected joint and the suspected dental focus of infection, many of the organisms isolated at the arthroplasty were not common oral flora, and some of the patients had active periodontal disease (20).

Patients with bacterial infections at distant sites should be treated promptly and aggressively to prevent late prosthetic joint infection. Antimicrobial prophylaxis for procedures that induce transient bacteremia remains controversial. Much of the literature addresses antimicrobial prophylaxis for dental procedures. One survey (15) showed that most of the orthopedic surgeons (81%, n = 44) and dentists (66%, n = 36) polled believed that patients with prosthetic joints should receive antimicrobial prophylaxis before dental procedures. Three approaches to antimicrobial prophylaxis for dental procedures are outlined in the literature. Some groups do not recommend routine prophylaxis before dental procedures, because of a lack of clear cause and effect, the adverse effects of antimicrobial agents, potential emergence of antimicrobial resistance, and cost (20). Because of the consequences of late prosthetic joint infection, other authors recommend routine prophylaxis before dental and other procedures known to induce transient bacteremia, until further research is completed. Still others recommend prophylaxis only in patients at high risk for hematogenous infections when undergoing dental procedures with a high incidence of bacteremia (23). Patients at high risk include those with conditions that predispose to infection (rheumatoid arthritis, insulin-dependent diabetes mellitus, and use of immunosuppressive agents), first two years following joint replacement, previous complications of joint replacement, and periodontal disease or infection that may cause chronic bacteremia. Because the risk for late prosthetic joint infection after a dental procedure is unknown, it is difficult to determine the risk-to-benefit ratio of antibiotic prophylaxis. It has been pointed out, however, that the risk for severe impairment or death from a reaction to an antibiotic may be greater than the risk for infection (8,18).

When prophylaxis is used for dental procedures, oral first-generation cephalosporins are an appropriate choice. Their antimicrobial spectrum includes most organisms found in the oral cavity, and these drugs have stability against β lactamase–producing organisms such as *Staph. aureus* (11). Cephalexin 1 to 2 g 1 hour before the procedure and 0.5 to 1 g 4 to 6 hours after the initial dose is recommended. Another option is amoxicillin 2.0 g 1 hour before the procedure and 1.5 g 6 hours after the initial dose. Patients with a β-lactam allergy should receive clindamycin 600 mg orally 1 hour before the procedure and 6 hours after the first dose or erythromycin 0.5 1 hour before the procedure and 4 to 6 hours after the first dose (11). Others recommend deletion of the second dose (23).

ANTIBIOTIC RESISTANCE

Resistance, caused by the indiscriminant use of antibiotics, is increasingly important in the management of all infections. The existence of resistance in organisms that previously were relatively sensitive to antibiotics increases the challenge of managing infection of a prosthetic hip if the culture result is negative or if epidemiologic patterns must be relied on to direct antimicrobial therapy.

SYSTEMIC ANTIMICROBIAL THERAPY FOR INFECTED TOTAL HIP ARTHROPLASTY

The goal of therapy for infection of a total hip replacement is to provide a stable, pain-free joint with adequate function to meet the patient's lifestyle needs. This is achieved through débridement, exchange or resection arthroplasty, and antibiotic therapy. Although antibiotic therapy plays an important role in eradicating the infection, no discussion of antibiotic therapy would be complete without an introductory statement concerning the importance of surgical débridement. Aggressive surgical débridement is the mainstay of treatment and is essential if the goal is to eradicate the infection. Without complete débridement, no antibiotic regimen is likely to be curative. Antibiotics alone cannot completely eradicate bacteria adherent to the surface of implants or large fragments of necrotic bone.

Selecting an Antibiotic

Long-term parenteral administration of antibiotics traditionally has been combined with one or two-stage revision arthroplasty. The Coventry classification system is used to describe total hip infections and to make general recommendations regarding therapy (5) (Table 1). Selecting a systemic antibiotic regimen is a complex process based on multiple, interrelated factors. Culture and susceptibility reports, surgical technique, and host factors all influence selection and therapeutic outcome (Table 2). Drugs of choice for selected pathogenic organisms are listed in Table 3. Often a clinical microbiology laboratory does not test all antibiotics against the organism or reports a class susceptibility. Consultation with a clinical microbiologist or infectious diseases specialist therefore may be helpful in interpretation and extrapolation of susceptibility reports.

Agents for the Management of Methicillin-Resistant *Staphylococcus Aureus* and *Staphylococcus Epidermidis* Infections

Clinical microbiology laboratories typically do not use the term *Methicillin-resistant staphylococcus.* Most often the laboratory tests staphylococci with an oxacillin disk and

Table 1. *Coventry classification system*

I. Positive intraoperative culture
  Treatment with 6 weeks of parenteral antibiotics
II. Early post operative infection
  Occurring within 1 month of the operation
  Débridement, exchange of liners, retention of components
  Parenteral administration of antibiotics for 4 weeks
III. Late chronic infection
  Occurring more than 1 month postoperatively, insidious
  Débridement, removal of components
  "Appropriate antibiotics", various other options (antibiotic-impregnated materials)
IV. Acute hematogenous infection
  If no loosening, treatment as early postoperative infection
  If loosening is present, treatment as late chronic infection

reports the organism as resistant to oxacillin. Oxacillin is the commonly used class disk for all penicillinase-resistant penicillins. Although not specifically stated, this indicates resistance to all other penicillinase-resistant penicillins, including methicillin, dicloxacillin, nafcillin, and cloxacillin. These "methicillin-resistant" organisms usually are also resistant to all available cephalosporins. *Staph. aureus* organisms are less likely to be methicillin resistant than are coagulase-negative staphylococci, including *Staph. epidermidis.* In our institution, 12% of outpatient and 32% of inpatient *Staph. aureus* isolates are methicillin resistant compared with 72% and 65%, respectively, of coagulase-negative staphylococci. Infections caused by methicillin-resistant staphylococci are troublesome because parenteral vancomycin is the only reliably effective antibiotic available in the United States. Oral vancomycin cannot be used because it is not absorbed. Teicoplanin, another glycopeptide antibiotic active against these organisms, is not available in the United States at this time. Trimethoprim-sulfamethoxazole (Bactrim, Septra, cotrimoxazole) is active against some strains of methicillin-resistant *Staph. aureus*. However, there is not much controlled experience with the use of the drug in this setting. If the organism is susceptible, trimethoprim-sulfamethoxazole may be used to manage selected infections, if high doses are used and patients are closely observed. The most appropriate use of this drug is long-term oral follow-up or suppression therapy after a long course of parenteral vancomycin.

Agents for the Management of Infection Caused by *Pseudomonas Aeruginosa*

Pseudomonas aeruginosa is another troublesome organism. Although there are several effective parenteral antibiotics (see Table 3), the only oral agents with systemic

Table 2. *Factors that affect selection of and response to an antibiotic regimen*

Pathogen
Antibiotic susceptibility pattern
Surgical issues
  One-stage arthroplasty
  Two-stage arthroplasty
  Resection arthroplasty
  Débridement and retention
  Use of antibiotic-impregnated materials
  Retained bone cement
  Number of prior operations
  Early postoperative infection after arthroplasty without cement
Host Factors
  Age
  Desired functional status
  Surgical risk factors
  Immune suppression

Table 3. *Pathogenic organisms and selected treatment options*

Pathogen	Selected antibiotic options	Alternatives
Gram-positive organisms		
Staphylococci		
Staphylococcus aureus, methicillin-sensitive	Nafcillin i.v.	Dicloxacillin p.o.
	Cefazolin i.v.	Clindamycin
	Trimethoprim-sulfamethoxazde i.v., p.o.	Fluoroquinolone[a] with or without rifampin[b]
		Ampicillin-sulbactam
		Amoxicillin-clavulanate
Staph. aureus, sulfamethoxazole- and methicillin-resistant[c]	Vancomycin (i.v. only)	Trimethoprim-sulfamethoxazole, high dose, i.v. or p.o., for some strains
Staphylococcus epidermidis (coagulase-negative staphylococci)	Vancomycin (i.v. only)	Trimethoprim-sulfamethoxazole, high dose, for some strains
		If sensitive, cefazolin, nafcillin or dicloxacillin
Streptococci		
Streptococcus faecalis (group D enterococci)	Penicillin G plus gentamicin	Vancomycin (i.v. only) plus gentamicin
	Ampicillin plus gentamicin	
Streptococcus faecium	Highly resistant organisms reported; no definitive therapy at this time	Chloramphenicol for some strains
		Tetracycline for some strains
		Quinupristin-dalfopristin for some strains (investigational)
Streptococcus pyogenes	Penicillin G or V	Most β-lactam agents active
Groups A, B, C, G, F enterococci	Cefazolin	Clindamycin
Gram-negative organisms		
Enterobacter sp.	Ceftriaxone	Piperacillin
	Trimethopim-sulfamethoxazole	Cefotaxime
		Fluoroquinolone
Escherichia coli	Cefazolin	Ceftriaxone
	Trimethoprim-sulfamethoxazole	Fluoroquinolones
		Many other agents
Pseudomonas aeruginosa	Piperacillin or mezlocillin plus an aminoglycoside	Ceftazidime plus aminoglycoside
		Cefepime plus aminoglycoside
		Fluoroquinolone plus aminoglycoside
		Imipenem or meropenem plus aminoglycoside
		Aztreonam plus aminoglycoside
Anaerobes		
Bacteroides fragilis	Metronidazole i.v. or p.o.	Clindamycin
		Ampicillin-sulbactam
		Amoxicillin-clavulanate
		Cefotetan, cefoxitin, piperacillin-tazobactam
Peptostreptococcus sp	Penicillin G	Clindamycin
Anaerobic streptococci		Doxycycline, vancomycin (i.v. only)
Corynebacterium jeikeium	Vancomycin	Ciprofloxacin, penicillin G plus aminoglycoside

These regimens represent the more commonly recommended medications for the indicated organism. However, the final selection should be based on patient-specific culture and susceptibility reports.

[a] Fluoroquinolones are ciprofloxacin, ofloxacin, and levofloxacin.

[b] Long-term use of fluoroquinolones as single agents in the management of staphylococcal infections may result in the development of resistance.

[c] Methicillin-resistant means resistant to oxacillin, nafcillin, cloxacillin, dicloxacillin, and vice versa.

antipseudomonal activity are the fluoroquinolones—ciprofloxacin, ofloxacin, trovofloxacin, and levofloxacin. Patients with an allergy to penicillin have few options—high-dose aztreonam, a fluoroquinolone, or desensitization. Imipenem, meropenem, and the cephalosporins should be avoided by patients with severe penicillin allergies characterized by evidence of immunoglobulin$_E$ (IgE) mediation (swelling, hives, angioedema) or an exfoliative, Stevens-Johnson rash. Another challenging aspect of *P. aeruginosa* infection is the need to administer combination therapy with an aminoglycoside. Aminoglycoside therapy requires careful dosing and close monitoring for renal, cochlear, and vestibular toxicity. Although monotherapy with agents such as ceftazidime, imipenem, and ciprofloxacin has been attempted with some success, treatment failures with and without development of resistance have occurred. Single-agent therapy and oral therapy for *P. aeruginosa* infection should be limited to step-down treatment after a long course of combination parenteral treatment that includes an aminoglycoside. There should be clear evidence of clinical response, no evidence of residual infection, and a likely small burden of organisms before monotherapy is attempted. As with use of oral agents for methicillin-resistant staphylococcal infections, the most appropriate use of monotherapy is in the setting of chronic suppression.

The Role of Oral Antimicrobials

Most studies were performed before the availability of the oral fluoroquinolone antibiotics. Therefore very few data are available on the efficacy of oral therapy for total hip arthroplasty infection. Most authorities continue to recommend 4 to 6 weeks of parenteral therapy and caution against the use of oral agents in this setting until more data are available.

Duration of Treatment

Most clinicians recommend 4 to 6 weeks of parenteral therapy for infected total hip arthroplasty. Some state that the empirical selection of a 6-week duration may be critical for efficacy, whereas other sources admit that there are no authoritative data on the most appropriate duration. Most recommendations for duration of treatment are based on older literature generated during a time when antibiotic-impregnated materials and the more potent antimicrobial agents were not available. A study by McDonald et al. (13) supported the need for at least 4 weeks of intravenous treatment. The failure rate was significantly higher among patients who underwent two-stage revision for infection caused by virulent organisms who received less than 4 weeks of parenteral antibiotic therapy. At our institution, most clinicians prescribe 4 to 6 weeks of parenteral therapy. If the organism is susceptible to a well-absorbed oral antibiotic and the infection appears quiescent, some physicians begin with intravenous therapy and change to oral treatment toward the end of the 4 to 6 week course.

Parenteral Administration of Antibiotics in the Home

Home antibiotic therapy can play an important role in the prolonged treatment regimens required for the infected total hip arthroplasty. In the past, only parenteral antibiotics with long serum half-lives, which could be administered once or twice daily, were considered for home administration. Vancomycin, ceftriaxone, cefoperazone, and cefonicid composed the relatively meager formulary. However, newer programmable, portable home infusion pumps have enabled prescription of home antibiotics that require administration every 8, 6, or 4 hours. These pumps, carried in a belt pack, have cassettes that hold a 24 to 48 hour supply of antibiotic. They infuse the required dose automatically at the programmed intervals. Antibiotics such as penicillin G, nafcillin, and cefazolin can now be administered easily in the home. For more information on medication stability and feasibility of administering a particular drug in the home setting, one should consult a home infusion pharmacist or physician.

Monitoring Therapy

Patients receiving long-term antibiotic therapy should be observed for efficacy and toxicity. Measurements of efficacy include pain, loosening, function, drainage, temperature, cultures, erythema, erythrocyte sedimentation rate, and radiographic changes. Toxicity monitoring varies with the antibiotic selected and the possible toxicities (16). The aminoglycosides require close monitoring of serum concentration and renal, cochlear, and vestibular function. β Lactam drugs require much less rigorous monitoring. The only laboratory test that need be ordered on an ongoing basis for most of these agents is a complete blood cell count with differential. Nafcillin, other penicillins, cephalosporins, and vancomycin can cause neutropenia with or without leukopenia and thus the complete blood cell count with differential should be monitored at least once a week (12). Oxacillin can cause cholestatic hepatitis with long-term use, so liver function tests and clinical signs and symptoms of hepatitis should be monitored.

Drug Interactions

There are several relevant drug interactions of which one should be aware when prescribing antimicrobial agents. The interaction between trimethoprim-sulfamethoxazole and warfarin is one of the most important. Trimethoprim-sulfamethoxazole can increase the hypoprothrombinemic effects of warfarin, resulting in bleeding. Several other important interactions can occur with rifampin. Rifampin can accelerate the metabolism of many drugs, including oral contraceptives, theophylline, oral hypoglycemic agents and prednisone, resulting in subtherapeutic levels of these agents. Oral absorption of ciprofloxacin, ofloxacin, and levofloxacin can be dramatically reduced if they are ingested with antacids, sucralfate, iron-containing products, magnesium, zinc, or other divalent cations.

To reduce the likelihood of drug interactions, a thorough medication history is obtained before antimicrobial therapy is begun, and the regimen is evaluated for potential drug interactions. A medication history is obtained when antimicrobial agents are discontinued. If an interaction occurred at initiation of the offending drug, a rebound reaction may occur when the offending antimicrobial agent is discontinued (e.g., supratherapeutic levels of oral hypoglycemic agents when rifampin is discontinued, subtherapeutic response to warfarin when trimethoprim-sulfamethoxazole is discontinued). Patients are counseled to ask about drug interactions before beginning any new prescription or over-the-counter medication during the antibiotic treatment period.

Response Rates to Treatment

A review of the literature on infected total hip arthroplasty reveals widely varying treatment response rates. There have been few controlled trials of specific antimicrobial regimens, and the surgical procedure, local antibiotics, pathogens, duration of infection, and follow-up period are variable. Under ideal circumstances primary revision of an infected total hip arthroplasty might be considered. However, most contemporary studies suggest that the best response rates are achieved with two-stage procedures combined with 4 to 6 weeks of parenteral therapy.

Two-Stage Revision of Infected Total Hip Arthroplasty

In a report of two-stage revision in which patients received intravenous antibiotics for 4 weeks and gentamicin-impregnated cement was used, there was a 93% response rate. The mean time between operations was 27 weeks (5). Brandt et al. (1) reported on the 1980 to 1991 Mayo Clinic experience with *Staph. aureus* prosthetic joint infections treated with two-stage arthroplasty and intravenous antimicrobial therapy. Parenteral antibiotic therapy was administered for a median of 33 days (23 to 77 days), and the median time to reimplantation was 133 days (8 to 4436 days). Antimicrobial agent–impregnated bone cement was used to treat 61% of patients. Only 1 of 22 (4.5%) reimplanted hips failed.

Débridement with Retention of Infected Total Hip Arthroplasty

Débridement with retention of the prosthesis and parenteral antibiotic therapy generally produces lower response rates, which range from 15% to 60% (22). However, this may be acceptable for patients for whom microbiologic cure is not necessary and for whom suppression may be appropriate. The infecting organism can affect response rate. Infections caused by methicillin-resistant staphylococci, enterococci, organisms with a glycocalyx, and gram-negative bacteria can be difficult to eradicate. Although *P. aeruginosa* infections have been difficult to cure in the past, Tsukayama et al. (19) reported favorable outcomes with gram-negative infections. They suspected that their success may have been related to use of newer antibiotics with greater gram-negative activity, and to intraoperative use of aminoglycoside-containing materials. In a review of 30 patients with *S. aureus* prosthetic joint infection in whom the arthroplasty was debrided and retained, Brandt et al. found treatment failure was common; 54% and 69% failed at one and two years respectively. Patients debrided more than two days after the onset of symptoms were more likely to fail than those debrided within two days (relative risk, 4.2; 95% CI, 1.6–10.3) (1).

Revision of "Aseptic" Total Hip Arthroplasty with Positive Results of Intraoperative Cultures

At the time of direct-exchange arthroplasty performed for presumed aseptic loosening the clinician occasionally obtains unanticipated positive results of intraoperative cultures. A reasonable approach for dealing with this phenomenon was articulated by Garvin et al. (5) and Tsukayama (19). Both cautioned that cultures should be positive from *at least two* different sites within the operative field and that cultures that grow in broth only should be disregarded. Patients with growth in two specimens are given 6 weeks of antibiotic treatment without further operative intervention. The authors conceded that some of these patients may not need treatment at all but point to their own experience with treatment failures in spite of this approach to indicate that these cultures should be taken seriously. Further validating this point, Dupont (4) reported on 98 cases of revision arthroplasty. Only 1 of the 83 patients with sterile cultures at the operation had subsequent infection compared with 6 of the 15 who had positive intraoperative culture results.

ANTIBIOTIC THERAPY FOR LONG-TERM SUPPRESSION OF TOTAL HIP ARTHROPLASTY INFECTION

The goal of most orthopedic surgeons caring for a patient with an infected hip prosthesis is eradication of infection and revision of the prosthesis to a functional and sterile state. However, clinical conditions may sometimes make this goal impossible to reach. First, some patients are too old or frail from other medical conditions to consider surgical revision. Others may refuse because they believe that the prosthesis is functioning adequately and they fear surgery. In such cases long-term antibiotic suppression may be attempted to control the local and systemic effects of the infection and to maintain function of the joint. A second situation in which chronic antibiotic suppression is attempted is to treat patients whose hips have been revised for infection but in whom infection continues. Although excellent results for single-stage and two-stage revisions of infected prostheses are described in Chapter 25, residual infection rates of 9% to 15% are to be expected (6,19). In these situations, postoperative antibiotics often are continued indefinitely to control signs and symptoms of infection. Moreover, although some protocols suggest that postrevision antibiotic treatment be limited to a defined period of 4 to 6 weeks (6,10,19), other physicians are more comfortable continuing treatment for an indefinite time in the hope of preventing relapses caused by residual organisms. A third situation in which antibiotics are used for extended periods is when the revision is routine but intraoperative cultures suggest the possibility of infection.

In each situation the clinician must adjust the goals on the basis of the individual patient's response to treatment. Pragmatism is required. The ideal response is complete resolution of all local (pain, induration, drainage) and systemic (fever, anorexia) signs of infection with correction of white blood cell count, hemoglobin level, and erythrocyte sedimentation rate. When this occurs, our approach is to continue oral antibiotic treatment (barring drug toxicity) for 6 to 12 additional months before considering a recommendation to discontinue therapy. At that time the relative risks of continuing antibiotics unnecessarily versus relapse at discontinuation are weighed by clinician and patient, and an individualized decision is made. Two studies from Europe showed that long-term administration of combinations of rifampin and a fluoroquinolone in cases of prosthesis infection by *Staph. aureus* organisms resulted in resolution of clinical, biologic, and radiologic evidence of residual infection among three fourths of patients 6 months after the antibiotic treatment was stopped (3,21). The range of oral agents with excellent absorption, broad spectrum, and low incidence of intolerance is now quite extensive, generally failing to inhibit only methicillin-resistant staphylococci (coagulase-positive and coagulase-negative) and vancomycin-resistant enterococci.

More often in our experience, total elimination of the signs and symptoms of infection in this patient population is not achievable. Then the goal becomes *control* of the infection at a level that allows continued function of the prosthesis without debilitating symptoms or drug toxicity. The effectiveness of control is usually decided within the first 30 to 60 days of treatment. Either the systemic and local signs and symptoms (defervescence, decreased local inflammation, wound healing, and not infrequently development of a draining sinus tract) slowly improve to a manageable level or the infection continues with fever, anorexia, painful local symptoms, and loss of function of the hip. If control is achieved, maintenance of a patent draining sinus tract can be important for continued function. Closing off of the tract is often the harbinger of recurrence of local pain and cellulitis accompanied by a fever that progress until the sinus reopens either spontaneously or surgically, followed by reestablishment of chronic drainage and the resolution of symptoms. In the event that control cannot be maintained with chronic antibiotic administration, the remaining options are surgical revision, a Girdlestone procedure, or in extremely rare instances amputation.

Use of antibiotics for chronic suppression of infection has several potential disadvantages. First, resistant organisms can emerge over time under the selective pressure of the antibiotic in the environment. This is a serious problem with infections in sites that are constantly being inoculated with environmental organisms (gastrointestinal tract, urinary bladder with indwelling catheter) and less of a problem in osteomyelitis, where the organism numbers are small and suprainfection uncommon. In contrast to deep-seated bone, sinus tracts are in close communication with the skin and commonly become colonized with resistant organisms in conditions of long-term antibiotic administration. Culture of such organisms from sinus tracts should not mislead the clinician to believe that the bone is necessarily similarly infected. A second disadvantage of long-term antibiotic administration is adverse drug experiences. In general, these occur relatively early in the course of drug use (30 to 60 days) and present a small risk for ongoing problems thereafter. Moreover, the wide range of antibiotics with excellent oral absorption improves the likelihood that chronic antibiotic suppression can be continued with another effective drug if the first choice must be abandoned. A third risk of chronic suppression is the possibility that chronic low-grade inflammation around the prosthesis will lead to loosening, bone resorption, and loss of function. Goulet et al. (7) reported that approximately half of infected hip prostheses left in place and treated with chronic antibiotic suppression failed over a 4 year period of observation and required replacement. Other groups have reported similar failure rates (4). A final concern is that the presence of a chronic bacterial infection will result in long-term sequelae such as secondary amyloidosis or a tumor at the site of infection. Although these complications have been reported, there are no good data regarding their frequency.

Our approach to observation of patients undertaking chronic suppressive antibiotic regimens is as follows. For the first 6 months, or until the infection has reached an acceptable steady state, patients are examined monthly with measurement of a complete blood cell count, including white blood cell differential and erythrocyte sedimentation rate, and a chemistry panel, including creatinine and liver enzymes. Thereafter they are examined and blood tests monitored at 3-month intervals.

As the reader can see, infection in total hip arthroplasty can be a devastating problem. This complication is among the most challenging of all the infectious diseases. Although the armamentarium of antibiotics available has increased over the years, further research is needed to determine the optimal therapeutic approach.

REFERENCES

1. Brandt CM, Sistrunk WW, Duffy MC, Steckelberg JM, Hanssen AD, Osmon DR. Staphylococcus aureus prosthetic joint infections treated with two stage revision arthroplasty. Presented at the 34th Annual Meeting of the Infectious Diseases Society of America; 1996 Sep. 18–20, New Orleans. In: *Abstracts of the Infectious Diseases Society of America.* 1996: abstract 182.
2. Brandt CM, Sistrunk WW, Duffy MC, Steckelberg JM, Hanssen AD, Ilstrup DM, Osmon DR. Staphylococcus aureus prosthetic joint infections treated with debridement and prosthesis retention. *Clin Infect Dis* 1997;24:914–919.
3. Drancourt M, Stein A, Argenson JN, Aznnier A, Curvale G, Raoult D. Oral rifampin plus ofloxacin for treatment of staphylococcus-infected orthopedic implants. *Antimicrob Agents Chemother* 1993;37:1214–1218.
4. Dupont JA. Significance of operative cultures in total hip arthroplasty. *Clin Orthop* 1986;211:122–127.
5. Garvin KL, Fitgerald RH, Salati E, et al. Reconstruction of the infected total hip and knee arthroplasty with gentamicin impregnated palacos bone cement. *Instr Course Lect* 1993;42:293–302.
6. Garvin KL, Hanssen AD. Infection after total hip arthroplasty. *J Bone Joint Surg Am* 1995;77:1576–1588.
7. Goulet JA, Pellicci PM, Brause BI, Salvati EM. Prolonged suppression of infection in total hip arthroplasty. *J Arthroplasty* 1988;3:109–116.
8. Jacobson JJ, Schweitzer SO, Kowalski CJ. Chemoprophylaxis of prosthetic joint patients during dental treatment: a decision-utility analysis. *Oral Surg Oral Med Oral Pathol Oral Radiol Endod* 1991;72:167–177.
9. Kloos WE, Bannerman TL. Update on clinical significance of coagulase negative staphylococci. *Clin Microbiol Rev* 1994;7:117–140.
10. Lieberman JR, Callaway GH, Salvatti EA, Pellicci PM, Brause BD. Threatment of the infected total hip arthroplasty with a two-stage reimplantation protocol. *Clin Orthop* 1994;301:205–214.
11. Little JW. Managing dental patients with joint prostheses. *J Am Dent Assoc* 1994;125:1374–1378.
12. McCluskey WP, Esterhai J, Brighton CT, Heppenstall RB. Neutropenia complicating parenteral antibiotic treatment of infected nonunion of the tibia. *Arch Surg* 1989;124:1309–1312.
13. McDonald DJ, Fitgerald RH, Ilstrup DM. Two stage reconstruction of a total hip arthroplasty because of infection. *Jone Bone Joint Surg Am* 1989;71:828–834.
14. Nasser S. Prevention and treatment of sepsis in total hip replacement surgery. *Orthop Clin North Am* 1992;23:265–277.
15. Shrout MK, Scarbrough F, Powell BJ. Dental care and the prosthetic joint patient: a survey of orthopedic surgeons and general dentists. *J Am Dent Assoc* 1994;125:429–434.
16. Stiefeld SM, Graziani AL, MacGregor R, Esterhai JL. Toxicities of antimicrobial agents used to treat osteomyelitis. *Orthop Clin North Am* 1991;22:439–465.
17. Stout RD, Ferguson KP, Li YN, Lambe DW Jr. Staphylococcal exopolysaccharides inhibit lymphocyte proliferative responses by activation of monocyte prostaglandin production. *Infect Immun* 1992;60:922–927.
18. Tsevat J, Durand-Zaleski I, Pauker SG. Cost-effectiveness of antibiotic prophylaxis for dental procedures in patients with artificial joints. *Am J Public Health* 1989;79:739–743.
19. Tsukayama DT, Estrada R, Gustilo RB. Infection after total hip arthroplasty: a study of the treatment of one hundred and six infections. *J Bone Joint Surg Am* 1996;78:512–523.
20. Wahl MJ. Myths of dental-induced prosthetic joint infections. *Clin Infect Dis* 1995;20:1420–1425.
21. Widmer AF, Gaechter A, Ochsner PE, Zimmerli W. Antimicrobial treatment of orthopedic implant-related infections with rifampin combinations. *Clin Infect Dis* 1992;14:1251–1253.
22. Wilde AH. Management of infected knee and hip prosthesis. *Curr Opin Rheumatol* 1994;6:172–176.
23. American Dental Association, American Academy of Orthopaedic Surgeons. Antibiotic prophylaxis for dental patients with total joint replacements, advisory statement. July 1997.

Revision Total Hip Arthroplasty,
edited by Marvin E. Steinberg and Jonathan P. Garino,
Lippincott Williams & Wilkins, Philadelphia © 1999.

28

Surgical Techniques

Robert H. Fitzgerald, Jr.

The surgical treatment of a patient with an infected total hip arthroplasty has mirrored the advances within the field of total joint surgery. Whereas in the past treatment was rather straightforward (7,8), the treatment options today are extensive. They depend on the individual patient's overall health and response to the infectious process and microbiologic diagnosis (14). Surgical treatment of a patient with an infected total hip arthroplasty can be associated with extensive surgical dissection, considerable blood loss, and an extended operative time. Unless the patient exhibits symptoms consistent with septicemia, the first step after establishment of the diagnosis of deep periprosthetic infection is performance of a thorough history interview and physical examination by an internist to identify any associated medical conditions that might influence the extent and duration of operative intervention. Patients with septicemia need immediate surgical intervention (14) (Fig. 1). Equally as important is complete microbiologic evaluation of the causal organism, because this information is influential in the decision making that is instrumental in achieving the desired outcome (5).

INFECTED TOTAL HIP ARTHROPLASTY WITH SEPTICEMIA

Fortunately, septicemia from a periprosthetic infection is uncommon (17,31). However, when a patient with a deep infection around a total hip arthroplasty is seen with systemic signs and symptoms of sepsis, it is a medical emergency (32). Even though the symptoms may be mild, they can progress very rapidly, producing cardiopulmonary instability and central nervous system toxicity, which commonly precipitates a coma. Emergency surgical treatment should include removal of the prosthetic components and other foreign materials if the patient's condition allows. Invariably, the surgeon encounters an abscess of some magnitude that envelops the femur, acetabulum, or both. An astute surgeon may elect either to pack the wound open or to loosely close the wound over gauze soaked in an antibiotic solution or half-strength iodophor solution.

R. H. Fitzgerald: Department of Orthopaedic Surgery, University of Pennsylvania, Philadelphia, Pennsylvania 19104.

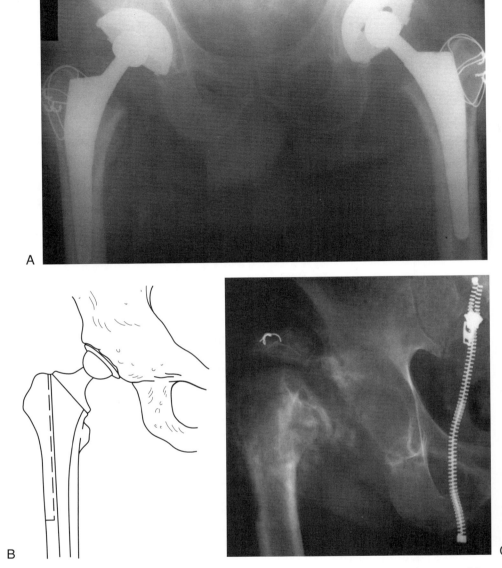

Figure 1. A well-fixed cementless total hip arthroplasty in an elderly man whose condition became septic and obtunded 4 months after the operation. **A:** Anteroposterior (AP) radiograph of the pelvis shows bilateral cementless hip arthroplasties, air in the fascial planes, and soft-tissue swelling of proximal aspect of the right thigh. The femoral and acetabular components appear to be well fixed. **B:** Drawing shows cuts made in the proximal femur for extended trochanteric osteotomy. **C:** AP radiograph of the right hip reveals a Girdlestone resection arthroplasty with evidence of extended trochanteric osteotomy to allow excision of a well-fixed femoral component.

Skeletal traction with a Steinmann pin placed in the proximal tibia allows greater control of the extremity for nursing needs, control of postoperative hematoma, and reduction of postoperative pain. Parenteral antimicrobial therapy can be begun on the basis of findings for intraoperative clinical material submitted to the microbiology laboratory for Gram stain. Therapy later can be modified on the basis of isolation of the causal microorganisms and findings of susceptibility studies. The patient can be returned to the operating room for additional débridement once his or her condition is stabilized. If the abscess has not recurred, definitive wound closure with or without a local muscle flap can be performed depending on the degree of the remaining dead space.

INFECTED TOTAL HIP ARTHROPLASTY WITHOUT SEPTICEMIA

If the condition of a patient with an infected total hip arthroplasty is not septic, the first major decision that both the surgeon and the patient must address is the intended outcome of the treatment plan. Although medical treatment alone would be the preference of all patients, experience with antimicrobial therapy without concomitant surgical intervention has been ineffective (18,38). A combination of antimicrobial therapy administered for an extended period has been proposed as effective in the management of infections from which *Staphylococcus aureus* organisms have been isolated (11,40). The investigators extended application of this technique to the treatment of patients with *Pseudomonas aeruginosa* infection of arthroplasties and substituted fusidic acid for fluoroquinolone (3,10). Unfortunately, the follow-up period is extremely short, precluding any comment as to the efficacy of this modality. Some patients want the infectious process and associated pain to be alleviated without reconstruction of the hip (34). Most patients find the instability associated with a Girdlestone resection arthroplasty unacceptable. Kostulk et al. (23) demonstrated that it is possible although often difficult to obtain arthrodesis of the proximal femur to the pelvis. However, most patients want eradication of the infection and reconstruction of the hip to achieve a level of function of the lower extremity consistent with the premorbid state. The options that must be considered include débridement without component removal, one-stage exchange arthroplasty, two-stage exchange arthroplasty, two-stage exchange arthroplasty with an intervening step with a prosthesis of antibiotic-loaded acrylic cement (Prostalac), and three-stage exchange arthroplasty. Most patients disdain two operations. However, a two-staged procedure is the treatment of choice for most patients with an infected total hip arthroplasty, because it provides time for the patient's immune system to become an active participant with surgical débridement and antimicrobial therapy in eradication of the infectious process before introduction of additional foreign material (21,29,35). Although any decision made during the preoperative evaluation of a low-grade infectious process around a total hip arthroplasty can be altered by intraoperative findings or the patient's response to treatment, it is usually wise to have a plan before initiation of surgical treatment.

INFECTED POSTOPERATIVE HEMATOMA AND LATE HEMATOGENOUS INFECTION

Infected postoperative hematoma and late hematogenous infection have traditionally been treated with surgical débridement and parenteral antimicrobial therapy without component removal (14) (Fig. 2). An acutely infected postoperative hematoma is usually a colonized hematoma and rarely a true infection. Thus thorough débridement and parenteral antimicrobial therapy have an excellent chance of successfully eradicating the infectious process. Certainly, administration of antimicrobial therapy by itself to a patient with a draining hematoma that emanates from deep to the fascia will most likely lead to deep infection with eventual loss of the implants. When a patient who has had a well-functioning arthroplasty for several years has an acute infection of the implant, it is difficult to consider Girdlestone resection arthroplasty as the initial therapeutic option. Many surgeons believe that surgical débridement and parenteral antimicrobial therapy without component removal is the treatment of choice (7,21,29,31). Although there are anecdotal reports of long-term success with this procedure, most surgeons experienced in the treatment of patients with an infected total hip arthroplasty have found that patients with late hematogenous infections of the implant treated with débridement and parenteral antimicrobial therapy without component removal have ultimately required Girdlestone resection arthroplasty. In my experience such treatment suppresses the infectious process but fails to eradicate it. When this group of patients has been followed for at least 5 years, all have ultimately been treated with Girdlestone resection arthroplasty. In Europe orthopedic surgeons have been attempting to treat this group of patients with aspiration of the hip. If *S. aureus* or *P. aeruginosa* organisms are isolated, these surgeons have been treating the patients with 6 months of fluoroquinolone and rifampin with surprising effectiveness (10,11,34). Unfortunately, long-term follow-up findings have not been reported. Thus this technique remains experimental at this time.

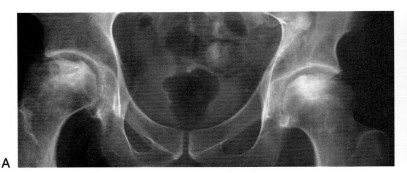

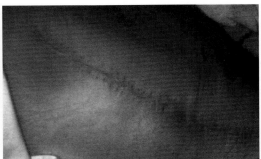

A

B

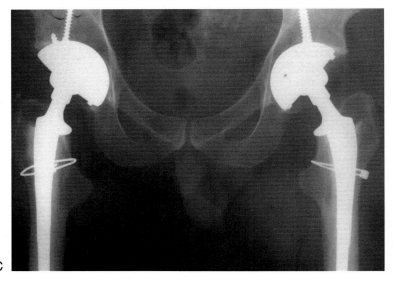

C

Figure 2. Postoperative hematoma after total hip arthroplasty. **A:** Anteroposterior (AP) radiograph reveals bilateral osteonecrosis of the femoral head in a 41-year-old man. **B:** Three days after total hip arthroplasty swelling with cellulitis is evident. A large hematoma was surgically evacuated. **C:** AP radiograph of the pelvis reveals bilateral hybrid total hip arthroplasty 4 months after an operation on the right and 2 months after an operation on the left. The patient has no symptoms.

ONE-STAGE ARTHROPLASTY

One-stage exchange arthroplasty, introduced by Buchholz et al. (4,5) allowed surgeons to manage the infectious process and reconstruct the hip during the same operation (Fig. 3). The operation was based on the fact that high local concentrations of antimicrobial agents could be achieved in the area of the infection through the addition of antimicrobial agents to bone cement (polymethyl methacrylate; PMMA) (39). It was fortuitous that German orthopedic surgeons were using Palacos bone cement, because this substance has subsequently been shown to have superior leaching properties compared with Simplex P or CMW bone cement (20). All antimicrobial agents studied appear to leach from Palacos without inhibition of their antimicrobial properties by the exothermic reaction that occurs with curing of the bone cement. The kinetics of the leaching from Palacos bone cement do seem to vary with the different classes of antibiotics (20). Gentamicin and other aminoglycosides appear to have sustained leaching properties for prolonged periods of time. Selection of antimicrobial agent to include within the PMMA is based on the susceptibility pattern of the microorganisms isolated from preoperative aspiration of the hip rather than the customary agent selected for primary arthroplasty (1,19,28).

The success of one-stage exchange arthroplasty is influenced by the virulence of the causal organism. When one analyzes the large experience of Buchhoz et al., the success of the procedure appears to have a direct correlation with the microorganism recovered (29) (Table 1). Patients with an infected total hip arthroplasty from which a more virulent microorganism was isolated had a greater chance of the procedure's being complicated by recurrent infection. In fact a gram-negative bacillary infection was complicated by recurrent infection among more than 50% of the patients. In contrast, infections associated with isolation of an anaerobic microorganism or coagulase-negative staphylococci were associated with recurrent infections less than one-fourth of the time. Glycocalyx may play an important role in the incidence of

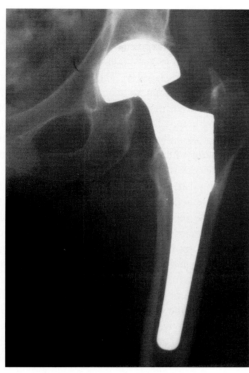
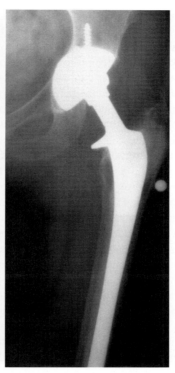

A   B

Figure 3. One-stage exchange arthroplasty on a 68-year-old English professor with a painful bipolar cementless arthroplasty 2 years after implantation. **A:** Anteroposterior (AP) radiograph of the left hip with a porous coated anatomic (PCA; Howmedica, East Rutherford, N.J.) cementless femoral component and a bipolar acetabular component. Her erythrocyte sedimentation rate was 53 mm in 1 hour (Westergren). A preoperative aspirate was sterile. **B:** AP radiograph of the left hip 1 year after one-stage exchange arthroplasty. Group D streptococci and enterococci were isolated from multiple surgical specimens. Tobramycin- and erythromycin-incorporated Palacos bone cement was used for fixation of the long-stemmed femoral component. The patient had no symptoms 8 years after the one-stage procedure.

recurrent sepsis (9,13,27). Patients with causal microorganisms that elaborate gylcocalyx probably should be treated with two-stage exchange arthroplasty.

Thorough surgical débridement is fundamental to the success of one-stage exchange arthroplasty. All foci of microabscess must be excised, or recurrent infection will complicate the procedure. A transtrochanteric exposure is advantageous because trochanteric osteotomy affords greater visualization of both the femoral canal and periacetabular tissues. The type of trochanteric osteotomy varies with the type of prosthetic device to be excised. Well-fixed femoral components that require visualization of the intramedullary canal to the level of the isthmus require that the proximal femur be delivered out of the wound. Otherwise the straight instruments used to remove cement (osteotomes, currettes, Midas Rex cutting tools, or

Table 1. *One-stage arthroplasty*

Microorganism	Success rate
Sterile	89%
Corynebacterium sp	85%
Peptococcus sp	76%
Staphylococcus aureus	72%
Gram-negative bacilli (*Pseudomonas aeruginosa,*	
Klebsiella sp, *Escherichia coli*)	<50%

ultrasonic tools) can perforate the femoral canal, and produce a stress riser that can precipitate a postoperative fracture. In attempts to remove a cemented femoral component of standard length, routine trochanteric osteotomy allows sufficient exposure for safe extirpation of the component. In attempts to excise an extensively coated femoral component that is well fixed, extended trochanteric osteotomy can be most useful (see Fig. 1B). The trochanteric osteotomy should be extended the length of the femoral component unless one plans to cut the device at the metaphyseal and diaphyseal junction and trephine the diaphyseal portion of the component. Unfortunately, this technique produces considerable metallic debris that can lead to persistent sepsis. If the component to be removed is a proximally coated and well-fixed cementless device, a trochanteric slide or standard osteotomy may allow the proximal femur to be delivered sufficiently into the wound to allow access with flexible osteotomes.

Once thorough débridement has been accomplished with removal of all of the foreign material, the patient's clinical situation can be assessed with the anesthesiologist to determine the appropriateness of proceeding with immediate reconstruction of the hip with antibiotic-incorporated PMMA (15,41). The presence of abscess formation precludes performance of one-stage exchange arthroplasty. If the microorganism isolated during preoperative evaluation does not elaborate glycocalyx and is susceptible to antimicrobial agents, one-stage exchange arthroplasty can be considered. If the proximal femur is intact and the endosteal surface will provide fixation of PMMA, a standard length femoral component can be implanted. If the proximal femur was damaged during removal of the original component and associated cement, a long-stemmed femoral component with or without a calcar replacement may be required to restore the femur. If the patient has exhibited any signs of cardiovascular instability during removal of the acetabular and femoral components, injection of several batches of PMMA and insertion of a long-stemmed femoral component can cause additional embolization of marrow contents with resultant hypotension and cardiac instability (15,41). Thus the patient's condition and type of implant both play important roles in intraoperative decision making. Palacos bone cement has an extremely short low viscous state. The entire operative team must be highly organized and ready to cement before mixing of antibiotic-loaded Palacos bone cement because the cement must be taken from the refrigerator, mixed with the appropriate antimicrobial agent, and injected without unnecessary delay. The usual mixing time for other types of cement is too long for Palacos bone cement, allowing it to become quite doughy and difficult to inject.

TWO-STAGE EXCHANGE ARTHROPLASTY

Most patients are best treated with a two-stage exchange arthroplasty (21,29,35) (Fig. 4). If this decision is made before surgical intervention, trochanteric osteotomy is avoided if at all possible because reattachment of the trochanteric fragment to the proximal femur necessitates introduction of foreign bodies and may lead to trochanteric nonunion. On completion of thorough débridement with removal of all foreign material, the would is closed in layers with resorbable sutures. Nonresorbable sutures can act as foreign bodies, providing a nidus for the formation of microabscesses. Insertion of a traction pin for application of skeletal traction helps control both postoperative pain and hematoma formation. A Steinmann pin is best inserted in the proximal tibia. Although the pin can introduce some stiffness of the knee, insertion into the distal femur can introduce microorganisms into this site, which can compromise reconstruction, especially if a long-stemmed femoral component is implanted at reconstruction. Skeletal traction once was continued for up to 6 weeks. Traction now is continued until the wound demonstrates healing without formation of a large hematoma, which is usually about 7 days after Girdlestone resection arthroplasty. Parenteral antibiotics specific for the causal microorganisms isolated from surgical tissue specimens are administered for a minimum of 4 weeks. Oral antibiotics can be administered for an additional 4 to 6 weeks.

The most difficult aspect of two-stage exchange arthroplasty is the timing of reconstruction. Ideally reconstruction is not done in the presence of active infection. Much of the information that has been used to select the appropriate time is empiric

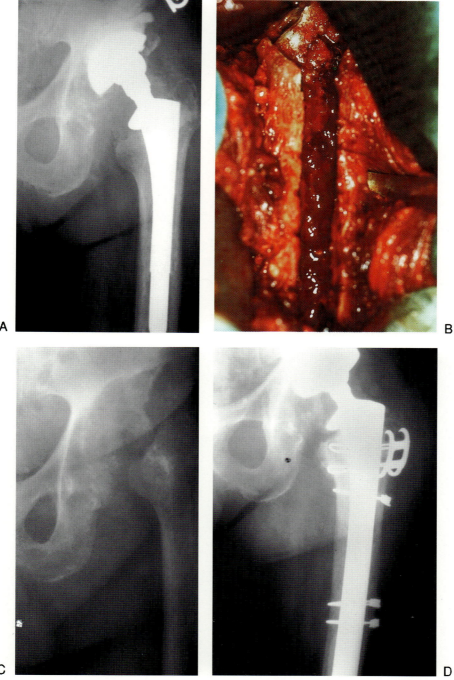

Figure 4. Hematogenous infection of an extensively coated cementless total hip arthroplasty in a 68-year-old accountant who had persistent infection after Girdlestone resection arthroplasty. **A:** Anteroposterior (AP) radiograph shows a cementless anatomic medullary locking (AML; DePuy, Warsaw, Ind.) total hip arthroplasty 4 years after implantation. The patient was febrile and had left hip pain. Grossly purulent material was obtained with aspiration of the hip. **B:** Intraoperative photograph of the slot made in the femoral canal for surgical extraction of the well-fixed femoral component. **C:** AP radiograph of left hip reveals Girdlestone arthroplasty. Group D streptococci, subspecies enterococci were isolated from multiple surgical specimens and the hip aspirate. The patient was treated with 13 weeks of parenteral antimicrobial therapy and three surgical débridements. **D:** AP radiograph of the left hip 14 months after reconstruction with a fully coated solution femoral component with structural allograft over the femoral defect. The reconstruction was performed 16 months after the original Girdlestone procedure. The patient was free of symptoms 60 months after reconstruction of the hip.

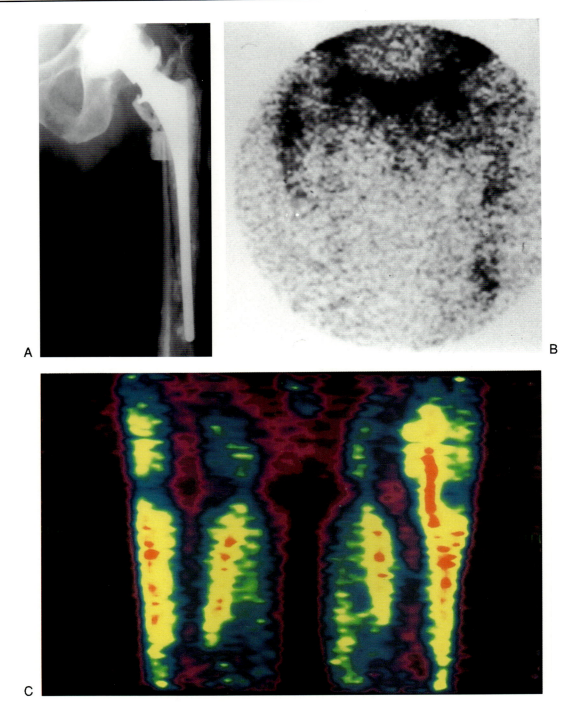

Figure 5. A 79-year-old man originally sustained an intracapsular hip fracture in 1979 after an automobile accident. He was initially treated with Austin Moore arthroplasty, which was converted to total hip arthroplasty in 1986. Three years later revision total hip arthroplasty was performed with an allograft. The prosthesis was painful, and the erythrocyte sedimentation rate was 35 mm in 1 hour (Westergren). **A:** Anteroposterior (AP) radiograph reveals a long-stemmed femoral component with a medially placed femoral allograft. A circumferential radiolucent line is visible. **B:** Indium-III autologous white blood cell image reveals equivocal increased uptake around the femoral component. **C:** Positron emission tomographic image of the right hip reveals increased uptake around the proximal femur in the area of the allograft. Group D streptococci enterococci were isolated during Girdlestone resection arthroplasty.

information. McDonald et al. (29) demonstrated that the incidence of recurrent infection was reduced if a 3-month interval elapsed between Girdlestone resection arthroplasty and reconstruction when a less virulent causal organism was isolated and the patient received at least 4 weeks of antimicrobial therapy. Patients in whom a more virulent causal organism was isolated had a lower incidence of recurrent infection if a year elapsed between the two procedures. Unfortunately, the database was not large enough to allow one to determine whether a delay of 4 to 12 months would be as effective. Thus considerable clinical judgment is involved in making this decision. Erythrocyte sedimentation rate and C reactive protein determination can be helpful in the decision (2,36). If these laboratory examinations of peripheral blood are monitored monthly, they can provide useful information. If both parameters return to normal and the wound has healed without evidence of inflammation 6 weeks after cessation of antimicrobial therapy, it would seem appropriate to proceed with reconstruction of the hip. If the erythrocyte sedimentation rate is slightly elevated, the use of nuclear radiologic studies to evaluate the hip can be helpful. The use of indium-III-labeled autologous white blood cell images can be diagnostic in 80% to 94% of instances (26,30). Positron emission tomography has proved to be effective in the identification of residual infections or infections around painful arthroplasties (24,25,37,42) (Fig. 5). New immunologic and genetic laboratory evaluations may in the future provide even more accurate results (6). Parenteral administration of prophylactic antibiotics is continued until aerobic and anaerobic cultures of intraoperatively obtained tissue specimens are found to be sterile rather than the short duration associated with primary arthroplasty (19,28). The agent selected should be effective against the causal organism isolated at the time of the index infection. If these cultures have positive results, prolonged antibiotic treatment may be indicated.

Restoration of leg-length inequality can be difficult during the second stage. A trochanteric slide osteotomy with a long, thin fragment allows lengthening, mobility, and union of the trochanter (Fig. 6).

Although the second stage of reconstruction has traditionally been done with cemented components and antibiotic-impregnated PMMA, the use of cementless components has not been associated with an increased incidence of recurrent sepsis (33) (Fig. 7). The incidence of recurrent sepsis in my practice has been lower with the use of cementless devices in recent years.

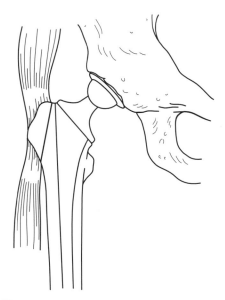

Figure 6. Trochanteric slide osteotomy. The gluteus medius and vastus lateralis muscles remain attached to the trochanteric fragment to provide vascularity and stability.

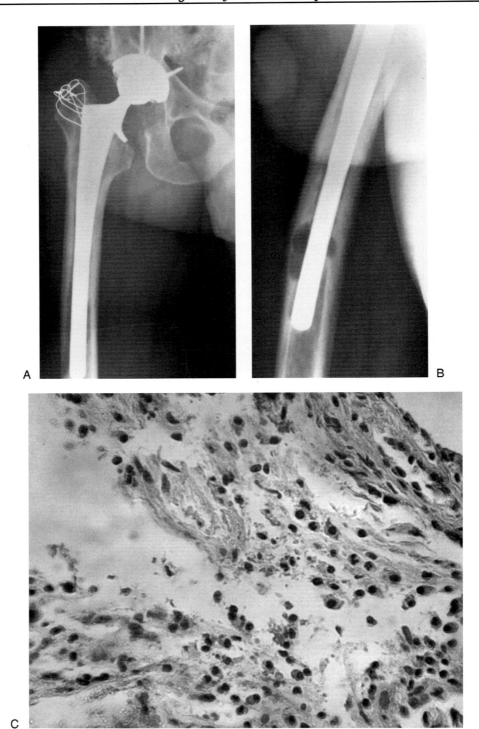

Figure 7. Painful total hip arthroplasty 1 year after two-stage exchange arthroplasty for an infection from which *Staphylococcus epidermidis* organisms were isolated. Although the patient has a lytic lesion in the distal femur, his erythrocyte sedimentation rate was 25 mm in 1 hour (Westergren), and a hip aspirate was sterile. A biopsy proved that the lytic lesion represented recurrent infection. **A:** Anteroposterior (AP) radiograph reveals cementless total hip arthroplasty with thinning of the cortex about the distal third of the femoral component. **B:** Table-down lateral view demonstrates a large lytic lesion. **C:** Histologic examination of the biopsy specimen revealed infiltration by many polymorphonuclear leukocytes consistent with a low-grade infection. *Staphylococcus epidermidis* organisms were isolated with aerobic incubation of the surgical specimen.

ANTIBIOTIC-IMPREGNATED SPACERS AND PROSTHESES

Duncan and Beauchamp (12) introduced the concept of insertion of a temporary prosthesis after thorough débridement of the wound. This prosthesis is coated with antibiotic-impregnated PMMA. However, during introduction of the cement and the prosthetic component, the cement is introduced in such a way as to not create an intimate bone–cement interface. Although Duncan and Beauchamp made a specialized prosthesis for this procedure, the PROSTALAC, it is possible to sterilize the recently removed femoral component and reimplant it (Fig. 8). An all-polyethylene acetabular component can be cemented into the bony acetabulum with antibiotic-impregnated PMMA. Although the PROSTALAC concept was promulgated as temporary prosthesis, most patients find that their pain is alleviated, and they often are able to function with this device in place until loosening takes place. Other types of antibiotic-impregnated spacers and beads have been inserted temporarily to help eradicate infection and preserve tissue planes.

THREE-STAGE EXCHANGE ARTHROPLASTY

Occasionally there is sufficient destruction of the acetabulum and femur by the infectious process that reconstruction of the hip requires structural allograft bone to

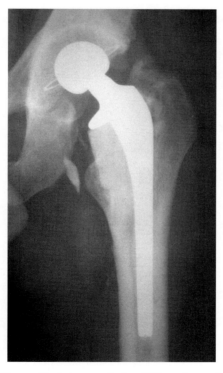

Figure 8. Anteroposterior (AP) radiograph of the left hip reveals a cemented total hip arthroplasty with an all-polyethylene acetabular component. Prosalac reconstruction with tobramycin and erythromycin incorporated Palacos bone cement for management of a methicillin-resistant coagulase-negative staphylococcal infection. The components were implanted without pressurization of the bone cement. This radiograph reveals minimal evidence of loosening 1 year after implantation. The patient had no symptoms.

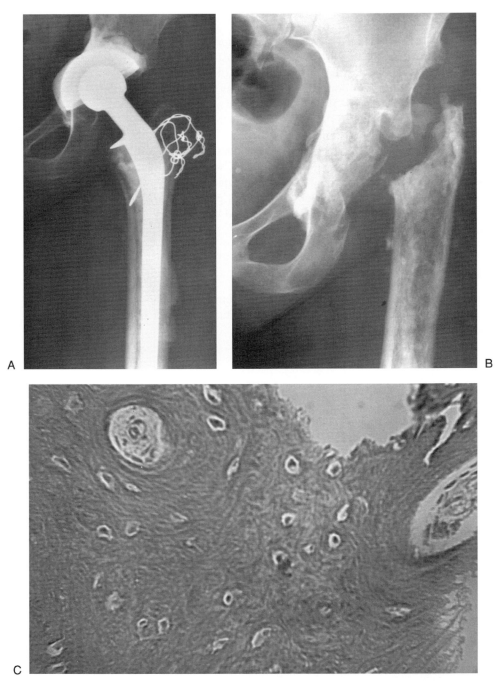

Figure 9. *Pseudomonous aeruginosa* infection of a revision total hip arthroplasty in a 25-year-old beautician treated with three-stage exchange arthroplasty. **A:** Anteroposterior (AP) radiograph of cemented total hip arthroplasty. The lateral femoral cortex is quite thin and the medial wall of the acetabulum is deficient. **B:** AP radiograph 3 months after bone grafting of the bony acetabulum (second stage). A combination of particulate autograft and allograft was placed in the acetabulum and proximal femur 3 months after Girdlestone arthroplasty. **C:** Histologic section of the bone in the acetabulum 8 months after implantation of the mixture of autograft and allograft. The bone is viable with nuclei in all of the lacuna visualized.

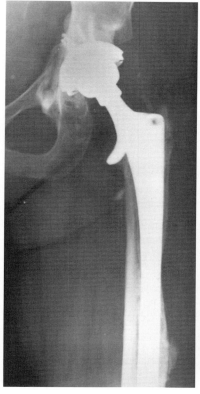

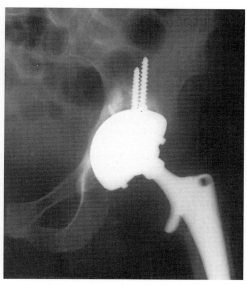

D   E

Figure 9. *Continued.* **D:** AP radiograph 2 years after reconstruction of the hip with cementless total hip arthroplasty (third stage). **E:** AP radiograph 11 years after revision of the acetabular component. The femoral component with titanium wire mesh pads proximally was well fixed when examined during the operation.

reconstitute the anatomic features (22). Although this is acceptable to older patients, for young patients insertion of allografts carries high risk to the longevity of the prosthesis. Implantation of modular components can be an alternative to use of structural allografts. Three-stage exchange arthroplasty with reconstruction of the bony deficits with a mixture of particulate autograft and allograft is another alternative (16) (Fig. 9). Although the stress on the graft is indirect, healing occurs and provides support for implantation of cementless components at reconstruction 6 months after insertion of the graft. The overall application of this technique is limited because there are few young patients with an infected total hip arthroplasty.

CONCLUSIONS

A variety of techniques can be applied to treatment of patients with perioprosthetic infection of a total hip arthroplasty. Application of each technique depends on the patient, the virulence of the causal organism, and the natural history of the infectious process. Most patients are best treated with two-stage exchange arthroplasty.

REFERENCES

1. Barrack RL, Harris WH. The value of aspiration of the hip joint before revision total hip arthroplasty. *J Bone Joint Surg Am* 1993;75:66–76.
2. Bauer TW, Saltarelli M. Infection versus aseptic loosening in revision arthroplasty: predictive value of frozen sections and other laboratory tests. *Orthop Trans* 1993;17:1054.

3. Brouqui P, Rousseau MC, Stein A, Drancourt M, Raoult D. Treatment of *Pseudomonas aeruginosa*–infected orthopedic prostheses with ceftazidime-ciprofloxacin antibiotic combination. *Antimicrob Agents Chemother* 1995;39:2423–2425.
4. Buchholz HW, Elson RA, Englebrecht E, et al. Management of deep infection of total hip replacement. *J Bone Joint Surg Br* 1981;63:342–353.
5. Buchholz HW, Gartmann HD. Infections prophylaze and operative Behandlung der sjchleichenden tiefen Infektion bei der totlen Endoprosthes. *Chirurg* 1972;43:446.
6. Chada HS, Wooley PH, Fitzgerald RH Jr. Cellular proliferation and cytokine responses to polymethyl-methacrylate (PMMA) following joint arthroplasty. *Orthop Trans* 1993;17:600.
7. Charnley J. The future of total hip arthroplasty. In: Nelson JP, ed. *The hip.* St. Louis: CV Mosby, 1982:198–210.
8. Charnley J. Low friction arthroplasty of the hip: theory and practice. New York: Springer-Verlag, 1979:152–168.
9. Christensen GD, Simpson WA, Bisno AL, et al. Adherence of slime-producing strains of *Staphylococcus epidermidis* to smooth surfaces. *Infect Immun* 1982;37:318–326.
10. Drancourt M, Stein A, Argenson JN, Roiron R, Groulier P, Raoult D. Oral treatment of *Staphylococcus* spp. infected orthopaedic implants with fusidic acid or ofloxacin in combination with rifampicin. *J Antimicrob Chemother* 1997;39:235–240.
11. Drancourt M, Stein A, Argenson JN, Zannier A, Curvale G, Raoult D. Oral rifampin plus ofloxacin for treatment of *Staphylococcus* infected orthopedic implants. *Antimicrob Agents Chemother* 1993;37:1214–1218.
12. Duncan CP, Beauchamp CP. A temporary antibiotic-loaded joint replacement system for management of complex infections involving the hip. *Orthop Clin North Am* 1993;24:751–759.
13. Dunne WM, Mason EO, Kaplan SL. Diffusion of rifampin and vancomycin through a *Staphylococcus epidermidis* biofilm. *Antimicrob Agents Chemother* 1993;37:2522–2526.
14. Fitzgerald RH Jr. Diagnosis and management of established infections of total hip arthroplasty. *J Am Acad Orthop Surg* 1995;3:249–262.
15. Fitzgerald RH Jr, Johnson C, Mason L. Embolic phenomena during revision total hip arthroplasty: diagnosis with transesophageal monitoring. *University Pennsylvania Orthop J* 1997;10:18–23.
16. Fitzgerald RH Jr, Jones DR. The infected implant: treatment with resection arthroplasty and late total hip arthroplasty. *Am J Med* 1985;78:225–228.
17. Fitzgerald RH Jr, Peterson LFA, Washington JA II, Van Scoy RE, Coventry MB. Bacterial colonization of wounds and sepsis in total hip arthroplasty. *J Bone Joint Surg Am* 1973;55:1242–1250.
18. Goulet JA, Pellicci PM, Brause BD, Salvati EM. Prolonged suppression of infection in total hip arthroplasty. *J Arthroplasty* 1988;3:109–116.
19. Hill C, Mazas F, Flamont R, Eorard J. Prophylactic cefazolin versus placebo in total hip replacement. *Lancet* 1981;1:795–797.
20. Hoff SF, Fitzgerald RH Jr, Kelly PJ. The depot administration of penicillin G and gentamicin in acrylic bone cement. *J Bone Joint Surg Am* 1981;63:798–804.
21. Hunter G, Dandy DJ. The natural history of the patient with an infected total hip replacement. *J Bone Joint Surg Br* 1976;1977;58,59:134,293.
22. Jasty M, Harris WH. Salvage Total Hip Reconstruction in patients with major acetabular bone deficiency using structural femoral head allografts. *J Bone Joint Surg Br* 1990;72:63–67.
23. Kostulk J, Alexander D. Arthrodesis for failed arthroplasty of the hip. *Clin Orthop* 1984;188:173–181.
24. Kubota R, Yamada S, Kubota K, Ishiwata K, Tamaahashi N, Ido T. Intratumoral distribution of fluorine-18-fluorodeoxyglucose in vivo: high accumulation in macrophages and granulation tissues studied by microautoradiography. *J Nucl Med* 1992;33:1972–1980.
25. Lewis PJ, Salma A. Uptake of fluorine-18-fluorodeoxyglucose in sarcoidosis. *J Nucl Med* 1994;35:1647–1649.
26. Magnuson JE, Brown ML, Hansen MF, Fitzgerald RH Jr, Klee GG. Indium-111 WBC scintigraphy versus other imaging tests in suspected orthopedic prosthesis infection: a comparison. *Radiology* 1988;168:235–239.
27. Marshal KC. Biofilm: an overview of bacterial adhesion, activity, and control at surfaces. *ASM News* 1992;58:202–207.
28. Mauerhan DR, Nelson CL, Smith DL, et al. Prophylaxis against infection in total joint arthroplasty: one day of cefuroxime compared with three days of cefazolin. *J Bone Joint Surg Am* 1994;76:46–59.
29. McDonald DJ, Fitzgerald RH Jr, Ilstrup DM. Two-stage reconstruction of a total hip arthroplasty because of infection. *J Bone Joint Surg Am* 1989;71:828–834.
30. Merkel KD, Brown ML, Dewanjee MK, et al. Comparison of indium-labeled leukocyte imaging with sequential technetium-gallium scanning in the diagnosis of low-grade musculoskeletal sepsis. *J Bone Joint Surg Am* 1985;67:465–476.
31. Nelson CL, Evarts CM, Andrish J, et al. Results of the infected total hip replacement arthroplasty. *Clin Orthop* 1980;147:258–261.
32. Nelson JP. Deep infection following total hip arthroplasty. *J Bone Joint Surg Am* 1977;59:1042–1044.
33. Nestor BJ, Hanssen AD, Ferrer-Gonzales R, Fitzgerald RH Jr. The use of porous prostheses in delayed reconstruction of total hip replacements that have failed because of infection. *J Bone Joint Surg Am* 1994;76:349–359.
34. Petty W, Goldsmith S. Resection arthroplasty following infected total hip arthroplasty. *J Bone Joint Surg Am* 1980;62:889–896.
35. Salvati EA, Brause BD, Chekofsky KM, Wilson PD Jr. Reimplantation in infection: an eleven year experience. *Orthop Trans* 1981;5:370.
36. Sanén L, Carlsson AS. The diagnostic value of C-reactive protein in infected total hip arthroplasties. *J Bone Joint Surg Br* 1989;71:638–641.

37. Som P, Atkins HL, Bandoypadhyay D, et al. A fluorinated glucose analog, 2-fluoro-2-doxy-D-glucose (F-18): nontoxic tracer for tumor detection. *J Nucl Med* 1980;21:670–675.
38. Tsukayama ET, Wickland B, Gustillo RB. Suppressive antibiotic therapy in chronic prosthesis joint infections. *Rev Orthop* 1991;14:841–844.
39. Wahlig H, Dingeldein E, Bergmann R, Reuss K. The release of gentamicin from polymethylmethacrylate beads. *J Bone Joint Surg Br* 1978;60:270–275.
40. Widmer AF, Gaechter A, Ochsner PE, Zimmerli W. Antimicrobial treatment of orthopedic implant-related infections with rifampin combinations. *Clin Infect Dis* 1992;14:1251–1253.
41. Woo R, Minster GJ, Fitzgerald RH Jr, Mason LD, Lucas DR, Smith FE. Pulmonary fat embolism in revision hip arthroplasty. *Clin Orthop* 1995;319:41–53.
42. Yamada S, Kubota K, Kubota R, Ido T, Tamahashi N. High accumulation of fluorine-18-fluorodeoxyglucose in turpentine-induced inflammatory tissue. *J Nucl Med* 1995;36:1301–1306.

Revision Total Hip Arthroplasty,
edited by Marvin E. Steinberg and Jonathan P. Garino,
Lippincott Williams & Wilkins, Philadelphia © 1999.

29

Results

Robert H. Fitzgerald, Jr. and Marvin E. Steinberg

At present approximately 200,000 total hip replacements are performed annually in the United States alone. Infection occurs in nearly 1% of these. Therefore orthopedic surgeons are called on to treat approximately 20,000 patients with infected total hips each year. These operations are among the most challenging of all revisions. They encompass all of the possible problems described earlier in this book, there is often more destruction of bone and soft tissue caused by the infection itself, and there is the prerequisite that the infection be completely eradicated before the revision can take place.

The preceding chapters discuss the diagnosis and evaluation of an infected total hip, infecting organisms, and the surgical techniques most commonly used. This chapter focuses on the results of the various methods used to manage an infected total hip. We do not have a prospective, parallel series of studies designed to evaluate the effectiveness of each of these techniques and to compare them with controls. We must therefore draw on the vast literature on this topic. This often makes it difficult to compare the results of the different forms of treatment because of the many variables involved. These include the method for diagnosing infection, the infecting organisms, the timing of treatment, patient selection, specifics of surgical technique, devices used, the type of antibiotic used and the means of administration and duration of its use, the method of evaluating results, and the duration of the follow-up period. The goal of treatment is to eradicate infection when possible, provide a hip with good function and pain relief, and achieve durable results with a low incidence of recurrent infection or mechanical failure.

R. H. Fitzgerald, Jr., and M. E. Steinberg: Department of Orthopaedic Surgery, Hospital of the University of Pennsylvania, Philadelphia, Pennsylvania 19104.

CLASSIFICATION

The use of an effective system of classification is extremely helpful both in comparing the results of treatment and in determining the best method of management. Tsukayama et al. (19) defined four clinical settings as follows:

1. A positive intraoperative culture result obtained at the time of revision of a hip for aseptic loosening with no obvious clinical infection either before or at the time of revision.
2. An early postoperative infection that developed and was diagnosed less than 1 month after a hip replacement.
3. A late, chronic infection that developed more than 1 month after the index operation and had an insidious clinical course.
4. An acute hematogenous infection associated with documented or suspected antecedent bacteremia and characterized by an acute onset of symptoms some time after the initial operation.

ANTIBIOTIC TREATMENT WITHOUT SURGICAL TREATMENT

One of the earlier forms of managing an infected total hip was use of systemic antibiotics without concomitant surgical intervention. In certain cases these drugs were used for a finite period, usually between 3 and 6 months, and then stopped. In other instances, they were used on a continuous basis in an attempt to suppress rather than eradicate the infection. The use of antibiotics alone as definitive treatment did not meet with a great deal of success in older reports. Canner et al. (3) achieved successful results with only 2 of 9 patients treated with this technique. Goulet et al. (10) initially reported that 12 of 19 patients treated with antibiotics alone retained their prostheses with satisfactory function after a mean follow-up period of 4 years. Drancourt et al. (5) reported their results with the use of oral rifampin plus oral ofloxacin for the treatment of staphylococci-infected orthopedic implants. Antibiotics were continued orally for 6 months. The investigators found infection to be eradicated from 8 of the 12 joints that had a retained prosthesis after a follow-up period of 12 to 57 months. These patients were carefully selected, and sensitivity of the infecting organism to both antibiotics was a requirement for inclusion in the study. The results in most other reports have been less encouraging.

Among the problems encountered by patients treated with prolonged administration of antibiotics are the development of resistant organisms, antibiotic intolerance caused by various side effects, and a high recurrence rate among patients who stop the antibiotics after a certain interval. The use of systemic antibiotics without operative treatment, either for a specific period of time or as a means of chronic suppression, plays a limited role in management of an infected total hip. It is reserved for the small group of patients with serious medical problems among whom the risks of major surgical intervention are unacceptable and for those who refuse surgical treatment.

DÉBRIDEMENT WITHOUT REMOVAL OF COMPONENTS

Débridement without removal of components has been met with a certain degree of success in studies in which specific indications have been followed closely. Tsukayama et al. (19) reported successful eradication of infection from 25 of 35 (70%) type 2 hips when the infection was diagnosed and the patient treated within the first month of the index procedure. At the time of the operation the polyethylene liner was replaced, the operative field carefully débrided and washed, and a new polyethylene liner inserted. Patients were treated for at least 4 weeks with intravenous antibiotics. At follow-up examinations the mean Harris hip score was 70 (range 40 to 93) among the 25 hips in which the infection had been eradicated. All failures in this group were associated with components that had been inserted without cement. These authors treated six hips with late, acute hematogenous infections (type 4). Infection was eradicated in only 3 of these 6.

Although some degree of success has been reported with débridement without component removal in treating patients with acute infection, there is general agreement that the results are poor in the treatment of patients with chronic infection (type 3). Crockarell et al. (4) reported that none of 19 chronic infections was successfully managed with this technique compared with successful management of four of 19 early postoperative infections and 2 of 4 acute hematogenous infections. Successful results were associated with débridement at a mean of 6 days compared with 23 days for unsuccessful results. Canner et al. (3) achieved successful results in only 1 of 23 cases.

Débridement with retention of the prosthetic components should be limited to the treatment of patients with a mechanically sound prosthesis for whom acute infection, either soon after the operation or as a result of later hematogenous spread, is diagnosed and managed promptly. The best results are obtained in treating organisms sensitive to antibiotics, that do not form glycocalyx, or in which treatment has been instituted before the organisms have had time to produce glycocalyx (8,9,14,19).

TREATMENT AFTER POSITIVE RESULTS OF INTRAOPERATIVE CULTURES

At most institutions intraoperative cultures are obtained routinely at the time of revision total hip arthroplasty. If there is any indication of sepsis either preoperatively or during the procedure, the surgeon often obtains several specimens of tissue that are examined immediately by means of Gram stain and culture and perhaps by means of histologic evaluation of frozen sections. If the findings indicate that there is a high likelihood of infection, the surgeon must decide whether to do a one-stage of a two-stage revision.

In certain instances, however, there is no indication of infection as a result of either preoperative or intraoperative evaluation. The prosthesis is then assumed to have loosened aseptically, and a new prosthesis is inserted before the results of the final intraoperative cultures are known. If the culture result is positive, it may be difficult to determine whether this is a false-positive finding or whether the hip is truly infected. The likelihood of infection is greater if the same organism is cultured from more than one specimen taken from different locations and if the microscopic indications of acute inflammation are present. Consultation with the infectious disease service often is helpful. If it is believed that the culture results is falsely positive, the surgeon must decide whether to administer or withhold postoperative antibiotics. If it is believed that the result indicates true infection, postoperative treatment with antibiotics is indicated. Although the route and duration vary considerably, 6 weeks of parental antibiotics usually is recommended.

Tsukayama et al. (19) identified 31 hips with the diagnosis of infection on the basis of positive intraoperative culture results at revision operations on hips being revised for what was presumed to be aseptic loosening (type 1). Accordingly, a new prosthesis was inserted in all cases. Ninety percent (28 of 31) of these procedures were successful. Patients were observed for a mean of 3.5 years (range 0.5 to 8.6 years). In three instances the infection was not eradicated despite 6 weeks of parental antibiotic therapy. Two patients had evidence of recurrent infection within 2 years after the completion of treatment. Three components showed evidence of loosening on follow-up radiographs.

ONE-STAGE REVISION OR PRIMARY EXCHANGE ARTHROPLASTY

Interest in one-stage revision stems from the early work of Bucholz et al. (2). In 1981 they reported on their first 10 years of experience with primary exchange arthroplasty for treatment of 583 patients with infected total hip replacements. Their success rate with this procedure, without parental antibiotics, was 77% after the first exchange. The overall success rate after subsequent surgical procedures was 90%. The authors stated that their morbidity was significant but acceptable and considered this approach the treatment of choice of most patients with deep total hip infections. Most other investigators, however, would take a more cautious approach to this technique. A failure rate of 23% is quite high, and re-revision of these procedures can be formidable and accompanied by a high rate of complications.

In 1995 Raut et al. (17) reported that 154 of 183 patients (84%) were free of infection after a mean follow-up period of more than 7 years. These patients received oral antibiotics for between 6 weeks and 3 months. In an excellent review of the literature, Garvin and Hanssen (9) found an average of 82% successful results in 16 reports of primary exchange with the use of antibiotics. However, they found only 58% successful results in four older reports in which this technique was used without antibiotics.

Today one-stage revision has a limited role and only when specific prerequisites are met. It is generally reserved for patients with an identifiable organism that is sensitive to antibiotics and does not produce glycocalyx, when complete débridement can be performed, when there is adequate and healthy bone stock remaining, and when the patient is not at increased risk for re-infection. It also may be used to treat elderly patients who would not tolerate the long recovery and need for a second operation, which would be required if two-stage reimplantation were performed. There are thus several advantages to achieving reimplantation in a single stage if possible.

TWO-STAGE REVISION OR DELAYED EXCHANGE

Although single-stage revision is frequently done in Europe, in North America most patients with infected hips are treated with two-stage or delayed reconstruction. The interval between the two stages may vary from 6 weeks to 1 year. Systemic antibiotics are routinely used, and frequently antibiotic-laden beads or spacers, such as the prosthesis of antibiotic-loaded acrylic cement (PROSTALAC) are used (6,12). A number of reports have concerned the effectiveness of two-stage revision. McDonald et al. (15) reported on 82 hips treated by means of this technique between 1969 and 1985. Components were inserted with cement that did not contain antibiotics. After an average follow-up period of 5.5 years the investigators found a recurrence rate of 13%. They found a high rate of failure in cases in which cement had been retained at resection arthroplasty, in which reimplantation took place less than 1 year after the initial resection, and in which systemic antibiotics were used for less than 28 days. Masri and Duncan (12) reported a 93% rate of successful revisions with temporary use of a PROSTALAC (12).

There are currently differences of opinion concerning the optimum interval between the two procedures, the prognostic importance of the specific bacteria identified, the temporary use of antibiotic-containing cement spacers or beads, and the use of cemented versus uncemented prostheses (6,8,9,14). There does, however, seem to be general agreement that the overall rate of success of delayed reimplantation is greater than that of primary or one-stage reimplantation. Elson (7) found a fourfold greater failure rate among primary versus delayed revisions when both recurrent infection and mechanical failure were considered. Salvati et al. (18) found a 6% recurrence rate after two-stage revision compared with a recurrence rate of 10% to 15% after primary revision. In a review of 12 separate reports, Garvin and Hanssen (9) found an average rate of 91% successful results with two-stage revision when antibiotics were used compared with 82% successful results in 9 reports in which antibiotics were not used. These were compared with 82% and 58% success rates, respectively, for one-stage revision with and without antibiotics (7–9,12–14,18).

THREE-STAGE REVISION

Not infrequently the surgeon is faced with a substantial loss of bone stock in either the acetabulum or the proximal femur. Bone grafting techniques, which have been used successfully in nonseptic revision total hip arthroplasty generally should be avoided if there is any question of residual sepsis. In a limited number of cases use of three-stage reconstruction may be indicated. This entails removal of the components and thorough débridement of the wound followed by parental antibiotic therapy. At a later date, when it is determined that infection is no longer present, the appropriate bone grafts can be inserted in a second stage. Still later, once the graft has become incorporated, the definitive reconstruction can take place in a third stage. Experience with this technique is too limited to generate meaningful data regarding the rate of success or failure (8).

PERMANENT RESECTION ARTHROPLASTY

Before the successful development of modern total hip replacement arthroplasty, resection arthroplasty or Girdlestone pseudarthrosis was frequently used as definitive arthroplasty in the treatment of patients with a variety of hip disorders, both infectious and noninfectious. In the case of bacterial and tuberculosis infections of the hip, eradication of the infection usually was accomplished. Range of motion and relief of pain were satisfactory, although the patient was left with a short, unstable hip, an abductor lurch, and the need to use a single cane or other walking support. With optimum surgical technique and follow-up care, and with realistic expectations, both patient and surgeon were generally satisfied with this procedure (see Chapter 36). With the advent of total hip replacement, the Girdlestone pseudarthrosis was essentially abandoned as a primary arthroplasty. Today it is used most frequently as an intermediate stage in the treatment of patients with infected total hip replacement.

Under certain circumstances, however, resection arthroplasty may be used as a definitive procedure. We have found that a number of patients were satisfied with resection arthroplasty and elected not to proceed with second-stage reimplantation, even though offered the opportunity. Among 33 patients who underwent pseudoarthrosis as the definitive surgical procedure, the infection was eradicated from 27, but clinical results were satisfactory for only 20. However, among 10 patients who underwent true Girdlestone arthroplasty, none had a recurrence of infection and all had a clinically satisfactory outcome (3).

Most surgeons have not been completely satisfied with resection arthroplasty as a definitive procedure and prefer to reserve this for special circumstances. These include the case of a patient with a high chance of reinfection caused by immunosuppression or intravenous drug use, the case of a patient who is noncompliant, the case of a patient with considerable deficiency of acetabular or femoral bone stock, circumstances in which there is reasonable doubt that infection has been completely eradicated, and the case of a patient who is satisfied with the outcome. Under these circumstances resection arthroplasty may play an important role. We urge that strict attention be paid to the operative technique and postoperative care and that both physician and patient have a realistic understanding of the advantages and disadvantages of this procedure (1,11,16, see Chapter 36).

MISCELLANEOUS PROCEDURES

In rare instances a surgeon has to resort to other procedures in the treatment of patients with an infected total hip. Patients who do not achieve wound closure after removal of infected components at times need a local muscle flap to eliminate dead space and obtain wound healing. Hip disarticulation may be indicated in the face of chronically recurrent or life-threatening infection or severe loss of function of the extremity. Arthrodesis has been resorted to infrequently although the results in a small series of seven patients were considered acceptable (11).

SUMMARY

Management of infected total hip arthroplasty is one of the greatest challenges faced by orthopedic surgeons. Several alternatives are available. The indications for each are based on several factors, including the category of infection being dealt with. Other considerations are the health and age of the patient, whether the components are mechanically sound, the infecting organisms, the acuteness or chronicity of the infection, and the status of bone and local tissues. Rarely can an infected prosthesis be managed definitively with antibiotics alone: at times suppressive antibiotic therapy may be chosen. Under ideal circumstances in which infection is diagnosed and treated promptly, débridement and retention of the components may be possible. Occasionally primary exchange or single-stage revision may be indicated. Under most circumstances, however, the best results are obtained with a delayed or two-stage revision, which if performed properly should yield approximately 90% success.

REFERENCES

1. Bourne TB, Hunter GA, Rorabeck CH, Macnab JJ. A six-year follow-up of infected total hip replacements managed by Girdlestone's arthroplasty. *J Bone Joint Surg Br* 1984;66:340–343.
2. Buchholz HW, Elson RA, Engelbrecht E, Lodenkämper H, Röttger J, Siegel A. Management of deep infection of total hip replacement. *J Bone Joint Surg Br* 1981;63:342–353.
3. Canner GC, Steinberg ME, Heppenstall RB, Balderston R. The infected hip after total hip arthroplasty. *J Bone Joint Surg Am* 1984;66:1393–1399.
4. Crockarell JR, Hanssen AD, Osmon DR, Morrey BF. Treatment of infected hip arthroplasty with debridement and retention of components. Presented at the 65th Annual Meeting of the American Academy of Orthopaedic Surgeons; 1998, Mar 19–23; New Orleans.
5. Drancourt M, Stein A, Argenson JN, Zannier A, Curvale G, Raoult D. Oral reifampin plus ofloxacin for treatment of *Staphylococus*-infected orthopaedic implants. *Antimicrob Agents Chemother* 1993;37:1214–1218.
6. Duncan CP, Beauchamp C. A temporary antibiotic-loaded joint replacement system for management of complex infections involving the hip. *Orthop Clin North Am* 1993;24:751–759.
7. Elson RA. Sepsis: one-stage exchange. In: Callaghan JJ, Rosenberg AG, Rubash HE, eds. *The Adult Hip.* Philadelphia: Lippincott-Raven, 1998:1307–1315.
8. Fitzgerald RH Jr. Infected total hip arthroplasty: diagnosis and treatment. *J Am Academy Orthop Surg* 1995;3:249–262.
9. Garvin KL, Hanssen AD. Current concepts review: infection after total hip arthroplasty—past, present, and future. *J Bone Joint Surg Am* 1985;77:1576–1588.
10. Goulet JA, Pellicci PM, Brause BD, Salvati EM. Prolonged suppression of infection in total hip arthroplasty. *J Arthroplasty* 1988;3:109–116.
11. Kostuik J, Alexander D. Arthrodesis for failed arthroplasty of the hip. *Clin Orthop* 1984;188:173–182.
12. Masri BA, Duncan CP. Sepsis: antibiotic loaded implants. In: Callaghan JJ, Rosenberg AG, Rubash HE, eds. *The Adult Hip.* Philadelphia: Lippincott-Raven, 1998:1331–1342.
13. Masri BA, Salvati EA. Sepsis: two-stage exchange. In: Callaghan JJ, Rosenberg AG, Rubash HE, eds. *The Adult Hip.* Philadelphia: Lippincott-Raven, 1998:1317–1330.
14. Masterman EL, Masri BA, Duncan CP. Treatment of infection at the site of total hip replacement. *J Bone Joint Surg Am* 1997;79:1740–1749.
15. McDonald DJ, Fitzgerald RH Jr, Ilstrup DM. Two-stage reconstruction of a total hip arthroplasty because of infection. *J Bone Joint Surg Am* 1989;71:828–834.
16. McElwaine JP, Colville J. Excision arthroplasty for infected total hip replacements. *J Bone Joint Surg Br* 1984;66:168–171.
17. Raut VV, Siney PD, Wroblewski BM. One-stage revision of total hip arthroplasty for deep infection: long-term follow-up. *Clin Orthop* 1995;321:202–207.
18. Salvati EA, Chekofsky KM, Brause BD, Wilson PD Jr. Reimplantation in infection: a 12-year experience. *Clin Orthop* 1982;170;62–75.
19. Tsukayama DT, Estrada R, Gustilo RB. Infection after total hip arthroplasty: a study of the treatment of one hundred and six infections. *J Bone Joint Surg Am* 1996;78:512–523.

Complications

Revision Total Hip Arthroplasty,
edited by Marvin E. Steinberg and Jonathan P. Garino,
Lippincott Williams & Wilkins, Philadelphia © 1999.

30

Intraoperative Complications

Ohannes A. Nercessian

GENERAL CONSIDERATIONS

Revision total hip arthroplasty is a complex surgical procedure that requires great expertise. A surgeon performing revision total hip arthroplasty must have the proper training and experience to successfully execute such a difficult procedure and achieve a successful outcome. Many complications have been reported during primary total hip arthroplasty. These and other complications are encountered more frequently and with higher degrees of severity during revision total hip arthroplasty. The time required for completion of the procedure, the amount of bleeding, and the degree of osteoporosis and osteolysis are some causes of complications. Other causes, particularly health problems such as congestive heart failure, asthma, diabetes, hypertension, and systemic arthritis involving other joints, have been identified.

A thorough medical evaluation must be completed before a revision procedure. Both surgeon and the evaluating internist must discuss the possible risks and complications with the patients and the family. All appropriate modalities of evaluation should be completed before the revision procedure. The examination must include an assessment of prerevision leg length and the neurovascular status of the limbs. Any circulatory compromise must be evaluated and corrected by a competent vascular surgeon to avoid possible disastrous consequences.

After the general assessment of the patients condition, surgical planning must include evaluation radiographs. If possible, the cause of the failure of the total hip arthroplasty is determined. Not every failed total hip arthroplasty is the result of aseptic loosening. An indolent or low-grade infection can be the cause of such failure. All appropriate

O. A. Nercessian: Department of Orthopaedic Surgery, Columbia Presbyterian Medical Center, New York, New York 10032.

evaluations, including radionucleotide study and aspiration biopsy, must be done before the surgical procedure if infection is suspected. If infection is present, plans for the operation bust be altered accordingly.

Bone defects or osteolysis must be evaluated before the revision procedure. Assessment of a large acetabular or femoral deficit can be a difficult task and may require studies such as radiographic special views, or computed tomography. Careful planning of revision total hip arthroplasty must include reconstruction of the deficits. If special equipment, prostheses, or bone grafts are needed, they must be available before the start of the operative procedure. By careful assessment of the patient's condition and with careful planning, the revision procedure will be completed successfully.

To avoid or minimize intraoperative difficulties and complications in revision total hip arthroplasty, the procedure must be properly planned by the surgeon and rehearsed by the surgical team. The procedure can be difficult and challenging. Attention must be paid to the smallest detail of every step of the procedure. With this approach no or minimal time is wasted in intraoperative decision making.

One of the factors that makes revision total hip arthroplasty challenging is that despite many radiographic similarities between two patients, the intraoperative findings can be very dissimilar. Therefore no two revision procedures require the same steps for completion. In addition to planning and rehearsal, alternative plans should be developed to manage unforeseen intraoperative finding and technical difficulties. Revision procedures should be performed only in specialized centers by experienced teams.

Preoperative planning includes the equipment needed to perform the procedure, the type of prosthesis, and the availability of bone autograft and allograft. If a special or custom-made prosthesis is needed, this should be ordered in advance and available for the operation. If bone grafting is contemplated, adequate bone must be available (ordered if allograft) for the desired procedure. Availability of surgical equipment, the prosthesis, and bone must be confirmed the day before the operation. If the items required are not available, it is prudent to postpone the revision procedure until the equipment and bone are ready for use.

STEPS DURING WHICH INTRAOPERATIVE COMPLICATIONS CAN DEVELOP

Revision total hip arthroplasty can take many hours. Therefore, the choice of anesthetic involves anesthesiologist, patient, and surgeon. It is based on the findings at the preoperative evaluation, the length of the procedure, and the general health of the patient. The anesthesiologist makes the final recommendation. After induction of anesthesia, in most instances general anesthesia and endotracheal intubation, and indwelling Foley catheter is inserted by means of sterile technique. This aids the anesthesiologist in monitoring hemodynamic status of the patient. It is also helpful to the patient postoperatively, especially male patients who may experience difficulty voiding while in the supine position. The anesthetized patient must be moved carefully to avoid injury. If the patient is in the lateral position, an adjustable arm support with sponge padding is placed in no more than 90 degrees of forward flexion and slight abduction. Overzealous abduction and forward elevation of the ipsilateral arm has been reported to lead to stretching injury to the brachial plexus and other neurologic compromise.

A soft roll or contralateral axillary pad is placed by means of slightly lifting the patient's chest. This avoids excessive pressure on the contralateral axilla. Because placement of the acetabular component depends on the overall position of the pelvis, positioning of the patient must be done carefully, the position must be held with two pelvic supports—one applied to the pubic symphysis and the other to the sacrum. The clamp must be well padded to prevent pressure necrosis of the skin and should be positioned directly against the pubic symphysis. Placement of the pad more inferiorly can cause occlusion or compromise of the femoral vessel of the opposite leg, which can remain unrecognized and may lead to severe and often disastrous complications (58). Placement of the pubic pad superiorly may compromise the ipsilateral femoral vessel and often prevents adequate flexion and adduction of the limb, which is needed during the operation. A direct check of the femoral triangle area and the distal pulses of the legs is essential before draping. The sacral pad must be positioned so as to not interfere with the skin incision, yet it must hold the patient securely on the table. The position of the pelvis is checked to be sure that it is perpendicular on the operating table and not tilted anteriorly or posteriorly. The table must be level. The leg must be handled gently and carefully during preparation. Fracture of the femur has occurred during forceful manipulation of the leg of a patient with severe osteoporosis (Fig. 1).

In making the surgical incision one should take into consideration the exposure of the hip and the acetabulum. The incision should be adequate in length for access and visualization of the anatomic features of the hip. For obese or muscular patients and patients with abnormal anatomic features, a longer incision may be necessary. Faulty draping or high placement of the sacral support may cover a portion of the incision area making it difficult to gain adequate exposure. A patient who has undergone many previous hip operations has more than one surgical scar. For such patients, placement of the skin incision must be done carefully. If only a single scar is present and its position is adequate, it can be used. This skin incision is carefully marked and may be excised. Excision of the old scar improves the blood supply and healing of the skin and may be cosmetically more acceptable to the patient. An old surgical scar not near the planned incision site should be left alone. As a rule, a new incision should not cross the old surgical scar. A narrow skin island is left between the old and the new incision, because these islands may be vulnerable to necrosis.

The approach to the hip joint must be well planned. In most revision procedures it is not necessary to osteotomize the trochanter. However, to treat patients with considerable

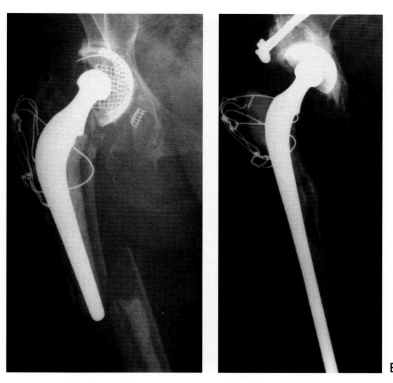

A   B

Figure 1. A: A 73-year-old woman with rheumatoid arthritis underwent revision total replacement of the right hip. During positioning of the patient on the operating table a crack was felt. Radiographs revealed fracture of the femoral shaft below the stem (**A**). Revision was performed with cemented long stem and acetabular bone grafting. **B:** Anteroposterior radiograph 7 years after the revision procedure.

stiffness or when it is to expose or mobilize the hip joint, a trochanteric osteotomy should be performed to improve exposure and prevent any possible risk for fracture of the femur. Dislocation of the hip joint can be difficult if adequate release of the capsule and soft tissue around the hip joint is not done. Care must be taken during the dislocation maneuver (flexion, abduction, and internal rotation) to prevent femoral fracture. This usually occurs among patients with severe osteoporosis and stiff hips. After dislocation of the hip, the femoral component is removed. Removal of the femoral component in revision operations can be difficult, particularly with well-fixed, porous ingrowth components. The technical difficulty in removal of the femoral component should be considered preoperatively and different instrumentation and techniques should be used to complete this task without undue damage to the proximal femur. Many reported complications have occurred during removal of the femoral component. In cemented revision, after removal of the component the cement must be similarly removed to accommodate a newly implanted femoral component. It is advisable not to proceed with the femoral cement removal before completion of acetabular preparation and acetabular fixation. Proceeding would lead to increased blood loss through oozing from the exposed medullary surfaces.

A cemented acetabular component is removed carefully, especially when there is osteolysis and substantial bone loss. For best exposure of the acetabulum in the posterolateral approach to the hip, retraction along the superior, inferior, anterior, and posterior aspects of the acetabulum is desired. Anterior retraction is done by means of placement of a Hohmann retractor along the anterior rim of the acetabulum. This retractor is applied directly against the bone of the anterior rim. This retractor also pulls the proximal femur anteriorly to gain access to the acetabulum. The femoral nerve and the vessels are about one finger-breadth away from the anterior rim of the acetabulum. Injudicious placement of the Hohman retractor can damage these neurovascular structures. Posterior retraction is important, but because of the sciatic nerve to the posterior rim of the acetabulum, careless and overzealous retraction or injudicious posterior placement of the retractor can traumatize the sciatic nerve. Some surgeons retract the posterior acetabulum with the Hohman retractor. I do not favor this method because if it is not applied properly, the tip of the retractor can be directly against the sciatic nerve and may cause direct trauma or stretch injury to the nerve. The anterior and inferior retractors applied at the interior inferior aspect of the acetabulum are held by the assistant during preparation and fixation of the acetabulum. In an operation on a patient with osteoporosis and marked osteolysis, overzealous retraction with the anterior retractor can lead to fracture of the anterior wall. After removal of the acetabular component, attention is paid to removal of the soft tissue and assessment of the degree of deficit. Soft-tissue removal must be thorough. It also should be gentle so if segments of the acetabulum are weakened, fracture or perforation is avoided. The surgeon should always be highly familiar with the anatomy of the acetabulum.

Reconstruction of the acetabulum must accommodate precise fixation of the acetabular component. If a cementless component is desired, the fit of the component into the reconstructed acetabulum must be snug. Fixation can be done with anchoring screws. The position of the screws is along the superior aspect of the acetabulum from 10 o'clock to 2 o'clock positions. Deviation from this zone can lead to perforation of the iliac vessels anteriorly or the sciatic nerve posteriorly. If a cemented acetabular component is to be used after reconstruction and bone grafting, adequate space must be left for the cement. A maloriented or malpositioned acetabular component can cause dislocation and instability of the hip joint.

After insertion of the acetabulum, attention should be paid to the femoral component. When a cemented femoral component was used, it is advisable that most or all of the cement be removed from the femoral canal. This can be an easy task if the cement is loose; however, if the femoral cement is well fixed, removal can be a real challenge, and perforation of the femoral shaft can occur. This perforation at times is unrecognized during the procedure and it is noted only after completion of the operation when radiographs are obtained (Fig. 2). Complete cement removal is required in revision of an infected hip and when cementless revision is being done. It is advisable to have good exposure of the proximal femur to facilitate removal of the cement and lessen the chance

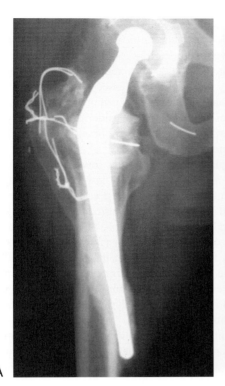 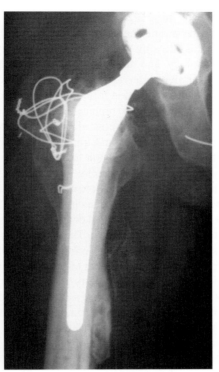

A   B

Figure 2. A: A 69-year-old man underwent revision total hip arthroplasty. Perforation of the femoral canal was found a postoperative radiograph (**A**). The patient was experiencing increasing pain in the thigh while walking. **B:** Radiograph 2 years after revision of the total hip arthroplasty.

of perforation. If the revision is being done with a cemented femoral component, it is not always necessary to remove well-fixed cement.

Proper positioning and fixation of the acetabular and femoral components are important because malposition of either can render the hip unstable and prone to dislocation. In revision total hip arthroplasty, there may be substantial acetabular and femoral bone loss, and reliable anatomic landmarks may not be present for positioning of the component. The surgeon must be well versed in anatomy of the pelvis and the acetabulum, the design of the implant, and the instrumentation needed. In implantation of a femoral component, the proper version must be selected. In addition, varus or valgus angulation should be avoided. In preparation of the femoral canal, the proximal femur must be well visualized. The surgeon must inspect the degree of bone loss and deficit at the neck of the femur and select the proper neck length femoral component to provide stability for the hip.

Trial reduction is done to ensure intraoperative stability of the joint. When the revision procedure is done through trochanteric osteotomy, soft-tissue tension usually can be established by means of reattachment or advancement of the greater trochanter. When the operation is performed through the posterolateral approach, soft-tissue tension must be achieved by means of adequate selection of neck length. If substantial proximal femoral bone loss is present, a customized stem might be required. Poor soft-tissue tension frequently leads to dislocation of the hip. Steps must be taken to provide adequate intraoperative soft-tissue tension and stability of the hip joint.

COMPLICATIONS

Infection

Although infection as a complication usually is manifested during the postoperative period, contamination usually occurs during the operative procedure. Operating room personnel must practice aseptic technique with respect to the patient, operating room instruments, and themselves. The orthopedic and other surgical literature is replete with reports addressing wound infection and preventive operating room technique. Progress in bacteriology and the use of antibiotics have considerably reduced the incidence of postoperative infection and the morbidity and mortality associated with infection. Nevertheless, infection following revision total hip arthroplasty is more frequent than after a primary total hip replacement and is associated with considerable morbidity and mortality and a high cost of treatment. Prevention of this complication is essential for successful short-term and long-term outcomes.

It is essential in revision total hip arthroplasty that indolent or low-grade infection be considered. Some surgeons suggest that all failed total hip arthroplasties must be considered infected until proved not to be infected by means of preoperative studies and intraoperative cultures. In a classic study, Charnley (11,12) suggested that in primary total hip arthroplasty, the wound could be infected by a much lower dose of infecting organisms than previously imagined. The experience of Elek and Cohen (24) classically demonstrated a cause-and-effect relation between foreign material in the surgical wound and increased risk for and extent of infection. The large mass of foreign body implanted during revision total hip arthroplasty and the wide exposure of the wound with a high degree of devascularization predisposes the patient to infection. The polymethyl methacrylate also appears to be a specific facilitator of infection.

As a rule, the first line of defense against infection during revision total hip arthroplasty is to control the site of entry of the organism, usually the surgical wound, and the operating room environment. Installation of special filteration units for the operating room to filter particles larger than 1 micrometer would decrease bacteria that carry particles into a surgical wound. Some particles, such as epithelial scales, are shed from operating room personnel. These particles come from an exposed part of the body, such as the face, upper neck, chest, perineum, and the nasopharynx. The larger the number of persons in operating room, the larger is the number of shed particles. Therefore, the number of personnel must be kept to the minimum required. The microorganism associated with wound colonization has been found to be predominantly the same organism found in skin and in infected postoperative total hip arthroplasty. Fitzgerald and Paterson (28) reported a high correlation between the presence of wound colonization and the development of deep wound sepsis. Lidwell et al. (39) reported on a multicenter prospective study in Britain of more than 8,000 total hip arthroplasties. The results are strong evidence that the use of ultraclean-air rooms during total hip arthroplasty reduces the incidence of postoperative wound infection. Use of a whole-body exhaust system may further increase protection against infection. The results also suggested that ultraclean air and antibiotic prophylaxis (5,39) had an independent but cumulative effect in preventing postoperative joint infection.

When revision total hip arthroplasty is performed, administration of antibiotic usually is held until adequate intraoperative cultures are obtained. This is done to increase the likelihood of growth and identification of indolent organisms. Intraoperative examination of the wound tissue by a pathologist can be of assistance to the surgeon if infection is suspected. In a study reported by Tsukayama et al. (64), the authors evaluated the results of management of 106 infected total hips. The results clearly indicated that factors associated with recurrence of infection were retained bone cement during revision, number of the previous operations, the potentional immunologic compromise of the patient, and early postoperative infection. It is therefore very important that adequate débridement of soft tissue and complete removal of cement be performed in revision of an infected total hip arthroplasty. Intraoperative frozen-section analysis and inspection of soft tissue during the procedure can be of great help in aiding the surgeon to determine whether infection is present.

Bleeding

All patients undergoing total hip arthroplasty must have a complete medical examination and laboratory evaluation before the planned operation including a coagulation profile. To minimize blood loss during hip arthroplasty, certain steps can be taken including careful planning of the operation to minimize operative time, use of hypotensive anesthesia (4) if not contraindicated, and meticulous surgical technique, including careful hemostatis. It has been estimated that the average patient undergoing revision total hip arthroplasty with normotensive anesthesia usually needs three to five units of blood during the perioperative period. With meticulous hemostasis and hypotensive anesthesia, the intraoperative blood loss can be reduced. The patient's position for revision total hip arthroplasty influences blood loss. For example, the lateral decubitis position decreases intraoperative blood loss caused by pooling of blood in the untreated limb. Reports have documented a considerable decrease in blood loss when general anesthesia is supplemented with epidural anesthesia. This decrease possibly results from lower blood pressure caused by vasodilatation that occurs with epidural anesthesia. These factors can be helpful in decreasing the likelihood of considerable blood loss with a concomitant reduction in the need for perioperative transfusions and the risks associated with them.

Many patients contemplating total hip arthroplasty have been chronic users of nonsteroidal antiinflammatory drugs or aspirin. These medications, particularly aspirin, can prolong bleeding time. The prothrombin time and partial thromboplastin time may be normal. It is important to have patients discontinue use of these medications at least 1 week before the planned date of the operation. More intraoperative blood loss can occur among patients who have not discontinued taking aspirin or other aspirin-containing medications. Connelly and Panush (16) studied the relation between perioperative use of nonsteroidal antiinflammatory drugs and postoperative bleeding. They examined patients who underwent total hip arthroplasty with respect to the postoperative complications of gastrointestinal bleeding and hypotension. Patients who had been taking non-steroidal anti-inflammatory drugs had more postoperative bleeding complications than patients not taking these medication. The authors recommended that patients undergoing elective procedures stop these medications and allow time for elimination of the drugs.

Intraoperative cell salvage and transfusion are used occasionally. The benefit has been reported by Turner et al. and others (3,63). Turner et al. advocate the use of preoperative autologous blood donation combined with a program of intraoperative salvage of blood. They reported that using this method eliminated transfusion of blood-bank blood in a large number of primary total hip arthroplasty procedures. Intraoperative cell salvage should not be used in infected revision procedures.

Vascular Injury

Intraoperative vascular injuries during total hip arthroplasty have been reported in many orthopedic studies (7,30) and occur more frequently in revision total hip arthroplasty than in primary total hip arthroplasty. Al-Salman et al. (1) reported that the cause of injury was medial displacement of the acetabular prosthesis, which led to iliac vessel injury. When cementless acetabular components are used in revision procedures, the use of screw fixation can injure the femoral and iliac vessels (33,36). Damage to intrapelvic vessels may result in profound bleeding and hypotension. These complications demand immediate identification and surgical repair of the vessel to prevent a catastrophic outcome.

Nachbar et al. (45) reported a 0.2% to 0.3% rate of vascular complications in an analysis of reconstructive hip procedures. They reported 15 cases of severe arterial injury in an 8-year period. The most commonly involved vessel was the femoral artery or one of its main branches (the lateral and medial femoral circumflex arteries). The injury was caused by the tip of a narrow, pointed Hohmann retractor used to exposed the hip joint. Other reported mechanisms include an intimal tear with appositional thrombosis probably caused by mechanical stress on the atherosclerotic artery giving rise to complete ischemia. Entry of bone cement into the pelvis through a defect in the acetabulum can cause thrombotic occlusion from the heat of polymerization and adhesion of cement to the external iliac artery. Direct arterial injury can be caused by surgical instruments of a sharp edge of protruding bone. This complication may be associated with the development of a false aneurysm. In the report by Nachbur et al. (45) 14 of the 15 involved extremities were salvaged, but above-the-knee amputation was performed on one patient.

Knowledge of the causative mechanism is important to prevent arterial injury during hip surgery operations. Nachbar et al. (45) suggested that the surgeon be sufficiently acquainted with exposure of the main vessels above and below the groin to be able to control life-threatening hemorrhage at all times. Lazarides et al. (38) reviewed the literature and found 22 vascular inquiries that had occurred after hip operations. They reported an additional 4 cases of iatrogenic arterial damage after total hip arthroplasty. Seventy-four percent of reported vascular injuries had occurred after total hip arthroplasty. The authors reported a 9% morbidity rate and 17% permanent disability rate after vascular operations. Revision hip operations were found to be the definite risk factor for vascular injury. Todd and Bintchcliffe (62) reported that injury to major vessels is a well-recognized, serious complication of total hip arthroplasty and that increased risk for such injury is found among patients with rheumatoid arthritis who undergo revision operations, especially with the injudicious use of instruments such as sharp Hohmann retractors. Feddian et al. (26) reported rupture of the femoral vein during attempted removal of a chain of beads after radical excision of a chronically infected Girdlestone arthroplasty. The patient later needed disarticulation of the hip. Matos et al. (42) reported on four patients who had ischemia in the ispilateral lower extremity after revision total hip arthroplasty. Three needed vascular operations and one needed lumbar sympathectomy for relief of pain. Each patient had undergone multiple previous procedures on the same hip, resulting in extensive scaring, shortening, flexion contracture, or fusion. The authors attributed the ischemia after revision total hip arthroplasty to interruption of the critical collateral circulation around the hip or traction on the femoral vessel tethered by scar and when the shortened limb was lengthened or the hip contracture was corrected. Doppler studies and careful preoperative evaluation and recognition of the signs of ischemia and institution of appropriate management were recommended to prevent catastrophic complications.

Shoenfeld et al. (57) reviewed the literature and found 68 cases and reported on 5 new cases of vascular injuries that had occurred during total hip arthroplasty. Among the 68 patients most injuries were sustained on the left side, and 39% underwent revision procedures. Complications were related to incorporation of the iliac vessel in cement, aggressive medial retraction, excessive traction on the atherosclerotic vessel, and improper technique in preparation of the acetabulum. The most commonly injured vessels were the external iliac artery (36 instances), femoral artery (17 instances), and iliac vein (6 instances). Twenty-seven of the patients needed emergency surgical treatment of hemorrhage. The complications included thrombosis with distal ischemia (47%), vessel laceration (26%), pseudoaneurysm (25%), and arteriovenous fistula (3%). The mortality rate was 7% and there was a 15% incidence of limb loss.

Other vascular complications related to revision total hip arthroplasty include embolic phenomena. Cerebral embolism during revision arthroplasty was reported by Rodriguez-Merchan et al. (52), who found an association with arteriosclerosis. A number of studies in the medical literature suggest that during implantation of cemented hip prostheses, pulmonary embolism of medullary contents, monomer, and air may occur. The proof was based on findings at histologic examination of lung tissue in animal experiments and postmortem examinations of human tissue. Ulrich et al. and other authors (14,37,65), using transesophageal echocardiography during total hip replacement demonstrated embolization of echogenic material during placement of the acetabular and femoral components and during relocation of the hip joint. If enough echogenic material is present, it may cause a clinical picture of pulmonary embolism, hypotension, cardiac arrest, and at times death (9,20). However, in most reported cases of hypotension, no severe sequelae resulted. These events seem related primarily to insertion of a cemented femoral component and may be caused by a rise in intramedullary pressure in the femoral cavity. Wenda et al. (67) suggested use of intramedullary plugs to restrict embolization of bone marrow. When the plugs were used, the authors found no marked drop in blood pressure compared with blood pressure when cementation was done without plugging of the distal canal. The authors also recommended venting of the canal in conjunction with plugging to avoid compression of the marrow.

Deep venous thrombosis is a well-documented complication of primary and revision total hip arthroplasty. Sharrock et al. (56) determined that longer surgical procedures and the type of anesthesia administered influence the rate of deep venous thrombosis after total hip arthroplasty. Other factors, such as a hypercoagulable state, obesity, immobility, and chronic illnesses also increase risk for deep venous thrombosis. Serious arterial occlusion during total hip arthroplasty is an uncommon complication. Stubbs et al. (60) reported total occlusion of the common femoral artery during total hip arthroplasty. The occlusion was attributed to the polymerization heat produced by methyl methacrylate cement. Parfenchuck and Young (48) reported on two patients who had intraoperative arterial occlusion during total hip arthroplasty. Both patients had severe peripheral vascular disease.

Neurologic Complications

Peripheral neurologic injuries following primary and revision total hip arthroplasty are troublesome complications and may leave both patient and surgeon disappointed. A review of the literature revealed an incidence ranging from 0.9% to 5.9% in primary arthroplasty and 2% to 7.6% in revision total hip arthroplasty (2,6,10,15,17,25,44,53,59). In a study (46) of 7,133 consecutive total hip arthroplasties performed between 1976 and 1989, the overall incidence of peripheral neurologic injuries was found to be 0.63%. In the upper extremity the incidence was 0.15%. Inflammatory arthritis was the diagnosis for most patients with neurologic injury to the upper extremity. The incidence of peripheral neurologic injury in the lower extremity was 0.48%. The peroneal branch of the sciatic nerve was the most commonly involved. The overall incidence of permanent neurologic injury in the study was 33%. The incidence in the lower extremity was 35%. A review of the literature indicated that most nerve injuries following primary and revision total hip arthroplasty were not explored because of the assumption that they were caused by stretch injury and would have a poor prognosis with exploration.

Although minor stretch injury may have a spontaneous recovery, prolonged traction or traumatic compression of the nerve at the hip level may show a less favorable prognosis. This fact could account for the high percentage of permanent neurologic palsies in revision procedures. Revision or reoperation requires prolonged and repeated retraction, especially along the posterior acetabulum for exposure and thus traction or traumatic compression of the main trunk of the sciatic nerve. The literature suggests a high predisposition among women for sustaining nerve injury. Johanson et al. (34) found that 27 of 34 nerve injuries (79%) occurred among women.

The cause of nerve injury among most patients described in the literature remains unknown. In the lower extremity most injuries were seen in the common peroneal nerve. The ulnar nerve was the most commonly involved in the upper extremity. Surgeons undertaking procedures such as revision total hip arthroplasty must be aware of these neurologic complications and use meticulous surgical technique to avoid them. Ratliff (49,50) in a review of 15 nerve injuries following total hip arthroplasty found 24 sciatic nerve injuries. Twelve occurred with the posterolateral approach, 7 with the transtrochanteric approach, and 5 with the anterior approach. The transtrochanteric approach is considered by many surgeons to be the safest approach because it may limit the need for retraction of the periacetabular structure, which can lead to traction injury to the sciatic nerve and its branches. Some authors advocate exposure of the sciatic nerve and retraction of the nerve away from the operative field to minimize neurologic injury. The literature is not clear on the effectiveness of this approach.

Other etiologic factors attributed to peripheral neurologic injury following revision or primary total hip arthroplasty included direct and indirect mechanical trauma to the sciatic nerve, thermal injury from polymerization of cement, paralysis caused by bleeding and hematoma formation, entrapment of the sciatic nerve by wire during reattachment of the greater trochanter, and migration of the trochanteric wires. Lengthening of the limb also has been frequently cited as a common etiologic factor. Edwards et al. (22) indicated in their study of 23 peroneal and sciatic nerve palsies that an average limb lengthening of 2.7

cm (range 1.9 to 3.7 cm) may lead to peroneal nerve injury; in comparison an average lengthening of 4.4 cm (range 4 to 5.1 cm) may lead to sciatic nerve injury. The authors advocated that limb lengthening be minimized to avoid this complication. Many authorities in neurophysiology estimate that the nerve may be safely elongated 15% to 20% of its length, and some estimate about 8% of the length of the nerve to be safe.

Leg-Length Equalization

The objective of primary and revision total hip arthroplasty is to restore the normal or nearly normal biomechanics of the hip joint. Equalization of leg length is therefore a very important consideration. Stability of the hip is likewise very important, and in some instances it is a distinct priority. Careful planning of the operation can be helpful to achieve both goals. In primary total hip arthroplasty, for example, careful templating of the acetabulum can help the surgeon determine the optimum position of the socket which influences tension on the myofascial sleeve. Templating the femur can assist in planning a proper neck osteotomy. In revision total hip arthroplasty templating is important, but intraoperative findings may dictate a change in the preoperative plan.

Some tall patients may tolerate a small degree of overlengthening. For short patients the same degree of discrepancy can become clinically significant. Preoperative planning should include leg-length measurement. Leg-length inequality can be a cause of great patient dissatisfaction after primary and revision total hip arthroplasty (21). Discrepancies more than 1 inch (2.54 cm) produce functional, cosmetic, and pain problems and possible nerve damage. It is valuable to discuss leg-length discrepancies with the patient. Some surgeons have found that a large amount of litigation is the result of leg-length inequality after primary and revision total hip arthroplasty.

Leg-length discrepancy is more of a problem when arthroplasty is performed through the posterolateral approach. It is usually not a commonly encountered problem in transtrochanteric total hip arthroplasty. Soft-tissue tension around the hip joint can be corrected by means of reattachment of the greater trochanter. In the posterolateral approach, however, myofascial sleeve tension is achieved with adjustment of the length of the femoral neck. Reliable intraoperative leg length assessment before hip dislocation and after implantation of the hip prosthesis is mandatory in all primary and revision total hip arthroplasties. Although no technique is exact, surgeons must develop a consistent approach to preoperative, intraoperatively, and postoperative evaluation of limb length and to reliable and convenient clinical and radiographic measurement (21).

Heterotopic Ossification

Although heterotopic ossification is a postoperative rather than an intraoperative complication, the stage may be set during the operative procedure itself. The incidence is variable, ranging from 8% to 70% (8,19,51). Brooker et al. (8) reported a classification commonly used to describe this complication. Most cases of heterotopic ossification are minimal and rarely cause marked limitation of hip motion, although complete joint ankylosis can occur. Morrey et al. (43) compared the incidences of heterotopic ossification with various surgical approaches. They found an incidence of 28% with the transtrochanteric approach, 29% with the anterolateral approach, and 22% with the posterior approach. They concluded that there was no statistically significant difference among the approaches. Hierton et al (32) found a very low incidence of heterotopic ossification among patients undergoing primary total hip arthroplasty with the diagnosis of rheumatoid arthritis and patients undergoing systemic steroid treatment. According to some reports (32,40) heterotopic ossification occurs as the result of a complex interaction of local factors. These include availability of calcium, soft-tissue edema, vascular stasis, tissue hypoxia, muscle damage, the presence of mesenchymal cells with osteoblastic activity, and unknown systemic factors. The basic defect in heterotopic ossification is inappropriate differentiation of fibroblasts to bone-forming cells. Urist et al. (66) isolated bone morphogenic protein and demonstrated that it can induce undifferentiated mesenchymal cells to form osteoblasts in vitro. Heterotopic bone is metabolically active, exhibiting about triple the normal rate of bone formation and double the normal number of osteoblasts.

Many risk factors are associated with heterotopic ossification. The most widely accepted risks factors are being a man and having hypertrophic osteoarthritis, history of heterotopic ossification, diffuse idiopathic skeletal hyperostosis, active ankylosing spondylolitis, and Paget's disease. High risk must be identified and prophylactic treatments instituted to prevent this complication. Tissue trauma should be minimized during the operation, and the wound must be free of bony debris. The most acceptable method of preventing heterotopic ossification is a single 600–700 millirad dose of radiation administered in the first 2 postoperative days (31). This produces good results. In revision operations in which uncemented components are used, no evidence of loosening was visualized after 1 year of follow-up study after this treatment. Radiation, however, may cause a delay in porous ingrowth and cause an increased incidence of delayed union or nonunion of a trochanteric osteotomy.

Perforation and Fracture

Perforation may occur in both the femur and the acetabulum (Fig. 2). Usually this takes place in a patient with osteoporosis or distorted anatomic features and when removal of well-osteointegrated cement is required for completion of the revision operation. After exposure of the acetabulum, removal of the acetabular component should be done with great care. Medial wall perforation or fracture, if they occur, must be recognized and repaired. Grafting with autologous bone or allograft can be used in the reconstruction. If the defect is large, as in intrapelvic migration of the acetabular component, revision may be done as a two-stage procedure. The first stage involves removal of the migrated component and bone grafting of the acetabulum. The second stage is carried out after bone incorporation has occurred. In one study (23), four revisions of complex intrapelvic acetabular migration were reported with good results with the two-stage procedure. Fracture of the posterior column and posterior wall can be very difficult to reconstruct. A large allograft may be needed. Special acetabular devices have been designed to assist the surgeon in such cases.

Fracture of the femoral shaft has been reported in numerous studies (27,30,35,41,55). The patients usually have severe osteoporosis or protrusio acetabuli and other difficult anatomic conditions. Femoral fractures usually are proximal; however, supracondylar fractures can occur among patients with osteopenia, particularly during dislocation of the hip. Fracture of the proximal femur has been reported during insertion of cementless femoral stems and during reaming and rasping for implantation of cemented components. When a cementless femoral component is used prophylactically, wiring the proximal femur may be considered. The wiring may protect against propagation of a small crack or creation of a major fracture of the proximal femur.

Fracture of the proximal femur can occur in the postoperative period when weight bearing is initiated. It is caused by hoop stresses. In a study reported by De Beer and Learmonth (18) ten patients with major femoral fractures complicating total hip arthroplasty were seen. Four had intraoperative fractures sustained at revision procedures, and 6 had late postoperative fractures of the femur associated with minimal trauma. In another study, by Schwartz et al. (54), of 1,318 consecutive uncemented total hip arthroplasties, 39 intraoperative fractures of the femur occurred for an incidence of 3%. Interesting was that only half of these fractures were diagnosed intraoperatively. The fractures occurred in the proximal femur or at the tip of the stem. Most were incomplete or minimally displaced and did not jeopardize the stability of the femoral component. Complete proximal fractures were stabilized with a four-fifths coated or fully coated cementless prosthesis to provide distal fixation. Circlage wires were used to stabilize the fracture fragments. Christensen et al. (13) reported 10 cases of fracture out of 159 revision total hip arthroplasties for a prevalence of 6.3%. Most necessitated surgical stabilization with compression plates and screws. All of the fractures healed. Only 6 patients, however, ultimately regained satisfactory hip function. Although intraoperative femoral fracture is a well-recognized technical complication of total hip arthroplasty, with careful surgical technique it can be minimized. Difficult anatomic conditions require good exposure. Overzealous traction and maneuvering of the femur can be significant factors in creation and propagation fractures.

Perforation of the femoral shaft has been reported as a complication of total hip revision (29,61). Perforation by the stem of the prosthesis is rare. Such perforation usually occurs during removal of well-fixed distal cement. The incidence of this complication can be decreased if meticulous attention is given to preoperative planning and intraoperative technique. The main predisposing factors for femoral perforation, according to a study by Talab et al. (61), are previous hip operations, revision total hip arthroplasty, dysplasia, osteoporosis, and poor exposure. Every attempt should be made to determine whether such perforation has occurred during the operation so that appropriate steps can be taken. If a perforation has occurred at the tip of the stem, a longer prosthesis can be used to bypass the perforation. Other techniques also may be used. If this complication has gone unrecognized and untreated, further problems often occur and require late surgical correction.

Hip Dislocation

Numerous factors lead to postoperative dislocation of a total hip. The incidence of dislocation ranges from 1% to 2% for primary arthroplasty to 25% for revision. Dislocation is most likely caused by malpositioning of the components or laxity of the soft tissues around the hip. During primary and more so during revision total hip arthroplasty, placement of acetabular and femoral components must be done carefully and in correct version. Restoring the stability of the hip depends on adequate tension on the myofascial sleeve, particularly if the procedure is done without trochanteric osteotomy. Achieving this at times may render the leg that is operated on slightly longer than desired. In such cases, however, leg-length equality may be less important than the necessity to establish a stable hip. If greater trochanteric osteotomy is performed, care must be taken to minimize the risk for trochanteric nonunion and migration. Such migration can lead to loss of myofascial sleeve tension, which can render the hip unstable and lead to dislocation. I have used a short course of immobilization of all patients undergoing revision total hip arthroplasty performed through the transtrochanteric approach. In a study (46) comparing such patients with those who were not immobilized, there were significant differences with respect to hip dislocation. Patients who were immobilized a brief period of 6 weeks had a lower rate of hip dislocation than those who underwent revision operations without immobilization.

Infrequent Complications

Other complications have been reported during primary and revision total hip arthroplasty. Sudden death has been reported during the insertion of a cemented femoral prosthesis. The exact cause of death was not clearly documented. Most postmortem studies have demonstrated that a large amount of femoral canal contents embolize to the pulmonary artery. To prevent this complication, plugging and venting of the femoral canal have been advocated.

Transient hypotension may develop during insertion of the cemented femoral component. It is advisable to keep the patient well oxygenated and replace blood loss to avoid further problems associated with transient hypotension.

Sudden blindness is a rare complication encountered during cementation of the femoral component. Although the exact cause is not clear, most experts have attributed the blindness to the transient hypotension. Elderly patients with atherosclerotic blood vessels may be more prone to this complication than are other patients.

REFERENCES

1. al-Salman M, Taylor DC, Beauchamp CP, Duncan CP. Prevention of vascular injuries in revision total hip replacements [Comment]. *Can J Surg* 1992;35:261–264.
2. Amstutz HC, Ma SM, Jinnah RH, Mai L. Revision of aseptic loose total hip arthroplasties. *Clin Orthop* 1982;170:21.
3. Ayers DC, Murrary DG, Duerr DM. Blood salvage after total hip arthroplasty. *J Bone Joint Surg Am* 1995;77:1347–1351.
4. Barbier-Bohm G, Desmonts JM, Couderc E, Moulin D, Prokocimer P, Oliver H. Comparative effects of induced hypotension and normovolaemic haemodilution on blood loss in total hip arthroplast. *Br J Anaesth* 1980;52:1039–1043.
5. Beck-Sague CM, Chong WH, Roy C, Anderson R, Jarvis WR. Outbreak of surgical wound infections associated with total hip arthroplasty. *Infect Control Hosp Epidemiol* 1992;13:526–534.
6. Beckenbaugh RD, Ilstrup DM. Total hip arthroplasty: a review of three hundred and thirty-three cases with long follow-up. *J Bone Joint Surg* 1978;60:306.
7. Bergqvist D, Carlsson AS, Ericsson BF. Vascular complications after total hip arthroplasty. *Acta Orthop Scand* 1983;54:157–163.
8. Brooker A, Bowerman J, Robinson R, et al. Ectopic ossification following total hip replacement: incidence and a method of classification. *J Bone Joint Surg Am* 1973;55:1629–1632.
9. Camann WR, Sacks GM, Schools AG, Heggeness ST, Reilly DT, Concepcion M. Nearly fatal cardiovascular collapse during total hip replacement: probable coronary arterial embolism. *Anesth Analg* 1991;72:245–248.
10. Charnley J. the long-term results of low friction arthroplasty of the hip performed as a primary intervention. *J Bone Joint Surg Br* 1972;54:61.
11. Charnley J. Postoperative infection after total hip replacement with special reference to air contamination in the operating room. *Clin Orthop* 1972;87:167.
12. Charnley J, Eftekhar N. Postoperative infection in total prosthetic replacement arthroplasty of the hip joint with special reference to the bacterial contact on the air in the operating room. *Br J Surg* 1969;56:641.
13. Christensen CM, Seger BM, Schultz RB. Management of intraoperative femur fractures associated with revision hip arthroplasty. *Clin Orthop* 1989;248:177–180.
14. Christie J, Robinson CM, Pell AC, McBirnie J, Burnett R. Transcardiac echocardiography during invasive intramedullary procedures. *J Bone Joint Surg Br* 1995;77:450–455.
15. Collis DK. Cemented total hip replacement in patients who are less than fifty years old. *J Bone Joint Surg Am* 1984;66:353.
16. Connelly CS, Panush RS. Should nonsteroidal anti-inflammatory drugs be stopped before elective surgery? *Arch Intern Med* 1991;151:1963–1966.
17. Coventry MB, Beckenbbaugh RD, Nolan DR, Ilstrup DM. 2012 total hip arthroplasties: a study of postoperative course and early complications. *J Bone Joint Surg Am* 1974;56:273.
18. De Beer JD, Learmonth ID. Pathological fracture of the femur: a complication of failed total hip arthroplasty. *South Afr Med J* 1991;79:202–205.
19. DeLee J, Ferrari A, Charnley J. Ectopic bone formation following low friction arthroplasty of the hip. *Clin Orthop* 1976;121:53–59.
20. Duncan JA. Intra-operative collapse or death related to the use of acrylic cement in hip surgery [Comment]. *Anaesthesia* 1989;44:694–695.
21. Edeen J, Sharkey PF, Alexander AH. Clinical significance of leg-length inequality after total hip arthroplasty. *Am J Orthop* 1995;24:347–351.
22. Edwards BN, Tullos HS, Nobel PC. Contributory factors and etiology of sciatic nerve palsy in total hip arthroplasty. *Clin Orthop* 1987;136:218.
23. Eftekhar NS, Nercessian OA. A combined femoral and retroperitoneal approach for safe removal of severely migrated total hip prosthesis. *J Bone Joint Surg Am* 1989;71:1480–1486.
24. Elek SD, Cohen PE. The virulence of *Staphylococus pyogenes* of man: a study of problems of wound infections. *Br J Exp Pathol* 1957;38:573.
25. Evarts CM, DeHaven KE, Nelson Cl et al. Interim results of Charnley-Müller total hip arthroplasty. *Clin Orthop* 1973;95:193.
26. Feddian NJ, Sudlow RA, Browett JP. Ruptured femoral vein: a complication of the use of gentamicin beads in an infected excision arthroplasty of the hip. *J Bone Joint Surg Br* 1984;66:493–494.
27. Fitzgerald RH Jr, Brindley GW, Kavanagh BF. The uncemented total hip arthroplasty: intraoperative femoral fractures. *Clin Orthop* 1988;235:61–66.
28. Fitzgerald RH Jr, Peterson LF. Wound colonization in deep wound sepsis. In: Eftekhar NS, ed. *Infection in total joint replacement surgery: prevention and management.* St. Louis: Mosby–Year Book, 1984.
29. Fredin H. Late fracture of the femur following perforation during hip arthroplasty: a report of 2 cases. *Acta Orthop Scand* 1988;59:331–333.
30. Freischlag JA, Sise M, Quinones-Baldrich WJ, Hye RJ, Sedwitz MM. Vascular complications associated with orthopaedic procedures. *Surg Gynecol Obstet* 1989;169:147–152.
31. Hedley A, Mead L, Hendren D. The prevention of heterotopic bone formation following total hip arthroplasty using 600 rad in a single dose. *J Arthroplasty* 1989;4:319–325.
32. Hierton C, Blomgren G, Lindgren V. Factors associated with heterotopic bone formation in cemented total hip prosthesis. *Acta Orthop Scand* 1983;54:698–702.
33. Hwand SK. Vascular injury during total hip arthroplasty: the anatomy of the acetabulum. *Int Orthop* 1994;18:29–31.
34. Johanson NA, Pellicci PM, Tsairis P, Salvati EA. Nerve injury in total hip arthroplasty. *Clin Orthop* 1983;179:214.
35. Kavanagh BF. Femoral fractures associated with total hip arthroplasty. *Orthop Clin North Am* 1992;23:249–257.

36. Kirkpatrick JA, Callaghan JJ, Vandemark RM, Goldner RD. The relationship of the intrapelvic vasculature to the acetabulum: implications in screw-fixation acetabular components. *Clin Orthop* 1990;258:183–190.
37. Lafont ND, Kostucki WM, Marchand PH, Michaux MN, Boogaerts JG. Embolism detected by trans-oesophageal echocardiography during hip arthroplasty. *Can J Anaesth* 1994;41:850–885.
38 Lazarides MK, Arvanitis DP, Dayantas JN. Iatrogenic arterial trauma associated with hip joint surgery: an overview. *Eur J Vas Surg* 1991;5:549–556.
39. Lidwell OM, Lowbury EJ, White W, et al. Effect of ultra-clean air in operating room on deep sepsis in the total knee replacement: a randomised study. *Br Med J* 1982;285:10.
40. Major P, Resnick D, Greenway G: Heterotopic ossification in paraplegia: a possible disturbance of the paravertebral venous plexus. *Radiology* 1980;136:797–799.
41. Mallory TH, Kras TJ, Vaughn BK. Intraoperative femoral fractures associated with cementless total hip arthroplasty. *Orthop* 1989;12:231–239.
42. Matos MH, Amstutz HC, Machleder HI. Ischemia of the lower extremity after total hip replacement. *J Bone Joint Surg Am* 1979;61:24–27.
43. Morrey B, Adams R, Cabanela M. Comparison of heterotopic bone after anterolateral transtrochanteric and posterior approaches for total hip arthroplasty. *Clin Orthop* 1984;188:160–167.
44. Murray WR. Results in patients with total hip replacement arthroplasty. *Clin Orthop* 1973;95:80.
45. Nachbur B, Meyer RP, Verkkala K, Zurcher R. The mechanisms of severe arterial injury in surgery of the hip joint. *Clin Orthop* 1979;141:122–133.
46. Nercessian O, McCaulay W, Stinchfield F. Peripheral neuropathies following total hip arthroplasty. *J Arthroplasty* 1994;9:645.
47. Nercessian O, Fernandez M. The effect of short term immobilization of the hip joint post revision on the rate of hip dislocations. In preparation.
48. Parfenchuck TA, Young TR. Intraoperative arterial occlusion in total joint arthroplasty. *J Arthroplasty* 1994;9:217–220.
49. Ratcliff AHC. Vascular and neurologic complications In: Ling RSM, ed. *Complications of total hip replacement* London: Churchill Livingstone 1984:18.
50. Ratcliff AHC. Vascular and neurologic complications following total hip arthroplasty. *Proceedings of the Ninth Open Scientific Meeting of the Hip Society*. St. Louis: Mosby, 1981:278–292.
51. Reigler H, Harrie C. Heterotopic bone formation after total hip arthroplasty. *Clin Orthop* 1976;117:209–216.
52. Rodriguez-Merchan EC, Comin-Gomes JA, Martinez-Chacon JL. Cerebral embolism during revision arthroplasty of the hip. *Acta Orthop Belg* 1995;61:319–322.
53. Salvati EA, Wilson PD, Jolley N, et al. A ten-year follow-up study of our first one hundred consecutive Charnley total hip replacements. *J Bone Joint Surg Am* 1981;63:753.
54. Schwartz JT Jr, Mayer JG, Engh CA. Femoral fracture during non-cemented total hip arthroplasty. *J Bone Joint Surg Am* 1989;71:1135–1142.
55. Sharkey PF, Hozack WJ, Booth RE Jr, Rothman RH. Intraoperative femoral fractures in cementless total hip arthroplasty. *Orthop Rev* 1992;21:337–342.
56. Sharrock NE, Ranawat CS, Urquhart B, Peterson M. Factors influencing deep vein thrombosis following total hip arthroplasty under epidural anesthesia. *Anesth Analg* 1993;76:765–771.
57. Shoenfeld NA, Stuchin SA, Pearl R, Haveson S. The management of vascular injuries associated with total hip arthroplasty. *J Vas Surg* 1990;11:549–555.
58. Smith JW, Pellici PM, Sharrock N, et al. Complications after total hip replacement: the cementless limb. *J Bone Joint Surg Am* 1989;71:528.
59. Solheim LF, Hagen R. Femoral and sciatic neuropathies after hip arthroplasty. *Acta Orthop Scand* 1980;51:531.
60. Stubbs DH, Dorner DB, Johnston RC. Thrombosis of the iliofemoral artery during revision of a total hip replacement: a case report. *J Bone Joint Surg Am* 1986;68:454–455.
61. Talab YA, States JD, Evarts CM. Femoral shaft perforation: a complication of total hip reconstruction. *Clin Orthop* 1979;141:158–165.
62. Todd BD, Bintcliffe IW. Injury to the external iliac artery during hip arthroplasty for old central dislocation. *J Arthroplasty* 1990;5[Suppl]:S53–S55.
63. Turner RH, Capozzi JD, Kim A, Anas PP, Hardman E. Blood conservation in major orthopedic surgery. *Clin Orthop* 1990;256:299–305.
64. Tsukayama DT, Estrada R, Gustilo RB. Infection after total hip arthroplasty: a study of the treatment of one hundred and six infections. *J Bone Joint Surg Am* 1996;78:512–523.
65. Ulrich C, Burri C, Worsdorfer O, Heinrich H. Intraoperative transesophageal two-dimensional echocardiography in total hip replacement. *Arch Orthop Trauma Surg* 1986;105:274–278.
66. Urist M, Mizutani H, Takagi, et al. A bovine low molecular weight bone morphogenetic protein (BMP) fraction. *Clin Orthop* 1982;162:219–232.
67. Wenda K, Degreif J, Runkel M, Ritter G. Pathogenesis and prophylaxis of circulatory reactions during total hip replacement. *Arch Orthop Trauma Surg* 1993;112:260–265.

Revision Total Hip Arthroplasty,
edited by Marvin E. Steinberg and Jonathan P. Garino,
Lippincott Williams & Wilkins, Philadelphia © 1999.

31

Controversies Associated with Thromboembolic Disease

Paul A. Lotke

The principles of prevention and management of thromboembolic disease continue to be controversial despite numerous recommendations and studies published in the last five decades. This chapter reviews the origin of these controversies and makes general recommendations with the understanding that there exists great diversity in opinions as to the best methods of prevention and management of thromboembolic disease. The origin of these controversies is multifactorial, but it is related to the assumptions on which many studies are designed and how the problem is defined. The importance of deep venous thrombosis in the postoperative period, as opposed to other medical conditions, is uncertain because it is yet to be shown that a reduction in deep venous thrombosis is associated with a reduction in fatal pulmonary embolism (20). To focus these controversies, the definition and diagnosis of deep venous thrombosis and pulmonary emboli and the currently available methods of prophylaxis and treatment are reviewed. This chapter is designed not to answer all questions about thromboembolic disease but to stimulate the reader appropriately to question the literature and stimulate interest to find the best solutions.

DEEP VENOUS THROMBOSIS

There is general agreement that the size and location of deep venous thrombi are important considerations in assessing risk for pulmonary embolism (19). Until recently, venography was the only diagnostic study capable of allowing one to both identify and

P. A. Lotke: Hospital of the University of Pennsylvania, Philadelphia, Pennsylvania 19104.

quantify clot. Techniques such as plethysmography, I-fibrinogen scans, and clinical assessment were widely used yet generally inaccurate in their ability to help one quantify thrombosis (15). Many of the reports in the literature that depended on these techniques may have led to inappropriate conclusions (29).

Venography is generally recognized as the most accurate method of confirming presence of a clot; it can help one diagnose, localize, and quantify the thrombosis. Although there are some inaccuracies related to nonfilling veins, this technique is currently still considered the most accurate method. Because of patient discomfort from this invasive examination and the potential for renal toxicity and allergic reactions, venography has not been used universally to diagnose deep venous thrombosis. In addition, in many studies in which venography was used, investigators inconsistently reported the size or location of clots and mixed data pertaining to distal and proximal clots to achieve statistical significance.

An interesting observation is the inexplicable variability among centers in the rates of deep venous thrombosis according to surgical site and treatment group. In one multicenter study on the use of low-molecular-weight heparin in total joint arthroplasty, the interinstitutional incidence of clot among patients using one treatment regimen ranged from 28% to 54% (11). Wille-Jorgenson et al. (29) found interobserver variability in venographic interpretations. From a primary individual reading to a consensus decision on a venogram, there was agreement for positive findings in only 70% to 90% of the cases. This factor of uncertainty was believed to be important enough to be considered in venographic studies. These differences are difficult to explain but indicate some of the variables in establishing the diagnosis of deep venous thrombosis and comparing treatment regimens.

B-mode duplex ultrasonography has become a popular method for diagnosis of deep venous thrombosis (9). This study has the potential to be very accurate, especially for proximal thrombosis. However, it is less accurate in the popliteal and calf areas and cannot show clots above the inguinal ligament. Because it is recognized to be technician dependent, with accuracy varying from 0% to 90%, the literature has shown great inconsistency in the reported sensitivity (6,8). Therefore reports that do not validate ultrasonographic results may lead to misleading conclusions.

SIGNIFICANCE OF DEEP VENOUS THROMBOSIS

In addition to the inconsistency and potential inaccuracy in reporting deep venous thrombosis, the importance of a clot has yet to be fully understood (10,17). Deep venous thrombi may occur in an array of sizes and locations in the postoperative period. There may be small clots in the calf, moderate clots in the popliteal area, small clots around femoral valve cusps, or large iliofemoral thrombi involving a substantial portion of the proximal venous system. It is believed that each of these clots has a different potential risk to the patient. However, because of inaccuracies in the diagnosis of clots and inconsistency in reporting size and location, the importance of deep venous thrombosis in a given location and size has not been well defined.

An example of the difficulty in determining the importance of a clot is the observation that calf thrombi are two and one half times more common after total knee arthroplasty than after total hip arthroplasty (17). Nevertheless, pulmonary embolism is much less common after total knee operations. Fatal pulmonary embolism after total hip operations is sevenfold more common. It is reported to occur among 0.35% of patients after total hip arthroplasty, whereas only 0.05% of patients experience pulmonary embolism after total knee operations (18). If calf thrombi represent high risk to a patient, then we should have noticed an increased incidence of pulmonary embolism after total knee arthroplasty. In fact, to date reduction in the incidence of deep venous thrombosis has not been shown to be associated with a reduction in fatal pulmonary embolism (21).

In addition to location, the size of a lower extremity clot is important. It appears that a large clot is necessary to produce a symptomatic pulmonary embolism (3,7). The exact size of a clot that causes pulmonary symptoms is as yet undetermined. In a study describing asymptomatic pulmonary embolism, there was a positive correlation between the size of the deep venous thrombus and the probability of development of asymptomatic pulmonary embolism as detected with a ventilation-perfusion scan. Although most ventilation-perfusion scan defects occurred among patients who had no symptoms, the data indicated that small clots embolize regularly but do not cause symptoms or appear to have clinical significance until they reach a large enough size (17).

The temporal sequence of postoperative deep venous thrombosis and embolic events has not been well defined. It is generally agreed that clots that adhere to the endothelium begin to organize and mature and are less likely to detach and become symptomatic emboli. Many clots form within the first 24 hours of an operation. One must then speculate on which clots are related to the pulmonary embolism and when they were formed. One study concluded that the clots formed very quickly in large veins and thus did not have the opportunity to adhere firmly. If large enough, the clots caused a fatal pulmonary embolism (25).

Part of the problem in establishing the importance of size, location, and timing of thromboembolic events is related to the assumption that data from the medical literature are equally valid for postsurgical patients. When nonsurgical patients have clots, for example, patients with congestive heart failure or carcinomatosis or those who take oral contraceptives, the clot demonstrates a coagulopathy that predisposes the person to thromboembolic disease (3). Although a calf clot itself may not be dangerous, it is a marker for the coagulopathy, and the patient is at risk. The importance of calf clots among medical patients has been transferred to postsurgical patients by many experts in the medical community. This may not be valid. However, after total hip and total knee operations, all patients should be assumed to have some degree of coagulopathy. In addition, extensive local endothelial injury may have occurred at the operation and encouraged local clot formation. Many patients have clots, but it is unclear which of these clots are reliable markers for the patient at increased risk for pulmonary embolism. Considering that 40% to 60% of patients have deep venous thrombosis after total hip and total knee operations and the incidence of fatal pulmonary embolism approximates only 0.1% to 0.3%, it is difficult to determine which patient with deep venous thrombosis is actually at risk for development of a fatal pulmonary embolism.

PULMONARY EMBOLISM

The presence of a pulmonary embolism should be clearly demonstrated. However, if the methods by which pulmonary embolism is diagnosed and reported are evaluated, it becomes clear that there may be serious inaccuracies in the data. If all patients believed to have a pulmonary embolism on the basis of clinical history and examination undergo a full evaluation, including blood gases, ventilation-perfusion scans, or angiography, only 5% to 20% of these patients actually have a pulmonary embolism (24). Therefore studies that depend on clinical evaluation alone may have inaccuracies in their databases.

Ventilation-perfusion scans have traditionally been considered the most accurate method of diagnosing pulmonary embolism. They also have been shown to have shortcomings (24). A large multiinstitutional study on pulmonary embolism concluded that a high-probability scan usually indicates a pulmonary embolism but that only a small number of patients with pulmonary embolism have a high-probability scan. A low-probability scan with a weak clinical impression of pulmonary embolism makes the possibility of pulmonary embolism remote, and an intermediate-probability scan is not of help in establishing a diagnosis. Therefore ventilation-perfusion scanning has considerable limitations. Angiography is probably the best way to determine the diagnosis of pulmonary embolism (24), but in general has not been used as an end point in the literature.

Considering that the clinical diagnosis of pulmonary embolism is unreliable, ventilation-perfusion scans are inconclusive, angiography is only rarely performed, and postoperative fat embolism has only recently been recognized and not considered in prior reports of pulmonary embolism, it is not surprising that pulmonary embolism has not been well defined in many studies.

FAT EMBOLISM

The recognition of fat embolism after total hip and knee operations has become particularly important (14). It is now recognized that this complication must be considered in the postoperative period when a patient has reduced oxygenation and does not thrive. In the past these patients were considered to have a pulmonary embolism, but in reality many had fat embolism syndrome. This entity has certainly affected conclusions in the literature regarding pulmonary embolism.

PROPHYLAXIS OF THROMBOEMBOLIC DISEASE

Pulmonary embolism still represents a threat to patients after total joint arthroplasty, although the incidence today is much lower than reported earlier. Many articles begin by citing old studies that found fatal pulmonary embolism occurred in as many as 1% to 7% of operations (27). However, with early mobilization and up-to-date surgical techniques, the incidence of fatal pulmonary embolism even among patients unprotected by pharmacologic agents is 0.1% to 0.3% after total hip arthroplasty and less after total knee arthroplasty (18,20). Accurate data on this risk are important in determining the choice of prophylactic agent.

Numerous studies in the literature concern prophylaxis of thromboembolic disease (13). There are two general types of prophylaxis—pharmacologic prevention with agents such as low-molecular-weight heparin (5,26), warfarin (1,22), and aspirin (2,16), and mechanical measures, such as use of calf or plantar compression devices (28). The more effective the chemoprophylaxis is in preventing clots, the greater is the risk for bleeding complications (4,11,12). Therefore agents such as low-molecular-weight heparin, which appear to be able to reduce substantially the incidence of deep venous thrombosis produce increased risk for bleeding. This observation was the topic of an editorial in the British *Journal of Bone and Joint Surgery* (21) in which the editors stated that the evidence to date did not warrant routine use of chemoprophylaxis because of the associated comorbidity of bleeding. It has been reported that none of the chemoprophylactic agents has made a difference in the incidence of fatal pulmonary embolism (20). Calf compression devices have not been shown to decrease the incidence of proximal deep venous thrombosis. However, use of plantar compressive devices has led to a reduction in proximal and distal thrombi.

MANAGEMENT OF THROMBOEMBOLIC DISEASE

The treatment of patients with thromboembolic disease is controversial. In general, patients who have documented pulmonary embolism or very large venous thigh clots should be treated. The current standard treatment is vigorous use of heparin followed by 3 to 6 months of warfarin therapy. However, if the same treatment recommendations are extended to patients who have undergone total joint replacement, there is a high incidence of bleeding complications. It has been reported (23) that if therapeutic levels of anticoagulation are initiated within the first week after total hip arthroplasty, there is a 45% chance of profuse bleeding. If initiated within the first 2 weeks, there is a 30% chance of bleeding (23). Hull et al. (12) reported a 10% chance of bleeding from therapeutic levels of heparin converted to warfarin in the perioperative period. They also found a 0.7% mortality rate with that regimen (12).

The decision to initiate treatment remains controversial. The risk for bleeding in the postoperative period is high, and the decision to anticoagulate to therapeutic levels should be made with caution.

PERSISTENCE OF CONTROVERSIES

When past literature is critically reviewed, some of the problems are appreciated. There are deficiencies in methods of diagnosis of deep venous thrombosis and in reporting the size and location of thrombi. There have been difficulties in defining pulmonary embolism and definitely confirming its presence. To solve the problem of statistical significance, there has been a tendency to pool patients with diverse causes of etiologic coagulopathies into single studies. This has only further confused the literature.

There have been dramatic changes in the pattern of orthopedic care of patients who undergo total joint arthroplasty. Originally patients stayed at bed rest for long periods of time, were mobilized slowly, and stayed in the hospital for weeks. Now patients are mobilized within 1 or 2 days of the operation and are discharged within the week. This appears to reduce the risk for thromboembolic disease and pulmonary embolism but as yet is only partially factored into current prophylactic recommendations.

AUTHOR'S PREFERENCE

At present I currently use aspirin and plantar foot pumps for prophylaxis against thromboembolic disease. Aspirin has been shown effectively to inhibit platelet function and in a metaanalysis (2) to reduce markedly the incidence of fatal pulmonary embolism. Mechanical foot pumps are well tolerated and can reduce early local deep venous thrombosis (28). I choose this regimen because it is safe and well tolerated and appears to be effective in preventing fatal pulmonary embolism. Other choices are available, very reasonable, and well accepted, including use of warfarin or low-molecular-weight heparin. However, the latter methods are more expensive and have higher rates of bleeding complications. In the current medical-legal environment, it is probably prudent to choose one or another prophylactic regimen. It will be many years before it can be determined which is the best regimen.

SUMMARY

Orthopedic surgeons should understand the genesis of the controversy regarding thromboembolic disease and appreciate the difficulties in finding solutions. Although there are numerous recommendations for the best method to diagnose, treat, and prevent thromboembolic disease, it will be several years before some of the more controversial issues are fully resolved.

REFERENCES

1. Amstutz HC, Friscia DA, Carney BT. Warfarin prophylaxis to prevent mortality from pulmonary embolism after total hip replacement. *J Bone Joint Surg Am* 1989;71:321–326.
2. Antiplatlet Trailists Collaboration. Collaborative overview of randomized trials of antiplatelet therapy, III: reduction in venous thrombosis and pulmonary embolism by antiplatelet prophylaxix among surgical and medical patients. *Br Med J* 1994;308:235–246.
3. Carson J, Kelley MA, Duff A, et al. The clinical course of pulmonary embolism. *N Engl J Med* 1992;326:1240–1245.
4. Collins R, Scrimgeour A, Yusuf S, Peto R. Reduction of fatal pulmonary embolism and venous thrombosis by perioperative administration of subcutaneous heparin. *N Engl J Med* 1988;318:1162–1173.
5. Colwell CS, Spiro TE. The efficacy and safety of enoxoparin to prevent deep venous thrombosis after hip arthroplasty. *Clin Orthop* 1995;319:215–222.
6. Davidson BL, Elliot CG, Lensing AWA. Radiographic analysis Heparin Arthroplasty Group: low accuracy of color doppler ultrasound in the detection of proximal leg vein thrombosis in asymptomatic high risk patients. *Ann Intern Med* 1992;117:735–738.
7. Foley M, Maslack MM, Rothman RH, et al. Course of pulmonary embolism. *Radiology* 1989;172:481–485.
8. Garino JP, Lotke PA, Kitziger K, Steinberg MD. Deep venous thrombosis after total joint arthroplasty: the role of compression ultrasonography and the importance of the experience of the technician. *J Bone Joint Surg Am* 1996;78:1359–1365.
9. Grady-Benson JC, Oishi CS, Hanssen PB, et al. Postoperative surveillance for deep venous thrombosis for duplex ultrasonography after total knee arthroplasty. *J Bone Joint Surg Am* 1994;76:1649–1657.
10. Haas SB, Tribus CB, Insall JN, Becker MW, Windsor RE. The significance of calf thrombi after total knee arthroplasty. *J Bone Joint Surg Br* 1992;74:799–802.
11. Hull R, Raskob G, Pineo G, et al. A comparison of subcutaneous low molecular weight heparin with warfarin sodium for prophylaxis against deep venous thrombosis after hip or knee implantation. *N Engl J Med* 1993;329:1370–1376.
12. Hull RD, Roskob G, Rosenberg D, et al. Heparin for 5 days as compared with 10 days in the initial treatment of proximal venous thrombosis. *N Engl J Med* 1990;322:1260–1264.

13. Imperiale TF, Sperof TE. A meta-analysis of methods to prevent venous thromboembolism following hip replacement. *JAMA* 1994;271:1780–1785.
14. Johnson JM, Lucas GL. Fat embolism syndrome. *Rev Orthop* 1996;19:41–49.
15. Lieberman JR, Geerts WH. Prevention of venous thromboembolism after total hip and knee arthroplasty: current concepts review. *J Bone Joint Surg* 1994;76A:1239–1250.
16. Lotke PA, Palevsky H, Keenan AM, et al. Aspirin and warfarin for thromboembolic disease after total joint arthroplasty. *Clin Orthop* 1996;324:251–258.
17. Lotke PA, Steinberg MD, Ecker ML. Significance of deep venous thrombosis in the lower extremity after total joint arthroplasty. *Clin Orthop* 1994;299:25–30.
18. Mohr DM, Silverstein MD, Earlstrup DM, Heit JA, Morrey BF. Venous thromboembolism associated with hip and knee arthroplasty: current prophylactic practices and outcome. *Mayo Clin Proc* 1992;67:861–870.
19. Moser KM, Lemoine JR. Is embolic risk conditioned by location of deep venous thrombosis? *Ann Intern Med* 1991;94:439–444.
20. Murray DW, Britton AR, Bulstrode CJK. Thromboprophylaxis and death after total hip replacement. *J Bone Joint Surg Br* 1996;78:863–879.
21. Murray DW, Carr AJ, Bulstrode CJK. Pharmacologic thromboprophylaxis in total hip replacement [Editorial]. *J Bone Joint Surg Br* 1994;77:3–5.
22. Paiment GD, Wessinger SJ, Hughes R, Harris WH. Routine use of adjusted low dose warfarin to prevent venous embolism after total hip replacement. *J Bone Joint Surg Am* 1993;75:893–898.
23. Patterson BM, Marshan R, Ranawat C. Complications of heparin therapy after total joint arthroplasty. *J Bone Joint Surg Am* 1989;71:1130–1134.
24. PIOPED Investigators. Value of the ventilation/perfusion scan in acute pulmonary embolism: results of the prospective investigation of pulmonary embolism diagnosis. *JAMA* 1990;263:2753–2795.
25. Priestly JT, Barker NW. Postoperative thrombosis and embolism. *Surg Gynecol Obstet* 1942;75:193–201.
26. Radiographic Analysis Heparin Arthroplasty Group. The RD-heparin compared with warfarin for prevention of venous thromboembolic disease following total hip or knee arthroplasty. *J Bone Joint Surg Am* 1994;76:1174–1185.
27. Warwick D, Williams MH, Bannister GC. Death and thromboembolic disease after total hip replacement. *J Bone Joint Surg Br* 1996;77:6–10.
28. Westrich GH, Sculco TP. Prophylaxis against deep venous thrombosis after total knee arthroplasty: pneumatic plantar compression and aspirin compared with aspirin alone. *J Bone Joint Surg Am* 1996;78:826–834.
29. Wille-Jorgenson P, Borris L, Jorgenson LN, et al. Phlebography as the gold standard in thromboprophylactic studies? A multicenter interobserver variation study. *Acta Radiol* 1992;33:24–28.

Revision Total Hip Arthroplasty,
edited by Marvin E. Steinberg and Jonathan P. Garino,
Lippincott Williams & Wilkins, Philadelphia © 1999.

32

Dislocation

Daniel J. Berry

Dislocation after total hip arthroplasty is a disturbing problem for both patient and surgeon. Despite innovations in surgical approach, surgical technique, and implant design, dislocation has not been eliminated. It remains one of the most frequent complications of total hip arthroplasty and one of the most frequent reasons for reoperation after total hip arthroplasty. When a reoperation is performed to correct recurrent dislocation, the reported failure rate is higher than for any other indication for revision surgery, including infection.

Fortunately, in the several decades since the introduction of the operation, much has been learned about hip instability after total hip arthroplasty. Application of this knowledge can lead to more effective prevention of the problem and much more successful treatment of recurrent dislocation than once was possible. This chapter reviews what is known about the incidence and causes of the problem, means of preventing the problem, and the nonoperative and operative methods available to treat patients with dislocation. The occurrence of the problem after revision total hip arthroplasty receives special attention.

INCIDENCE

A wide range of incidence figures for dislocation rate after primary total hip arthroplasty are reported in the literature (12,14); most cluster between 2% and 5% (15,21,25,30,34). A higher rate of dislocation has been identified following revision total hip arthroplasty (25,43). In an excellent review Morrey (34) combined the data in several large series and identified a 2% dislocation rate for 4,753 primary total hip arthroplasties compared with a 6.3% dislocation rate among 1,290 revision hip arthroplasties. Woo and Morrey (48) reviewed the Mayo Clinic experience and reported a 2.4% dislocation rate after 7,241 primary total hip arthroplasties compared with a 4.8% rate for patients with

D. J. Berry: Department of Orthopaedics, Mayo Medical School, Mayo Clinic, Rochester Methodist Hospital, St. Mary's Hospital, Rochester, Minnesota 55905.

previous hip operations, a statistically significant difference. A number of presumed factors lead to elevated risk for dislocation after revision surgery: poorer soft tissues, altered abductor muscle attachments, the use of extensile surgical exposures at revision, and nonanatomic component positioning necessitated by bone loss in the revision setting.

The incidence of dislocation varies as a function of time after the operation (22,34). The reduced risk for dislocation with time probably is attributable to healing of soft tissues, improved muscle tone, and formation of a pseudocapsule around the joint, all of which make the hip more difficult to dislocate. However, dislocations do continue to occur—albeit at a lower rate—indefinitely after total hip arthroplasty. First dislocations have been reported more than 20 years after the operation.

RISK FACTORS

A number of demographic factors are associated with a higher risk for dislocation after total hip arthroplasty (22). Although aggregate data on risk factors come from series composed either exclusively or mostly of primary total hip arthroplasties, many of the same risk factors can be assumed for the revision population. Women have a higher dislocation rate than men in a proportion of about 2:1 (25,35,43,48); the reason is not known, although more compliant soft tissues that allow greater range of motion may be implicated. Older patient age has been associated with a higher risk for dislocation (14,20), probably because of increased risk for falls, less ability to comply with hip dislocation precautions, and possibly poor soft tissues. Certain specific underlying diagnoses are also associated with an increased risk for dislocation. Patients with neuromuscular problems are probably at higher risk because of poor muscle control, contractures, and altered muscle balance and body mechanics (25).

Technical factors related to hip arthroplasty also affect risk for dislocation (4). Surgical approach has received the most attention: most publications demonstrate a higher risk for dislocation associated with posterior approaches than anterior lateral or direct lateral approaches (34,40,43,44,48). The higher rate of dislocation after use of a posterior approach has been attributed to violation of the posterior capsule and short external rotators and to increased risk of inadequate acetabular component anteversion. The transtrochanteric approach has been associated with increased risk for dislocation when nonunion with proximal trochanteric migration occurs. The effect on dislocation rates of more extensile exposures commonly used in revision surgery has not been specifically examined.

The diameter of the femoral head should affect the likelihood of hip dislocation. Larger head sizes have a higher prosthetic head size to neck size ratio and therefore a larger range of hip motion before the prosthetic neck impinges against the acetabular component. Furthermore, larger head sizes require greater displacement (because their radius is larger) before the hips dislocates. Despite the theoretic underpinning that suggests larger head sizes might reduce instability and smaller sizes might increase instability, this relation has not been proved clinically (11). Perhaps the large number of other factors involved in instability obscure any association. Many physicians still believe an association, yet to be proved, exists and act accordingly.

A final risk factor for dislocation is patient compliance. Even the most technically perfect total hip arthroplasty is less inherently stable than a native hip joint, and patients who routinely violate hip dislocation precautions are at increased risk for dislocation. Very poor compliance can be related to poor cognition (as the result of age, substance abuse (22), or other comorbidities or may be related to inability to control the extremity satisfactorily because of contractures, stroke, or other neuromuscular problems (34).

ETIOLOGIC FACTORS

The risk factors discussed place certain patient populations at increased or decreased risk for dislocation. But for an individual patient, a specific cause or combination of causes leads to the dislocation. Prevention and management of dislocation for individual patients—during either primary or revision total hip arthroplasty—are based on understanding the reasons that dislocation can occur. Fortunately the number of causes of dislocation is limited. Thus a systematic review of the possibilities usually leads to identification of the source or sources of the instability.

Component Malposition

Component malposition is one of the most frequent sources of recurrent hip instability and is almost certainly the one that surgeons can do the most to avoid. Malposition of either the acetabular component or the femoral component can lead to hip instability, although acetabular malposition is probably more common. Khan et al. (25) reviewed the cases of 142 patients with hip dislocations and found half had unsatisfactory acetabular component anteversion or abduction. Lewinnek et al. (29) found the safe zone of acetabular component position to be 15 degrees of anteversion plus or minus 10 degrees and 40 degrees of abduction plus or minus 10 degrees. These numbers are not inviolable, and ideal component position varies with specific circumstances. Nevertheless, extreme acetabular anteversion predisposes to anterior dislocation, whereas retroversion predisposes to posterior dislocation. Many surgeons believe that more anteversion of the socket is desirable when a total hip arthroplasty is performed through a posterior approach (because soft-tissue restraint to internal rotation is less) than after an anterior lateral approach, although this has not been proved. Excessively abducted sockets (too vertical) may lead to higher risk for lateral dislocation when the leg is adducted.

Undoubtedly femoral component position also affects risk for dislocation, but much less information is available on this subject, probably because accurate measurement of femoral component anteversion is difficult radiographically without computed tomography. Despite a paucity of hard data, most experts believe inadequate anteversion of the femoral component is associated with higher risk for posterior dislocation and excessive anteversion with a higher rate of anterior dislocation.

The positions of the acetabular component and the femoral component are additive. Thus a small amount of excess anteversion of *both* the femoral and the acetabular component may lead to anterior instability, whereas a small insufficiency of anteversion of both components may lead to posterior instability. Similarly, within limits an excess of acetabular anteversion may be compensated by less femoral anteversion and vice versa. Most experts agree the total anteversion of the femoral and acetabular components should be about 45 degrees when a posterior approach is used and perhaps a little less when an anterior approach is used.

Soft-Tissue Tension

Poor soft-tissue tension almost certainly predisposes a hip to dislocation, although the lack of objective methods of quantitating soft-tissue tension make this common-sense argument difficult to prove (9). Support for the theory that poor soft-tissue tension contributes to instability is provided by the knowledge that trochanteric advancement, which improves soft-tissue tension, has been proved effective in stabilizing unstable hips with well-positioned components. Poor soft-tissue tension may be caused by limb shortening, reduction of femoral offset, extensive soft-tissue dissection, and capsulectomy. Poor soft-tissue tension also can arise from trochanteric nonunion with subsequent proximal migration or from abductor muscle dysfunction or avulsion after an approach to the hip that involves abductor muscle release (46).

Impingement

Bony structures, soft-tissue structures, or the prosthesis itself can provide a fulcrum that allows the prosthetic head to be levered out of the socket; this process is known as *impingement*. Impingement of the greater trochanter or anterior proximal femur against the pelvis can occur with the hip in a flexed, internally rotated position. Likewise, redundant anterior capsule, scar, or other soft tissues can serve as a fulcrum when the hip is flexed and internally rotated, leading to posterior dislocation. Impingement of the femur against the ischium in extension and external rotation may lead to anterior dislocation.

Impingement of the prosthetic femoral neck against the wall of the socket can lead to dislocation. The range of motion that can occur before neck–liner impingement is governed by design features of both the femoral and acetabular components. The femoral head-to-neck ratio affects the likelihood of impingement. Small head sizes matched with large femoral neck diameters have the lowest head-to-neck ratio and provide the least range of motion before impingement. Modular components typically provide a less favorable head-to-neck ratio than monoblock components. This is particularly true for long-necked modular heads that are manufactured with skirts for strength but also increase the femoral neck diameter. Acetabular components with extended walls or elevated rims also may reduce the amount of hip motion that can occur before impingement. Socket position naturally has an effect on risk for impingement. Large amounts of anteversion can lead to posterior impingement when the hip is extended and externally rotated, and acetabular retroversion can lead to anterior impingement when the hip is flexed and internally rotated. Very horizontal socket position leads to earlier impingement in both flexion and extension.

Noncompliance

Extremes of hip position can be the sole cause of dislocation, even absent component malposition or poor soft-tissue tension.

PREVENTION

Surgeons are well aware that preventing dislocation is far preferable to having to manage the problem. Once dislocation occurs, patient and surgeon are always concerned that the problem may become recurrent. Chandler et al. (6) demonstrated that patients with dislocation have poorer functional status than those who do not have dislocation and that some of the poorer function may be related to apprehension about dislocation.

Preoperative Measures

Prevention of dislocation begins preoperatively. High risk patients can be identified on the basis of factors described earlier during the preoperative interview and examination, and may be treated differently with respect to surgical approach or special implants when primary or revision total hip arthroplasty is performed. A patient at exceptionally high risk may be considered for an alternative means of treatment, such as the Girdlestone procedure, or for nonoperative treatment.

Good preoperative planning for the surgical procedure can reduce the likelihood of dislocation by providing the surgeon with important information on expected component position relative to bony landmarks and expected prosthetic needs to restore hip biomechanics and soft-tissue tension. In revision surgery, in which bone loss and soft-tissue deficiencies often require special implants, preoperative planning assumes an especially important role.

Intraoperative Measures

Exposure

The choice of exposure during revision operations is predicated on many factors, including the magnitude of exposure needed to remove failed implants and to implant new ones. Exposures for revision operations are discussed in Chapter 12, but optimal choice of surgical exposure should take into account prevention of hip instability. Patients at high risk for posterior dislocation, such as those with large flexion and adduction contractures or those less able to comply with hip dislocation precautions, may be considered for an anterior lateral approach, possibly reducing the chance of posterior dislocation. When poor soft-tissue tension is expected at the conclusion of a procedure (for example, when the acetabulum is being revised and a femoral component is retained that does not allow addition of neck length) a transtrochanteric approach, which allows trochanteric advancement, may be considered. When a fixed acetabular component is being retained but the femoral component is revised, consideration of the existing acetabular component anteversion is helpful. If the acetabular anteversion is large, a posterior approach may be considered, leaving intact anterior structures that restrain external rotation and minimizing risk for anterior instability. Likewise, if the retained acetabular component has little anteversion, an anterior lateral or transtrochanteric approach may be considered to preserve the posterior capsule and restraints to internal rotation, minimizing the likelihood of posterior instability.

Component Position

Nothing is more difficult to perform reliably during total hip arthroplasty—and nothing is more important—than proper positioning of the acetabular component. When total hip arthroplasty is performed with the patient in the lateral decubitus position, careful positioning of the patient on the table with firm positioning devices is essential. When this step is not performed, the patient tends to roll forward, leading to an exaggerated sense of acetabular anteversion during the operation, but in reality to inadequate acetabular component anteversion. The pelvis tends to roll forward most frequently when a posterior approach is used, because internal rotation of the femur rolls the pelvis forward. This problem is compounded when a posterior approach is used in the revision setting. Noncompliant, scarred tissue necessitates vigorous anterior retraction of the femur to allow wide access to the acetabulum, almost invariably causing the pelvis to roll forward.

Bony acetabular landmarks help provide correct orientation of the socket. The best landmarks are the ischium posteriorly, the bottom of the fovea (the radiographic tear drop) inferiorly, the anterior wall, and the lateral acetabulum. One can be misled by bone deficiencies during revision operations when the usual bony landmarks are obliterated or distorted. During revision operations the position of the pelvis may be surmised by means of intraoperative comparison of the position of the acetabular component being removed with its known position on immediately preoperative radiographs. If the anteversion appears greater intraoperatively than the radiographs showed preoperatively, one concludes the pelvis has rolled forward. Especially during revision operations, an intraoperative radiograph to check the position of the newly implanted acetabular component is helpful. The apparent acetabular anteversion on intraoperative radiographs appears greater than actual if the pelvis has rolled forward. The surgeon can recognize this, and therefore take it into account, on intraoperative radiographs by observing whether the obturator rings are symmetric and whether the midline of the sacrum lines up with the symphysis pubis. Radiographs that resemble an obturator oblique Judet radiograph suggest the pelvis has rolled forward.

During revision operations the position of the acetabular component and thus the center of hip rotation plays an important role in hip stability. Medial bone deficiencies predispose the hip to a medial center of rotation. When possible this should be avoided by use of extra large cups, extra depth cups, eccentric socket liners, or medial bone grafts, because medialization of the hip center leads to increased risk for bony impingement between the femur and pelvis and thus increased risk for instability. Particularly during revision operations, a high center of hip rotation may be considered to optimize socket contact with native bone. In some circumstances this is needed to optimize the likelihood of long-term socket fixation. However, a high center of hip rotation does predispose to problems with hip instability (probably because of soft-tissue tension problems and femoral impingement against the pelvis in adduction). Thus when the center of hip rotation can be normalized without compromising socket fixation, the likelihood of dislocation may be reduced.

Elevated rim acetabular polyethylene liners are available for the modular uncemented sockets most commonly used in revision surgery. Cobb et al. (8) found that elevated liners lowered risk for dislocation after revision operations. Despite these data the authors did not advocate routine use of elevated liners because they recognized these devices do not by themselves impart a wider range of stable hip motion. Elevated liners do, however, allow the surgeon to fine tune effective socket position after shell implantation, a valuable resource in revision surgery.

The optimal femoral component and optimal position of the femoral component can reduce the chance of dislocation. Femoral component anteversion should be optimized with reference to the bony anatomic landmarks of the proximal femur and the patient's leg with the knee in flexion. Large varus or valgus knee deformities affect the perceived femoral anteversion. In the primary setting the femoral neck is osteotomized at an optimal level on the basis of preoperative plan. References include the ipsilateral greater trochanter, the ipsilateral lesser trochanter, and the ipsilateral center of the femoral head. In revision surgery, judging proper femoral length is more difficult. Femoral and pelvic bony landmarks may be obliterated or altered, and the center of hip rotation may no longer be anatomic. The femoral component chosen must provide stable and durable femoral fixation but must also provide sufficient neck length to restore soft-tissue tension and hip stability. The level of proximal femoral bone loss in revision operations is predetermined, thus the surgeon must decide whether special implants or bone grafts are needed to build up the proximal femur. Because of the poor track record of medial "napkin ring" allografts, most surgeons prefer calcar-replacing implants that rest on native bone for marked proximal femoral bone loss. When possible, implants should be chosen to reproduce hip mechanics without long modular necks with skirts that can cause prosthetic impingement and a smaller arc of stable hip range of motion.

Proper soft-tissue tensioning during the operation reduces the likelihood of dislocation. In primary operations simply choosing proper femoral neck length and offset usually provides satisfactory soft-tissue tension. In revision operations, soft-tissue tension cannot always be restored by means of changing neck length (for example, when a well-fixed femoral implant is being retained during an acetabular revision). In such circumstances one means of improving soft-tissue tension is trochanteric advancement.

Stability Testing

The ritual of checking hip stability is a critical part of every total hip arthroplasty. Hip stability should be checked in flexion and internal rotation and adduction (to test posterior stability), extension and external rotation (to test anterior stability), and in the position of sleep (adduction, partial flexion, and mild internal rotation). In each position any tendency toward instability or prosthetic or bony impingement should be identified and corrected.

Soft-Tissue Repair

Risk for dislocation rises dramatically with trochanteric nonunion and proximal trochanteric migration, probably because of decreased soft-tissue tension and poorer abductor muscle function. Woo and Morrey (48) reported an instability rate of 17.6% for patients with trochanteric nonunion compared with 2.8% for those with a united trochanteric osteotomy. Failure of abductor muscle repair after an anterolateral approach to the hip predisposes the hip to many of the same problems as trochanteric nonunion (46). Thus good repair of the abductor muscles after an anterolateral approach to the hip is important to provide optimal abductor function and to minimize hip instability related to poor soft-tissue tension and poor abductor function. The value of optimal soft-tissue repair after a posterior approach has not been fully recognized until recently. Careful preservation of posterior soft-tissue structures during exposure and meticulous, solid repair of those structures to bone at closure can provide a check-rein effect that reduces excessive internal rotation and thereby may reduce risk for dislocation. These structures can almost always be preserved and repaired during primary total hip arthroplasty, although some surgeons have questioned whether the soft-tissue repair remains intact over time (23).

During revision arthroplasty the posterior soft tissues can be preserved by means of taking them down as a single sleeve from the posterior proximal femur then carefully repairing them to bone at the close of the procedure.

Constrained Devices

Occasionally the surgeon preoperatively or intraoperatively identifies instability problems that cannot be solved with conventional implants. Such problems include severely compromised abductor muscles, absent abductor muscle attachments, and severe compliance problems. In these circumstances the surgeon may choose prophylactic use of a constrained acetabular implant or a bipolar acetabular implant—either of which provides more immediate hip stability than conventional implants. These devices can be very helpful, but trade-offs (discussed later) are associated with their use; thus use of these implants is probably best limited to infrequent circumstances. Lombardi et al. (31) reported routine use of a constrained S-ROM socket (Johnson & Johnson Orthopedics, Raynham, Mass.) reduced their dislocation rate in revision surgery from 19% in 176 revisions to 4.5%, a statistically significant improvement. Rather than use a constrained implant before postoperative instability has been demonstrated, some surgeons prefer to implant an uncemented socket with a conventional liner (but of a design with compatible modular constrained liners available). The reasoning is that if instability manifests itself postoperatively a second operation to place a constrained liner can be performed after the initially placed shell has osteointegrated.

Postoperative Treatment

Education about hip dislocation precautions helps prevent dislocation. Counseling about allowed and disallowed activities after the operation is important. A list of don'ts, such as "don't sit on low chairs," "don't attempt to cut your own toenails," for the early postoperative period is valuable. The patient should be shown how to avoid excessive hip flexion, adduction, and internal rotation. Demonstrating how to maintain proper hip position while rising from chairs, getting in and out of bed, and getting in and out of cars is helpful.

Some patients may benefit from prophylactic postoperative bracing or casting. Postoperative casts and braces operate on the principle that external immobilization prevents excessive hip motion during the early postoperative period when the risk for dislocation is highest. By externally restricting motion until the hip is stabilized by soft-tissue healing, dislocation may be avoided. More is said about bracing and spica casts in the section that follows on nonoperative management of hip dislocation. Because patients who undergo revision hip arthroplasty are recognized to be at increased risk for dislocation, many surgeons routinely provide prophylactic braces for several months after the operation.

MANAGEMENT OF HIP DISLOCATION

Immediate management of a dislocation after primary or revision operations is relocation, which in most instances can be affected by closed means. Good anteroposterior and true lateral views of the pelvis should be obtained with the hip dislocated. These radiographs provide the surgeon with unequivocal evidence of the direction of dislocation and thereby facilitate proper treatment. Reduction of an anterior dislocation usually is effected by means of traction followed by gentle internal rotation of the hip. Reduction of a posterior dislocation usually is effected by means of traction with the hip in a flexed, adducted position. Modifications of these reduction methods have been described (28). The choice of sedation or anesthesia for reduction is based on the individual patient's situation and on the surgeon's preference. Anesthesia with muscle relaxation is needed for some dislocations and should be used when the surgeon fears excessive force could cause a complication such as bony fracture or damage to the prosthesis (27,41). Open reduction of a hip dislocation occasionally is required. During the operation an effort should be made to identify the source of instability and if necessary manage it at the time of the open reduction (see later).

Nonoperative Treatment

After closed reduction of dislocation, most surgeons allow the patient to resume weight-bearing as tolerated, except when special circumstances dictate otherwise, such as in the immediately postoperative period. Most surgeons prefer to place the patient in a hip guide brace that restricts motion and allows soft-tissue healing. Most braces are designed to provide some abduction (about 15 degrees is the most tolerated by patients) and some restriction of hip flexion (Fig. 1). The surgeon should be aware that all braces allow some hip motion beyond the stated limits of the flexion stop (because of motion of the brace allowed by compliance of the soft-tissue envelope around the hip) so the surgeon should adjust stops accordingly (a flexion stop of 45 to 75 degrees is most common). The patient also should be counseled that the brace is a reminder and that braces are not rigid enough to restrict hip motion completely.

The results of bracing programs in several small series of dislocations have been reported. Stewart (42) reported on 13 hips treated with closed reduction followed by a hip guide brace and found no further instability in 8 cases and redislocation in 5. For patients with one dislocation the rate of success was 5 of 5, but for patients with recurrent dislocation, the rate of success was only 3 of 8. Clayton and Thirupathi (7) reported on 9 patients treated with a hip guide brace for 6 to 9 months. All had satisfactory implant position and most had had at least two dislocations. Seven of 9 patients avoided further dislocation using the bracing protocol. Dorr et al. (11) reported on the use of a hip guide brace with 10 degrees of abduction and a 60 degree flexion stop and found it effectively prevented further dislocation for 10 of 12 patients when worn for 4 to 6 weeks.

Some surgeons prefer a spica cast to a brace, at least in some circumstances, reasoning that a spica cast provides more complete, reliable, and rigid immobilization. Williams et

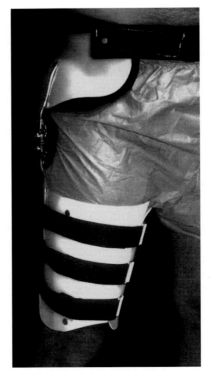

Figure 1. Hip guide brace provides hip abduction and a flexion stop.

al. (47) reported on the use of a spica cast for 6 weeks after either closed or open reduction by 16 patients (for 4 a revision procedure was combined with open reduction). After a mean of 32 months, only one hip had redislocated. Ritter (39) reported 3 of 5 hips managed with a spica cast for 6 weeks after a first-time dislocation became stable but 2 continued to subluxate anteriorly. Usually a one-half spica cast (an above-knee spica cast) is sufficient to restrict hip motion yet still allow the patient limited mobility. Providing a patient with a reclining wheelchair while the cast is being worn is helpful. As for any patient in a spica cast, personal hygiene and skin integrity require special attention. There are no published data that specifically address the efficacy of bracing or spica casts when dislocation follows revision hip arthroplasty, but one might anticipate that the efficacy would be similar to that identified after primary hip arthroplasty.

Operative Treatment

The decision to use operative management to restore hip stability requires consideration of many factors. How many times has the hip dislocated? How long after the operation did the dislocation occur? Is there a technical factor that can be rectified that explains the dislocation? What are the operative risks of another operation?

As a rule, most dislocations that occur in the first few months after an operation are treated nonoperatively. This principle is based on information showing that early dislocations have a relatively good chance of becoming stable as soft tissues heal. Khan et al. (25) found that 60% of 94 hips that dislocated within 5 weeks of an operation did not redislocate, whereas, this was true of only 40% of those that dislocated after 5 weeks. An exception to the aforementioned guidelines is a patient with a severe technical problem deemed certain to cause recurrent dislocation; such a patient usually is selected for earlier reoperation.

In most circumstances a first or second dislocation is managed nonoperatively. Khan et al. (25) showed an overall success rate of 62% for closed reduction after a single dislocation but only a 23% rate for recurrent dislocation. A third or fourth dislocation typically leads to consideration of surgical therapy, particularly if the dislocations have occurred in rapid succession. Exceptions include hopelessly noncompliant patients, patients with a technical problem considered too difficult to solve, or patients medically unable to tolerate another major procedure.

The historical rate of success of revision surgery for dislocation is lower than the success rate of revision total hip arthroplasty for any other single indication. Daly and Morrey (10) reported the hips of 58 of 95 patients (61%) were stabilized after one surgical procedure. Fraser and Wroblewski (17) reported that 16 of 21 hips (76%) with recurrent instability became stable after reoperation. As our understanding of dislocation improves and as improved devices to manage dislocation become available, the rate of success almost certainly can be improved (17). Nevertheless, before undertaking revision for instability, it is wise for the surgeon to make the patient aware that restoration of stability is not always successfully accomplished.

Preoperative Evaluation

To treat an unstable hip successfully the surgeon must know the direction of instability. This may be surmised from a description of the activity lending to dislocation (hip flexion and internal rotation leading to posterior instability, hip extension, and external rotation leading to anterior instability). However, the most certain knowledge comes from a true lateral radiograph of the pelvis while the hip is dislocated (Fig. 2). In addition to knowing the direction of dislocation, the surgeon should try to identify other factors that contributed to the instability. Issues of noncompliance or substance abuse may have to be solved before any further surgical treatment is undertaken, lest the operation be doomed to failure from the outset.

A physical examination can help identify factors that predispose to dislocation. Does the patient have abductor insufficiency? Does the patient have severe flexion or adduction contractures?

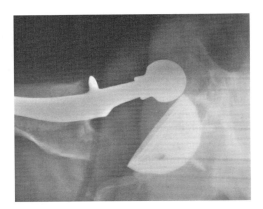

Figure 2. True lateral radiograph of total hip arthroplasty demonstrates anterior hip dislocation.

Radiographic evaluation of the arthroplasty provides information about the status of component fixation and implant position. A true lateral radiograph of the pelvis and hip is the most direct means of obtaining information on socket anteversion. More elaborate mathematical methods have been described (1,32). Computed tomographic scans can provide reliable information on socket and femur position. Interestingly, however, Pierchon et al. (37) reported computed tomography did not provide further helpful information when used as a routine diagnostic tool to find the source of dislocation in 36 of 38 cases.

Before the operation, review of the preoperative reports of previous procedures on the hip can provide information essential during revision. It is important to know with certainty the socket size, manufacturer, and design, the acetabular liner design (Is the rim elevated? If so where is the elevation?), and the femoral component manufacturer and design (Does the component have a modular neck? What is the neck length? What is the femoral head size?). This information is important for any revision but is critical in revision operations for instability, in which having proper matching implants (such as polyethylene liners and femoral heads) often allows the surgeon to retain well-fixed parts of the arthroplasty.

Choosing the Operation

Once a decision has been made to reoperate, the surgeon has the difficult task of choosing the best surgical procedure. The procedure chosen follows directly from a preoperative understanding of the etiology of the instability in the individual patient. Daly and Morrey (10), in their review of operative correction of an unstable hip arthroplasty, concluded that "the results of operative management for an unstable hip arthroplasty can be optimized when a precise determination of the cause of instability is made and appropriate measures applied." Component malposition requires component reorientation; soft-tissue tension problems require restoration of tension either by means of changing components or advancing the trochanter; impingement problems necessitate that the source of impingement be identified and removed. When a combination of these problems coexist, several problems must be solved at once. When problems are present that cannot be solved reliably with conventional implants or without solutions that carry unacceptable trade-offs, conversion of the arthroplasty to a system with more inherent stability, such as a constrained socket or bipolar design, may be needed.

Choosing the Approach

The surgical approach depends on the problem at hand and the surgeon's preference. If the surgeon anticipates that trochanteric advancement will be required, a transtrochanteric approach or a posterior approach (which allows easy conversion to a transtrochanteric approach) may be chosen. In these circumstances an anterolateral approach, which does not allow effective trochanteric advancement, is best avoided. Regardless of the approach chosen, some experts believe capsular preservation during exposure and plication at the close of the procedure may help restore hip stability.

Component Reorientation

When the primary problem or a large part of the problem is suboptimal component position, component reorientation is necessary (Fig. 3). Acetabular malposition is a more common source of instability than femoral malposition; thus acetabular reconstruction is more frequently required.

When a nonmodular acetabular component is malpositioned, in most cases the component must be removed and a new component placed. However, there exists a body of literature reporting the efficacy of mechanically affixing a separate piece of polyethylene to augment a well-fixed implant, in essence creating an elevated rim without removing the socket (33,35,45). Bradbury and Milligan (3) reported this method to be successful for 4 of 5 patients with recurrent anterior dislocation and 9 of 11 patients with recurrent posterior dislocation. Olerud and Karlström (36) found the method successful for 6 of 6 patients, though one patient needed the procedure twice.

When a modular acetabular component is malpositioned, the surgeon must decide whether a new modular liner with an elevated rim will provide sufficient stability or whether the whole implant must be removed. Elevated rims, though they differ in design by manufacturer, all provide the same effect. Placing an elevated rim posteriorly improves posterior stability at the expense of anterior stability. Placing an elevated rim anteriorly improves anterior stability at the expense of posterior stability. Elevated rim liners do not increase the safe arc of hip motion (unless placed directly laterally for lateral instability), but they reorient it (26). When acetabular position is not ideal but is not grossly unsatisfactory, an elevated rim liner may provide sufficient effective reorientation of the articulating surface. More severe malorientation of the socket usually necessitates exchange of the entire component. When a new component is placed, in most instances an uncemented porous coated modular socket is preferred. These implants provide the best fixation in most revision circumstances, and they have the advantage of allowing the surgeon to fine tune the effective socket position after placement of the metal shell.

Reorientation of the femoral component is required less frequently than acetabular reorientation. However, if the femoral component is extremely anteverted and the problem

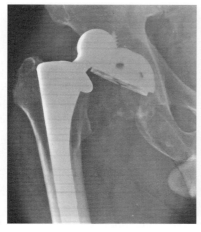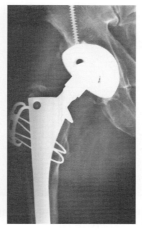

A   B

Figure 3. A: Recurrent posterior hip instability related to inadequate acetabular component anteversion. **B:** Acetabular reorientation to provide more anteversion with trochanteric advancement and a longer modular femoral head restored hip stability.

is anterior instability or if the component is extremely retroverted and the problem is posterior instability, exchange of the implant may be necessary. Because removal of a well-fixed femoral implant can be a major undertaking, some surgeons prefer to manage mildly suboptimal femoral version by compensating appropriately on the acetabular side of the arthroplasty.

Improving Soft-Tissue Tension

Unsatisfactory soft-tissue tension can be improved by means of lowering the hip center of rotation; lateralizing the hip center of rotation; increasing femoral neck length; placing a new femoral implant with more offset or more proximal body length; placing a femoral component in a more proximal position; or advancing the greater trochanter (Fig. 4).

When implants are well fixed and well positioned, greater trochanteric advancement alone, which improves soft-tissue tension by means of tightening the abductor mechanism, has proved effective. Ekelund et al. (13) demonstrated that 19 of 21 unstable total hips, all with satisfactory component position, became stable after trochanteric advancement alone, although two patients underwent reoperations for a second trochanteric fixation. Kaplan et al. (24) also reported on 21 patients with hip instability and satisfactory component position observed a mean of 2.7 years after reoperation. Seventeen of 21 hips had no further instability, 2 had one episode of instability, and 2 had ongoing recurrent instability. One of the patients with ongoing instability experienced trochanteric migration of more than 1 cm after the advancement.

When a femoral component with a modular head is in place, soft-tissue tension can be improved if a modular head of longer neck length is placed. It should be recognized that long modular heads in most systems have skirts that reduce the head-to-neck ratio and can cause earlier prosthetic impingement. For individual patients the advantages of improved tension have to be weighed against the possibility of earlier prosthetic impingement when this solution is used. If the femoral component must be exchanged, placement of a new implant with increased femoral offset or increased proximal femoral-component length (such as a head and neck prosthesis) can improve soft-tissue tension.

When the location or orientation of the acetabular component is suboptimal, placement of a new socket with the hip center in a more inferior or more lateral position also increases soft-tissue tension. Large-diameter uncemented sockets frequently lower and

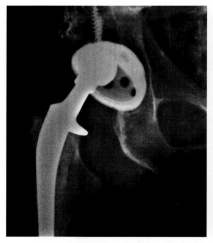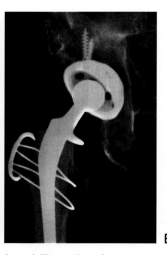

A   **B**

Figure 4. A: Recurrent anterior hip instability related to poor soft-tissue tension and prosthetic impingement of the femoral neck against the acetabular liner. **B:** Hip stability was restored by modular femoral head exchange to a shorter head with no skirt, solving the impingement problem, and trochanteric advancement to restore soft-tissue tension.

lateralize the center of hip rotation compared with the implant they replace. Some modular acetabular implants provide offset or eccentric liners that lower or lateralize the hip center and improve soft-tissue tension.

When soft-tissue tension is a main factor in instability, the decision to use one of the aforedescribed means of improving tension over another should be based on consideration of the desirability of leaving the existing socket in place; the desirability of leaving the existing femoral implant in place; the leg-length discrepancy; and the quality of the trochanteric bone. When the patient's leg lengths are equal or long on the side in question, when the socket and femur are well-positioned, and when the trochanteric bone is good, conditions are ideal for trochanteric advancement.

Removing Sources of Impingement

Whatever the presumed source of instability, careful examination of the hip at the time of any reoperation is made to exclude impingement as a contributing factor. When impingement is suspected as the primary cause of the instability, the cause of impingement must be identified and removed.

Impingement leading to posterior instability most commonly is caused by impingement of the trochanter or proximal femur against the pelvis in flexion and internal rotation. Thick soft tissues or heterotopic bone between the trochanter or proximal femur and pelvis also can be a source of impingement. In most cases resection of some of the anterior greater trochanter (sparing the abductors), removal of thickened anterior soft tissue, or removal of anterior osteophytes or heterotopic bone solves the impingement problem. A medialized socket can predispose to impingement of the femur on the socket. Revision of the socket with restoration of a more lateral hip center may be needed to solve this problem. Impingement of the femur against the ischium in extension and external rotation can lead to anterior instability, most often when the center of hip rotation is elevated. Resection of a portion of the lateral ischium can help solve this problem.

Impingement of the prosthetic neck against the socket requires a change in the prosthesis itself. If the impingement is caused by malposition, the offending component, usually the socket, must be repositioned. If components are reasonably well positioned but impingement still occurs, the usual problems are either an elevated rim liner that has to be repositioned or exchanged for a standard flat liner or a poor head-to-neck ratio (Fig. 5). In the latter circumstance something must be done to improve the head-to-neck ratio. Options include using a larger-diameter head or exchanging a modular head with a skirt for one without a skirt. When optimizing the head-to-neck ratio causes relative shortening of the limb, compensatory measures to regain soft-tissue tension should be considered.

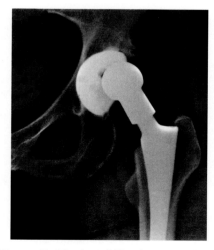

Figure 5. Hip instability in part related to impingement caused by modular femoral head with large skirt and poor head-to-neck ratio.

Combined Measures

Not infrequently instability occurs because of a combination of suboptimal component position, poor soft-tissue tension, and impingement. In such circumstances several measures must be undertaken at once. The troublesome components must be repositioned, soft-tissue tension must be improved with trochanteric advancement or component exchange, the sources of bony and soft-tissue impingement must be removed, and the head-to-neck ratio must be optimized (Fig. 6).

Special Implants

Bipolar implants and constrained sockets both provide more inherent stability than standard total hip arthroplasty and thus are powerful weapons against hip instability (5). Both categories of implant, however, have serious drawbacks. In the revision setting bipolar implants are liable to cause pain or migrate into the pelvic bone. Constrained implants provide better hip stability at the expense of transferring the forces (that would otherwise lead to dislocation) to other prosthetic or prosthesis–bone interfaces (16). For these reasons use of these implants is usually limited to problem cases that cannot readily be solved with more traditional methods.

Bipolar implants provide improved stability by virtue of the large outside diameter of the socket and the biarticular nature of the implant. Zelicoff and Scott (49) reported results for 11 patients and Ries and Wiedel (38) for 3 patients. Both sets of authors found a 100% rate of success in restoring hip stability to an unstable total hip arthroplasty by conversion to a bipolar implant. When used for revision surgery for other indications, bipolar components have been found to have a high rate of migration, particularly if large acetabular bone deficiencies are present. Thus the best indication for conversion to a bipolar implant may be recurrent instability that cannot be managed by more standard methods, is associated with little bone deficiency (less risk of migration), and affects a patient with low activity demands (probably less risk of pain) (Fig. 7). Grigoris et al. (19) showed the efficacy of a tripolar technique (a fixed socket into which a bipolar device is placed). They found 8 of 8 hips with a history of multiple dislocations converted to a tripolar device were rendered stable. Tripolar devices theoretically carry less risk for migration and pain but might generate more particulate debris.

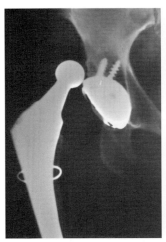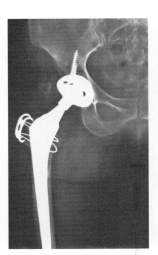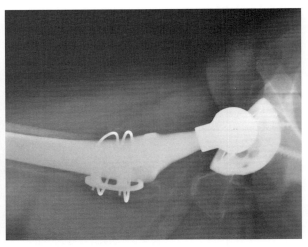

A,B   C

Figure 6. A: Recurrent posterior hip instability in patient with 22-mm head, poor soft-tissue tension (old partial trochanteric avulsion is visible). The socket is mildly underanteverted. **B,C:** Hip stability restore by means of changing the femoral head to 28-mm size and a longer neck to improve soft-tissue tension; advancing the trochanter to improve soft-tissue tension; and revising the socket to a more anteverted position.

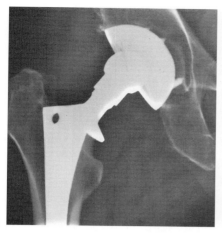 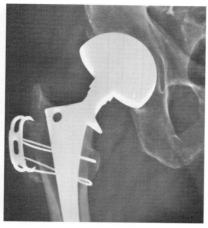

Figure 7. A: Elderly man with recurrent hip dislocation despite several previous surgical attempts to regain stability. The patient had good remaining acetabular bone. **B:** Conversion to bipolar hemiarthroplasty and trochanteric advancement restored hip stability.

Constrained acetabular implants vary greatly in design, but all provide some level of constraint to dislocation of the femoral head from the socket. The amount of constraint varies greatly from snap-fit sockets that provide little constraint to more rigid designs (Fig. 8). Higher levels of constraint make dislocation less likely but transmit greater forces to other interfaces of the implant in the event that the safe arc of hip motion is exceeded and impingement occurs. A further disadvantage of constrained implants is that once dislocation occurs, an operative procedure is usually needed to achieve reduction. Despite these disadvantages, constrained implants often can solve, with a high likelihood of pain relief, instability problems that cannot be solved by more traditional methods. They have become a very valuable tool to manage instability.

Obtaining data on the efficacy of implants is difficult as there are few reports on the use of these implants. Results with one implant design are not transferable to other designs, and the indications and circumstances under which a specific implant is used has a dramatic effect on the reported results. Many reports combine results of prophylactic use of these implants to prevent instability with use to manage established instability.

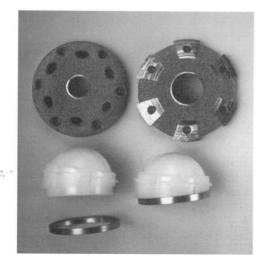

Figure 8. Modular constrained acetabular components with locking ring (S-ROM design, courtesy of Johnson & Johnson Orthopedics).

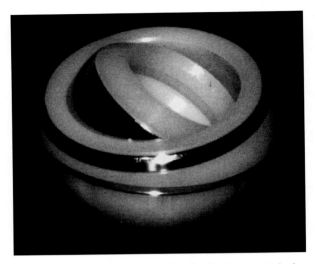

Figure 9. Modular constrained tripolar acetabular component. The construct shown snaps into a porous coated metal hemispheric shell. (Osteonics design, courtesy of Osteonics Corporation).

Lombardi et al. (31) and Anderson et al. (2) reported on the S-ROM implant, a device that has a constrained polyethylene liner with a locking ring fixed with screws to an uncemented porous socket. In the series of Lombardi et al. the device was used in 57 hips, 31 of which had a history of previous instability. By 24 to 37 months after implantation 5 hips had redislocated. Three of the dislocations occurred in the 31 hips with previous dislocation problems. Two of the uncemented sockets migrated and exhibited broken screws. In the series of Anderson et al. (2) 21 constrained sockets, 18 of which had been placed for recurrent dislocation, were followed 24 to 64 months. Six patients had dislocations after the operation. The modes of failure in this report illustrate the forces transferred to other interfaces in constrained implants. In 4 the liner disengaged from the metal shell, and in 2 the head disengaged from the liner when the metal reinforcing ring at the rim of the liner disengaged. None of the 19 uncemented sockets loosened at the prosthesis–bone interface.

A,B 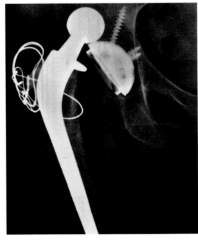 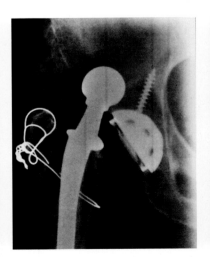 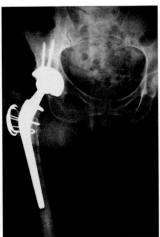 C

Figure 10. A,B: Elderly woman with recurrent anterior and posterior hip dislocations despite multiple surgical attempts to restore stability. **C:** Conversion to constrained socket and trochanteric advancement restored hip stability.

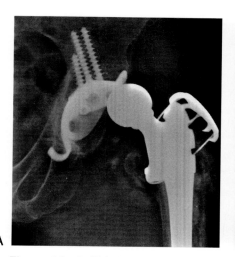
A
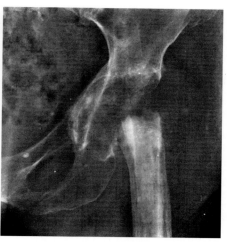
B

Figure 11. A: Elderly woman with recurrent hip instability and acetabular bone loss. Multiple operations to regain stability were unsuccessful. **B:** Definitive treatment with resection arthroplasty.

Goetz et al. (18) reported on the use of a constrained tripolar device (Osteonics, Allendale, N.J.). This device has a bipolar head locked into a polyethylene shell that itself locks into porous coated metal shell. In 56 consecutive revisions done for instability, the authors reported only 2 failures caused by instability, a success rate of 96%. Constrained devices of a tripolar design appear to have the theoretic advantage of allowing more hip range of motion before impingement and therefore may be especially effective in restoring hip stability (Fig. 9). The theoretic disadvantage of the design—multiple mobile metal on polyethylene bearing surfaces—is the potential for production of large amounts of particulate debris. Though osteolysis problems may be seen after longer follow-up periods, they were not identified at short time intervals.

Most experts agree that the typical indications for the use of constrained implants are limited to problems that cannot readily be solved by traditional methods. Patients include those with unsolvable soft-tissue problems (such as loss of abductors or presence of a proximal femoral replacement) and those for whom previous attempts to stabilize the arthroplasty without a constrained implant have failed (Fig. 10). Many experts also consider an older patient with an already osteointegrated modular socket in satisfactory position to be a good candidate for the procedure. When a compatible constrained socket is available, conversion to a constrained design may provide a quick and effective solution. As with all newer technology, the long-term results of using constrained implants are not available. Use of these devices should be tempered with the knowledge that a moderate number of problems have been reported after short follow-up periods, and more problems may arise with longer follow-up periods.

Resection Arthroplasty

Component removal is the final procedure available to patients with recurrent instability. Because resection arthroplasty provides less reliable pain relief and less satisfactory function than a well-functioning arthroplasty, this solution is usually reserved for patients whose instability cannot be resolved despite the measures described herein. Recalcitrant noncompliance or severe compromise of soft tissues or bone stock are the most common reasons that the many powerful methods available to manage hip instability ultimately fail, necessitating resection arthroplasty (Fig. 11).

CONCLUSIONS

A patient undergoing revision hip arthroplasty is at higher risk for hip instability than a patient undergoing primary hip arthroplasty. A thorough understanding of the factors that lead to dislocation allows effective management of the problem. Improved technology has made management of even the most difficult instability problems more likely to be a successful undertaking.

REFERENCES

1. Ackland MK, Bourne WB, Uhthoff HK. Anteversion of the acetabular cup: measurement of angle after total hip replacement. *J Bone Joint Surg Br* 1986;68:409–413.
2. Anderson MJ, Murray WR, Skinner HB. Constrained acetabular components. *J Arthroplasty* 1994;9:17–23.
3. Bradbury N, Milligan GF. Acetabular augmentation for dislocation of the prosthetic hip: a 3 (1–6) year follow-up of 16 patients. *Acta Orthop Scand* 1994;65:424–426.
4. Brien WW, Salvati EA, Wright TM, Burstein AH. Dislocation following THA: comparison of two acetabular component designs. *Orthopedics* 1993;16:869–872.
5. Cameron HU. Use of a constrained acetabular component in revision hip surgery. *Contemp Orthop* 1991;23:481–484.
6. Chandler RW, Dorr LD, Perry J. The functional cost of dislocation following total hip arthroplasty. *Clin Orthop* 1982;168:168–172.
7. Clayton ML, Thirupathi RG. Dislocation following total hip arthroplasty: management by special brace in selected patients. *Clin Orthop* 1983;177:154–159.
8. Cobb TK, Morrey BF, Ilstrup DM. The elevated-rim acetabular liner in total hip arthroplasty: relationship to postoperative dislocation. *J Bone Joint Surg Am* 1996;78:80–86.
9. Coventry MB. Late dislocations in patients with Charnley total hip arthroplasty. *J Bone Joint Surg Am* 1985;67:832–841.
10. Daly PJ, Morrey BF. Operative correction of an unstable total hip arthroplasty. *J Bone Joint Surg Am* 1992;74:1334–1343.
11. Dorr LD, Wolf AW, Chandler R, Conaty JP. Classification and treatment of dislocations of total hip arthroplasty. *Clin Orthop* 1983;173:151–158.
12. Eftekhar NS. Dislocation and instability complicating low friction arthroplasty of the hip joint. *Clin Orthop* 1976;121:120–125.
13. Ekelund A. Trochanteric osteotomy for recurrent dislocation of total hip arthroplasty. *J Arthroplasty* 1993;8:629–632.
14. Ekelund A, Rydell N, Nilsson OS. Total hip arthroplasty in patients 80 years of age and older. *Clin Orthop* 1992;281:101–106.
15. Fackler CD, Poss R. Dislocation in total hip arthroplasties. *Clin Orthop* 1980;151:169–178.
16. Fisher DA, Kiley K. Constrained acetabular cup disassembly. *J Arthroplasty* 1994;9:325–329.
17. Fraser GA, Wroblewski BM. Revision of the Charnley low-friction arthroplasty for recurrent or irreducible dislocation. *J Bone Joint Surg Br* 1982;63:552–555.
18. Goetz DD, Capello WN, Callaghan JJ, Brown TD, Johnston RC. Salvage of a recurrently dislocating total hip prosthesis with use of a constrained acetabular component: a retrospective analysis of fifty-six cases. *J Bone Joint Surg* 1998;80:502–509.
19. Grigoris P, Grecular MJ, Amstutz HC. Tripolar hip replacement for recurrent prosthetic dislocation. *Clin Orthop* 1994;304:148–155.
20. Grossmann P, Braun M, Becker W. Dislocation following total hip endoprosthesis: association with surgical approach and other factors. *Z Orthop Ihre Grenzgeb* 1994;132:521–526.
21. Hedlundh U, Ahnfelt L, Fredin H. Incidence of dislocation after hip arthroplasty: comparison of different registration methods in 408 cases. *Acta Orthop Scand* 1992;63:403–406.
22. Hedlundh U, Fredin H. Patient characteristics in dislocations after primary total hip arthroplasty: 60 patients compared with a control group. *Acta Orthop Scand* 1995;66:225–228.
23. Kao JT, Woolson ST. Piriformis tendon repair failure after total hip replacement. *Orthop Rev* 1992;21:171–174.
24. Kaplan SJ, Thomas WH, Poss R. Trochanteric advancement for recurrent dislocation after total hip arthroplasty. *J Arthroplasty* 1987;2:119–124.
25. Khan MAA, Brakenbury PH, Reynolds ISR. Dislocation following total hip replacement. *J Bone Joint Surg Br* 1981;63:214–218.
26. Krushell RJ, Burke DW, Harris WH. Elevated-rim acetabular components: effect on range of motion and stability in total hip arthroplasty. *J Arthroplasty* 1991;6:S53–S58.
27. Laughlin RT, Smith KL, Adair DM. Displacement of an uncemented acetabular component after dislocation of a total hip prosthesis: a case report. *J Arthroplasty* 1992;7:303–307.
28. Lefkowitz M. A new method for reduction of hip dislocations. *Orthop Rev* 1993;22:253–256.
29. Lewinnek GE, Lewis JL, Tarr R, Compere CL, Zimmerman JR. Dislocations after total hip replacement arthroplasties. *J Bone Joint Surg Am* 1978;60:217–220.
30. Lindberg HO, Carlsson AS, Gentz CF, Pettersson H. Recurrent and nonrecurrent dislocation following total hip arthroplasty. *Acta Orthop Scand* 1982;53:947–952.
31. Lombardi A, Mallory T, Krays T, Vaughn B. Preliminary report on the S-ROM™ constraining acetabular insert: a retrospective clinical experience. *Orthopedics* 1991;14:297–303.
32. Magilligan DJ. Calculation of the angle of anteversion by means of horizontal lateral roentgenography. *J Bone Joint Surg Am* 1956;38:1231–1246.
33. Mogensen B, Árnason H, Jónsson GT. Socket wall additional for dislocating total hip: report of two cases. *Acta Orthop Scand* 1986;57:373–374.
34. Morrey BF. Instability after total hip arthroplasty. *Orthop Clin North Am* 1992;N23:237–248.
35. Nicholas RM, Orr JF, Mollan RAB, Calderwood JW, Nixon JR, Watson P. Dislocation of total hip replacements: a comparative study of standard, long posterior wall and augmented acetabular components. *J Bone Joint Surg Br* 1990;72:418–422.

36. Olerud S, Karlström G. Recurrent dislocation after total hip replacement: treatment by fixing an additional sector to the acetabular component. *J Bone Joint Surg Br* 1985;467:402–405.

37. Pierchon F, Pasquier G, Cotten A, Fontaine C, Clarisse J, Buquennoy A. Causes of dislocation of total hip arthroplasty: CT study of component alignment. *J Bone Joint Surg Br* 1994;76:45–48.

38. Ries MD, Wiedel JD. Bipolar hip arthroplasty for recurrent dislocation after total hip arthroplasty: a report of three cases. *Clin Orthop* 1992;278:121–127.

39. Ritter MA. Dislocation and subluxation of the total hip replacement. *Clin Orthop* 1976;121:92–94.

40. Roberts JM, Fu FH, McClain EJ, Ferguson AB Jr. A comparison of the posterolateral and anterolateral approaches to total hip arthroplasty. *Clin Orthop* 1984;187:205–210.

41. Star MJ, Colwell CW Jr, Donaldson WF III, Walker RH. Dissociation of modular hip arthroplasty components after dislocation: a report of three cases at differing dissociation levels. *Clin Orthop* 1993;278:111–115.

42. Stewart H. The hip cast-brace for hip prosthesis instability. *Ann R Coll Surg Engl* 1983;65:404–406.

43. Turner RS. Postoperative total hip prosthetic femoral head dislocations: incidence, etiologic factors, and management. *Clin Orthop* 1994;301:196–204.

44. Vicar AJ, Coleman CR. A comparison of the anterolateral, transtrochanteric, and posterior surgical approaches in primary total hip arthroplasty. *Clin Orthop* 1984;188:152–159.

45. Watson P, Nixon JR, Mollan RAB. A prosthesis augmentation device for the prevention of recurrent hip dislocation: a preliminary report. *Clin Orthop* 1991;267:79–84.

46. Weber M, Berry DJ. Abductor avulsion after primary total hip arthroplasty: results of repair. *J Arthroplasty* 1997;12:202–206.

47. Williams JF, Gottesman MJ, Mallory TH. Dislocation after total hip arthroplasty: treatment with an above-knee hip spica cast. *Clin Orthop* 1982;171:53–58.

48. Woo RYG, Morrey BF. Dislocations after total hip arthroplasty. *J Bone Joint Surg Am* 1982;64:1295–1306.

49. Zelicoff SB, Scott RD. Conversion to bipolar arthroplasty for the treatment of recurrent total hip dislocations: a two to seven year follow-up study. Presented at the 59th Annual Meeting of the American Academy of Orthopaedic Surgeons, Washington, D.C.; 1992; Feb 20–25.

Revision Total Hip Arthroplasty,
edited by Marvin E. Steinberg and Jonathan P. Garino,
Lippincott Williams & Wilkins, Philadelphia © 1999.

33

Heterotopic Ossification

David G. Lewallen

Heterotopic ossification is a commonly observed radiographic finding associated with total hip arthroplasty, and it occurs among 20% to 90% of patients who have undergone arthroplasty (11,17,37). Less than 10% of patients have substantial amounts of bone formation, and not all of those so affected experience marked symptoms. However, heterotopic ossification can cause disability due to restriction of joint motion or ankylosis and pain that for a small subgroup of patients results in reoperation.

The pathogenesis of heterotopic ossification associated with hip arthroplasty is incompletely understood. As early as 1977 it was postulated that short-range diffusion of bone inductive substances in the region of the hip wound was responsible for bone formation by mesenchymal cells lines (24). Over the past two decades the complex cascade of cellular events responsible for new bone formation has been studied intensively. Transforming growth factors isolated from bone have been identified that exhibit chondrogenic and osteogenic affects (43,45,46). Although bone morphogenic protein, as originally described by Urist (43), has been demonstrated to consist of a collection of polypeptide substances, including at least seven different bone morphogenic proteins, it is clear that these growth factors have a role in mediating bone formation and likely participate in both normal and pathologic bone-formation processes. Transformation of muscle flaps into mature cancellous bone has been accomplished experimentally as a result of exposure to bone morpholgic protein and demineralized bone matrix providing an experimental model of heterotopic bone formation from muscle, suggesting the possibility that the substances play a role in clinical forms of this disorder (26). Although it seems reasonable to assume that the family of peptides referred to as bone morphogenic protein participate in a central way

D. G. Lewallen: Mayo Graduate School of Medicine, Mayo Clinic and Mayo Foundation, Rochester, Minnesota 55905.

in the induction of heterotopic ossification, the details of the underlying cellular events and interaction of factors that stimulate and inhibit this process remain incompletely understood.

CLINICAL PRESENTATION

Heterotopic ossification is usually first diagnosed with radiographs. Subsequent symptoms vary from none at all to disabling pain and marked limitation of motion of the hip. Heterotopic ossification becomes radiographically visible as a haze of new bone formation within the soft tissues beginning 3 to 6 weeks after arthroplasty. The extent of involvement may not be completely clear before 3 months of maturation, and an increase in density may be seen radiographically for as long as 1 year post arthroplasty (Fig. 1). Intense activity is observed on a bone scan in areas of new bone formation in the months after arthroplasty with a gradual decline in uptake over many months. These findings suggest persistent, elevated bone blood flow and increased new bone formation for as long as 1 year or more after initiation of the process by the surgical insult.

Most patients with evidence of heterotopic ossification on radiographs have limited amounts of bone formation. The bone consists of small foci of calcification within the soft tissues that do not produce any clinically significant symptoms. More extensive bone formation has the potential to result in restricted range of motion, pain, or both with variability in the degree of effect produced by similar amounts of ossification on radiographs. Some patients' symptoms are of sufficient severity to require excision of the heterotopic bone in an effort to improve motion or reduce the pain associated with the process.

Although questions have been raised about the effect of heterotopic ossification on component loosening rates, no clear interrelation has been documented. Isolated cases of persons with recurrent dislocation after arthroplasty associated with heterotopic ossification and the observation of apparent edge impingement of heterotopic bone against the rim of the acetabular component raise the possibility that this process may predispose patients to instability after total hip arthroplasty (Fig. 2).

A,B 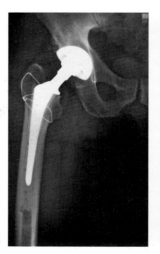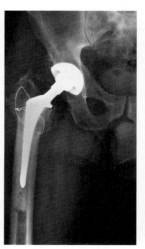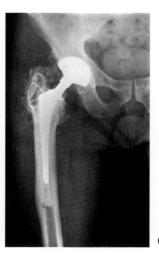 C

Figure 1. A 50-year-old man after hybrid total hip arthroplasty with an uncemented cup and cemented stem. **A:** Initial postoperative radiographic appearance. **B:** Same patient 8 weeks postoperatively with fluffy calcification caused by heterotopic ossification. **C:** Radiograph 1 year postoperatively shows mature heterotopic bone with distinct margins. The patient had mild occasional pain and restricted motion with flexion to 85 degrees and occasionally uses antiinflammatory drugs because of these symptoms.

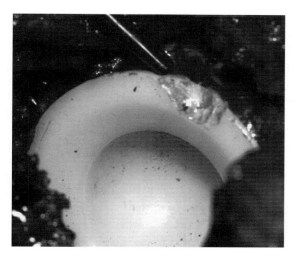

Figure 2. Intraoperative photograph of acetabular component rim damage caused by edge impingement of heterotopic bone excised from area immediately adjacent to superior rim of cup.

CLASSIFICATION

Brooker et al. (8) described four classes of heterotopic ossification. Class I represents small isolated flecks of bone visible radiographically. Class II consists of bone spurs with a gap between the areas of at least 1 cm or more. Class III consists of near complete bridging with a gap between the areas of ossification measuring less than 1 cm. Class IV is apparent ankylosis (8). Morrey et al. (32) suggested an alternative system with four grades similar to those provided by Brooker et al. but with percentage area between the trochanter and pelvis used to discriminate between grade II (less than 50% bridging) and grade III (greater than 50% bridging).

RISK FACTORS FOR HETEROTOPIC OSSIFICATION

A number of potential risk factors have been identified as associated with heterotopic ossification after total hip arthroplasty. Previous heterotopic bone formation in the same patient whether involving the opposite hip or the same hip after prior arthroplasty carries a definite increased risk for heterotopic ossification. After any proposed additional surgical intervention in the hip represents a clear-cut indication for clinical prophylaxis. If a patient has formed heterotopic bone after hip arthroplasty the incidence of heterotopic bone formation after contralateral total hip arthroplasty is 60% to 100% (14,29). The amount or severity of heterotopic bone formation tends to mirror that observed after the first hip replacement (36). Hypertrophic osteoarthritic changes also have been associated with an increased incidence of heterotopic bone formation after hip arthroplasty (20). Diffuse idiopathic skeletal hyperostosis (DISH syndrome) and spinal hyperostosis (Forestier's disease) have been associated with increased risk for postoperative heterotopic ossification. Fahrer et al. (16) associated the DISH syndrome with a twofold increase in heterotopic ossification. However, other investigators did not substantiate increased risk among this patient population (9). It is the more severe grades of heterotopic bone formation that achieve clinical significance. Among patients with spinal hyperostosis who did not receive prophylaxis, one study showed an incidence of 38% to 50% grade III to IV heterotopic bone formation (5).

Active ankylosing spondylitis has been cited as a risk factor for heterotopic ossification. Attempts have been made to correlate disease activity with relative risk for development of this problem after arthroplasty. However, in a study correlating erythrocyte sedimentation rate and incidence or extent of heterotopic ossification among a group of arthroplasty patients with ankylosing spondylitis, Sundaram and Murphy (40) did not find a correlation between this measure of disease activity and incidence of bone formation (40). In one study 60% of patients with ankhylosing spondylitis were observed to form heterotopic bone after arthroplasty. The risk for grade III or IV heterotopic bone formation reached 39% among patients not receiving any form of prophylaxis (4). In contrast, clinically important heterotopic ossification was observed among only 11% of patients with ankylosing spondylitis undergoing total hip arthroplasty in another series (27).

Men have roughly a twofold greater prevalence of heterotopic bone formation than women (32,36). This has been postulated to be caused by the increased bulk of the abductor musculature in men and perhaps increased soft-tissue trauma related to surgical exposure. However, the exact explanation for this observation remains uncertain.

Spinal or head injuries produce a much increased risk for heterotopic ossification around the hip, both after arthroplasty or in some cases spontaneously. These injuries are associated with some of the most severe instances of heterotopic ossification observed clinically. It would be most unusual for an arthroplasty candidate to have an associated serious head or spine injury, though it is possible this clinical situation could arise. An example might be a patient who as part of multiple trauma has a fracture that splits the head of the femur and necessitates arthroplasty for initial reconstruction. Clinical scenarios of this sort certainly produce high risk for heterotopic bone formation and seem to justify aggressive efforts at prophylaxis.

Mode of implant fixation appears to influence the prevalence of heterotopic bone formation. In one series the prevalence and severity of heterotopic bone formation after arthroplasty among a group of patients with osteoarthritis was greater among those receiving an uncemented femoral component than among those for whom the stems were implanted with cement (30).

Additional potential risk factors that have been implicated but are less definitely established in the literature as associated with heterotopic ossification after arthroplasty include limited hip motion before arthroplasty, trochanteric osteotomy, postoperative hematoma around the hip, and recent fracture, including intraoperative fractures (15,32). It is also possible that at the time of bone grafting, either on the socket side or the stem side, excessive spillage of bone-graft material into the soft tissues might exert an adverse effect with regard to heterotopic bone formation. Thus it seems reasonable to avoid contamination of the surrounding soft tissues by bone reamings or bone graft during the course of the surgical procedure.

PREVENTION OF HETEROTOPIC BONE FORMATION

Prevention of complications is always preferred to management of the residuals of that same complication. There has been a great deal of interest in preventive measures for patients considered at risk for heterotopic ossification. Prophylactic efforts can be grouped into three categories: surgical technique, medication, and radiation treatment.

Surgical Technique

Gentle handling of soft tissues and avoidance of excessive damage to the muscle envelope around the hip are worthwhile. Extent of surgical exposure and degree of damage to the musculature around the hip do seem to correlate with the prevalence of new bone formation after a hip operation (1,7,25). Trochanteric osteotomy has been reported as increasing the risk for development of heterotopic bone compared with the posterior approach though this effect may not be as large as has been previously claimed (15,32). Use of wound drainage has become somewhat controversial, though discussion regarding the pros and cons of use of wound drains have tended to center on wound healing and blood loss concerns. Formation of heterotopic bone around the hip has been observed in instances in which excessive wound hematoma formation has been observed clinically. Thus use of a drain would seem reasonable in the care of patients deemed to be at increased risk for heterotopic bone formation if such drains are not used routinely to treat all patients.

Medication

Among the initial medications used in an effort to suppress heterotopic bone formation after hip arthroplasty were the diphosphonates. Because diphosphonates inhibit growth of hydroxyapatite crystals, it was believed that they might be of benefit in preventing ectopic bone formation after hip surgery. Although the medications do inhibit hydroxyapatite crystal growth, their effect is only to delay the appearance of new bone on radiographs; osteoid formation continues uninhibited. Once the medication was stopped the osteoid present calcified, explaining why the drug has been ineffective clinically in preventing symptomatic heterotopic ossification after total hip arthroplasty (41). After a comprehensive review Thomas and Amstutz (41) recommended that diphosphonates no longer be used for prophylaxis against heterotopic bone formation.

Nonsteroidal antiinflammatory drugs (NSAIDs) have proved effective in preventing heterotopic ossification. Numerous authors have demonstrated the efficacy of indomethacin in this regard (10,28,31,35,38,39,42). Indomethacin has been studied more extensively than other NSAIDs for this indication. A prospective doubled-blinded, randomized study demonstrated 0% grade III or IV heterotopic bone formation among treated patients compared with an 18% incidence among patients who took a placebo. The same investigators documented prevention of any heterotopic ossification among 85% of those treated, whereas only 25% of the placebo group were free of any ectopic bone formation (38). Shorter and shorter courses of indomethacin treatment have been shown to be effective, from 6 weeks initially down to a 2-week course of therapy (10,31,35,38,39,42). Demonstration that shorter and shorter treatment courses are effective is helpful in this clinical setting. As many as 37% of patients have gastrointestinal side effects severe enough to require discontinuation of treatment when indomethacin is used for 6 weeks (10). Other NSAIDs investigated and found to be effective in reducing the prevalence and severity of heterotopic ossification after hip arthroplasty include aspirin, ibuprofen, naproxen, and diclofenac (18,19,28,35,39,43).

One potential concern related to use of NSAIDs for prevention of heterotopic ossification is the documented effect of this class of medication on the fracture repair process (2). Impairment of fracture healing by NSAIDs has lead some surgeons to avoid use of these medications to treat patients with extensive bone grafts, trochanteric osteotomy, periprosthetic fractures when union is being attempted, or in some instances porous ingrowth components. These surgeons are concerned about bone formation and attachment to the uncemented implant. Documentation of an adverse effect of these medications in these specific clinical settings is lacking.

Low-Dose Radiation Therapy

Since the initial report by Coventry and Scanlon (13) on the beneficial effects of low-dose irradiation in preventing recurrence of heterotopic bone after excision, a number of studies have investigated the issue of effective dosage for prevention of heterotopic bone formation in the postoperative setting. The initial regimen recommended by Coventry and Scanlon was 2000 rad in ten fractions. Grade III or IV heterotopic ossification was prevented among all 48 hips so treated. Treatment of a patient with ten fractionated doses of radiation is logistically difficult in an era of increasingly short hospital stays. One thousand rad given in five fractions has been shown to be as effective as 2,000 rad in 10 fractions (3). A single dose of 800 centigray (or rad) was shown to be as effective as 1,000 centigray in five fractions (34). Studies by Healy et al. (21) of 700 vs. 500 centigray on postoperative day 1 and by Hedley et al. (22) on the efficacy of 600 centigray given as a single dose up to postoperative day 3 suggest that the threshold for effectiveness in radiation treatment is somewhere around this 600 to 700 centigray figure.

Preoperative radiation treatment has been shown to limit formation of heterotopic bone just as effectively as postoperative treatment (33). Pelligrini et al. (33) conducted a prospective, randomized study of 86 hips. One group was treated 4 hours before with a single 800-centigray dose, and the other group was treated with a similar radiation dose

72 hours after arthroplasty. There was no difference in prevalence of heterotopic ossification and no grade III or IV heterotopic bone in any of the patients treated preoperatively (33). The implications of this study are that heterotopic ossification arises from osteoprogenator cells derived locally rather than from a circulating cell population transported to the surgical site.

The disadvantage of radiation treatment relates to the possible adverse effect of therapy on bone attachment to uncemented implants or healing of areas of bone grafting or trochanteric osteotomy. These concerns have led to the routine use of custom lead shields to prevent irradiation of bone-ingrowth regions on components or other areas of concern with regard to bone healing (Fig. 3). This allows irradiation of only the soft tissues adjacent to the arthroplasty (6,23).

Choice of Prophylactic Method

Although both low-dose radiation treatment and use of NSAIDs have been shown to be effective in preventing heterotopic ossification, the clinical decision about which modality to use can be difficult. Certain clinical situations, however, seem to lend themselves to one form of treatment versus the other. Because of concerns regarding the systemic effects on bone healing of indomethacin or other NSAIDs, it has been my practice to favor radiation treatment in this clinical setting. Custom-designed lead shields are used to block any ingrowth areas of the components or bone grafts (Fig. 4). If the patient is a woman of childbearing age, however, the relative risk shifts to favor use of NSAIDs despite the presence of grafts or uncemented implants. Satisfactory results in the short term have been reported among patients receiving porous ingrowth components and using indomethacin (31). Among patients undergoing cemented arthroplasty indomethacin or an alternative NSAID would seem a reasonable choice, particularly because a 2- or 3-week course of treatment is effective

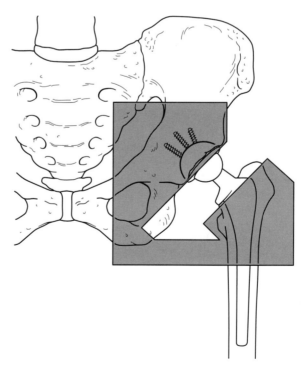

Figure 3. Diagram of custom lead shield to protect porous coated portions of uncemented implants during low-dose radiation therapy to prevent heterotopic bone formation.

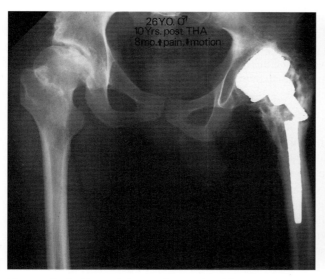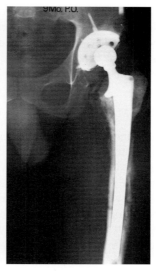

Figure 4. A: Prerevision radiograph with extensive heterotopic bone formation and fractured femoral stem. **B:** Radiograph 9 months after revision and radiation therapy to prevent recurrent heterotopic ossification. Uncemented implants, femoral cortical window, and bone graft were shielded.

in simplifying management with regard to gastrointestinal effects. However, routine use of warfarin sodium or low-molecular-weight heparin for prophylaxis against deep venous thrombosis does raise concerns about concomitant use of NSAIDs, particularly by frail, elderly patients with multiple medical problems. Bleeding complications can be catastrophic for these patients. Thus in some clinical situations, such as active peptic ulcer disease, radiation therapy might be preferable. In the end the choice of prophylactic modality must rest with the clinician. It hinges on the individual patient's circumstances, associated medical problems, and relative risk for heterotopic ossification. For patients deemed to be at extremely high risk for heterotopic bone formation, NSAIDs and low-dose radiation have been combined in some instances.

SURGICAL EXCISION OF HETEROTOPIC OSSIFICATION

Surgical excision of grade III or IV heterotopic ossification may be indicated in the care of some patients when the process has produced considerable pain and restriction of motion. However, the most common clinical setting in which heterotopic bone is excised is in revision of an arthroplasty for other reasons when heterotopic bone also is present. Isolated excision of heterotopic ossification can be attempted when the amount of pain present and limitations imposed by the pain and restricted motion make surgery a worthwhile undertaking in the eyes of the patient. Some form of postoperative prophylaxis should be used to treat all such patients to prevent reformation of heterotopic bone around the hip. Surgical excision should be delayed until the bone that has formed around the hip has matured. This process may take as long as 1 year and can be assessed by the use of bone scanning, particularly if excision is entertained earlier than 1 year after arthroplasty. Although the success of excision of heterotopic bone with postoperative prophylaxis historically has been judged radiographically, it is not the radiographic findings but pain and limited motion that drive patients to surgery. Thus it is by these criteria that success should be judged. Cobb et al. (12) reviewed 53 cases of excision of isolated heterotopic ossification a mean of 3.5 years after the operation and found that range of motion increased significantly by a mean of 33 degrees of flexion. However, pain relief was unpredictable even when reformation of heterotopic bone was effectively prevented by means of prophylaxis with either radiation therapy or NSAIDs, both of which were used separately in the series in question (12). The study suggested that patients should be cautioned that isolated excision of heterotopic bone after total hip arthroplasty may or may not produce appreciable relief of pain, even when radiographs show that reformation of bone has been prevented. The procedure can be depended on, however, to improve range of motion. This study also drives home the importance of prevention of this complication after hip arthroplasty among patients recognized to be at increased risk.

SUMMARY

Heterotopic ossification commonly occurs after total hip arthroplasty. In most instances it is limited in amount and does not produce important clinical symptoms. Among the subgroup of patients who have larger amounts of heterotopic bone formation, the process may be symptomatic. In some cases it may even require repeat surgical intervention to try to relieve pain and limited range of motion. Clinical subgroups recognized to be at risk for heterotopic ossification should be treated with prophylaxis. Low-dose radiation or NSAIDs both have been shown to be effective. The choice between these two modalities rests with the surgeon. It is based on patient status, associated medical problems, necessity for bone grafting, osteotomies or repair of fracture lines, and availability of radiation therapy support, including fabrication of custom shielding for areas of critical bone healing. Use of NSAIDs, particularly indomethacin, is a reasonable and acceptable alternative to radiation treatment, is more cost effective, and may be preferred in cemented arthroplasties or in many routine uncemented arthroplasties in which large bone grafts, osteotomies, or fracture lines are not a concern. Surgical excision of heterotopic bone when highly symptomatic should not be performed before 6 to 12 months after arthroplasty and then only once it is established that the process has reached full maturity. Waiting reduces the risk for reformation of heterotopic bone after excision. Bone scanning is a useful adjunct in assessing the maturity of ossification and can help to guide timing of excision, particularly if this procedure is entertained earlier than 1 year after arthroplasty. After excision of heterotopic bone, all patients should receive some form of prophylaxis with the expectation that reformation of heterotopic bone can be successfully prevented, range of motion improved, and pain improved for some but not all patients.

REFERENCES

1. Ahrengart L. Periarticular heterotopic ossification after total hip arthroplasty: risk factors and consequences. *Clin Orthop* 1991;263:49–58.
2. Allen HL, Wase A, Bear WT. Indomethacin and aspirin: effect of nonsteroidal anti-inflammatory agents on the rate of fracture repair in the rat. *Acta Orthop Scand* 1980;51:595–600.
3. Ayers DC, Evants CM, Parkinson JR. Prevention of heterotopic ossification in high-risk patients by low-dose radiation therapy after total hip arthroplasty. *J Bone Joint Surg Am* 1986;68:1423–1430.
4. Bisla RS, Ranawat CS, Inglis AE. Total hip replacement in patients with ankylosing spondylitis with involvement of the hip. *J Bone Joint Surg Am* 1987;58:233–238.
5. Blasingame JP, Resnick D, Coults RD, Danzig LA. Extensive spinal osteophytosis as a risk factor for heterotopic bone formation after total hip arthroplasty. *Clin Orthop* 1981;161:191–197.
6. Blount LH, Thomas BJ, Tran L, Selch MT, Sylvester JE, Parker RG. Postoperative irradiation for the prevention of heterotopic bone: analysis of different dose schedules and shielding considerations. *Int J Radiat Oncol Biol Phys* 1990;19:577–581.
7. Bosse M, Poka A, Reinhardt C, Elwanger F, Slosson R, McDevit E. Heterotopic ossification as a complication of acetabular fracture. *J Bone Joint Surg Am* 1988;70:1231–1237.
8. Brooker AF, Bowerman JW, Robinson RA, Riley LH. Ectopic ossification following total hip arthroplasty: incidence and method of classification. *J Bone Joint Surg Am* 1973;55:1629–1632.
9. Bunderick JJ, Cook DE, Resnik CS. Heterotopic bone formation in patients with DISH following total hip replacement. *Radiology* 1985;155:595–597.
10. Cella JP, Salvati EA, Sculco TP. Indomethacin for the prevention of heterotopic ossification following total hip arthroplasty: effectiveness, contraindications, and adverse effects. *J Arthroplasty* 1988;3:229.
11. Charnley J. Long-term results of low friction arthroplasty of the hip performed as a primary intervention. *J Bone Joint Surg Br* 1972;54:61–76.
12. Cobb TK, Berry DJ, Morrey BF, Wallrichs SL, Ilstrup MS. Functional outcome of excision of heterotopic ossification after total hip arthroplasty. Presented at the 61st Annual Meeting of the American Academy of Orthopaedic Surgeons; 1994 Feb 2–Mar 1; New Orleans.
13. Coventry MB, Scanlon PW. The use of irradiation to discourage ectopic bone: a nine year study in surgery about the hip. *J Bone Joint Surg Am* 1981;63:201–208.
14. DeLee J, Ferrari A, Charnley J. Ectopic bone formation following low friction arthroplasty of the hip. *Clin Orthop* 1976;121:53–59.

15. Errico TJ, Fetto JF, Waugh TR. Heterotopic ossification: incidence and relation to trochanteric osteotomy in 100 total hip arthroplasties. *Clin Orthop* 1984;190:138–141.

16. Fahrer H, Koch P, Ballmer P, Enzler P, Gerber N. Ectopic ossification following total hip arthroplasty: is diffuse idiopathic skeletal hyperostosis a risk factor? *Br J Rheumatol* 1988;27:187–190.

17. Frassica FJ, Frassica DA, Coventry MB. Ectopic bone. In: Morrey BF, ed. *Joint Replacement Arthroplasty.* New York: Churchill Livingstone, 1991:867–876.

18. Freiberg AA, Cantor R, Freiberg RA. The use of aspirin to prevent heterotopic ossification after total hip arthroplasty: a preliminary report. *Clin Orthop* 1991;267:93–96.

19. Gebuhr P, Soelberg M, Orsnes T, Wilbek H. Naproxen prevention of heterotopic ossification after hip arthroplasty: a prospective control study of 55 patients. *Acta Orthop Scand* 1991;62:226–229.

20. Goel A, Sharp DJ. Heterotopic bone formation after hip replacement: the influence of the type of osteoarthritis. *J Bone Joint Surg Br* 1991;73:255–257.

21. Healy WL, Lo TC, Covall DJ, Pfeifer BA, Wasilewski SA. Single-dose radiation therapy for prevention of heterotopic ossification after total hip arthroplasty. *J Arthroplasty* 1990;5:369–374.

22. Hedley AK, Mead LP, Hendren DH. The prevention of heterotopic bone formation following total hip arthroplasty using 600 rad in a single dose. *J Arthroplasty* 1989;4:319–325.

23. Jasty M, Schutzer S, Tepzer J, Willet C, Stracher MA, Harris WH. Radiation-blocking shields to localize periarticular radiation precisely for prevention of heterotopic bone formation around uncemented total hip arthroplasties. *Clin Orthop* 1990;257:138–145.

24. Jowsey J, Coventry MB, Robins PR. Heterotopic ossification: theoretical consideration, possible etiologic factors, and a clinical review of total hip arthroplasty patients exhibiting this phenomenon. In: *The hip: proceedings of the Fifth Open Scientific Meeting of the Hip Society, 1977.* St. Louis: Mosby, 1977:210–221.

25. Kaempffe FA, Bone LB, Border JR. Open reduction, internal fixation of acetabular fractures: heterotopic ossification and other complications of treatment. *J Orthop Trauma* 1991;5:439–445.

26. Khouri RK, Koudsi B, Reddi H. Tissue transformation into bone in vivo: a potential practical application. *JAMA* 1991;266:1953–1955.

27. Kilgus DJ, Namba RS, Gorek JE, Cracchiolo A III, Amstutz H. Total hip replacement for patients who have ankylosing spondylitis. *J Bone Joint Surg Am* 1990;72:834–839.

28. Kjaersgaard-Andersen P, Ritter MA. Short-term treatment with nonsteroidal anti-inflammatory medications to prevent heterotopic bone formation after total hip arthroplasty: a preliminary report. *Clin Orthop* 1992;279:157–162.

29. Kromann-Andersen C, Sorenson TS, Hougaard K, et al. Ectopic bone formation following Charnley hip arthroplasty. *Acta Orthop Scand* 1980;61:633–638.

30. Maloney WJ, Krushell RJ, Jasty M, Harris WH. Incidence of heterotopic ossification after total hip replacement: effect of the type of fixation of the femoral component. *J Bone Joint Surg Am* 1991;73:191–193.

31. McMahon JS, Waddell JP, Morton J. Effect of short-course indomethacin on heterotopic bone formation after uncemented total hip arthroplasty. *J Arthroplasty* 1991;6:259–264.

32. Morrey BF, Adams RA, Cabanela ME. Comparison of heterotopic bone after anterolateral, transtrochanteric and posterior approaches for total hip arthroplasty. *Clin Orthop* 1984;188:160–167.

33. Pellegrini VD, Gregoritch SJ. Preoperative irradiation for prevention of heterotopic ossification following total hip arthroplasty. *J Bone Joint Surg Am* 1996;78:770–781.

34. Pellegrini VD, Konski AA, Gastel JA, Rubin P, Evarts CM. Prevention of heterotopic ossification with irradiation after total hip arthroplasty. *J Bone Joint Surg Am* 1992;74:186–200.

35. Ritter MA, Gioe TJ. The effect of indomethacin on para-articular ectopic ossification following total hip arthroplasty. *Clin Orthop* 1982;167:113.

36. Ritter MA, Vaughan RB. Ectopic ossification after total hip arthroplasty: predisposing factors, frequency and effect on results. *J Bone Joint Surg Am* 1977;59:345.

37. Rosendahl S, Christoffersen JK, Norgaard M. Para-articular ossification following hip replacement. *Acta Orthop Scand* 1977;48:400–404.

38. Schmidt P, Kjaersgaard-Andersen P, Pedersen NW, Kristensen SS, Pedersen P, Nielsen JB. The use of indomethacin to prevent the formation of heterotopic bone after total hip arthroplasty: a randomized, double-blinded clinical trial. *J Bone Joint Surg Am* 1988;70:834–838.

39. Sodemann B, Persson PE, Nilsson OS. Prevention of periarticular heterotopic ossification following total hip arthroplasty: clinical experience with indomethacin and ibuprofen. *Archives Orthop Trauma Surg* 1988; 107:329–333.

40. Sundaram NA, Murphy JC. Heterotopic bone formation following total hip arthroplasty in ankylosing spondylitis. *Clin Orthop* 1986;207:223–226.

41. Thomas BJ, Amstutz HC. Results of the administration of diphosphonate for the prevention of heterotopic ossification after total hip arthroplasty. *J Bone Joint Surg Am* 1985;67:400–403.

42. Tozun R, Pinar H, Yesiller E, Hamzaoglu A. Indomethacin for prevention of heterotopic ossification after total hip arthroplasty. *J Arthroplasty* 1992;71:57–61.

43. Urist MR. Bone: formation by autoinduction. *Science* 1965;150:893–899.

44. Walstrom O, Risto O, Djerf K, Hammerby S. Heterotopic bone formation prevented by diclofenac. *Acta Orthop Scand* 1991;62:419–421.

45. Wozney JM, Rosen V, Byrne M, et al. Growth factors influencing bone development. *J Cell Sci Suppl* 1990;13:149–156.

46. Wozney JM, Rosen V, Celeste AJ, et al. Novel regulators of bone formation: molecular clones and activities. *Science* 1988;242:1528–1534.

Revision Total Hip Arthroplasty,
edited by Marvin E. Steinberg and Jonathan P. Garino,
Lippincott Williams & Wilkins, Philadelphia © 1999.

34

Fractures of the Femur

Donald S. Garbuz, Bassam A. Masri, and Clive P. Duncan

Fracture of the femur during or after hip arthroplasty is a serious complication that can be difficult to treat. In recent years there has been an increased frequency of this serious complication. This increase is caused in part by the increased number of hip arthroplasties being done, especially revision procedures, in which loss of bone stock can lead to periprosthetic fracture (1).

The incidence of periprosthetic fractures depends on whether the fracture occurs intraoperatively or postoperatively, whether the femoral implant was cemented or cementless, and whether the arthroplasty was the index operation or a revision arthroplasty. The rate of intraoperative fractures with primary cemented stems has been reported to be less than 1% (12,21) and between 3% and 20% with primary uncemented stems (7,20,23). In revision arthroplasty there is an increased rate of intraoperative fracture with both cemented and cementless revisions. Rates vary depending on the series. Cemented revisions have a rate of intraoperative fracture of 3% to 6.3% (4,11), whereas the rate for revisions with cementless implants ranges between 17.6% and 46% (7).

Postoperative fractures can occur days to years after hip arthroplasty. Most series in the literature combine cases of primary and revision arthroplasty making it difficult to study selectively the incidence of postoperative fractures between revision and primary operations. In the Mayo clinic series (14) the overall incidence of fracture following primary hip arthroplasty was 0.6%. Fractures following revision arthroplasty were seen in 2.4% of all cases. The increased incidence in revision surgery was seen with both cemented and cementless implants. The true incidence of this complication for an

D. S. Garbuz and B. A. Masri: Division of Reconstructive Orthopaedics, Department of Orthopaedics, University of British Columbia, Vancouver Hospital and Health Sciences Center, Vancouver, British Columbia, Canada V5Z 4E3.

C. P. Duncan: Department of Orthopaedics, University of British Columbia, Vancouver Hospital and Health Sciences Center, Vancouver, British Columbia, Canada V5Z 4E3.

individual hip arthroplasty is unknown, because in all series the data were examined in a retrospective manner. Löwenhielm et al. (15) estimated an accumulated risk of 25.3 fractures per 1,000 hip replacements over 15 years, whereas Beals and Tower (1) estimated that the incidence over the lifetime of a prosthesis is less than 1%.

As the frequency of revision operations increases, the number of intraoperative and postoperative periprosthetic fractures will continue to rise. Because management of these fractures often is complex, prevention is becoming increasingly important. Intimate knowledge of the risk factors, causation, and outcome are needed to prevent or manage these injuries.

ETIOLOGIC FACTORS AND PREVENTION

To prevent fractures it is important to know the factors that increase the risk for this complication. Factors that predispose to fracture can be classified in three broad categories: factors related to the patient, to the surgical technique, and to the specific implant being used. Although these three groups help in understanding the cause of a periprosthetic fracture, for any patient multiple factors may be present. Clearly in any case the more risk factors present the higher is the incidence of fracture. The risk factors for intraoperative and postoperative fracture also differ somewhat.

Intraoperative Fractures

Patient factors usually are related to the quality and mechanical strength of the host femur. Revision surgery carries an increased risk for fracture (14). Osteolysis is probably the single most important factor that increases intraoperative fracture risk in revision surgery. Decreased bone strength due to osteoporosis or rheumatoid arthritis (12) also puts the femur at risk. Deformities of the proximal femur, as seen among patients with developmental dysplasia of the hip and previous operations on the proximal femur other than arthroplasty (21), have been associated with increased risk for intraoperative fracture. It is important to recognize these factors preoperatively, because careful preoperative planning and attention to operative technique help prevent intraoperative fracture of the femur at risk.

Intraoperative fractures occur at specific times during the procedure, and this time varies between the primary and the revision operations. During surgical exposure excessive torque at the time of dislocation or during delivery of the proximal femur out of the wound may result in an intraoperative fracture if the femur has been previously weakened. This is especially true in the revision situation, in which the femur can be weakened focally by osteolysis or diffusely by osteopenia. To avoid this complication, any hip that has a plate on the femur should be dislocated before plate removal. When the femur is at high risk for fracture during exposure, trochanteric osteotomy and proximal femur skeletonization should be considered before dislocation and delivery of the femur from the wound.

After exposure has been completed, fracture can occur during implant removal or cement removal in revision procedures. To prevent fracture during cement removal and reaming, adequate visualization of the femoral canal is required. Use of an extended trochanteric osteotomy (26) facilitates cement removal and reaming. Other techniques for cement removal include use of cortical windows, but these always should be protected with a femoral stem that bypasses the window by at least two cortical diameters or with a cortical onlay allograft.

Intraoperative fractures commonly occur during canal preparation and stem insertion in both primary and revision operations. In primary hip arthroplasty, intraoperative fracture occurs most often with cementless implants. In the preparation stage fracture can occur during reaming or broaching. Eccentric reaming in particular may weaken the femur and predispose it to fracture during reduction or dislocation of trial components (20). Insertion of the final prosthesis or broaching may cause a fracture owing to the wedging effect proximally as the surgeon tries to achieve a press fit (12,20). Underreaming distally or insertion of a straight stem into a normal femoral bow can lead to fracture during final insertion of the prosthesis. To reduce the incidence of intraoperative fracture in cementless arthroplasty, careful preoperative templating to select an appropriately sized implant is recommended (7,20). It is important not to undersize the broach, which can lead to a proximal fracture caused by wedging of the final prosthesis. Care has to be taken to avoid varus reaming, particularly if the greater trochanter overhangs the medullary canal. If there is doubt about the direction of reaming, an intraoperative radiograph should be obtained to ensure adequate centering of the reamer in the canal. Last, during final insertion of the prosthesis, if significant resistance is met, the surgeon should check to be certain the levels of the rasp and prosthesis are the same. If one attempts to insert the final prosthesis farther than the rasp, a fracture can occur (11).

If the surgeon believes that the femur is at risk for fracture, cerclage wire can be used as prophylaxis before broaching or reaming. This has been shown to increase the force required to fracture the proximal femur (8). Cerclage fixation also has been shown to be effective in preventing crack propagation (9). This is very useful clinically because a small crack caused by a femoral broach can be prevented from propagating by use of proximal cerclage wires before insertion of the definitive femoral component. Preventing propagation of this crack reduces the chance of instability of the implant interface.

In revision surgery, to decrease the incidence of fracture during stem insertion, implant design is important. The use of long stems with smaller proximal cross sections and bowed stems that match the patient's femoral bow helps decrease the fracture rate.

Prevention of intraoperative fracture always should be planned. The surgeon should pay close attention to patient factors that put the femur at risk for fracture during the surgical procedure. Preoperative planning should include clear documentation of the direction of the old stem and any focal areas of osteolysis. Great care should be taken during exposure in operations on patients at high risk. During cement removal, the surgeon should point all instruments away from these weak areas to avoid perforation or fracture. Moreover, power instruments for cement removal should be used with great care to avoid perforation. Knowing which femurs are at risk and paying close attention to surgical technique should help prevent this complication intraoperatively.

Postoperative Fractures

Postoperative fractures are caused by both patient and surgical factors. The common feature of all risk factors is a decrease in the mechanical strength of host bone. This can be generalized, such as osteopenia, or localized, such as osteolysis. Osteolysis only recently has been recognized as a risk factor for fracture (12). These fractures usually occur in association with a loose prosthesis. Recognition of this impending pathologic fracture and early intervention make revision easier than when a fracture is associated with a loose prosthesis (Fig. 1).

Surgical factors that put the femur at risk for postoperative fracture usually are a cortical defect or perforations. Cortical defects have long been recognized as a risk factor for postoperative periprosthetic fracture (1,16,21,25). These defects can be unintentional perforations during cement removal, reaming, or insertion of the femoral prosthesis. The presence of cortical windows made for cement removal (2,10) also can put the femur at risk.

Cortical perforation is a problem the frequency of which has been increasing. Early reports estimated the incidence to be between 0.4% and 4% (19,25). However, with the increase in the number of revision operations, the rate of this complication has increased; it is estimated to complicate between 13% and 18% (3,11) of operations. Prevention of cortical perforation involves careful surgical technique in removing cement at the time of revision. If the surgeon anticipates that the cement mantle is well fixed and may be difficult to remove, extended trochanteric osteotomy facilitates exposure and cement removal, thus avoiding unintentional penetration (26). Another technique used to improve the ease of cement removal is controlled perforation of the anterior femoral cortex (24). Because this perforation is always recognized during the operation, it is bypassed with a long femoral stem. Thus the stress riser effect is eliminated, and fracture risk is decreased.

Cortical defects, be they perforations, windows, or screw holes, should be anticipated or recognized during the operation. When recognized, they should be bypassed with a long femoral stem (1,11,16). Experimental work has shown (13) that bypassing the defect by

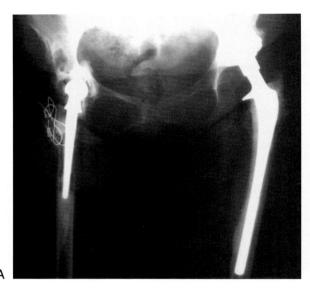 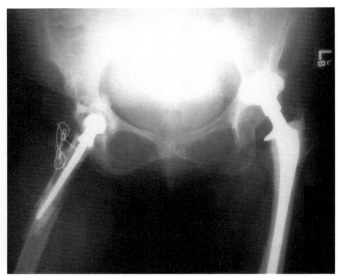

Figure 1. A: Marked osteolysis and femoral loosening of right hip. **B:** Early revision would have prevented the periprosthetic fracture that occurred after a minor fall.

two cortical diameters increases bone strength to 80% of normal. This is the current recommendation for managing cortical defects. In addition to using longer stems, cortical strut grafts have been suggested as a prophylactic measure against stress risers. These struts have been shown to be effective in increasing cortical strength in animal fracture models (6). At present it is generally agreed that all substantial defects be grafted as well as bypassed with longer femoral stems.

CLASSIFICATION

Most fracture classification systems have addressed the location and fracture pattern. Most systems are based on postoperative fractures. The relation of the tip of the femoral prosthesis to the fracture often receives the most attention because it is considered to have the most important implications for treatment and prognosis.

The classification system of Johannson et al. (10) is the most commonly used system for both intraoperative and postoperative periprosthetic fractures. Type I fractures are proximal to the stem tip. Type II fractures are located around the stem tip and commonly extend below it. Type III fractures are entirely distal to the stem tip.

The Johansson system is just one of many classifications in the literature. It is becoming increasingly clear that fracture location although important is only one of several factors important in determining treatment and predicting outcome in periprosthetic fractures. Factors believed to be important in determining treatment include fracture location and stability, implant stability, quality of bone stock, patient age, and surgeon experience. The Vancouver classification was developed in 1991 and published in 1995 to address factors crucial in decision making. These factors are the location of the fracture, the stability of the implant, and the quality of the host bone (5). This system divides fractures into three categories on the basis of location (Fig. 2). Type A fractures occur in the trochanteric region. Type B fractures are around the stem or extend just below it. Type C fractures are well below the stem. Type A fractures are subdivided into fractures involving the greater trochanter (A_G) or the lesser trochanter (A_L). Type B fractures are subdivided on the basis of implant stability and host bone stock. In type B_1 fractures the femoral component is well fixed; in type B_2 the stem is loose; and in type B_3 the stem is loose and there is marked loss of bone stock due to osteolysis, osteopenia, or fracture comminution. Any classification system should describe factors important in determining treatment and prognosis and should be shown to be reliable and valid if it is to be used. The Vancouver classification system has been tested for reliability and validity (unpublished data) since

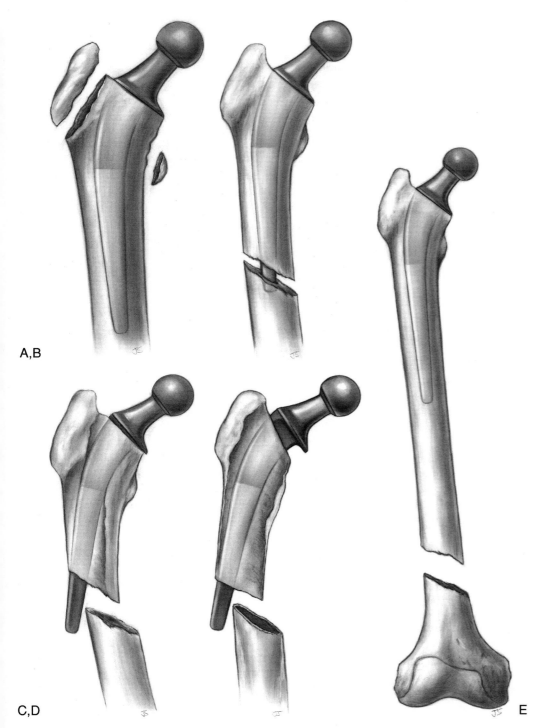

Figure 2. Vancouver classification of periprosthetic fractures. **A:** Type A. **B:** Type B₁. **C:** Type B₂. **D:** Type B₃. **E:** Type C.

it was originally described by two of us (C. P. D., B. A. M.). Both intraobserver and interobserver reliability were assessed, and kappa analysis showed high agreement beyond chance for both. Validity testing showed substantial agreement beyond chance when preoperative assessment was compared with intraoperative findings. Because the Vancouver classification addresses factors known to be important in the management of periprosthetic fractures and has been shown to be valid and reliable, we favor this classification when planning management of periprosthetic fractures.

TREATMENT METHODS

Intraoperative fractures are not always recognized at the time of the operation (20). When they are recognized, treatment depends on the location, configuration, and stability of the femoral component. With cementless implants most fractures occur proximal to the lesser trochanter (17,20). These fractures usually occur as a result of aggressive rasping and broaching or during final insertion of the femoral component. Various treatment options have been suggested, including cerclage wiring (17,20) or use of a collared component (11,22) to prevent subsidence. In all series, if the prosthesis was stable, a good final result was obtained. Fractures that occur around the stem tip that are recognized intraoperatively present a greater challenge. The surgeon must define the extent of the fracture. These fractures can range from small fissures to perforations and spiral fractures. Distal perforations and fractures should be managed whenever possible by the use of a longer stem to bypass the weakened area (12). Supplemental bone grafting should be considered. Fractures not recognized intraoperatively often are stable and may be managed conservatively with restricted weight bearing. If the fracture is not stable or is at risk for propagation, internal fixation with cerclage wires and cortical onlay allografting should be considered.

Numerous case series on the management of postoperative fractures have been reported in the literature, and there is little agreement on the optimum management. The goals of management of these fractures should include a united fracture in near anatomic alignment, a stable prosthesis, return to prefracture function, and early mobilization. Numerous options have been described. These include nonoperative management, open reduction and internal fixation, revision arthroplasty with a long-stemmed component, or proximal femoral replacement. The choice of treatment depends on the location of the fracture, the stability of the prosthesis, available bone stock, and the age and medical status of the patient.

Early reports in the literature favored nonoperative treatment, including traction or a hip spica cast (16,21). The authors stated that the risk of surgical treatment may be too high. However, conservative treatment is fraught with complications for the patient, the fracture, and the arthroplasty. Most nonoperative regimens involve a long period of traction. For elderly patients bed rest can be complicated by skin ulcers, pneumonia, and fat embolism syndrome, to name a few. It would seem advantageous to avoid recumbency for these patients, and this is one of the goals of modern fracture treatment.

In addition to medical risks to the patient, nonoperative treatment has been associated with a high incidence of subsequent revision for femoral loosening of between 19% and 100% (1,2,10). Nonunion rates of 25% to 42% and a malunion rate of 45% have been reported with nonoperative treatment. Although nonoperative treatment should be avoided in most cases, there are situations in which it may be effective. These usually are cases in which the fracture is stable and the femoral implant is well fixed. In a recent series, Beals and Tower (1) showed equally good results with nonoperative management of fractures that were proximal to the stem tip with a stable prosthesis. In their series this situation accounted for only 15% of the total number of periprosthetic fractures.

As is the case for femoral fractures in general, it is becoming increasingly clear that unstable periprosthetic fractures usually do better with operative stabilization. This can take the form of intramedullary fixation, extramedullary fixation, or a combination of the two. In extreme cases proximal femoral replacement may be indicated when bone loss is severe.

Intramedullary fixation is revision with a longer-stemmed component. Periprosthetic fractures often are associated with loose femoral components. When the femoral prosthesis is loose, most authors recommend revision with a long-stemmed prosthesis. This addresses the prosthetic stability and provides optimum management of the femoral shaft fracture with intramedullary fixation. With the use of this technique the combined nonunion rate, refracture rate, and revision rate have been reported to be 12% to 20% (12). Whereas most reports in the literature concern long-stemmed, cemented revisions, more recent literature favors uncemented revision in the fracture situation (1,12). In their report, Beals and Tower found a significantly improved outcome ($p = .01$) with the use of ingrowth prosthesis versus cemented revision for the management of periprosthetic fractures. In addition to the use of long-stemmed revisions, many authors advocate the addition of bone grafting to stimulate fracture healing (11). When a long-stemmed prosthesis does not provide sufficient stability, supplementary fixation can be achieved with cerclage wires, plates, or cortical strut allografting.

Open reduction and internal fixation would seem an attractive alternative when the prosthesis is well fixed and the fracture is distal. Using standard AO techniques, Serocki et al. (22) had good to excellent results. When the fracture is distal to the stem tip, it is possible to achieve rigid fixation with standard plates and screws. However, with periprosthetic fractures proximal to the stem tip, there is the disadvantage that the screws may violate the cement mantle or may not gain sufficient purchase if a canal-filling device is in place. With cementless devices there may not be adequate bone in which to place the screws. For this reason plates, such as the Ogden plate, were introduced that allow fixation with either screws or cerclage techniques (18). Such devices are fixed distally with screws and proximally with cerclage wires, bands, or cables. The union rate has been excellent with this device, approaching 100% in many series (18). Although these results with plating are encouraging, some authors (10) have reported that as many as 50% of patients treated by means of open reduction and internal fixation needed revision procedures. Most authors would agree that open reduction and internal fixation should be reserved for instances in which the femoral stem is solidly fixed (1,11,12). Cerclage wiring alone has been shown to be a poor technique (14). Its use should be limited in the management of postoperative fractures and be combined to supplemental fixation.

Another technique for fixation of fractures with a stable femoral component is use of cortical onlay allograft. This technique is attractive because it requires no screw fixation and has the ability to restore bone stock and bone strength (6). Emerson et al. (6) showed in animal models that strut grafting is an effective technique to restore cortical strength in the presence of a fracture. In a finite element analysis this technique was found to be as effective as use of Ogden plates in restoring strength to the femur. Although union rates of 90% of cortical struts to host bone have been reported for revision surgery, there is limited clinical experience with

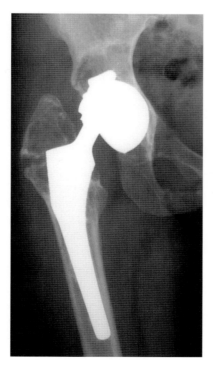

Figure 3. Vancouver A$_G$ periprosthetic fracture. Osteolysis of the greater trochanter and the acetabulum is present. Polyethylene wear debris was the cause of this fracture.

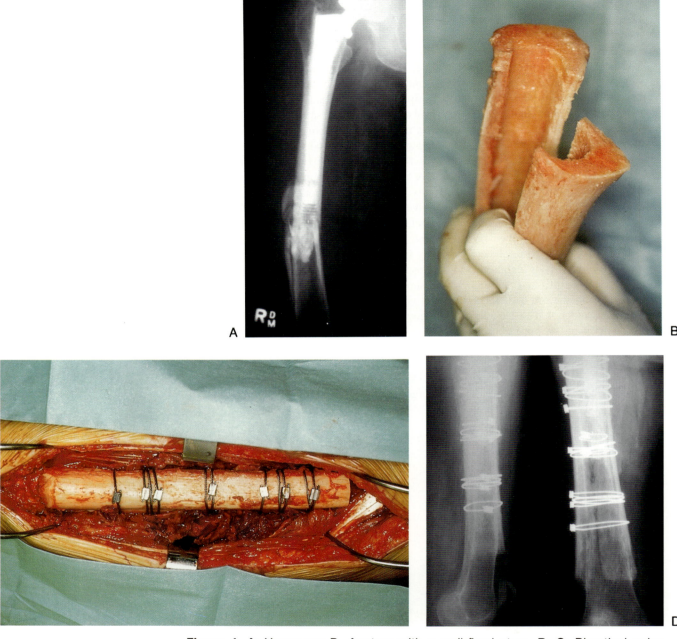

Figure 4. A: Vancouver B$_1$ fracture with a well-fixed stem. **B, C:** Bicortical onlay allografting is an attractive technique to fix this fracture. **D:** Incorporation of the allograft with healing of the fracture.

the use of this technique for the management of periprosthetic fractures. We have found this technique very effective in the treatment of a limited number of patients. Another alternative is to use both a plate and a cortical onlay graft in combination.

AUTHORS' PREFERRED METHOD

Many options exist for the management of postoperative periprosthetic fractures. The goals of treatment should be a healed fracture in near anatomic position, a stable

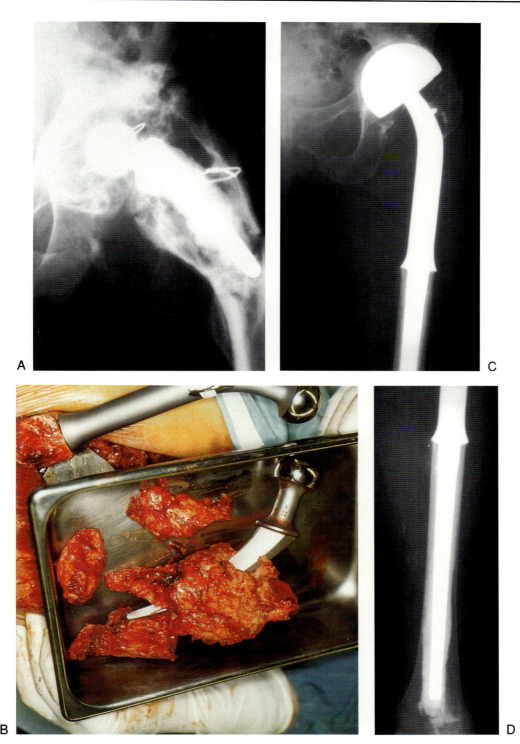

Figure 5. A, B: Periprosthetic fracture (B$_3$) in an elderly woman with poor proximal bone stock. **C, D:** Prosthetic femoral replacement was used to replace the deficient proximal femur and allowed immediate mobilization.

prosthesis, a return to prefracture functional status, and early mobilization. We use the Vancouver classification system of periprosthetic fractures to guide treatment.

Proximal fractures of type A are generally stable, and most series support nonoperative treatment with protected weight bearing (1,12). A large number of these fractures are caused by avulsion of bone weakened by osteolysis associated with severe polyethylene

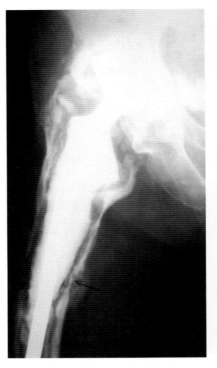
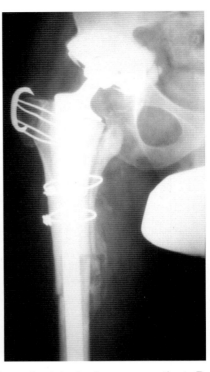

A   B

Figure 6. A: Vancouver B₃ fracture in a physiologically young patient. **B:** Treatment in these cases involves replacement of the proximal femur with an allograft prosthetic composite. A step cut at the graft–host junction gives rotational stability. With this technique the greater trochanter can be reattached to improve function and stability.

wear (Fig. 3). Revision of the socket may have to be considered. Type B fractures in most large series represent the highest proportion of cases. In type B fractures the first decision to be made is whether the implant is stable. Prefracture radiographs and prefracture clinical status may help categorize a fracture as B_1 (prosthesis stable) or B_2 or B_3 (prosthesis unstable). For patients with B_1 fractures open reduction and internal fixation is the best treatment. We believe that cortical onlay allografting has several theoretical advantages over conventional open reduction and internal fixation, and we advocate this as the management of most B_1 fractures (Fig. 4). For B_2 fractures, revision with a medium-length or long-stemmed component with or without cortical strut supplementation is recommended. The method of stem fixation depends on the preference of the surgical team and the physiologic age of the patient. For elderly patients for whom immediate, full weight bearing is desirable, a cemented stem is the best option. Type B_3 fractures are the most difficult to treat and often necessitate replacement of the proximal femur with a structural allograft–prosthesis composite or custom prosthesis. Proximal femoral replacement prostheses are used to treat elderly patients to whom early mobilization is important (Fig. 5). Allograft–prosthesis composites are favored in the care of younger patients. They allow reattachment of soft tissues, specifically the greater trochanter, which improves the function and stability of the construct (Fig. 6). Although preoperative evaluation may allow differentiation between those femurs with good and those with poor bone stock, the final decision can only be made intraoperatively. It is important for anyone managing these difficult fractures to have an adequate inventory of femoral components and access to allograft bone. Type C fractures can be managed with standard plates or plates and cerclage. Even when the stem is loose in Type C fractures, the stem can be addressed after fracture union is obtained.

SUMMARY

Periprosthetic fractures of the femur are a complex problem to solve. With the increasing number of both primary and revision hip arthroplasties being done and the advancing age of the population, the numbers of fractures will continue to increase. Prevention of these fractures is the best form of management. Intimate knowledge of the risk factors outlined herein will help to decrease the incidence of this serious complication. When these fractures do occur, careful planning should involve multiple factors in the decision about a treatment regimen. These include patient factors, surgeon factors, and factors related to the implant and residual bone stock. Use of the Vancouver classification scheme allows a logical approach to deal with this difficult problem.

REFERENCES

1. Beals R, Tower SS. Periprosthetic fractures of the femur: an analysis of 93 fractures. *Clin Orthop* 1996;327:238–246.
2. Bethea JS, DeAndrade JR, Fleming LL, et al. Proximal femoral fractures following total hip arthroplasty. *Clin Orthop* 1982;170:95–106.
3. Callaghan JJ, Salvati EA, Pellicci PM, et al. A result of revision from mechanical failure after cemented total hip replacement. *J Bone Joint Surg Am* 1985;67:1074–1085.
4. Christensen CM, Seger BM, Schultz RB. Management of intraoperative femur fractures associated with revision hip arthroplasty. *Clin Orthop* 1989;248:178–180.
5. Duncan CP, Masri BA. Fractures of the femur after hip replacement. *Instruct Course Lect* 1995;45:293–304.
6. Emerson RH, Malinin IT, Cueaar AD, et al. Cortical strut allografts in the reconstruction of the femur and revision in total hip arthroplasty: a basic science and clinical study. *Clin Orthop* 1992;285:35–44.
7. Fitzgerald RH, Brindley GW, Kavanagh BF. The uncemented total hip arthroplasty: intraoperative femoral fractures. *Clin Orthop* 1988;235:61–66.
8. Herzwurm PJ, Walsh J, Pettine KL, et al. Prophylactic cerclage: a method of preventing femur fracture in an uncemented total hip arthroplasty. *Orthopedics* 1992;15:143–146.
9. Incavo SJ, DiFazio F, Wilder D, et al. Longitudinal crack propagation in bone around femoral prosthesis. *Clin Orthop* 1991;272:175–180.
10. Johansson JE, McBroom R, Barrington TW, et al. Fracture of the ipsilateral femur in patients with total hip replacement. *J Bone Joint Surg Am* 1981;63:1435–1442.
11. Kavanagh BF. Femoral fractures associated with total hip arthroplasty. *Orthop Clin North Am* 1992;23:249–257.
12. Kelley SS. Periprosthetic femoral fractures. *J Am Acad Orthop Surg* 1994;2:164–172.
13. Larson JE, Chao EYS, Fitzgerald RH. Bypassing femoral cortical defects with cemented intramedullary stems. *J Orthop Res* 1991;9:414–421.
14. Lewallen, DG, Berry DJ. Femoral fractures associated with hip arthroplasty. In: Morrey BF, ed. *Reconstructive surgery of the joints.* New York: Churchill Livingstone, 1996:1273–1288.
15. Löwenhielm G, Hansson LI, Kärrholm J. Fracture of the lower extremity after total hip replacement. *Arch Orthop Trauma Surg* 1989;108:141–143.
16. McElfresh EC, Conventry MB. Femoral and pelvic fractures after total hip arthroplasty. *J Bone Joint Surg Am* 1974;56:483–492.
17. Mont MA, Maar DC. Fractures of the ipsilateral femur after hip arthroplasty: a statistical analysis of outcome based on 487 patients. *J Arthroplasty* 1994;9:511–519.
18. Ogden WS, Rendall J. Fractures beneath hip prosthesis: a special indication for Parham bands in plating. *Orthop Trans* 1978;2:70 [abstract].
19. Pellicci PM, Inglis AE, Salvati EA. Perforation of the femoral shaft during total hip replacement: report of twelve cases. *J Bone Joint Surg Am* 1980;62:234–240.
20. Schwartz JT, Mayer JG, Engh CA. Femoral fracture during non-cemented total hip arthroplasty. *J Bone Joint Surg Am* 1989;71:1135–1142.
21. Scott RD, Turner RH, Leitzes SM, Aufranc OE. Femoral fractures in conjunction with total hip replacement. *J Bone Joint Surg Am* 1975;57:494–501.
22. Serocki JH, Chandler RW, Dorr LD. Treatment of fractures about hip prosthesis with compression plating. *J Arthroplasty* 1992;7:129–135.
23. Stuchin SA. Femoral shaft fracture in porous and press-fit total hip arthroplasty. *Orthop Rev* 1990;2:153–159.
24. Sydney SV, Mallory TH. Control perforations: a safe method of cement removal from the femoral canal. *Clin Orthop* 1990;253:168–172.
25. Talab YA, States JD, McCollister Evarts C. Femoral shaft perforation: a complication of total hip replacement. *Clin Orthop* 1979;141:158–165.
26. Younger TI, Bradford MS, Magnus RE, et al. Extended proximal femoral osteotomy: a new technique for femoral revision arthroplasty. *J Arthroplasty* 1995;10:329–338.

Revision Total Hip Arthroplasty,
edited by Marvin E. Steinberg and Jonathan P. Garino,
Lippincott Williams & Wilkins, Philadelphia © 1999.

35

Trochanteric Nonunion and Abductor Compromise

Russell G. Cohen and Aaron G. Rosenberg

After total hip arthroplasty, strength of the periarticular musculature is vital to ensure stability of the hip and restore the patient's gait to as near normal as possible. Abductor compromise, either through intrinsic weakness of the gluteus medius and minimus muscles or as a result of an ununited, proximally migrated greater trochanter can affect the results of total hip arthroplasty. A variety of problems exist that can compromise muscle function and leave the patient with weakness of the abductors. When the problem exists preoperatively, careful planning can prevent disastrous results that may otherwise be encountered. Quite frequently, however, the weakness arises out of a surgical complication and has to be addressed postoperatively to prevent premature failure of the reconstruction.

The subject of abductor weakness can best be divided into two categories—problems present preoperatively and factors related to the technical aspects of surgery. Neurologic problems such as hemiplegia, postpolio syndrome, cerebral palsy, myelomeningocele, spinal stenosis, and spinal cord injury are diagnoses that typically exist preoperatively. Other diagnoses associated with weakness include neuropathic joints and disorders that alter the normal resting length of muscle (developmental dysplasia of the hip, coxa vara, and arthroplasty after a Girdlestone operation or arthrodesis).

More typically, however, weakness arises from a complication related to either surgical technique or postoperative complications. These may be associated with the surgical approach used, use of trochanteric osteotomy and union of the osteotomy, restoration of soft-tissue tension, and damage to the musculature or muscular attachments during the

R. G. Cohen: Tucson Orthopedic Institute, Tucson, Arizona 85712.
A. G. Rosenberg: Rush–Presbyterian–St. Lukes Medical Center, Chicago, Illinois 60612.

operation (7,28–30,33–36,40). These issues have been addressed at great length in the literature and can be reviewed in greater detail.

Although the literature remains devoid of an organized approach to abductor compromise around total hip arthroplasty, it is important for the hip surgeon to understand the implications, causes and solutions to the problems presented by these patients. Early recognition of the problem and careful preoperative planning assist both patient and surgeon in attaining a successful result.

IMPLICATIONS

Since the inception of hip replacement surgery, numerous publications have addressed instability and dislocation after total hip arthroplasty (10,11,15,21–23,41,42). After reviewing 35,000 cases in the literature through 1987, Morrey (29) found the incidence to be 2.2%; a similar incidence was found in a Mayo Clinic study (43). Although preoperative diagnosis has not been found to correlate with the development of dislocation, numerous factors relating to dislocation have been found, including femoral offset, component malposition, surgical approach, and head size of the femoral component (29). Most reviews, however, address only such common diagnoses as osteoarthritis, rheumatoid arthritis, avascular necrosis, and congenital hip dysplasia. Few articles address comorbid neuromuscular conditions, such as Parkinson's disease, poststroke status, and cerebral palsy; status after arthrodesis or Girdlestone arthroplasty; coxa vara or other associated deformities and their specific correlation with the development of hip instability.

Abductor compromise is one of several potential causes of hip instability and dislocation that should be recognized preoperatively, dealt with intraoperatively, and specifically addressed during rehabilitation. However, once the problem of weakness is known to exist, there is not always an easy way to compensate for the problem, as is the case among patients with primary neuromuscular involvement. If the problem is discovered preoperatively, methods to compensate for the weakness can help to prevent recurrent dislocation.

Another sequela of postarthroplasty weakness around the hip is the development of a limp. This most often relates to abductor weakness and may result in an abductor lurch or Trendelenburg gait due to inability to fully support the hemipelvis during single-leg stance (27). This produces a noticeable limp, which may ultimately affect the degree of patient satisfaction. It also may increase the incidence of component loosening. Proximal migration of the greater trochanter after fracture or nonunion may similarly leave the abductors functioning at a suboptimal level, resulting in a limp. These issues and several surgical factors relating to development of abductor weakness are discussed in greater detail in this chapter.

CAUSES OF ABDUCTOR COMPROMISE

Preoperative Factors

Several comorbid conditions exist in conjunction with degenerative arthritis of the hip that may ultimately progress to total hip arthroplasty. Patients with hemiplegia resulting from a cerebrovascular insult may have degenerative joint disease. Although the two diagnoses are not codependent, both typically occur among the aging population and may be present concurrently. Similarly, patients with cerebral palsy may have degenerative hip disease as a result of long-standing hip dysplasia or dislocation (9,37). In both patient groups, the abductors and extensors are preferentially weaker than the abductors and flexors, leading to a flexion deformity with scissoring of the legs.

Treating patients with cerebral palsy with arthritis of the hip is a complicated issue, in part as a result of the muscle imbalances. However, the literature supports treating them with hip arthroplasty to alleviate pain and maximize care and function (9,37). Root et al. reported their 6-year follow-up findings for 15 patients treated with total hip replacement.

Thirteen of 15 were free of pain and functioning at a level consistent with their degree of involvement; only two needed revision. The authors later reported the 10-year survivorship of the prostheses in these patients to be 86%.

Even with these results, performing hip arthroplasty on patients with cerebral palsy remains a viable option. However, recognizing the muscle imbalances around the hip and relative abductor weakness, one must carefully plan the approach and choose the appropriate implant to avoid complications related to the muscle imbalances. Use of the anterolateral approach with preservation of the posterior capsule adds stability to these patients, who may spend more time sitting than the typical total hip patient.

Patients with myelomeningocele have varying needs for surgical intervention around the hip depending of the level of the neural defect (4). The midlumbar levels have the highest incidence of dislocation in childhood and usually have the greatest need for intervention at a young age. Third, fourth, and fifth lumbar levels typically have intact flexor and adductor muscles without functioning abductors and extensors. As a result, they have the greatest propensity to dislocate over time. Surgical therapy to correct this usually involves open reduction, capsulorrhaphy, or derotational osteotomy on either the femoral or acetabular side of the joint. The age at which the diagnosis of dislocation is made can influence the procedure performed. It is unrecognized dislocations that may ultimately lead to osteoarthritis of the hip.

Although total hip arthroplasty to treat this population of patients has not been reported, many patients maintain some degree of sensation. For patients left with dislocation or subluxation, hip degeneration and pain may become an issue later in life. Reconstructive surgery in adulthood would require joint replacement, and muscle balancing to avoid problems with instability and dislocation.

Hip arthritis frequently is seen in conjunction with spinal stenosis. Patients tend to lose muscle tone from the inability to walk, because of the hip disease and neurogenic claudication. The hip musculature is not typically weakened as a result of stenosis, but patients tend to become quite deconditioned from the combination of spinal stenosis and hip arthritis. A complete neurologic examination and preoperative evaluation of the supporting muscles is imperative to avoid missing the occasional instance in which the abductors are weakened as a result of high-level stenosis. This allows the surgeon to address the problem at the operation by choosing a more stable approach and focusing specifically on the abductors during postoperative rehabilitation.

Conditions such as postpolio syndrome and spinal cord injury occasionally are associated with hip arthritis. Although no literature exists on outcome for and treatment of these patients who undergo hip replacement surgery, management presents similar problems. Recognizing the diagnosis and associated lack of muscle support preoperatively enables the surgeon to modify the technique and choice of components in an effort to avoid chronic instability.

Patients who have undergone arthrodesis and those with spontaneous ankylosis of the hip, as in ankylosing spondylitis, present challenges at the time of hip reconstruction. In both instances, the patients lose muscle strength as a result of disuse, sometimes for more than 20 years. Surgically ankylosed hips may have considerable abductor muscle abnormality or loss of the trochanter as a result of the technique used for arthrodesis, leaving the abductors scarred or weakened.

The early results of hip arthroplasty to treat patients with abductor compromise seemed favorable, with few problems at early follow-up evaluations. In separate studies, Lubahn et al. (26) and Brewster et al. (8) reported good results after takedown of a hip fusion and conversion to total hip arthroplasty. Complication rates were acceptable, and 50% of patients did not need an assistive device for ambulation at 1-year follow-up examinations. However, Strathy and Fitzgerald (40) reported their results after average follow-up period of 10 years to be much less favorable. They reported a 25% failure rate and an additional 11% rate of poor clinical results. Most failures were attributed to mechanical loosening and some to deep infections. Only one hip replacement was revised because of recurrent dislocation. These results imply that although these patients initially do well, altered mechanics and weakness of the supporting musculature may lead to earlier failure than among a control population.

Patients with developmental dysplasia of the hip have altered mechanics around the hip (12,19), and preoperative motor testing can be performed. Besides the problem of compromised abductors, several other issues need to be addressed in the care of these patients. Transtrochanteric osteotomy has frequently been used to aid in exposure of the acetabulum. This too may predispose the hip area to weakening of the abductors, particularly if nonunion occurs. In addition, the center of rotation of the hip is not always in the usual location, and altered mechanics and forces result around the hip. Linde et al. (24), reported a cumulative survivorship of 89% after 10 years but a significantly higher failure rate when the acetabulum was placed high rather than low (42% versus 13%). One may not always have the luxury of placing the acetabulum in the original position, and in these situations the long-term results may be compromised.

Operative and Postoperative Factors

Surgical Approach

An important factor contributing to instability and abductor compromise is the effect of the approach on the surrounding muscles. Three standard approaches to the hip, anterolateral (Hardinge), transtrochanteric (trochanteric osteotomy), and posterior (Kocher-Langenbach) all have been critically evaluated regarding the incidence of instability and dislocation. Robinson et al. (36) found a significant difference in dislocation rate between hips exposed through a posterior approach and those exposed through trochanteric osteotomy. A lower incidence of dislocation was found among subjects who underwent trochanteric osteotomy as opposed to a posterior approach (0 vs 7.5%). Other studies found similar findings, including the Mayo report of a 2.3% dislocation rate with an anterior approach in comparison to 5.8% using the posterior approach (43). Roberts et al. (35) found a threefold increase in dislocation with the posterior approach compared with the anterior approach.

In a technique recently described by Poss (32) the piriformis and conjoined tendons are resected from their base, the bursa and quadratus femoris are removed from the posterior femur leaving a soft-tissue pedicle for closure, and a rectangular flap is made in the posterior capsule. These structures are tagged and then reapproximated during closure through drill holes in the greater trochanter and the quadratus is reattached to its soft-tissue base. This technique produces a check rein effect on internal rotation and has reduced the dislocation rate after posterior exposure to less than 1%.

The anterolaral approach of Hardinge, although considered an intrinsically more stable approach, is not without its complications. The technique involves detachment of the anterior fibers of the gluteus medius and minimus muscles with proximal splitting of the fibers. This places the inferior branch of the superior gluteal nerve at risk for injury and potentially leaves the muscle denervated if excessive muscle splitting is performed. Baker and Bitounis (3) performed nine cadaveric dissections of the superior gluteal nerve and found it to course from 3 cm to 5 cm proximal to the anterior edge of the trochanter. This approach depends on sound technique when reattaching the tendinous insertions of the gluteus minimus and medius muscles to the greater trochanter to avoid permanently weakened abductors.

If denervation or disruption of the repaired abductors occurs, the resultant weakness may lead to a limp or hip instability. In the study by Baker and Bitounis (3) 10 hips approached through an anterolateral exposure demonstrated abductor denervation 10 weeks after the operation, and 56% of patients continued to have a positive Trendelenburg sign 12 months after the operation. Minns et al. (28) compared results for patients who underwent an anterolateral approach by means of their technique with results for undergoing trochanteric osteotomy. They found their method safe and effective, and no difference was found in strength-test results for the abductors.

In both primary and revision surgery, variability in surgical technique may account for the substantial differences in complications reported. Recognizing the potential hazards of a given approach is important when deciding on a preferred approach to the hip. It is important to remember that no technique is free of complications.

The concern about trochanteric osteotomy and its relation to development of instability remains a controversial subject. When there is union of the trochanter without proximal migration beyond 2 cm (43), this technique aids greatly in exposure without compromising muscle strength (7,28,30). Most surgeons today have abandoned the technique of transtrochanteric osteotomy except in more complex operations in which exposure is not adequate without its use. The main concern over such a technique, particularly in revision surgery, is the high number of nonunions associated with repair of the small fragment (17). Variations of the technique, such as the trochanteric slide, in which the soft-tissue sleeve is kept in continuity with the bony fragment, and the use of the extended trochanteric osteotomy, are both excellent alternatives to separation of the proximal trochanteric fragment from the remaining femur (Fig. 1).

Several authors have described factors attributable to nonunion and its effect on gait pattern, pain, hip instability, and clinical outcome. Robinson et al. (36) found trochanteric osteotomy to be safe and effective with no dislocations when that technique was used. Ritter et al. (34) found both a higher incidence of pain associated with trochanteric nonunion and a greater ability to walk in the presence of a well-united fragment. Fraser and Wroblewski (16), on the other hand, cited loss of the abductor mechanism as a factor contributing to dislocation after trochanteric osteotomy, not only from nonunion of the fragment but also as a result of the approach.

When the trochanter migrates proximally, allowing the abductor lever arm to shorten, instability and dislocation may become a problem for the patient. Although some authors consider migration of more than 1.5 cm to result in abductor weakness (6), most consider more than 2.0 cm of migration to lead to functional impairment (1,2,20,31). Patients with more than 1 cm of separation, however, usually have a positive Trendelenburg sign (20).

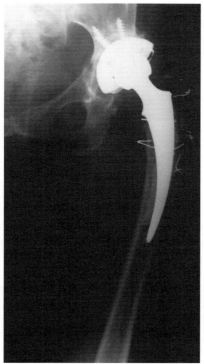

Figure 1. Transtrochanteric approach resulting in trochanteric nonunion with hardware failure.

Although the effect of releasing the trochanter for exposure of the hip is desirable in select situations, its contribution to abductor compromise is not universally accepted. Murray et al. (30) performed a controlled study involving 82 patients. Half underwent total hip replacement through trochanteric osteotomy and the other half by the anterior approach described by Müller. At 2-year follow-up evaluations, there was no difference between the two groups in muscle strength as measured by means of kinesiologic testing. Borja et al. (7) in a similar study, found no difference in isometric and isokinetic muscle strength measurements between two groups of patients undergoing either trochanteric osteotomy or a standard posterolateral approach.

Soft-Tissue Tensioning

The success of hip arthroplasty depends to some degree on the structural integrity of the soft tissues around the joint, particularly in revision surgery in which the normal tissue architecture has been altered. Restoring length to the extremity, achieving the appropriate degree of offset, and finding the center of rotation of the femoral head relative to the revised acetabulum are more complex in this setting. However, reaching these goals is crucial to the success of both primary and revision surgery.

Every muscle has an optimum resting length and tension that maximize its efficiency during contraction. An overstretched muscle does not have overlap between the thick and thin myofilaments within the sarcomere, whereas a muscle that is overly shortened has abutment of thick bands between adjacent sarcomeres (39). Similarly, a muscle that has improper innervation undergoes changes at the neuromuscular junction and muscular atrophy that result in alteration of the contractile properties of skeletal muscle and the efficiency of muscle function.

Failure to restore adequate tension of the soft tissues around the hip has two deleterious effects on the function of the abductors and outcome of arthroplasty. The first relates to stability of the reconstruction and subsequent increased risk for dislocation. Although many authors have addressed the issue, no consensus exists that restoring limb length alone affects hip stability. Morrey (29) found that in a series of unstable hips, the limb was 1.6 mm longer than the untreated limb. Coventry (11) reported similar findings; 75% of 32 patients had limbs equal in length. Only 25% had a shorter limb on the unstable side. Carlsson and Gentz (10), however, found a statistically significant correlation between limb shortening and dislocation. Kristiansen et al. (22) observed that the unstable hip was slightly more proximal than the control limb, but the differences found were not statistically significant.

The distance from the center of the femoral head to the greater trochanter is referred to as *femoral offset*. Although it does not add length to the extremity, femoral offset provides clearance of the trochanter from impinging on the acetabulum by bringing it laterally and maximizes the efficiency of the abductors. As a result, it also affects the amount of force generated by the muscles as the dynamic stabilizing elements cross the joint. The amount of offset for any given patient is highly variable, and restoring this offset is an important goal of hip reconstruction. In the revision setting in which the femoral component has loosened and subsided within the femur, offset is lost, and inadequate abductor function is present preoperatively. Patients with coxa vara, on the other hand, have a greater degree of offset to begin with, and choosing an appropriate prosthesis to match this offset is critical. Failure to do so leaves the abductors relatively loose and inefficient, increasing the likelihood of limp, instability, and dislocation postoperatively.

In a study by Kaplan et al. (21) of offset in a population of patients with unstable hips, a strong correlation was found between a shorter distance from the tip of the trochanter to the center of the femoral head. The authors demonstrated the importance of lateralization and distal advancement of the trochanter to restore the efficiency of the abductor mechanism.

In the revision setting and certain primary situations, the degree of offset is limited from the outset. Patients with protrusio acetabuli, for example, have a shortened acetabular-trochanteric distance and consequently lose the efficiency of the abductors to some degree.

Adding offset by means of appropriate prosthesis selection adds tension to the muscles, improves the abductor lever arm, and provides clearance of the trochanter from the pelvis. In revision settings in which the cup has eroded into the pelvis and migrated proximally, restoration of offset during the operation provides the same advantage in optimizing the clinical result.

Resection arthroplasty (Girdlestone procedure) is most commonly performed for sepsis and subsequent removal of implants in an effort to eradicate the infection. However, there are instances in which it is done for aseptic reasons such as cerebral palsy, multiple failures of hip arthroplasty, fractures in debilitated patients, and neuropathic joints. Among patients who have undergone a Girdlestone procedure, conversion to an arthroplasty remains an option if the underlying problem has been resolved. These patients frequently have shortened, fibrotic, soft tissues that are markedly atrophied, resulting in compromise of the supporting musculature. Surgical treatment requires careful attention to restoration of offset, orientation of the components and diligent postoperative rehabilitation to minimize postoperative fatigability, limp, and dislocation.

TREATMENT

Instability and dislocation resulting from weakening of the abductors or trochanteric migration are challenging problems often not easily resolved. Recognizing the potential complications associated with periarticular muscle weakness and planning accordingly may help alleviate some of these difficulties. There is no literature to guide the surgeon in these circumstances, but avoiding certain situations that can accentuate the problem may reduce the potential for complications. Such measures include using an anterior approach when possible, meticulous closure of the posterior structures when feasible, selection of a prosthesis with adequate offset, and restoration of limb lengths. These goals are no different from those of routine primary arthroplasty, but the margin for error is so narrow that the extra attention to detail is vital if one is to avoid potentially catastrophic results.

When instability develops, the treatment plan should follow a logical sequence for dislocated total hip replacement. Closed reduction is performed, and the patient is placed in either an abduction brace or hip spica cast and then allowed to resume usual activities. For patients with known abductor weakness, physical therapy should be added as an adjunct after bracing to strengthen the abductors and extensors. This is particularly important among patients who have undergone conversion of an arthrodesis or Girdlestone arthroplasty to total hip replacement. Therapy should be instituted routinely at the appropriate postoperative juncture (usually 6 weeks after a Hardinge approach) and not after the complication has already occurred.

For patients who have weakness and a limp but not recurrent dislocation, the use of a cane is an easy measure and potentially avoids long-term complications and wear of the prosthesis. With use of a cane, the forces across the hip joint can be reduced and abnormal wear patterns avoided.

For patients with recurrent dislocations, several treatment options exist. The first is to place the patient in a hip spica cast for 6 weeks while the periarticular soft tissues are allowed to heal. Williams et al. (42) reported on use of an above-knee hip spica cast after dislocation and saw only one redislocation among 16 patients. For patients who do go on to have recurrent dislocation, a permanent brace to maintain reduction and function of the hip is a reasonable alternative. Patients who cannot undergo surgical treatment for medical reasons, the brace may provide enough stability to the hip to allow limited activity without the need for additional surgical intervention. However, patients generally feel a brace is cumbersome and restrictive to wear and difficult to apply.

When trochanteric nonunion contributes to recurrent dislocation, surgical options are available when nonoperative treatment has failed. An attempt should be made to obtain union of the trochanter in the normal anatomic position. This is not always easy to accomplish because the nonunited fragment frequently is a shell of thin cortical bone, and the bone on which it lies is typically less than ideal. Nonetheless, numerous fixation devices are available to hold the fragment in place while an attempt is made at union.

These have included use of monofilament wires in an array of orientations, a Volz bolt, wire mesh, braided cables, and cable grip systems, to name a few of the devices that have been used to secure the trochanter (38).

In primary settings in which trochanteric osteotomy is performed, reattachment with three or four monofilament wires frequently is used. Sixteen or 18 gauge wire is simple to use, provides adequate strength, and is the least expensive material available for this technique (38). On the other hand, in revision settings in which the bony fragment often is a small shell of bone or in the case of a nonunion, the cable grip system provides additional means of securing the fragment while union is achieved.

Supplementing a poor bony bed with bone graft may increase the likelihood of achieving successful union of a nonunited fragment. If the trochanter is advanced to improve hip stability or fixation of the fragment is less than optimal, a spica cast with the leg held in abduction is recommended. This helps to relieve tension on the repair while the bone is allowed to unite in the desired position (36).

On rare occasions, releasing the origin of the abductors from the ilium is necessary to allow enough distal transfer of the trochanter to prevent excessive tension on the repair. This requires a subperiosteal dissection of the abductors off the ilium to their origin at the iliac crest. Electrocauterization is used to aid in the dissection. Careful avoidance of the superior gluteal neurovascular bundle as it courses anteriorly from the sciatic notch is imperative. A separate incision along the iliac crest may be necessary to release the abductors from their origin. The use of a postoperative spica cast with the leg held in abduction for 6 weeks is recommended for the muscle to scar down to its new bed (Fig. 2).

When inadequate tension on the soft tissues around the joint results in chronic instability, trochanteric advancement is one surgical option to restore tension. The trochanter is osteotomized and advanced distally to restore myofascial tension on the periarticular abductor sleeve. Ecklund (13) performed such a procedure on 21 patients for recurrent dislocation and stabilized 17 patients with this procedure alone. Three others needed additional operations to gain stability, and the fourth patient underwent resection of the components. Kaplan et al. (21) had similar success with 17 of 21 patients and deemed such a procedure indicated when other factors such as component malposition and impingement have been ruled out.

Another option gaining popularity is use of a constrained capture cup mechanism. Unlike the bipolar prosthesis, this allows the acetabular component to be fixed to the pelvis with a constrained interface within the cup. This affords added stability to the reconstruction through a greater range of motion but adds additional stresses on the

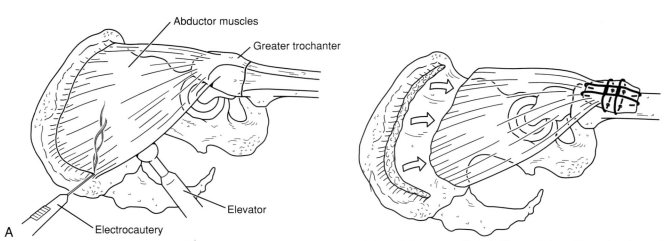

Figure 2. Proximal dissection of the abductors off their iliac origin with reattachment of the trochanter is sometimes necessary to avoid excessive tension on the ununited trochanter. **A:** Subperiosteal dissection of abductors off ilium with trochanteric advancement. **B:** Reattachment of advanced trochanter without excessive tension on repair.

acetabular prosthesis–bone interface. No results of long-term studies have been reported to date, but an article by Lombardi et al. (25) using the S-ROM constraining acetabular insert (Joint Medical Products, Stamford, Conn.) showed a reduction in dislocation rate for revision procedures from 19% to 4.5%. The follow-up period was 30 months, and as yet a significantly higher loosening rate has not been found. Five of the 50 patients had redislocations an additional eight times, one because of improper neck length and the others because of underlying neurologic problems.

Goetz (18) used a constraining acetabular component to treat 100 patients undergoing revision for recurrent dislocations. The average number of documented dislocations before revision was 5 and the mean number of prior hip replacements was 3. After a mean follow-up period of 4 years, 4 hips had redislocated (4%). Although it remains an option, this technique does not always definitively solve the problem, and the long-term results of increased interfacial stresses are not yet known.

Less commonly used solutions to the problems of instability around the hip caused by muscle weakness and abductor insufficiency include muscle transfers and soft-tissue slings. Besser (5) reported on use of the tensor fascia lata sling to the bed of the greater trochanter to provide stability to the hip. He reported use of this operation on a patient who underwent conversion from arthrodesis and had poor abductor function from long-term immobility. Tenodesis was performed of the tensor fascia to the bed of the greater trochanter to allow the proximal portion to function as an abductor. The hip was stable 2 years postoperatively.

On rare occasions, we have used the gluteus maximus as a sling that is rotated anteriorly and sutured to fascia lata, transferring the pull of the deficient abductors to the fascia lata. In addition, the tensor fascia femoris may be attached to the trochanter, providing anterior support as the hip rotates externally. This technique gives an additional option to a revision surgeon who may otherwise be left with an unstable reconstruction despite judicious use of all other options.

Enneking (14) described another method to replace or augment absent or deficient abductors in the tumor setting. It also can be used to treat patients undergoing revision who may need additional means to compensate for weakness resulting from prior reconstructive surgery. A 5-cm-wide strip of tensor fascia is peeled from distal in the thigh to the level of the trochanter and kept in continuity with its proximal extension. With the leg held in abduction, this strip is reattached to its bed and acts as an abductor sling through the tensor fascia lata. The limb is then maintained in a spica cast while the soft tissues heal (14).

A rare situation may arise in which the hip cannot be stabilized with any of the aforementioned methods and conversion to a Girdlestone arthroplasty is the only feasible option. Although this limits the patient in many ways, it is a solution that affords patients peace of mind and enables them to move forward in their lives without the constant fear of their hips dislocating without warning.

Patients undergoing revision arthroplasty and in certain primary operations when deficiency of the abductors exists either through muscular dysfunction, inadequate soft-tissue tension, or proximal migration of the greater trochanter, careful planning and early recognition of such a situation is vital to the success of hip reconstruction. The surgeon may change the operative approach, select an appropriate prosthesis, or change the postoperative protocol to achieve a stable reconstruction without recurrent instability or dislocation. Although the desired outcome may not always be achieved, recognizing these unique conditions should help prevent complications and allow both patient and surgeon to enjoy a successful surgical outcome.

REFERENCES

1. Amstutz H, Mai L, Schmidt I. Results of interlocking wire trochanteric reattachment and technique refinements to prevent complications following total hip arthroplasty. *Clin Orthop* 1984;183:82–89.
2. Amstutz H, Maki S. Complications of trochanteric osteotomy in total hip replacement. *J Bone Joint Surg Am* 1978;60:214–216.
3. Baker AS, Bitounis VC. Abductor function after total hip replacement. *J Bone Joint Surg Br* 1989;71:47–50.
4. Benton L, Salvati E, Root L. Reconstructive surgery in the myelomeningocele hip. *Clin Orthop* 1975;110:261–268.

5. Besser M. A muscle transfer to replace absent abductors in the conversion of a fused hip to a total hip arthroplasty. *Clin Orthop* 1982;162:173–174.

6. Boardman K, Bocco F, Charnley J. An evaluation method of trochanteric fixation using three wires in the Charnley low-friction arthroplasty. *Clin Orthop* 1978;132:31–38.

7. Borja F, Latta L, Stinchfield F, et al. Abductor performance in total hip arthroplasty with and without trochanteric osteotomy. *Clin Orthop* 1985;197:181–190.

8. Brewster R, Coventry M, Johnson E. Conversion of the arthrodesed hip to a total hip arthroplasty. *J Bone Joint Surg Am* 1975;57:27–30.

9. Bully R, Huo M, Root L, et al. Total hip arthroplasty in cerebral palsy. *Clin Orthop* 1993;296:148–153.

10. Carlsson A, Gentz C. Postoperative dislocation in the Charnley and Brunswick total hip arthroplasy. *Clin Orthop* 1977;125:177–182.

11. Coventry M. Late dislocations in patients with Charnley total hip arthroplasty. *J Bone Joint Surg Am* 1985;67:832–841.

12. Crowe J, Mani J, Ranawat C. Total hip replacement in congenital dislocation and dysplasia of the hip. *J Bone Joint Surg Am* 1979;61:15–23.

13. Ecklund A. Trochanteric osteotomy for recurrent dislocation of total hip arthroplasty. *J Arthroplasty* 1993;8:629–632.

14. Enneking W. *Musculoskeletal tumor surgery.* New York: Churchill Livingstone, 1983.

15. Fackler CD, Poss R. Dislocation in total hip arthroplasty. *Clin Orthop* 1980;151:169–178.

16. Fraser G, Wroblewski B. Revision of the Charnley low-friction arthroplasty. *J Bone Joint Surg Br* 1981;63B(4):552–555.

17. Glassman A. Complications of trochanteric osteotomy. *Orthop Clin* 1992;23:321–333.

18. Goetz D. Salvage of total hip instability with a constrained acetabular component. Presented at the Harris Hip Course; 1996; Oct, Boston, Mass.

19. Herold H. Congenital dislocation of the hip treated by total hip arthroplasty. *Clin Orthop* 1998;242:195–200.

20. Johnston R. Clinical follow up of total hip replacement. *Clin Orthop* 1973;95:118–126.

21. Kaplan S, Thomas W, Poss R. Trochanteric advancement for recurrent dislocation after total hip replacement. *J Arthroplasty* 1987;2:119–124.

22. Kristiansen B, Jorgensen L, Holmich P. Dislocation following total hip arthroplasty. *Arch Orthop Trauma Surg* 1985;103:375–377.

23. Lindberg H, Carlsson A, Gentz C, et al. Recurrent and non-recurrent dislocation following total hip arthroplasty. *Acta Orthop Scand* 1982;53:947–952.

24. Linde F, Jensen J. Socket loosening in arthroplasty for congenital dislocation of the hip. *Acta Orthop Scand* 1988;59:254–257.

25. Lombardi V, Mallory T, Kraus T, Vaughn B. Preliminary report on the S-ROM constraining acetabular insert. *Orthopedics* 1991;153:147–152.

26. Lubahn J, Evarts M, Feltner J. Conversion of ankylosed hips to total hip arthroplasty. *Clin Orthop* 1980;153:147–152.

27. McLeish RD, Charnley J. Abduction forces in the one legged stance. *J Biomech* 1970;3:191–209.

28. Minns RJ, Crawford B, Porter M, et al. Muscle strength following total hip replacement. *J Arthroplasty* 1993;8:625–627.

29. Morrey B. Instability after total hip replacement. *Orthop Clin North Am* 1992;23:237–247.

30. Murray P, Gore D, Brewer B, et al. Comparison of Müller total hip replacement with and without trochanteric osteotomy. *Acta Orthop Scand* 1981;52:345–352.

31. Nutton R, Checketts R. The effects of trochanteric osteotomy of abductor power. *J Bone Joint Surg Br* 1984;66:180–183.

32. Poss R. Factors contibuting to a marked decrease in the incidence of dislocation following THA. Presented at the Vail Total Knee and Hip Replacement Symposium; 1997; Jan; Vail, Colo.

33. Reikeras O, Bjerkheim I, Gundersson R. Total hip arthroplasty for arthrodesed hips. *J Arthroplasty* 1995;10:529–531.

34. Ritter M, Groe T, Stringer E. Functional significance of nonunion of the greater trochanter. *Clin Orthop* 1981;159:177–182.

35. Roberts J, Fu F, McClain E, et al. A comparison of the dislocated hip and anterolateral approach to total hip arthroplasty. *Clin Orthop* 1983;187:205–209.

36. Robinson R, Robinson H, Salvati E. Comparison of the transtrochanteric and posterior approaches for total hip replacement. *Clin Orthop* 1980;147:143.

37. Root L, Goss J, Mendes J. Treatment of painful hip in cerbral palsy by total hip arthroplasty or hip arthrodesis. *J Bone Joint Surg Am* 1986;68:590–598.

38. Silverton C. In: *The adult hip (in press).*

39. Simon S. Anatomy, physiology, and mechanics of skeletal muscle. In: *Orthopedic basic science.* American Academy of Orthopaedic Surgeons, 1994:106.

40. Strathy G, Fitzgerald R. Total hip arthroplasty in the ankylosed hip. *J Bone Joint Surg Am* 1988;70:963–966.

41. Vicar A, Coleman C. A comparison of the anterolateral, transtrochanteric, and posterior surgical approaches in primary total hip arthroplasty. *Clin Orthop* 1984;188:153–159.

42. Williams J, Gottesman M, Mallory T. Dislocation after total hip arthrplasty. *Clin Orthop* 1982;171;53–58.

43. Woo R, Morrey B. Dislocations after total hip arthroplasty. *J Bone Joint Surg Am* 1982;64:1295–1306.

Special Considerations

Revision Total Hip Arthroplasty,
edited by Marvin E. Steinberg and Jonathan P. Garino,
Lippincott Williams & Wilkins, Philadelphia © 1999.

36

Resection Arthroplasty

Marvin E. Steinberg and Jonathan P. Garino

Resection arthroplasty of the hip, often referred to as a Girdlestone pseudarthrosis, is a procedure that was used initially to manage tuberculous or septic arthritis of the hip. Before the development of total hip replacement, it was also used as a primary arthroplasty for patients with advanced stages of osteoarthritis and rheumatoid arthritis. After the development of total hip replacement, resection arthroplasty rarely was used as a primary arthroplasty. Today it serves primarily to salvage a failed and usually infected total hip replacement or endoprosthesis.

BACKGROUND

Resection arthroplasty was initially described by Smaltz in 1817 and later by White in 1821, both of whom used it for the treatment of children with tuberculosis of the hip. In 1861 Fock described this procedure for the management of severe osteoarthritis of the hip. It was introduced into the United States in 1871 by Sayre. G. R. Girdlestone, professor of orthopaedic surgery at the Nuffield Orthopaedic Centre, Oxford, England, gained considerable experience with resection arthroplasty and used it to treat patients with a variety of infectious and noninfectious conditions. He published his findings in 1943 and 1945. Eventually this procedure came to bear his name (8,9).

Before the development of total hip replacement, resection arthroplasty or Girdlestone pseudarthrosis was used not infrequently in England and on continental Europe as a primary arthroplasty for the treatment of patients with advanced stages of osteoarthritis and rheumatoid arthritis. It consisted of resection of the entire femoral head and neck at the intertrochanteric line, and the projecting edges of the acetabulum to leave two

M. E. Steinberg and J. P. Garino: Department of Orthopaedic Surgery, Hospital of the University of Pennsylvania, Philadelphia, Pennsylvania 19104.

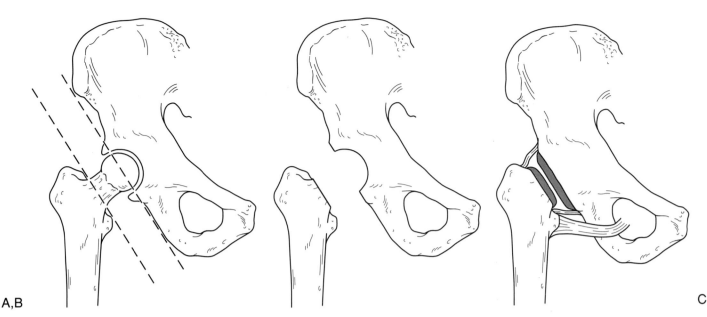

A,B   C

Figure 1. Resection arthroplasty. **A:** Location of bone resection is indicated by *dotted lines.* **B:** Resection should produce smooth, parallel surfaces on the pelvis and proximal femur. **C:** After healing, a pseudarthrosis develops, and dense, fibrous tissue or fibrocartilage covers the articulating surfaces of the pelvis and femur. The iliopsoas tendon, capsule, and scar tissue prevent excessive proximal migration.

relatively smooth parallel surfaces (Fig. 1A and 1B). Patients were placed in skeletal traction for 6 weeks after the operation and then into an ischial weight-bearing brace for an additional 6 months. The goal was to keep the femur in a distal position to preserve as much length as possible and to allow development of fibrocartilage on the opposing surfaces of the proximal femur and the acetabulum that would act as a false joint or pseudarthrosis. (Fig. 1C). It is important not to leave prominent bony projections from the margins of the acetabulum or the femoral neck because these would impinge on each other, prevent formation of a smooth articular surface covered with fibrocartilage, and cause pain and disability. After the operation, patients usually develop a good range of motion and satisfactory relief of pain; however, most hips are grossly unstable and are an average of $1\frac{1}{2}$ inches short. Patients routinely have a marked abductor lurch and normally require the use of at least one cane. The results generally do not deteriorate with time (8,9,13,14,20–23).

INDICATIONS AND PATIENT SELECTION

Resection arthroplasty of the hip rarely is used today as a primary arthroplasty, although it still has a limited role in special circumstances in which hip reconstruction is needed but total hip replacement is contraindicated. Resection arthroplasty is used most often in the management of a failed and often infected total hip or endoprosthesis. The most common cause of failure of a total hip is aseptic loosening. These patients generally are treated with one-stage total hip revision. Less than 10% of hip revisions are done for sepsis. Under ideal circumstances, this revision might be performed as a one-stage procedure or exchange arthroplasty. In most instances, however, a two-stage procedure is indicated. The first step is resection arthroplasty to remove all devitalized soft tissue and foreign material so that the infection can be eradicated and a total hip reimplanted a later date. The interval usually ranges from 6 weeks to 1 year.

Not infrequently, resection arthroplasty serves as a definitive procedure. This may be indicated in managing a septic hip in which virulent and resistant organisms are present and there is no assurance that the infection has been eradicated. It might also be indicated in managing both septic and nonseptic hips in which extensive bone loss, usually in the acetabulum, has occurred, making reimplantation of a new prosthesis technically difficult and prone to early failure (12). In other cases general medical debility, neurologic disorders, and poor potential for rehabilitation might be contraindications to total hip replacement. In such instances realistic goals might be limited to relief of pain and control of infection with limited potential for walking. In still other circumstances, the patient may be satisfied with the outcome of resection arthroplasty and prefer not to undergo additional surgical treatment.

SURGICAL TECHNIQUE

The surgical technique in large part is determined by the specific problems being addressed and the short- and long-term goals of surgery. Among the most important considerations are whether the hip is septic, how much bone stock is available, and whether the resection arthroplasty is to serve as a temporizing or a permanent procedure (3,15,22).

Septic Joints

If the joint is infected, the immediate goal must be eradication of infection. This can be best accomplished by means of aggressive débridement of devitalized soft tissue and removal of all foreign material. Most studies have shown that the chance for eradicating infection is best if all cement is removed. There are circumstances, however, in which it might be prudent to leave behind a small amount of well-fixed cement rather than risk gross destruction of bone or damage to vital structures. If possible, the greater trochanter and abductor mechanism are left intact. Bone grafting generally is not done in the presence of active infection. The procedure can be performed through a number of surgical approaches. It is usually best to use the previous incision if possible.

Most of the time the goal is to reinsert a total hip at some point in the future, after the infection has been eradicated. Under these circumstances, certain modifications are made in the technique described for a classic primary Girdlestone procedure. The margins of the acetabulum are left in place to be available to support a new acetabular component. The remaining femoral neck is preserved.

Not infrequently resection arthroplasty serves as a definitive procedure. If this is anticipated, it is advisable to perform a classic resection arthroplasty, removing projecting margins of the acetabulum and resecting the femoral neck at the intertrochanteric line to provide two smooth articulating surfaces for the pseudarthrosis (Figs. 2 and 3). Some surgeons have advocated leaving the remaining femoral neck intact. Although this may provide increased stability, it usually leads to increased pain and decreased patient satisfaction with the procedure (4,10,18). At times it is uncertain whether the resection arthroplasty will serve only a temporary function or be a definitive procedure. In such cases the amount of bone resected should fall between the two extremes described earlier. In general the margins of the acetabulum are left intact, whereas a prominent femoral neck is resected close to the lesser trochanter.

To deliver a high concentration of antibiotic to the region, antibiotic-impregnated beads or spacers can be inserted before wound closure. Spacers also have the theoretical advantage of preserving limb length and tissue planes for delayed prosthetic insertion. The use of a modified femoral prosthesis coated with antibiotic-impregnated cement also provides a functional joint while the patient awaits the definitive procedure. The disadvantages of using such large spacers are that they provide a lower concentration of antibiotic than do beads because of the decreased surface area; they remain in place and act as foreign bodies until a second major operative procedure is performed; and they eliminate the possibility that resection arthroplasty will serve as a definitive procedure. Antibiotic-impregnated beads, on the other hand, provide a higher dose of local antibiotic and can be removed at any time with a minor procedure performed under local anesthesia. If adequate débridement of foreign material and devitalized tissue has been accomplished,

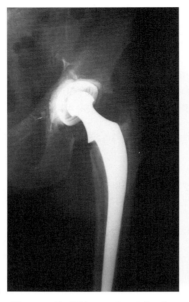
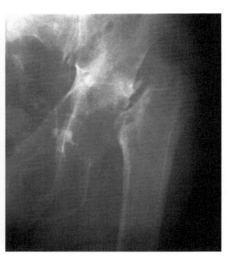

A

B

Figure 2. This patient had a postoperative infection that did not respond to incision and drainage and prolonged antibiotic treatment. **A:** Radiograph obtained before removal of components. **B:** Radiographs 2 years after resection arthroplasty. Ten years after the operation, the patient's functional result was so good that he refused conversion to a total hip replacement.

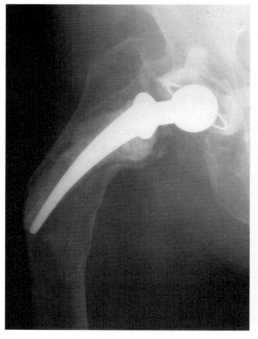
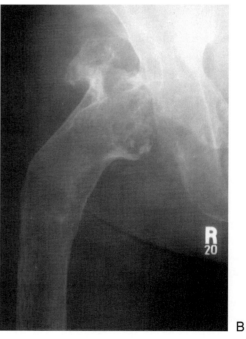

A

B

Figure 3. After total hip replacement, this patient sustained a fracture of the proximal femur, which healed in varus. The femoral component became loose and painful. At the revision operation the hip was found to be infected, and resection arthroplasty was performed. **A:** Before resection arthroplasty. **B:** After resection arthroplasty. The patient had essentially no pain and reasonable function and declined conversion to a total hip replacement, which would have required osteotomy of the proximal femur.

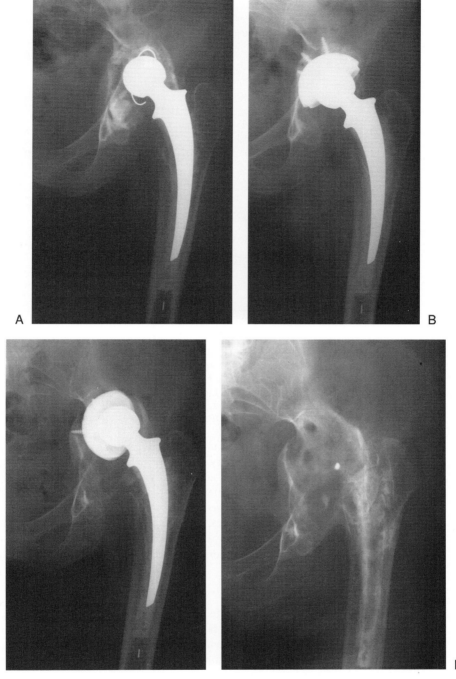

Figure 4. A 38 year old nurse with severe generalized rheumatoid arthritis underwent revision of a loose cemented acetabular component. **A:** Before revision. **B:** Loss of acetabular bone stock at the time of revision was managed with grafting and insertion of an uncemented acetabulum. **C:** The acetabulum continued to migrate medially and superiorly and spun into retroversion. **D:** At the time of the operation, substantial loss of acetabular bone stock was found, and it was elected to perform a resection arthroplasty rather than attempt another revision. This option had been discussed with the patient preoperatively. The patient continued to function well after the operation and preferred not to undergo another attempt at total hip replacement.

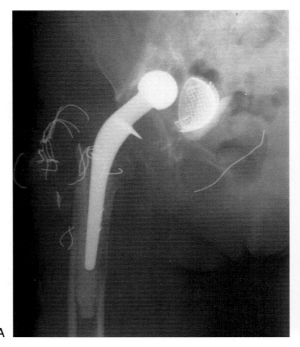
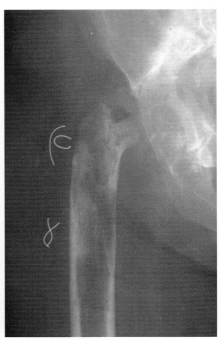

A
B

Figure 5. After total hip replacement, this patient had loosening of the femoral component, avulsion of the greater trochanter, and fracture of the medial wall of the acetabulum with marked protrusion. The acetabular component was removed through a retroperitoneal approach. **A:** Prior to component removal. **B:** After two-stage resection arthroplasty. A large defect in the acetabulum was found at the operation, and the patient's medical status was such that attempts to reinsert a total hip replacement were contraindicated.

it is best to close the wound primarily leaving a suction drain in place. Rarely is it advisable to do a secondary closure or pack the wound open for granulation (18).

Postoperatively patients are treated with appropriate antibiotics. Some surgeons prefer to maintain the limb in skeletal or skin traction initially and then protect the joint with an ischial weight-bearing brace. In most instances the advantages of early mobilization outweigh the disadvantages, and the joint can be protected by minimal weight bearing with the use of crutches or a walker rather than use of a brace. In revision surgery, there is no evidence that postoperative traction or bracing effectively alters the end result.

Aseptic Joints

When treating a noninfected hip with resection arthroplasty, measures specifically designed to eradicate infection are not required. Complete removal of cement, especially that well fixed distally within the femoral canal, is not necessary, and soft tissue débridement can be more limited. If it is anticipated that a prosthesis will be reinserted at a later time, defects in the acetabulum and proximal femur can be reconstituted with appropriate grafts placed at the time of initial resection. These require several months to mature before they are ready to accept the insertion of a new prosthesis. If a secondary procedure is not anticipated, grafting is less indicated, although some surgeons prefer to graft the proximal femoral canal to provide a broad, smooth surface for the pseudarthrosis. However, because the proximal femur often comes to lie in the soft tissues lateral and proximal to the hip rather than articulating with the lateral wall of the pelvis, this may not be necessary (Figs. 4 and 5).

RESULTS

Opinions vary as to the effectiveness of resection arthroplasty as a definitive procedure. It is generally agreed that the results when this operation is used to salvage a failed total hip are not as good as those achieved when it is used as a primary procedure. If infection is present, it is controlled or eradicated in more than 90% of cases. Passive range of motion is good, although active motion is limited. Limbs generally are 1 to 2 inches short with a mean shortening of $1\frac{1}{2}$ inches. A shoe lift is needed. These hips are unstable, and virtually all patients have a marked limp. Some are able to walk short distances without support, but most patients need at least one cane. Occasionally two canes, crutches, or even a walker are needed for longer distances. With careful surgical technique and postoperative care, most patients have no pain at rest and little pain with activity. The reported degree of patient satisfaction varies widely. This is, of course, a highly subjective evaluation of outcome by both patient and physician and is determined in large part by preoperative expectations. Good relief of pain usually can be achieved by more than 80% of patients, whereas hip function per se often is considered unsatisfactory because of the inherent shortening and instability that result. If the hip on which resection arthroplasty has been performed is compared with a normal hip or even a well-functioning total hip replacement, the outcome will be considered disappointing. If, however, the procedure is put into proper perspective and is viewed as a necessary compromise with the advantages and disadvantages kept clearly in mind, there will be a much greater degree of satisfaction on the part of both patient and physician (1,3,4,10,13–15,20,22).

CONVERSION OF RESECTION ARTHROPLASTY TO TOTAL HIP REPLACEMENT

Under most circumstances resection arthroplasty is only temporary, and a total hip is reinserted after eradication of infection or maturation of bone graft. Resection arthroplasty should not be undertaken lightly, because many intraoperative and postoperative complications can be encountered. The operation may be technically difficult, time consuming, and associated with large blood loss. Anatomic features are distorted, and it is often difficult to identify important neurovascular structures. Pains therefore must be taken to avoid injury to the sciatic and femoral nerves and to major regional vessels.

Some degree of limb shortening will be present, although with a moderate amount of soft tissue dissection enough length can be restored so that a hip can be inserted without undue difficulty. Trochanteric osteotomy and abductor compromise should be avoided. Loss of bone stock and considerable osteoporosis of both the proximal femur and acetabulum are frequently encountered, and all the bone must be treated with extreme care to avoid intrapelvic perforation or femoral fracture. These complications have been reported both during insertion of components and during reduction of the hip after component insertion. It is frequently advisable to use bone graft to supplement deficient bone stock in the acetabulum or proximal femur. At times a proximal femoral replacement prosthesis may be needed. Perhaps the most frequent and most serious complication encountered is reactivation of infection. This often leads to a poor outcome (17). It is therefore mandatory that previously infected hips be evaluated thoroughly both before and during prosthesis reinsertion to be certain that residual infection is not present. If cemented components are to be used, it is generally accepted that appropriate antibiotics be placed in the cement. Some surgeons favor revision with uncemented components; it has not been established which technique results in a lower incidence of postoperative sepsis (7,19). Because of soft-tissue laxity and poor muscle tone, postoperative dislocation may be encountered (Fig. 6). If there is any question about the stability of the hip at the time of closure, an abduction brace should be worn postoperatively for at least 6 weeks.

Careful preoperative planning, surgical technique, and postoperative care are required to minimize the many possible complications attendant with reinsertion of a total hip after resection arthroplasty. Complications are considerably more frequent, and results are not as good as after primary total hip replacement arthroplasty. Therefore both surgeon and patient should give serious thought to whether it is advisable to proceed with conversion to a second total hip if the patient has a well-functioning resection arthroplasty. However,

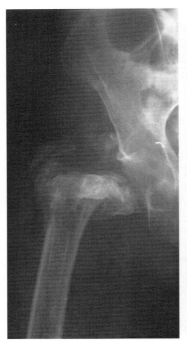
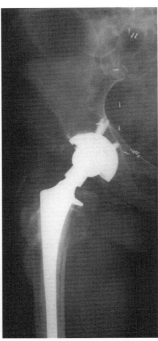

A   B

Figure 6. A bipolar endoprosthesis was inserted for a femoral neck fracture. It became infected and necessitated removal and wide débridement. The patient was dissatisfied with her status and requested total hip replacement. **A:** Status before reinsertion of total hip replacement. Avulsion and fragmentation of the greater trochanter are present. **B:** Status after reinsertion of total hip replacement. Soft-tissue laxity was found at the operation, and the patient sustained a dislocation postoperatively. This was managed with an abduction brace. The final outcome was satisfactory.

with thorough preoperative planning and careful surgical technique, satisfactory results should be achieved for at least 85% to 90% of patients (2,5,6,7,11,16,17,19).

SUMMARY

Before the development of successful total hip replacement arthroplasty, resection arthroplasty or Girdlestone pseudarthrosis was used not only for management of a septic hip but also as primary arthroplasty for the treatment of hips afflicted with advanced stages of arthritis. With careful attention to operative and postoperative details, satisfactory results could usually be achieved provided that both patient and physician understood the advantages and disadvantages of this procedure and had realistic expectations. Today primary resection arthroplasty has only limited use in selected circumstances. Its main role is salvage of a failed and usually infected total hip replacement or endoprosthesis. If used to treat an infected hip, resection arthroplasty most often is a temporizing procedure used to eradicate infection with the anticipation that it will be converted to a total hip replacement at a later time. Under selected circumstances, resection arthroplasty may be the definitive procedure. These include inability to eradicate infection, substantial loss of bone stock, and treatment of an ill and debilitated patient with a poor chance of rehabilitation. Not infrequently a patient finds that the pain relief and functional results afforded by resection arthroplasty are quite acceptable and questions whether he or she should undergo further surgical treatment. The surgeon must place these alternatives into perspective and acknowledge the possibility of intraoperative or postoperative complications and a less than optimum outcome. The surgeon then can help this patient determine whether to accept resection arthroplasty as a definitive procedure or proceed with an attempt to improve the results by means of insertion of a second total hip replacement.

REFERENCES

1. Ballard WT, Lowry DA, Brand RA. Resection arthroplasty of the hip. *J Arthroplasty* 1995:10:772–779.
2. Berman AT, Mazur D. Conversion of resection arthroplasty to total hip replacement. *Orthopedics* 1994;17:1155–1158.
3. Bourne RB, Hunter GA, Rorabeck CH, Macnab JJ. A six-year follow-up of infected total hip replacements managed by Girdlestone's arthroplasty. *J Bone Joint Surg Br* 1984;66:340–343.
4. Canner GC, Steinberg ME, Heppenstall RB, Balderston R. The infected total hip prosthesis. *J Bone Joint Surg Am* 1984;66:1393–1399.
5. Carlsson AS, Josefsson G, Lindberg L. Revision with gentamicin-impregnated cement for deep infections in total hip arthroplasties. *J Bone Joint Surg Am* 1978;60:1059–1064.
6. Engelbrecht E, Siegel A, Kappus M. Total hip endoprosthesis following resection arthroplasty. *Orthopade* 1995;24:344–352.
7. Fitzgerald RH Jr. Treatment of the infected THA: indirect exchange arthroplasty. In: Galante, JO, Rosenberg, AG, Callaghan, JJ, eds. *Total hip revision surgery.* New York: Raven Press, 1995:495–587.
8. Girdlestone GR. Acute pyogenic arthritis of the hip: an operation giving free access and effective drainage [Reprinted]. *Clin Orthop* 1982;170:3–7.
9. Girdlestone GR. Pseudarthrosis: discussion on the treatment of unilateral osteoarthritis of the hip joint. *Proc R Soc Med* 1945;38:363.
10. Grauer JD, Amstutz HC, O'Carroll PF, Dorey FJ. Resection arthroplasty of the hip. *J Bone Joint Surg Am* 1989;71:669–678.
11. Hanssen AD, Mariani EM, Kavanagh BF, Coventry MB. Resection arthroplasty. In: Morrey BF, ed. *Joint replacement arthroplasty.* New York: Churchill Livingstone, 1991:891–897.
12. Harris WH, White RE, Resection arthroplasty for nonseptic failure of total hip arthroplasty. *Clin Orthop* 1982;171:62–67.
13. Kantor GS, Osterkamp JA, Dorr LD, et al. Resection arthroplasty following infected total hip replacement arthroplasty. *J Arthroplasty* 1986;1:83–89.
14. Marchetti PG, Toni A, Baldini N, et al. Clinical evaluation of 104 hip resection arthroplasties after removal of a total hip prosthesis. *J Arthroplasty* 1987;2:37–41.
15. McElwaine JB, Colville J. Excision arthroplasty for infected total hip replacement. *J Bone Joint Surg Br* 1984;66:168–171.
16. Nestor BJ, Hanssen AD, Ferrer-Gonzalez R, Fitzgerald RH. The use of porous prothesis in delayed reconstruction of total hip replacements that have failed because of infection. *J Bone Joint Surg Am* 1994;76:349–359.
17. Pagnano MW, Trousdale RT, Hanssen AD. Outcome after reinfection following reimplantation hip arthroplasty. *Clin Orthop* 1997;338;192–204.
18. Petty W, Goldsmith S. Resection arthroplasty following infected total hip arthroplasty. *J Bone Joint Surg Am* 1980;62:889–896.
19. Salvati EA. Primary exchange of the infected total hip replacement. In: Galante JO, Rosenberg AG, Callaghan JJ, eds. *Total Hip Revision Surgery.* New York: Raven Press, 1995:487–493.
20. Scalvi A, Campacci A, Marcer M, et al. Girdlestone arthroplasty for loosening of the total hip prosthesis: evaluation and results. *Chir Organi Mov* 1995;80:279–285.
21. Somerville EW. Girdlestone pseudarthrosis of the hip. In: Rob C, Smith R, eds. *Operative surgery: orthopaedics.* Part I. Philadelphia: Lippincott, 1969.
22. Steinberg ME, Steinberg DR. Resection arthroplasty of the hip. In: Steinberg ME, ed. *The hip and its disorders.* Philadelphia: WB Saunders, 1991:770–787.
23. Taylor RG. Pseudarthrosis of the hip joint. *J Bone Joint Surg Br* 1950;32:161–165.

Revision Total Hip Arthroplasty,
edited by Marvin E. Steinberg and Jonathan P. Garino,
Lippincott Williams & Wilkins, Philadelphia © 1999.

37

Conversion of the Arthrodesed Hip to Total Hip Replacement

Ohannes A. Nercessian

Surgical arthrodesis of the hip joint is being performed less frequently nowadays. Before the development and popularization of total hip arthroplasty, hip arthrodesis was a commonly performed orthopedic procedure for a variety of diseases and conditions affecting the hip joint. Septic arthritis, posttraumatic arthritis, and painful pseudoarthrosis were primary indications for hip arthrodesis. Orthopedic residents nowadays are infrequently exposed to the surgical arthrodesis of the hip joint because most patients prefer a painless mobile hip over a painless arthrodesed hip. Although a variety of surgical techniques have been described in the literature, some of the newer techniques have been advocated to maximize the success rate of arthrodesis. A cobra plate is used to achieve a stable compression across the hip joint and improve the rate of arthrodeses. However, use of a cobra plate can cause considerable damage to the great trochanter and abductor mechanism of the hip joint. Most residents during their training have been exposed to only a few hip arthrodesis procedures, and few have developed the technical expertise to perform a hip fusion comfortably. However, surgical arthrodesis of the hip joint despite its limitations remains a valid alternative for a selected group of patients even in modern times. This is especially true among young and very active patients who place tremendous loads on their hips such as manual laborers and farmers. Arthrodesis should be performed in a way that causes the least possible damage to bone and soft tissues so that possible future conversion to total hip arthroplasty can be done without technical problems and complications.

Patients who have obtained many years of satisfactory painless hip function from an

O. A. Nercessian: Department of Orthopaedic Surgery, Columbia Presbyterian Medical Center, New York, NY 10032.

arthrodesed hip frequently become dissatisfied later in life because of symptoms associated with secondary degenerative changes that develop in the lower back, both knees, and the contralateral hip. In one study (3) it was reported that close to 60% of patients who underwent surgical arthrodesis of the hip had considerable low back pain later in life because of degenerative changes. A larger percentage of patients have ipsilateral knee pain and contralateral hip pain. Similar findings have been observed by other authors (13,14,20). In some instances spontaneous hip fusion developed, such as after a hip infection ankylosing arthritis, or traumatic injury to the hip joint. Hip arthrodesis in these conditions may not be in the optimal position and can lead to severe functional disability and gait pattern disturbances. In these conditions disability from low back pain or ipsilateral knee pain can be more dramatic. Most orthopedic surgeons advocate that during surgical fusion the hip be placed at 30 degrees of flexion, 5 degrees of adduction, and neutral rotation. The literature suggests that spontaneous fusion of the hip can result in deformity and an abnormal position of the hip joint (4,9,10). This condition often times becomes more symptomatic with respect to lower back pain and ipsilateral knee pain.

INDICATIONS

The most common symptoms that lead a patient to consider conversion of an arthrodesed hip to total hip arthroplasty are low back pain, generalized functional disability, ipsilateral knee pain, and contralateral hip pain. No hip fusion should be converted to total hip arthroplasty without objective clinical findings of pain and functional disability. Prior infection in the ipsilateral hip for which a fusion was undertaken also must not be taken lightly. Although some reports (13) suggest there is no correlation between the old infection and total hip arthroplasty, regardless of the time elapsed between fusion and the contemplated total hip arthroplasty, activation of an old infection can be a real possibility. Low back pain associated with an arthrodesed hip is caused by the degenerative changes in the lumbosacral spine that can develop over a period of many years (Fig. 1). Among patients with an ankylosed hip, these changes may be related to alterations in body mechanics that develop to compensate for the immobilized hip. In a gait analysis study (8) of patients with an arthrodesed hip, it was demonstrated that there is increased pelvic tilt in the anteroposterior plane that appears to be one of the causes of the increased stress on the lumbosacral spine. There is also increased pelvic rotation, which is an apparent attempt to increase stride length. Some of this limitation of rotation of the hip is translated to the ipsilateral knee, foot, and ankle. It has been demonstrated that the ipsilateral knee remains relatively more flexed throughout the stance phase. All these accommodations can lead to degenerative changes in the ipsilateral knee (3,20–22) and at times the contralateral hip. Callaghan et al.(3) reported that 60% of patients with an arthrodesed hip have a symptomatic contralateral hip due to degenerative changes.

Follow-up studies have indicated that conversion of hip arthrodesis to total hip arthroplasty is desired by many patients for restoration of the hip motion. Although postconversion motion is less than achieved after routine total hip arthroplasty, the motion is greatly appreciated by patients who have had functional limitation from the immobile hip. Many studies (1,2,5,10,12,15–19,22) have indicated that the end result of conversion of hip arthrodesis to total hip arthroplasty is not as good as after primary operations and that the result takes longer to achieve. Conversion of a surgically arthrodesed hip to total hip arthroplasty also is more prone to complications than conversion from spontaneous arthrodesis.

Regardless of the type of arthrodesis performed, several technical details must be considered in the care of patients who undergo hip arthroplasty. The most important considerations for patients with arthrodesed hip undergoing conversion arthroplasty are the physical condition of the greater trochanter, the status of the abductor muscles, the limitation of motion, the persistence of limp, and possible use of a walking aid. A concern about the physiologic status of the abductor muscle is a real one.

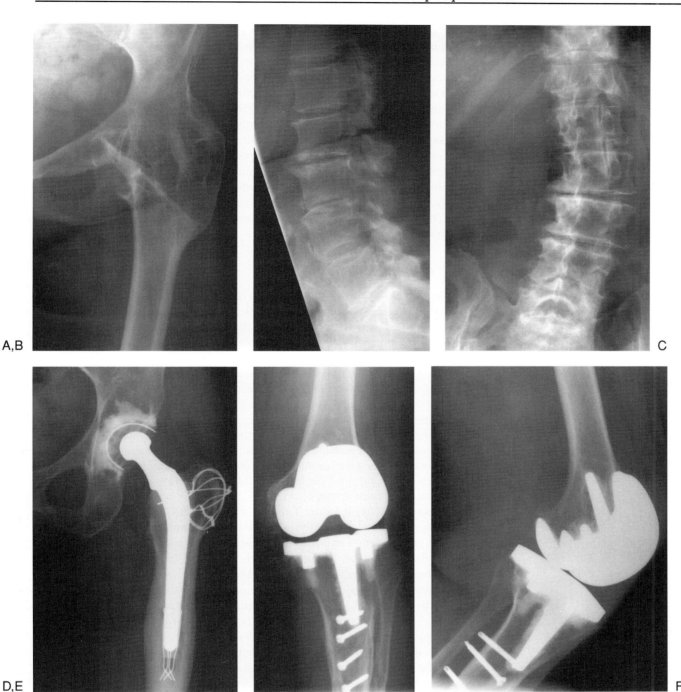

Figure 1. A: A 73-year-old woman underwent arthrodesis of the left hip for arthritis at the age of 37 years and did well for many years. **B,C:** At the age of 60 years she began to have pain in the upsilateral knee and lumbosacral region. **D:** Conversion of the arthrodesed hip to total hip replacement was performed. Radiograph of the left hip 13 years after conversion arthroplasty. **E,F:** The patient subsequently needed left total knee replacement. Radiograph of the left total knee 11 years after replacement.

Preoperative electromyographic evaluation of the abductor muscles has been performed on patients who have undergone hip fusion. The studies, however, did not prove to be of sufficient value, and their routine use is not warranted. An overall clinical and radiographic examination is important. It is not always possible to determine the degree of muscle function when the hip has been arthrodesed. The function and the strength of the abductor muscle usually are compromised in arthrodesed hips. Abductor muscle strength gradually returns to most patients, however, over several years after conversion to total hip arthroplasty, providing the abductors were not excised during the original arthrodesis and their attachments to the greater trochanter have remained intact. It is important to evaluate preconversion radiographs to determine whether the abductor mechanism and the greater trochanter have been violated. Careful planning of the procedure is warranted to achieve a successful outcome. Although limited range of motion of the hip is expected after conversion of hip arthrodesis to total hip arthroplasty, relief of back, knee, and contralateral hip pain is substantial, and most patients are pleased with the outcome despite residual stiffness and limping after conversion. The best clinical result after conversion of hip fusion to total hip arthroplasty occurs among patients who had a spontaneously fused hip. Patients who have undergone repeated operations before the hip fusion have been reported to have more complications and poorer outcome after conversion to total hip arthroplasty (14,22).

SURGICAL CONSIDERATIONS

Many factors influence the technical aspects of conversion of a hip fusion to a total hip arthroplasty. These factors include the patient's age and diagnosis at the time of fusion, the position of the fusion, the state of the greater trochanter and the abductor mechanism, and the presence of previous infection. Conversion of fused hip to total hip arthroplasty is a complex surgical procedure with many inherent potential complications. It is advisable that surgeons without extensive experience with surgery of the hip joint not undertake this type of reconstructive procedure. The principle goals in conversion are to improve range of motion of the hip, alleviate strain on the back and ipsilateral knee, and in hips with malunion or nonunion correct the deformity and relieve pain. Careful planning is mandatory before such complex procedures. Correct placement of the acetabular component in the true acetabulum is important in restoring the normal biomechanics of the hip joint (11,23). Many important landmarks may have been lost, and the surgeon should make every effort and place the component in near-anatomic position.

Important technical consideration must be observed during conversion total hip arthroplasty. Most surgeons advocate use of the transtrochanteric approach (6,8). This is important to provide good exposure to the acetabulum and the neck of the femur. Trochanteric osteotomy also minimizes further damage to an already weakened abductor mechanism. After osteotomy of the greater trochanter, the abductor mechanism is retracted superiorly for exposure of the neck of the femur. The next step is to clear the tissue around the neck of the femur and perform an osteotomy on the femoral neck. The osteotomy of the neck is done carefully to not damage the surrounding neurovascular structures, especially the sciatic nerve. Osteotomy of the femoral neck is done *in situ* with meticulous technique close to the acetabulum. After osteotomy of the neck of the femur the proximal soft tissue around the neck is released for exposure of the acetabulum. The exact location and the site of the original acetabulum are determined. This can be difficult because of the type of fusion and hardware and extraarticular bone graft used in fusion. Error in selection of the site of the acetabulum may lead to complications such as perforation and fracture. After the location of the acetabulum is identified, the acetabulum is excavated. A variety of techniques can be used. Gouges may be used initially followed by progressively larger reamers. Despite the method selected, care must be exercised not to perforate the acetabulum. Reaming eccentically can damage the anterior or posterior wall (Fig. 2). Proper reaming and opening of the acetabulum is required for correct placement of the acetabular component, which is necessary to assure stability of the hip joint. Maximum clearance between the upper end of the femur and the pelvis must be achieved to provide good range of motion. In a similar manner recanalization of the upper femur is done carefully. To prevent fracture, maneuvering of the hip joint should not be overzealous. Stability of the hip must be achieved during trial reduction

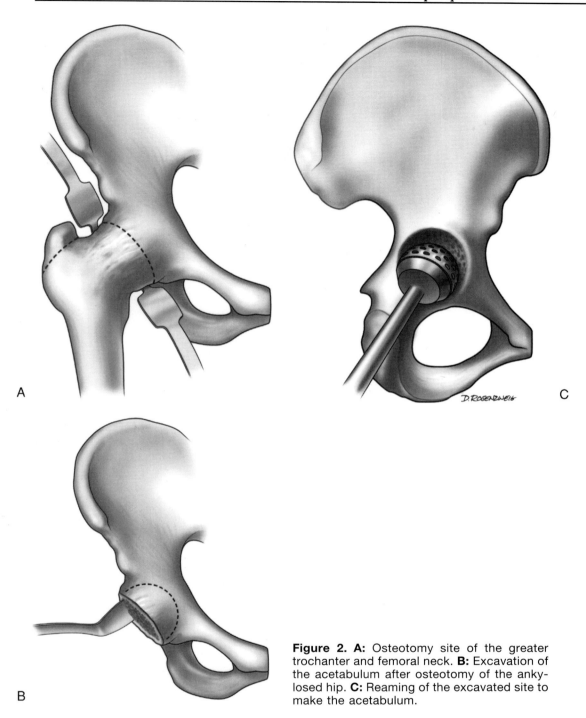

Figure 2. A: Osteotomy site of the greater trochanter and femoral neck. **B:** Excavation of the acetabulum after osteotomy of the ankylosed hip. **C:** Reaming of the excavated site to make the acetabulum.

by establishing good myofascial sleeve tension. Reattachment of the greater trochanter at the appropriate level also is essential to restore proper myofascial tension.

POSTOPERATIVE CARE

Two important factors are important after conversion of hip arthrodesis to total hip arthroplasty—abductor weakness and trochanteric complications. The abductors can remain weak for long periods after conversion of hip arthrodesis to total hip arthroplasty. Many patients, however, demonstrate improvement in strength postoperatively over

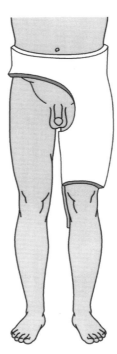

Figure 3. Short single-leg spica cast. Patients are immobilized for 6 weeks. The cast allows the patient to walk and sit on a raised chair and toilet seat. Immobilization improves healing of the soft tissue and osteotomized greater trochanter.

several years. Some surgeons advocate hip flexion, extension, and abduction exercises immediately after the operation and until hip strength is adequate. However, starting the exercises immediately after the operation can jeopardize fixation of the greater trochanter and may lead to trochanteric nonunion and migration with loss of myofascial tension and possible dislocation. Six weeks of immobilization with a short single- leg spica cast can protect the greater trochanter and increase the chance of trochanteric union (Fig. 3). Physical therapy is started after this short period of immobilization. Therapy focuses on improving the strength of the flexors and abductors and increasing range of motion.

RESULTS

Pain Relief

Conversion arthroplasty is undertaken in most instances to alleviate pain in the lumbosacral region, ipsilateral knee, and contralateral hip. Most reports indicate that most patients who undergo conversion arthroplasty have marked improvement in the low-back symptoms and, to a lesser degree, the ipsilateral knee pain (Fig. 4). Reikeras et al. (19) reported on 55 arthrodesed hips converted to total hip arthroplasty. Of 24 patients who had severe low back pain, most had marked improvement after arthroplasty. In a report by Kilgus and Amstutz (13), 20 of 25 patients with severe back pain preoperatively reported complete or near complete pain relief. With respect to knee pain, two thirds of patients who underwent conversion arthroplasty who had had severe knee pain before the operation reported improvement of the pain; one third did not have any evidence of improvement. Persistent low back pain was attributed to advanced degenerative changes in the lumbosacral spine that was aggravated with activity. Some of the patients with knee pain who did not have improvement chose total knee arthroplasty to relieve the symptoms.

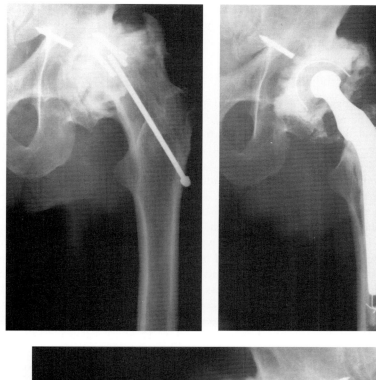

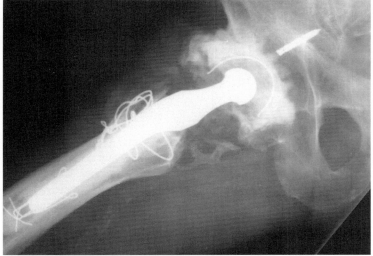

Figure 4. A: A 78-year-old man who had undergone left hip fusion for posttraumatic osteoarthritis needed conversion to left total hip replacement. **B,C:** Anteroposterior and lateral radiographs 16 years after conversion to total hip replacement.

Other studies (4,8), however, indicated that improvement of pain after conversion arthroplasty depended on the severity of the degenerative changes and duration of symptoms.

Hip Motion

The principle goal of conversion arthroplasty is to gain motion of the arthrodesed hip to alleviate strain on the back and ipsilateral knee. Many reports indicate that hip motion after conversion arthroplasty ranges between 70 and 90 degrees of flexion. Kilgus and Amstutz (13) reported a flexion arc of 87 degrees a range of 25 to 135 degrees, an abduction arc of 46 degrees, and adduction of 33 degrees. The average rotation was 46 degrees with 18 degrees of internal rotation and 28 degrees of external rotation. Although the range of motion achieved after conversion arthroplasty is less than the range obtained after primary total hip arthroplasty, the restored range of motion is highly appreciated by the patient.

Pain Function and Mobility Scores

Different scoring systems have been used in the cases reported in the literature. Kilgus and Amstutz (13) reported that with the UCLA hip rating system, preoperative pain, walking, and function scores averaged 6.9, 6, and 5.7 and improved to 8.5, 7.5, and 7.2 postoperatively. This improvement was not statistically significant. Reikeras et al. (19) reported improvement in Harris hip score from 51 to 83 preoperatively to 53 to 93 at follow-up examinations after conversion arthroplasty. Interestingly was that 34 of 55 patients in the study needed walking aids: 24 used one crutch and 12 patients used two crutches after conversion arthroplasty. None of the patients had used walking aids before conversion arthroplasty. Other reports also indicated that after arthroplasty dependency on walking aids increased. Dependency on walking aids is important after conversion arthroplasty. Abductor muscle is weakened because of the arthrodesis status of the hip. After restoration of hip motion, most patients benefit from use of a walking aid, such as a single crutch or cane, because of weakness in the abductor muscle. Lubahn et al. (15) reported that the duration of fusion before conversion ranged from 5 to 60 years among 17 patients who underwent conversion of ankylosed hips to total hip arthopasty. Relief of preoperative pain in the lower back was achieved by 12 of 13 patients. Knee pain was relieved for 4 of 4 patients. Complications included infection, perforation of the posterior shaft of the femur, and failure of trochanteric fixation with subsequent dislocation. Among 15 patients with surgically arthrodesed hips converted to total hip arthroplasty at our institution , 8 resorted to using a cane after conversion arthroplasty (7). Pain related to the lumbosacral spine improved, but 10 of 15 patients had occasional low back pain after prolonged activity.

Patient Satisfaction

Many factors determine patient satisfaction after conversion arthroplasty. These include relief of pain in the lumbosacral spine, ipsilateral knee, and contralateral hip, restoration of hip motion, and correction of a limp and leg-length inequality. Kilgus and Amstutz (13) reported on 38 patients, 32 of whom thought they were much improved after conversion arthroplasty. Four indicated some improvement. In a report of Reikeras et al. (19) on 55 patients, 13 reported they were very much satisfied, 19 were much satisfied, and 7 were satisfied. Seven of 55 patients reported less satisfaction or were not satisfied with the procedure. In our study of 15 conversions, 10 patients were satisfied with the conversion, and 5 were less satisfied or dissatisfied. One patient had a serious vascular complication in the contralateral hip caused by faulty placement of the pubic support during positioning of the patient.

Few studies report on survivalship of a total hip arthroplasty after conversion of an arthrodesed hip. Strathy and Fitzgerald (22) reported on 80 conversion total hip arthroplasties on 74 patients who had either spontaneous or surgical arthrodesis of the hip. Follow-up evaluations took place to 15 years (average 10.4 years) after conversion. Among the 20 patients who had spontaneous ankylosis and underwent conversion total hip arthroplasty, there was one failure. In contrast, 20 of the 60 patients who had surgical ankylosis had complications associated with the arthroplasty. Mechanical loosening developed in 11 patients, infection in 8, and recurrent dislocation in 1 patient. Failures of total hip arthroplasty were more common among patients who had a previous surgical arthrodesis than among patients with spontaneous arthrodeses among patients who were 50 years old or younger at arthroplasty. Risk for failure was not related to the length of time that the hip had been ankylosed. In a study by Kilgus et al. (14), a higher failure rate was found among patients who were 50 years of age or younger at arthroplasty and among patients who had had two or more surgical procedures.

Magyar and Gschwend (16) reported on 11 patients with hip arthrodesis who underwent conversion to total hip arthroplasty and were observed 1 to 21 years. Long-term survival rate proved to be slightly better than the overall survival rate for all patients with arthroplasties performed in their clinic. Duration of the arthrodeses did not influence the long-term results.

COMPLICATIONS

Conversion of an ankylosed hip to total hip arthroplasty is a complex surgical undertaking. The reported incidence of complications in the literature varies. It is considerably higher than after primary total hip arthroplasty. Amstutz and Sakai (1) reported four instances of complications (infection in 2 patients, subluxation in 1 patient, death of 1 patient) among 16 patient who underwent conversion arthroplasty for an incidence of (25%). Kilgus et al. (14) reported 10 major complications and nine minor complications among 41 patients after conversion arthroplasty. They included 3 instances of sepsis, 1 of nerve palsy, and 6 of component loosening. In the minor complication group the authors found trochanteric wire breakage requiring removal in 4 patients, trochanteric nonunion requiring reattachment in 1 patient, heterotopic ossification requiring excision in 1 patient, dislocation of the hip in 2 patients, and necrosis of the skin of 1 patient. The complications were more frequent among young patients and among patients with a history of trauma and two or more previous operations. Hardinge et al. (10) reported that among 54 patients undergoing conversion arthroplasty, 3 had pulmonary emboli, 2 had trochanteric nonunion, 3 had heterotopic ossification, and 1 patient had sciatic nerve palsy. Strathy and Fitzgerald (22) reported a 26.3% failure rate among 80 patients, 11.3% due to sepsis. The complications included a 50% rate of sepsis when conversion arthroplasty was performed within 5 years after surgical arthrodesis. Fernandez and I (7) reviewed the results of 15 conversion arthroplasties performed on surgically arthrodesed hips at our institution. One patient had vascular compression at the femoral triangle of the contralateral hip caused by faulty placement of the pubic support, 1 patient had a pelvic fracture caused by excessive reaming of the acetabulum, 2 patients had trochanteric nonunion with subsequent hip dislocation, 1 patient had peroneal nerve palsy, and 1 patient had an infection.

SUMMARY

Conversion of an ankylosed hip to total hip arthroplasty is a demanding procedure that should be performed on selected patients with disabling pain in the lower spine, ipsilateral knee or contralateral hip. A patient with an asymptomatic unilateral hip fusion without other disabilities is not a candidate for conversion to total hip arthroplasty. The role of this procedure is to alleviate pain in the lumbosacral spine and ipsilateral knee, and to restore motion at the hip joint. The abductor muscles in most instances are weak and need a long period of rehabilitation after the operation. The outcome of the procedure depends on the integrity of the greater trochanter and the abductor mechanism. Patients who have undergone repeated prior operations to ankylose the hip and younger patients appear to have poor outcomes after conversion arthroplasty. Patients with spontaneously fused hips appear to have better outcomes and far fewer complications than patients who have undergone surgical ankylosis.

REFERENCES

1. Amstutz HC, Sakai DN. Total joint replacement for ankylosed hips. *J Bone Joint Surg Am* 1975;57:619–625.
2. Brewster RC, Coventry MB, Johnson EW Jr. Conversion of the arthrodesed hip to a total hip arthroplasty. *J Bone Joint Surg Am* 1975;57:27–30.
3. Callaghan JJ, Brand RA, Pedersen DR. Hip arthrodesis. *J Bone Joint Surg Am* 1985;67:1328–1335.
4. Courpied JR, Kerboul M, Bellier G, Postel M. Arthroplastie totale sur hanche ankylosee. *Rev Chir Orthop* 1981;67:289.

5. Dorr LD, Takei GK, Conaty JP. Total hip arthroplasty in patients less than forty-five years old. *J Bone Joint Surg Am* 1983;65:474.

6. Eftekhar NS. Total hip arthroplasty. St Louis: Mosby, 1993:1000–1010, 1140–1159.

7. Fernandez M, Nercessian O. The result of conversion of surgically arthrodesed hip to total hip arthroplasty (*in preparation*).

8. Gore DR, Murray MP, Sepic SB, Gardner GM. Walking patterns of men with unilateral surgical hip fusion. *J Bone Joint Surg Am* 1975;57:759–765.

9. Hardinge K, Murphy JC, Frenyo S. Conversion of hip fusion to Charnley low friction arthroplasty. *Clin Orthop* 1986;211:173–179.

10. Hardinge K, Williams D, Etienne A et al. Conversion of fused hips to low friction arthroplasty. *J Bone Joint Surg Br* 1977;59:385–392.

11. Johnston RC, Brand RA, Crowninshield RD. Reconstruction of the hip: a mechanical approach to determine optimism, geometric relationship. *J Bone Joint Surg Am* 1979;61:639–652.

12. Kempf I, Jenny JY. Total prothesis after ankylosis of the hip joint: report of 22 cases [French]. *Int Orthop* 1991;15:239–243.

13. Kilgus DJ, Amstutz HC. Conversion of ankylosed hips to total hip replacements. In: Amstutz HC, ed. *Hip Arthroplasty* New York: Churchill Livingstone, 1991:799–811.

14. Kilgus DJ, Amstutz HC, Wolgin MA, Dorey FJ. Joint replacement for ankylosed hips. *J Bone Joint Surg Am* 1990;72:45–54.

15. Lubahn JD, Evarts C, Feltner TB. Conversion of ankylosed hips to total hip arthroplasty. *Clin Orthop* 1980;153:146–152.

16. Magyar A, Gschwend N. Total prosthesis implantation in arthritic hip. [Total prothesen Implantation bei de arthrodesierten Hufte.] *Orthopade* 1989;18:493–497.

17. Perugia L, Santori FS, Mancini A, Manili M, Falez F. Conversion of the arthrodesed hip to a total hip arthroplasty: indications and limitations. *Ital Traumato* 1992;18:145–153.

18. Ranawat CS, Atkinson RE, Salvati EA, Wilson PD. Conventional total hip arthroplasty for degenerative joint disease in patients between the ages of forty and sixty years. *J Bone Joint Surg Am* 1984;66;745–752.

19. Reikeras O, Bjerkrein I, Gundersson R. Total hip arthroplasty for arthrodesed hips: 5 to 13 year results. *J Arthroplasty* 1995;10:529–531.

20. Sponseller PD, McBeath AA, Perpich M. Long-term follow-up of hip arthrodesis performed in young patients. In: *The hip: proceedings of the Twelfth Open Scientific Meeting of The Hip Society.* St. Louis:CV Mosby, 1984:43–53.

21. Stinchfield FE, Cavallaro WU. Arthrodesis of the hip joint. *J Bone Joint Surg Am* 1950;32:48–58.

22. Strathy GM, Fitzgerald RH Jr. Total hip arthroplasty in the ankylosed hip. *J Bone Joint Surg Am* 1988;70:963–966.

23. White RE Jr. Arthrodesis of the hip. In: The hip: proceedings of the Twelfth Open Scientific Meeting of The Hip Society. St. Louis: CV Mosby, 1984, 54–67.

Revision Total Hip Arthroplasty,
edited by Marvin E. Steinberg and Jonathan P. Garino,
Lippincott Williams & Wilkins, Philadelphia © 1999.

38

Conversion of Cup Arthroplasty and Femoral Endoprostheses to Total Hip Arthroplasty

Miguel E. Cabanela

Conversion of cup arthroplasty to total joint replacement is a relatively uncommon operation today. Some patients, however, have old cup arthroplasties that have functioned reasonably well for more than 20 years and eventually come to need total hip replacement. Stiffness, contractures, and defects of acetabular bone both in quality and in stock are common in this situation. The femur, however, although often osteoporotic usually does not present a problem unless there has been previous trauma.

Conversion of a femoral endoprosthesis to a hip replacement has a completely different set of problems. The simplest conversion today would be that of a modular or bipolar prosthesis that is well fixed in the femur but has produced acetabular wear with resulting groin pain. This type of revision usually presents no serious problem. A different situation is conversion of a cemented unipolar femoral endoprosthesis. This often has the same set of problems as revision of a cemented total hip prosthesis, cement removal with avoidance of femoral shaft perforation being the most important concern. Perhaps the most common situation is conversion of an uncemented prosthesis to total hip arthroplasty. The problems can be very different depending on how long the prosthesis has been in place and the status of its fixation to bone. These situations are analyzed separately because they present different sets of problems.

M. E. Cabanela: Department of Orthopedics, Mayo Medical School, Rochester, Minnesota 55905.

BACKGROUND

The initial publications on conversion of cup arthroplasty or femoral endoprosthesis to total joint replacement emphasized the transtrochanteric approach and usually reported only problems with extraction of uncemented femoral endoprostheses of the Moore type. In the case of previous cup arthroplasties, presence of sclerotic bone and osseous deficiencies frequently were reported in the acetabulum. The advice provided was that after complete capsulectomy the acetabular component should be placed as far medially and inferiorly as possible. Some authors (1) emphasized the avoidance of bone grafts in this instance and preferred to fill any defect with cement. In the case of previous femoral endoprostheses it was believed that potential difficulties included detachment of a fragment of greater trochanter of proper size and shape, the difficulty in extracting the prosthesis even when it was loose in the medullary canal, and the fact that the track left by the prosthesis in the canal often was lined with either endosteal sclerotic bone or fibrous tissue, which made anchoring a new prosthesis with cement difficult. It was thus suggested (6) that thorough curettage of the medullary canal was needed to remove all fibrous membrane and the shell of reactive bone around the prosthetic stem.

INDICATIONS AND PATIENT SELECTION

As with any hip arthroplasty, the main indication for conversion of a cup arthroplasty or femoral endoprosthesis to total hip arthroplasty is pain of sufficient intensity to alter the patient's daily life and thus justify surgical intervention. A second indication present perhaps about 10% of the time is considerable stiffness. In the case of cup arthroplasty this often acquires the form of severe adduction contractures, which can make personal hygiene difficult or nearly impossible.

In the case of a failed femoral endoprosthesis the most common indication is pain in the groin. This is related to the acetabular wear caused by metal articulating with cartilage. With an uncemented prostheses or less commonly with loose cemented prostheses, thigh pain also can be a reason for revision. A third indication is progressive acetabular bone loss and protrusio acetabuli.

Before revision surgery is undertaken, one must ensure that the patient's general condition allows him or her to tolerate the procedure without excessive risk. Complete preoperative medical evaluation, particularly for older patients, is essential.

PREOPERATIVE PLANNING

Conversion of a cup arthroplasty necessitates primarily assessment of acetabular bone stock and quality. Often there is marked sclerosis, lateralization of the center of rotation of the hip, and presence of a medial osteophyte (Fig. 1). Proper templating must be carried out, and a preoperative prediction must be made regarding the need for medialization of the center of rotation of the hip or the potential need to move the center of rotation upwards to ensure adequate support on native bone of good quality. Seldom is there a need for augmentation acetabular allografting but this need can be predicted preoperatively. On the femoral side conversion of cup arthroplasty usually does not entail serious problems. Most of the time, because of the marked osteoporosis of the femur, cemented fixation of the femoral component is advisable. Not infrequently adduction contracture is present, which is predictive of the need for intraoperative adductor tenotomy.

Conversion of a femoral hemiarthroplasty to total hip replacement usually necessitates preoperative planning similar to that of revision total hip replacement. Depending on the quality of the residual bone stock and the age of the patient, predictions can be made for selection of cemented or uncemented fixation of the femoral component. If uncemented fixation is chosen, most frequently it means diaphyseal fixation with a fully coated prosthesis (Fig. 2). Proper preoperative templating is essential. One essential step in preoperative planning is assessment of the greater trochanter. If there is marked medial overhang of the trochanter over the proximal end of the prosthesis, trochanteric osteotomy

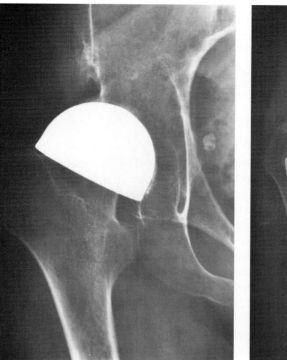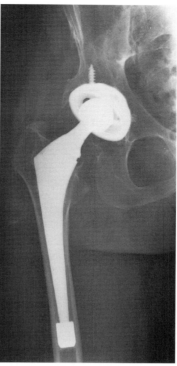

A B

Figure 1. A: A 35-year old man with a 15-year-old cup arthroplasty that is painful. Lateral subluxation of the cup is present with marked adduction deformity. **B:** Six years after revision arthroplasty. The uncemented acetabular component is in the anatomic position. An uncemented femoral component was used because of the young age of the patient.

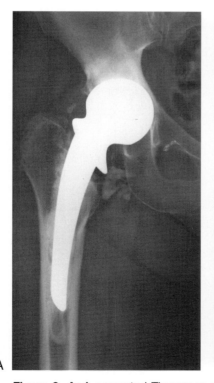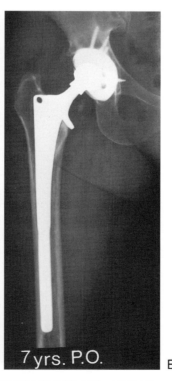

A 7 yrs. P.O. B

Figure 2. A: A cemented Thompson prosthesis with early protrusio, acetabular sclerosis, and marked groin pain in a 60-year-old woman. **B:** Same patient 7 years after revision with an uncemented proximally coated, prosthesis. A fully porous coated femoral prosthesis would probably have been used today in the same situation, if an uncemented component were used.

might be needed. Extended proximal femoral osteotomy occasionally may be necessary if one anticipates that removal of conventional fragment of trochanter would be followed by difficulties at reattachment because of an anticipated very poor trochanteric bed or if there is angular, often varus deformity of the femoral shaft.

SURGICAL TECHNIQUE

Conversion of Cup Arthroplasty

Stiffness, contractures, and heterotopic ossification around a cup arthroplasty can make exposure difficult. With patience, adequate exposure for revision can be accomplished without trochanteric osteotomy. A standard trochanteric osteotomy might be necessary. Preoperative templating ensures adequate placement of the acetabular component. This, however, necessitates attention to the usual landmarks. Definition of the anterior, posterior, and inferior borders of the acetabulum is helpful before one proceeds with acetabular reaming. Reaming can be difficult, particularly if sclerotic bone is present. Careful attention to reamer placement and avoidance of translational motions during reaming are important. If cemented acetabular fixation is planned, multiple small holes anchoring are preferred to the large fixation cement holes that were used in the past (Fig. 3). Today uncemented fixation is used most often, and I prefer an acetabular component with an enlarged peripheral rim to ensure proper press fitting. I also prefer to augment acetabular fixation with two or three screws, one placed into the ilium in a straight superior direction, and the other directed posteriorly and perforating the posterior cortex to achieve bicortical fixation. Preparation of the femur usually is not a problem after cup arthroplasty and is basically the same as for primary total hip arthroplasty. At the time of exposure attention should be paid to avoiding extreme rotational maneuvers. Not infrequently the femur is rather osteoporotic, and intraoperative fractures can occur with injudicious use of force.

Revision of a Femoral Hemiarthroplasty to Total Hip Replacement

The problem in revision of a femoral hemiarthroplasty is more frequent on the femoral side than in the acetabulum. Three situations can occur, as follows.

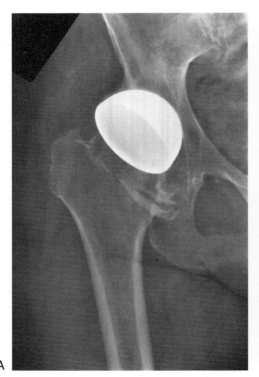
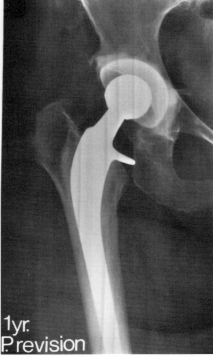

A   B

Figure 3. A: 60-year old woman with a 20-year-old cup arthroplasty that has been very painful for the last 5 years. **B:** One year after revision with a cemented prosthesis.

Conversion of Cemented Monoblock Femoral Prosthesis to a Total Hip Replacement

This situation is comparable on the femoral side to revision of total hip arthroplasty, because the femoral component must be removed. If the component is loose, removal of the cement may not present much of a problem. If, on the other hand, the component is firmly cemented and revision is necessary because of acetabular symptoms (groin or buttock pain) and radiographic changes in the acetabulum (loss of acetabular cartilage, sclerosis, or migration), revision can be fraught with risk for perforating or fracturing the femur. If this situation is present use of extended femoral osteotomy might facilitate cement removal. However, most of the time modern methods of cement removal can help avoid osteotomy. In general, revision of the acetabulum is not fraught with problems unless there has been considerable prosthetic migration into pelvic bone. In this instance careful and judicious reaming, use of morselized bone to fill the back and medial aspects of the acetabular cavity, and anchoring of an uncemented acetabular prosthesis on the periphery of the acetabulum is the preferred technique. When marked prosthetic protrusio is present, exposure might be very difficult and necessitate trochanteric osteotomy and even removal of a thin rim of peripheral acetabular bone to facilitate dislocation.

Revision of an Uncemented Prosthesis

The most common prosthesis necessitating revision is an Austin-Moore uncemented prosthesis or one of its variants. The reason for revision usually is thigh pain caused by loosening of the prosthesis or, less frequently, groin or buttock pain.

The danger in this procedure is fracturing the greater trochanter in the process of removing the femoral prosthesis. The lateral aspect of the metaphysis of the prosthesis often is embedded into the substance of the greater trochanter, and forceful blows on the extractor can jam the lateral aspect of the prosthesis against the trochanter and fracture it off. During exposure, one should remember to visualize the lateral most aspect of the

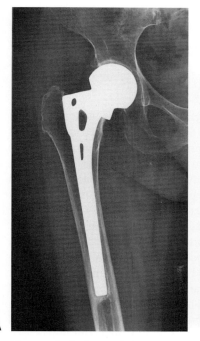
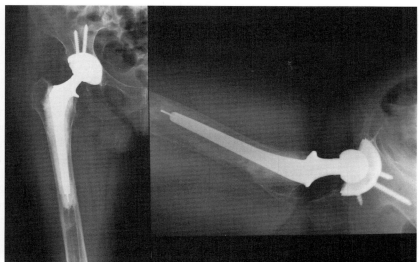

A   B

Figure 4. A: A painful uncemented Austin-Moore prosthetic hemiarthroplasty done for femoral neck fracture on a 63-year-old woman $1\frac{1}{2}$ years before this radiograph was obtained. Patient never had satisfactory pain relief and continued to have groin and thigh pain. **B:** Anteroposterior and lateral radiographs of the same patient 3 months after revision to hybrid arthroplasty. Excellent pain relief was obtained.

prosthesis and make sure that there is no bone in the path to extraction by hollowing the medial aspect of the greater trochanter with a burr. An alternative solution is trochanteric osteotomy, but this might leave a very poor trochanteric bed for subsequent reattachment. If the prosthesis is well fixed by bone that was grown through the fenestrations, freeing its anterior and posterior surfaces with flexible osteotomes between the prosthesis and the endosteal surface of the femur may be necessary. In general, this does not present a problem. If protrusio is present (and this is less frequent than in the case of a cemented prosthesis), tricks can be used that are similar to those mentioned for a cemented prosthesis.

Once the prosthesis is extracted, preparation of the medullary canal of the femur demands removal of the endosteal neocortex that often surrounds the stem of the Austin-Moore prothesis. Use of a small burr to make irregularities in the medullary canal might facilitate and enhance cement fixation. Revision of an uncemented femoral prosthesis most commonly is done with cement (Fig. 4).

Revision of a Bipolar Prosthesis to Total Hip Replacement

This can be the simplest type of revision, particularly in the case of a well-fixed modular, bipolar component. Exposure seldom is a problem once the femoral prosthetic head has been removed. In the case of a monolithic bipolar prosthesis, the femoral component may be left in place if the head size can be accommodated by a standard acetabular component. A problem with instability may occur because of poor myofascial tension because neck length cannot be adjusted. This problem can be solved with greater trochanteric osteotomy and advancement.

POSTOPERATIVE CARE

There is little difference between care after conversion of a cup arthroplasty or femoral hemiarthroplasty to total hip replacement and that after primary hip replacement. If instability is present, use of a hip orthosis might be advisable. Use of assistive devices for walking and partial to full weight bearing might be predicated depending on the type of arthroplasty used.

RESULTS

Early reports of revision of failed cups and failed femoral prostheses were included in general follow-up studies of total hip replacements. Stauffer (8) reported on 42 failed femoral prostheses and 19 failed cups converted to Charnley hip replacement arthroplasty. Conversion of failed cups produced a high incidence of loose acetabular components, whereas conversion of failed femoral prostheses produced a high incidence of femoral component loosening. Dupont and Charnley (3) reported on 51 femoral prostheses converted to low-friction Charnley total hip replacements for 49 patients. Clinical 1-year follow-up results were satisfactory but not as good as those after primary arthroplasty. Sarmiento and Gerard (6) reported on 95 total hip arthroplasties performed on 85 patients for failed femoral endoprostheses and followed for about 3 years. In this short follow-up period, there was one case of acetabular loosening and possibly 6 of femoral component loosening. Results were reported to be satisfactory. Stambough et al. (7) in 1986 reported on 140 conversions of previous procedures to total hip arthroplasty with a 40-month radiographic and clinical follow-up period. This group included 32 failed femoral endoprostheses, all of them uncemented. A group of 17 patients with failed cup arthroplasties or surface replacement arthroplasties also was included. The overall results showed that the complication rate for this group was similar to that of a group with primary arthroplasties performed contemporaneously. Again, the incidence of radiologic demarcation in the socket was higher after cup arthroplasy. The incidence of femoral bone–cement demarcation and subsidence also was higher for replacements done after failure of a femoral endoprosthesis. Overall clinical results, however, were comparable with those of primary arthroplasty.

Llinas et al. (5) reviewed their experience with secondary hip replacements after failed uncemented hemiarthroplasty and failed cup arthroplasty. When they compared the results of 99 cemented hip replacements after failed uncemented hemiarthroplasty and 21 after failed cup arthroplasty with those of 825 primary cemented total hip arthroplasties with a mean follow-up period of 7.6 years, the incidence of radiologic loosening was higher for femoral components implanted after failed hemiarthroplasty and for acetabular components implanted after failed cup arthroplasty. They also found that the incidence of continuous radiolucent lines was lower for acetabular components inserted after failed hemiarthroplasty than those after primary hip replacement. The authors speculated that previous exposure of an unreamed acetabulum to the articulated metallic femoral head of a hemiarthroplasty might have had a beneficial effect on performance of the subsequently placed cemented socket. They suggested that perhaps a structural modification such as trabecular hypertrophy of subchondral bone brought about by nonphysiologic load transfer imposed by the metallic hemiarthroplasty might provide better support for the subsequently placed cemented cup. Ash et al. (1) reviewed 96 cup arthroplasties converted to cemented total hip arthroplasties. Of these, 58 hips in 50 patients were followed for at least 10 years. There was a 16% revision rate caused by aseptic loosening of the acetabular component. No hip was revised because of loosening of the femoral component. Kaplan-Meier survivorship analysis with revision for any reason, including infection as the end point, showed a survival rate of 92% at 10 years and 74% at 20 years. In this study patients younger than 50 years were significantly more likely to have aseptic loosening of the acetabular component necessitating revision.

At my institution the first 333 Charnley total hip arthroplasties were reported on at 5 years by Beckenbaugh and Ilstrup (2), at 10 years by Stauffer (8), and at 15 years by Kavanagh et al. (4). In this group of 333 patients, 21 had failed cup arthroplasties converted to Charnley hip replacements and 55 had failed femoral endoprostheses converted to hip replacement.

We studied these two groups of patients separately for up to 20 years. For the 21 cup arthroplasty conversions, the 15-year survivorship free of acetabular revision was 73.6%. The 15-year survivorship free of femoral revision was 71%. The 15-year survivorship free of probable or definite acetabular loosening was 59.3%, and that for femoral loosening was 62.4%. The overall survivorship free of acetabular or femoral revision by 15 years was 59.5%. For the 55 femoral endoprostheses converted to cemented Charnley total hip arthroplasty, the same statistical analysis yielded the following results. The 15-year survivorship without acetabular revision was 98.2%. This figure was very similar for patients older and younger than 60 years. The 15-year survivorship without femoral revision was 91.8%. No significant difference was observed between patients older and younger than 60 years. The 15-year survivorship without acetabular or femoral revision was 90.1%. When we looked at survival without probable or definite acetabular loosening, the actual number was 96.4%, but the same 15-year survival rate for the femur was 62.9%.

It appeared that among our patients the revision and incidence rates of loosening after cemented Charnley replacement for failure of cup arthroplasty were similar for the acetabulum and the femur. However, the femoral component appeared to fail much more frequently after arthroplasty revision of a previous femoral endoprosthesis.

SUMMARY

Revision of Cup Arthroplasty

1. Because of stiffness, contractures, or heterotopic bone, exposure can be difficult and may require a trochanteric osteotomy.
2. Proper preoperative templating and attention to detail ensure adequate socket position.
3. Uncemented sockets are probably the best choice.

4. Because one often is dealing with porotic femora, cemented femoral components might be indicated more often than uncemented components.

5. Adductor tenotomy might be necessary in cases of marked adduction contractures.

Revision of a Femoral Endoprosthesis

1. Removal of a loose uncemented femoral prostheses can be difficult and might put the greater trochanter in jeopardy. Careful exposure with burring of the lateral aspect of the trochanter to facilitate prosthetic extraction is advisable. If bone has grown through the fenestrations in the prosthesis, it should be removed or divided before attempts are made to extract the component.

2. In revision of a uncemented femoral endoprosthesis, choice of acetabular fixation should follow the same philosophy as for primary arthroplasty.

3. In revision of a cemented femoral endoprostheses, particularly if there is acetabular protrusion, uncemented acetabular fixation with intraacetabular bone grafting might be the best choice.

4. Revision of an uncemented femoral endoprostheses demands careful preparation of the femoral canal with removal of the endosteal sclerotic prosthetic envelope.

5. Removal of cemented femoral endoprostheses can be followed by either cemented or uncemented fixation. This judgment should be made as with any other revision of a cemented femoral prostheses.

6. Conversion of a well-fixed bipolar prosthesis to a total hip arthroplasty usually is a simple procedure. If the bipolar prosthesis is monolithic, poor myofascial tension may necessitate trochanteric osteotomy and advancement to improve hip stability.

REFERENCES

1. Ash SA, Callaghan JJ, Johnston RC. Revision total hip arthroplasty with cement after cup arthroplasty. *J Bone Joint Surg Am* 1996;78:87–93.
2. Beckenbaugh RD, Ilstrup DM. Total hip arthroplasty: a review of three hundred and thirty three cases with long follow-up. *J Bone Joint Surg Am* 1978;60:306–313.
3. Dupont JA, Charnley J. Low friction arthroplasty of the hip for the failures of previous operations. *J Bone Joint Surg Br* 1972;54:77–87.
4. Kavanagh BF, Dewitz MA, Ilstrup DM, Stauffer RN, Coventry MB. Charnley total hip arthroplasty with cement: 15 year results. *J Bone Joint Surg Am* 1989;71:1496–1503.
5. Llinas A, Sarmiento A, Ebramzadeh E, Gogan WJ, McKellop HA. Total hip replacement after failed hemiarthroplasty or mould arthroplasty. *J Bone Joint Surg Br* 1991;73:902–910.
6. Sarmiento A, Gerard FN. Total hip arthroplasty for failed endoprostheses. *Clin Orthop* 1978;137:112–117.
7. Stambough JL, Balderston RA, Booth RE Jr, Rothman RH, Cohn JC. Conversion total hip replacement. *J Arthroplasty* 1986;1:261–269.
8. Stauffer RN. Ten year follow-up study of total hip replacement. *J Bone Joint Surg Am* 1982;64:983–990.

Revision Total Hip Arthroplasty,
edited by Marvin E. Steinberg and Jonathan P. Garino,
Lippincott Williams & Wilkins, Philadelphia © 1999.

39

Use of Custom Components and Robotics in Revision Total Hip Arthroplasty

William L. Bargar, Bill Williamson, and
Alan D. Kalvin

COMPUTED TOMOGRAPHY–BASED CUSTOM COMPONENTS IN REVISION TOTAL HIP REPLACEMENT

In revision total hip arthroplasty, a failing hip implant, typically cemented, is replaced with a new one by means of removal of the old implant, removal of the cement, and fitting a new implant into the enlarged femoral canal. As the installed base of orthopedic implants grows and ages, revision operations for total hip replacement are increasing in frequency. In 1992, 23,000 revision total hip arthroplasty procedures were performed in the United States with an annual growth rate of 10%. The average cost per procedure was $23,744 with an average hospital stay of 10.9 days (28). Estimates are that 18% of total hip replacements performed annually are revisions, both the number and the percentage increasing (National Center for Health Statistics, 1994). By the year 2000 we can expect to perform 175,000 hip replacements per year, 20% being revisions.

The reasons for revision are varied, but a common theme encountered at the time of revision is bone loss. Dealing with this bone loss means that one must address unique defects in each case and realize that the bone that remains may not be strong enough strength to support the new implant. Many authors (4,6,9–11,13,16,22,24) have resorted

W. L. Bargar: Department of Orthopaedics, University of California, Davis, and Sutter General Hospital, Sacramento, California 95816.
B. Williamson: Integrated Surgical Systems, Sacramento, California 95834.
A. D. Kalvin: Thomas J. Watson Research Center, Yorktown Heights, New York 10598.

to structural allografts and conventional implants to solve the problem of bone loss. Recent reports (14,15,18,21,27,30), however, show late collapse (5 to 10 years) of most structural allografts. Exceptions to this general tend are cemented stems with compaction allografting (8) and cementless implants with over 50% of ingrowth surface contacting host bone (24).

In addition to causing problems of implant sizing and fit, the bone defects encountered in revision surgery also generate problems of restoring offset, version, and leg length that make each case unique. To address these problems caused by individual anatomic variations and bone loss, we have chosen to use computed tomography (CT)–based custom-made cementless components.

Background

Custom-made implants have been used since the beginning of joint replacement surgery. All orthopedic implants usually began as custom devices. As these implants mature and the necessary elements of design and sizing ranges are defined, off-the-shelf systems develop. The use of any off-the-shelf implant constitutes a compromise, because rarely does an individual present the exact size and shape bone for a particularly sized implant. This is even more true for revisions with the unique bone defects described earlier.

The use of custom implants has problems caused by time for manufacture, inaccuracies of fit, and high cost. The development of linking CT-generated data with computer-assisted design and manufacturing (CAD/CAM) in the mid 1980s, however, shortened the time for manufacture and improved the fit of custom implants (1). Cost differentials also improved over time. Custom-made stems have decreased in cost from more than $5,000 each to approximately $3,800. In addition, the use of custom implants can eliminate the need for structural allografts, which range in cost between $700 and $2,500 each, thereby making use of custom implants potentially cost effective.

Obtaining a Custom Implant

To design and fabricate a custom implant, the manufacturer needs CT and radiographic data and the design criteria specified by the surgeon. Most companies provide a protocol for obtaining the CT scan. Because an implant usually is in place, some CT artifact is unavoidable (Fig. 1). Good CT data usually can be obtained from the region above and below the metal. In the region of the metal the periosteal contour can be visualized, but endosteal information has to be estimated from the radiographs. Ideally anteroposterior (AP) and lateral radiographs are 90 degrees apart with magnification markers. In the case of a custom femoral component, the AP view is obtained with 20-degree internal rotation at the knee. The lateral view is table-down frog lateral (Lauenstein) (23) with the knee flexed and resting on the table. Both views should be of the proximal two thirds of the femur. For a custom acetabular component, an AP pelvic view usually is sufficient, but Judet views may add important clinical information. The CT scan for an acetabular component encompasses the entire hemipelvis from the top of the iliac crest to the ischial tuberosity.

The manufacturer needs to know where the surgeon plans to locate the new joint center and what the desired leg-length change is to be. Once the initial design is completed by the manufacturer, a drawing and radiographic acetate templates at the appropriate magnifications are sent to the surgeon. Additional changes or modifications are made by means of discussion between the surgeon and design engineer. Required instrumentation also is discussed. Custom broaches or custom trial implants can be provided. The surgeon usually signs the final drawing, which constitutes a prescription for the device and is required to meet the U.S. Food and Drug Administration (FDA) exemption for custom devices).

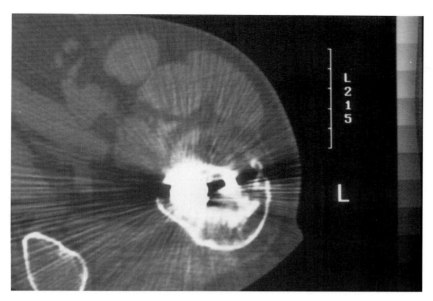

Figure 1. CT scan shows metal artifact.

Custom Femoral Components

Although custom-designed components can be obtained for use both with and without cement, we generally prefer the use of uncemented porous ingrowth devices. Our design specifications include the following:

1. Proximal body with rhomboidal cross section to best fit CT and radiographic data. (In areas of severe artifact from metal scatter, dimensions are estimated from radiograph).
2. Long, bowed, cylindrical, fluted distal stem with arc of bow and diameter determined from CT data.
3. Length of bow to bypass potential stress risers by three internal-canal diameters.
4. Proximal collar designed to lie 2 mm above the proximal medial bone to prevent excessive subsidence but allow wedging of the proximal body.
5. A transitional area of underfit at the junction of metaphysis to the diaphysis to force proximal load transfer.
6. Femoral head position designed to restore horizontal offset, anteversion and leg length.

Our minimum 5-year results for CT-based CAD/CAM cementless femoral components were presented at the 1996 meeting of the International Society for Technologies in Arthroplasty (ISTA; Amsterdam, August 1996). Specific bone defects, identified through preoperative CT and radiographic analysis, were addressed through implant design, optimization of proximal endosteal fit supplemented with collars, and stems designed to bypass segmental and cavitary defects. Initial press-fit fixation was augmented with proximal porous titanium mesh pads for ingrowth fixation (Fig. 2). The articular portion of the implant was designed to restore leg length and normal joint mechanics. One hundred five consecutive revision hips received this CAD/CAM implant 5 or more years ago (5 to 9 years). Included were 56 men and 49 women. Average weight at operation was 166 pounds (78 to 286 pounds). Average age was 60 years (29 to 85 years). At the operation all femoral reconstructions were completed without resorting to structural grafts. Leg-length discrepancy averaged 2 cm preoperatively (0 to 7 cm) and 0.7 cm postoperatively (0 to 5 cm). Ten patients died, and 14 were not available for the follow-up study, leaving 81 for complete analysis at 5 years. Thirteen hips needed revision. Four revisions were performed in the first 5 years (1 for deep infection, 1 for osteolysis, 7 for loosening, and 4 for pad separation with subsequent pain). Complications among all patients who did not undergo revision included 10 intraoperative femoral fractures, 1 late deep infection, 2

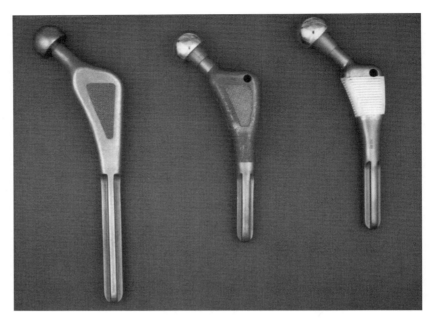

Figure 2. The evolution of custom implant designs. Left to right, 1985 to 1988, 1988 to 1990, 1990 to present.

dislocations, and 3 cases of late ingrowth pad separation (classified as material, not design, failures). At last follow-up evaluation of surviving hips, average Harris hip score was 84 (42 to 100) and average pain score was 39 (10 to 44). All revisions with pad separation were clinically successful until the material failure occurred. The other implants were mechanically stable without progressive subsidence. Radiographic analysis of fixation demonstrated ingrowth in 62% of patients, indeterminate findings in 16%, and no ingrowth in 21%. There was a 95% prosthesis survival rate after 5 years.

The incidence of pad failure in this early series was unacceptable, and the method of fixation was abandoned in 1990 in favor of circumferentially coated hydroxyapatite on a grooved surface over the proximal 3 to 5 cm of the implant. The 2- to 5-year results with this method of fixation have not been published, but mechanical loosening has occurred in only 1 case out of more than 100.

Custom Acetabular Components

Nowhere is loss of bone more critical than in the acetabulum. Cemented revisions have a high failure rate (26), and cementless revision must have more than 50% host-bone contact with excellent initial stability to be successful (24). Restoring the anatomic joint center is difficult in most revision operations.

Our early experience with custom cementless acetabular components was with oblong components (17) (Fig. 3). The specific indications for use of these implants were combined superior segmental plus superior cavitary defects with intact anterior and posterior columns. The design specifications for these implants were as follows:

1. An oblong shape determined by two hemispheres connected by parallel lines
2. The AP diameter obtained from the CT scan.
3. The superior to inferior distance and the anatomic joint center obtained from the AP pelvic radiograph
4. Screw holes for radial screws superiorly and in the ischim determined from CT scan or foam model
5. Version determined from CT to allow 20 degrees anteversion by use of a hemispheric hooded liner placed at the anatomic joint center.

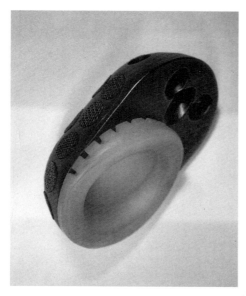

Figure 3. Custom oblong acetabular component.

Our 5- to 9-year results with 10 of these components were presented along with those of Amstutz at the 63rd Annual Meeting of the American Academy of Orthopaedic Surgeons (Feb. 22–26, 1996, Atlanta). At a mean follow-up period of 6.6 years (4 to 10 years), the average Harris hip score was 73 (62 to 86). One acetabular component at 9 years rotated from the pelvis inferiorly and was radiographically loose with revision pending. One patient underwent revision for a loose cementless femoral component at 7.3 years at another institution. Though the cup was judged to be well fixed, it was revised for compatibility. One patient had 4 mm of cup migration caused by collapse of a structural allograft, needed because the custom component at 80 mm was insufficient to fill the defect. The patient had no clinical symptoms at last examination. The remaining seven hips were radiographically well fixed without migration or rotation.

Since 1991, an off-the-shelf oblong implant has been available—the Arthropor II oblong acetabular cup (Joint Medical Products, Stamford, Conn.), which has obviated many custom acetabular components.

We still use some CT-based custom acetabular components to address two specific types of severe acetabular bone defects—a medial segmental defect with expanding inner walls (the so-called monkey trap defect) and a combined superior posterior cavitary and segmental defect such that the entire posterior column is absent. Both of these types of defects are impossible to reconstruct with off-the-shelf implants without use of large structural allografts and cement. For these types of defects we prefer a cementless hydroxyapatite-coated implant with custom contoured ilial and ischeal flanges and screws (Fig. 4). Our experience with this component is limited to only seven operations in 3 years with no failures to date, but it is too early to judge the efficacy of this device.

Results

We know of no other series of use of custom cementless implants for revision. We continue to pursue their use because we perceive limitations of techniques with off-the-shelf devices. Reasonable success has been reported by Engh and Lawrence et al. (5,19,20) for extensively coated femoral components that require endosteal press fit on good remaining host bone. Fortunately in many revisions there still is good diaphyseal bone. Engh and Lawrence et al. reported on 81 patients with a minimum 5-year follow-up period (mean 7.4 years). The rate of re-revision of the index femoral component was 10%.

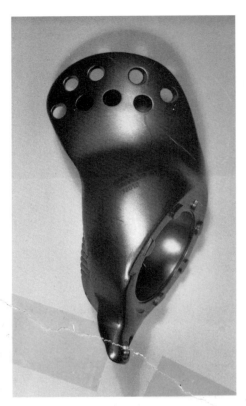

Figure 4. Custom flanged acetabular component.

Chandler et al. (3) also reported their results with a modular femoral implant (S-ROM; Joint Medical Products) used in 52 complex total hip revisions. Twenty-two required structural femoral allografts. There were 5 cases of mechanical loosening, 13 of intraoperative fracture, 12 postoperative dislocations, and 20 of trochanteric nonunion.

Head et al. (12) reported good midterm results for 174 revision total hips managed with onlay strut allograft and a proximally coated, long-stemmed titanium femoral component. The follow-up period was 2 to 9 years. Ninety-eight percent of grafts healed. Six hips were revised because of femoral failure. The authors emphasized that the implant must be stable on host bone.

Our results with custom-made femoral components compare favorably with those of Lawrence et al. (20) and Chandler et al. (3). The implants we have used have the advantage of being proximally coated, thereby avoiding severe stress shielding in already compromised bone. They also are one piece (as opposed to modular) and thereby avoid concerns about fretting and corrosion at the modular junction. Of course, all modern implants, including our custom-made ones, are modular at the head–neck junction.

Experience with customized acetabular components is too limited at this time to draw meaningful conclusions. The true efficacy of CT-based custom cementless implants for revision total hip replacement awaits long-term studies of 10 or 15 years' duration. Our initial experience appears to be favorable and cost effective even in the short term.

ROBOTICS IN REVISION TOTAL HIP ARTHROPLASTY

Revision total hip arthroplasty is a difficult procedure fraught with clinical and technical challenges and a high incidence of complications. Removal of as much of the old femoral cement as possible provides an optimal surface for bone support and interdigitation. Removing the cement mantle and plug in the distal area is the most tedious, time-consuming, and risky aspect because of the canal depth and bowing of the femur. The femur is fractured in about 18% of cases and the surgeon perforates the cortical wall of the femur in another 10% of cases. When errors occur, more time is required to repair the damage, additional blood is lost, and the infection rate increases.

None of the current techniques of cement removal is fully satisfactory. Osteotomes and flexible reamers are difficult to manipulate and have a tendency to follow the old canal. Handheld, high-speed drills require fluoroscopy for guidance to avoid perforating the femur walls. New technologies, such as cement softening with an ultrasonically driven tool (2,7) might lower the complication rate but are unlikely to improve accuracy or shorten the procedure. The growing numbers, greater difficulty, and reduced margin for error make revision total hip arthroplasty a natural focal point to develop robotic machining methods to remove old cement and prepare the new cavity in the femoral shaft. To date this technique has not been used on the acetabular side.

Methods

In traditional primary total hip replacement procedures, the abnormal femoral head is replaced by a stemmed metallic implant inserted into the medullary canal, which is broached or reamed manually. Our method involves the Robodoc computer-integrated system for primary hip replacement procedures (Integrated Surgical Systems, Davis, Calif.) (25,29). Robodoc was developed clinically by Integrated Surgical Systems from a prototype developed at IBM Research. Preclinical testing showed order-of-magnitude improvement in precision and repeatability in preparing the implant cavity compared with use of handheld broaches and reamers. To date about 800 operations have been performed on patients with very encouraging preliminary results.

The Robodoc system consists of an interactive presurgical planning system, called Orthodoc, and a robotic system for use in the operating room. A Robodoc primary total hip replacement starts with a minor surgical procedure in which three small pins are implanted in the femur. A CT scan of the patient shows the femur and pins, which are used to register the images to the robot. Next Orthodoc processes the CT data set, locates the three pins, and allows the surgeon to select three orthogonal planar slices through the three-dimensional image volume. Orthodoc superimposes cross-sectional displays of the implant model selected by the surgeon on the femoral views, allowing detailed examination of bone–implant interfaces.

In the operating room, the operation follows the established protocol up to the point where the femoral head is removed. The femur is then placed into a fixation device and attached to the robot base. The three pins are exposed and located in robot coordinates by a combination of force-compliant guiding and autonomous tactile search by the robot. The system then computes the transformation from CT to robot coordinates and machines out the desired shape in the femur while the surgeon follows the progress on an intraoperative display. Once the shape is cut, the robot is moved out of the way, and the procedure resumes manually.

Project Overview

To apply the existing Robodoc technology to revision total hip arthroplasty it is necessary to accommodate the artifact encountered when producing CT images of the implants in bone and to allow sufficient visualization of the cement–bone or implant–bone interface to allow surgeons to define a cut volume that will remove most or all of the cement and preserve the remaining bone for the new implant.

Events such as intraoperative fracture, cement removal problems and other unanticipated factors can occur intraoperatively that can alter the preoperative plan. To optimize the system, intraoperative imaging registered to a common coordinate system and incorporated into Orthodoc would be required. This would allow intraoperative modification of the plan in order to take full advantage of the capabilities of the Robodoc system to accurately remove the cement mantle and prepare the bone for the implant. The ability to use intraoperative imaging is not yet developed and is an area of research and development. Project goals are elimination of cement removal complications; reduction of cement removal labor and time required; improved positioning accuracy and fit of the new implant, and reduction of bone sacrificed to fit the new implant. In addition to direct patient benefits, these advantages can lower costs by potentially reducing operating room charges and by shortening hospital stay and recovery time.

Computed Tomographic Artifact Removal

The presence of a metal implant in the femur results in blooming and streaking of the CT image. CT images reconstructed from incomplete projection data contain artifacts, making it difficult to determine the boundary between the implant, the cement, and the bone. Because the quality of the CT images is key in determining the quality of the surgical plan, reducing artifact as much as possible is essential. The best approach for reducing artifacts is to correct the raw projection data before image reconstruction. We use 12 to 20 scout images to generate the simulated projections (Fig. 5).

The Orthodoc surgical planning workstation has been further augmented in the area of interactive cut volume definition. The surgeon now plans on separate AP and transaxial views which simplifies the process and does not interfere with normal implant selection and placement. The surgeon first segments out the bone cement by creating a contour that defines the bone–cement interface on several CT sections (Fig. 6). These contour data are fed into a cut-path generator algorithm, which outputs a second contour to identify the computed robot cut path on the basis of the cutter diameter. The cut path is made by means of examination of all the contours the user has entered and constructing a cut path that allows straight insertion along the vertical axis. The surgeon can edit each contour to maximize cement removal or minimize the removal of cortical bone.

Future versions of the cut-path generator will automatically compute the robot reorientation angle needed to machine out the user-defined cavity, effectively removing the constraint of a straight-line insertion path imposed by the current system.

We have begun the process of allowing the surgeon to plan with planar radiographs. This is the typical method of preoperative planning in both primary and revision operations and will allow greater flexibility in the preoperative planning system. A key element in this scenario is registering radiographs to each other to allow implant movements in one view to be simultaneously reflected in other views.

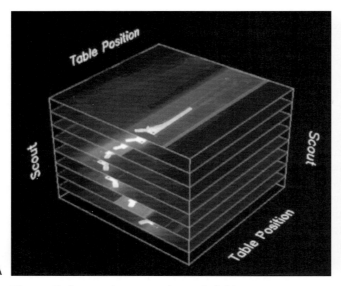 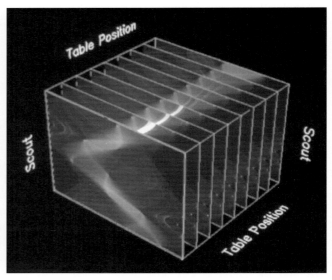

A   B

Figure 5. Interactive cut volume definition.

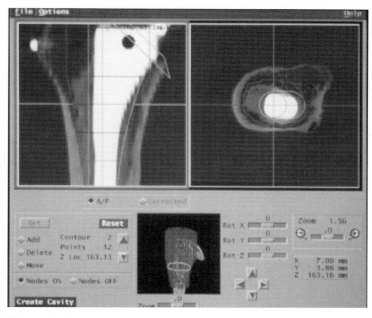

Figure 6. Example of interface surgeon uses to define interactively cut cavity for the robot.

Cement Machining

We have designed and conducted experiments to simulate as closely as possible bone-cement removal. We have tested whether the cutters currently used in Robodoc primary total hip replacement are adequate to cute bone cement by means of milling circular shapes in the actual cement used clinically. By means of direct measurement we confirmed that the cavities actually cut into bone were very close to those that had been programmed in regard to size, shape, and position. We also tested for compliance when cutting distally in the bone. This is necessary to remove the cement plug located deep within the femoral canal. With current instrumentation, the Robodoc system can be used to cut an implant cavity to a depth of about 225 mm (with a sleeve diameter of 12.5 mm) along the axis of the bone (Figs. 7 and 8).

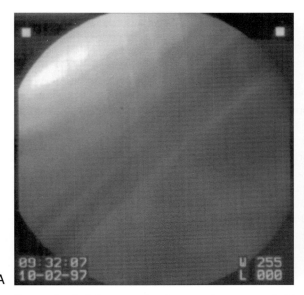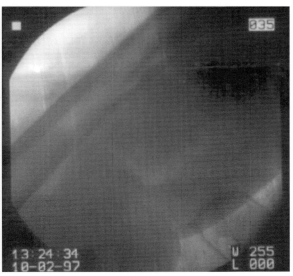

A   B

Figure 7. A: Intraoperative image after removal of implant. Cement mantle is still intact (patient 1). **B:** Intraoperative image after robotic removal of bone cement (patient 1).

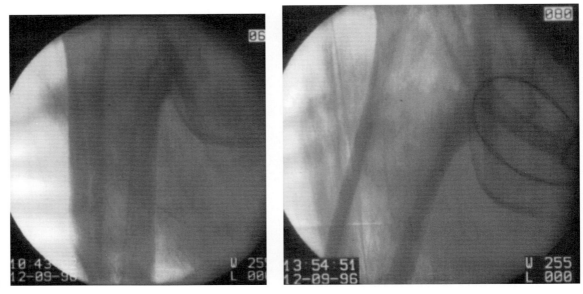

Figure 8. A: Intraoperative image after implant removal. Cement mantle is still intact (patient 2). **B:** Intraoperative image after robotic removal of bone cement (patient 2).

Clinical Results

The Robotic revision total hip replacement was used successfully to treat several patients at the Berufsgenossenschaftliche Unfallklinik in Frankfurt, Germany. Operating room time reached a mean of 164 minutes (incision to closure) for robotic revision total hip arthroplasty compared with a mean of 124 minutes for robotic primary total hip replacement with the Robodoc system. One possible reason for the increase in time is that the cut paths for revision total hip arthroplasty are patient specific and generated at the time of planning; The cut path is therefore not optimized for speed. In every case, an arthroscope was used to verify that the fibrous tissue was completely removed from the cavity. No fracture or any other complication occurred. After the operation or immediate full weight bearing was encouraged. In subsequent follow-up examinations, no subsidence or loosening was encountered.

Conclusion

Because revision total hip arthroplasty presents many problems even to skilled surgeons, use of a computer-guided, robotic system for removal of old cement and fibrous tissue is an enabling technology. We developed and clinically demonstrated a computer-integrated system to assist surgeons in revision total hip arthroplasty. These solutions developed specifically for revision total hip arthroplasty will extend to many orthopedic and other surgical problems. The indications for use of robotics as an alternative to conventional techniques for performing revision total hip arthroplasty have yet to be determined.

Dr. Roderick Turner, Dr. Joseph McCarthy, and Dr. James Bono provided early guidance during the conceptualization phase of the project. The National Institute of Standards' Advanced Technology Program (NIST/APT) provided partial funding for this project.

REFERENCES

1. Bargar WL. Shape the implant to the patient: a rationale for the use of custom-fit cementless total hip implants. *Clin Orthop* 1989;249:73–78.

2. Brooks AT, Nelson CL, Stewart CL, Skinner RA, Siems ML. Effect of an ultrasonic device of temperatures generated in bone and on bone-cement structure. *J Arthroplasty* 1993;8:413–418.
3. Chandler HP, Ayres DK, Tan RC, Anderson LC, Varma AK. Revision total hip replacement using the S-ROM femoral component. *Clin Orthop* 1995;319:130–140.
4. Chandler H, Clark J, Murphy S, et al. Reconstruction of major segmental loss of the proximal femur in revision total hip arthroplasty. *Clin Orthop* 1994;298:67–74.
5. Engh CA, Glassman AH, Griffin WL, Mayer JG. Results of cementless revision for failed cemented total hip arthroplasty. *Clin Orthop* 1988;235:91–110.
6. Garbuz D, Morsi E, Gross AE. Revision of the acetabular component of a total hip arthroplasty with a massive structural allograft: study with a minimum five year follow-up. *J Bone Joint Surg Am* 1996;78:693–697.
7. Gardiner R, Hozack WJ, Nelson C, Keating EM. Revision total hip arthroplasty using ultrasonically driven tools. *J Arthroplasty* 1993;8:517–521.
8. Gie GA, Linder L, Long RS, Simon JP, Slooff TJ, Timperley AJ. Impacted cancellous allografts and cement for revision total hip arthroplasty. *J Bone Joint Surg Br* 1993;75:14–21.
9. Gross AE, Allan DG, Lavoie GJ, Oakeshott RD. Revision arthroplasty of the proximal femur using allograft bone. *Orthop Clin North Am* 1993;24:705–715.
10. Gross AE, Hutchison CR, Alexeeff M, Mahomed N, Leitch K, Morsi E. Proximal femoral allografts for reconstruction of bone stock in revision arthroplasty of the hip. *Clin Orthop* 1995;319:151–158.
11. Head WC, Berklacich FM, Malinin TI, Emerson RH Jr. Proximal femoral allografts in revision total hip arthroplasty. *Clin Orthop* 1987;225:22–36.
12. Head WC, Wagner RA, Emerson RH Jr, Malinin TI. Revision total hip arthroplasty in the deficient femur with a proximal load-bearing prosthesis. *Clin Orthop* 1994;298:119–126.
13. Head WC, Wagner RA, Emerson RH Jr, Malinin TI. Restoration of femoral bone stock in revision total hip arthroplasty. *Orthop Clin North Am* 1993;24:697–703.
14. Hoikka V, Schlenzka D, Wirta J, et al. Failures after revision hip arthroplasties with threaded cups and structural bone allografts: loosening of 13/18 cases after 1-4 years. *Acta Orthop Scand* 1993;64:403–407.
15. Hooten JP Jr, Engh CA Jr, Engh CA. Failure of structural acetabular allografts in cementless revision hip arthroplasty. *J Bone Joint Surg Br* 1994;76:419–422.
16. Jasty M, Harris WH. Salvage total hip reconstruction in patients with major acetabular bone deficiency using structural femoral head allografts. *J Bone Joint Surg Br* 1990;72:63–67.
17. John JF, Talbert RE, Taylor JK, Bargar WL. Use of acetabular models in planning complex acetabular reconstructions. *J Arthroplasty* 1995;10:661–666.
18. Kwong LM, Jasty M, Harris WH. High failure rate of bulk femoral head allografts in total hip acetabular reconstructions at 10 years. *J Arthroplasty* 1993;8:341–346.
19. Lawrence JM, Engh CA, Macalino GE. Revision total hip arthroplasty: long-term results without cement. *Orthop Clin North Am* 1993;24:635–644.
20. Lawrence JM, Engh CA, Macalino GE, Lavro GA. Outcome of revision hip arthroplasty done without cement. *J Bone Joint Surg Am* 1994;76:965–973.
21. Martin WR, Suterhland CJ. Complications of Proximal femoral allografts in revision total hip arthroplasty. *Clin Orthop* 1993;295:161–167.
22. McGann WA, Welch RB, Iicetti GD. Acetabular preparation in cementless revision total hip arthroplasty. *Clin Orthop* 1988;235:35–46.
23. Merrill V, ed. *Atlas of roentgenographic positions.* 3rd ed. Vol 1. St. Louis: CV Mosby, 1967.
24. Paprosky WG, Magnus RE. Principles of bone grafting in revision total hip arthroplasty: acetabular technique. *Clin Orthop* 1994;298:147–155.
25. Paul H, Mittelstadt BD, Bargar WL, et al. A surgical robot for total hip replacement surgery. In: 606–611, Proceedings of the IEEE Intenational Conference on Robotics and Automation; May, 1992; Nice, France.
26. Pellicci PM, Wilson PD Jr, Sledge CB, et al. Long-term results of revision total hip replacement: a follow-up report. *J Bone Joint Surg Am* 1985;67:513–516.
27. Pollock FH, Whiteside LA. The fate of massive allografts in total hip acetabular revision surgery. *J Arthroplasty* 1992;7:271–276.
28. Schurman DJ, Maloney WJ. Segmental cement extraction at revision total hip arthroplasty. *Clinical Orthop* 1992;285:158–163.
29. Taylor RH, Mittelstadt BD, Paul HA, et al. An image-directed robotic system for precise orthopedic surgery. *IEEE Trans Robotics Automation* 1994;10:261–275.
30. Wilson MG, Nikpoor N, Aliabadi P, Poss R, Weissman BN. The fate of acetabular allografts after bipolar revision arthroplasty of the hip: a radiographic review. *J Bone Joint Surg Am* 1989;71:1469–1479.

Revision Total Hip Arthroplasty,
edited by Marvin E. Steinberg and Jonathan P. Garino,
Lippincott Williams & Wilkins, Philadelphia © 1999.

40

Blood Conservation and Replacement

Carl L. Nelson and Jess H. Lonner

A noticeable paradigm shift has occurred in the last several decades regarding the use of allogeneic blood transfusion after orthopedic procedures. This change in attitude was a direct response to emerging statistics regarding the incidence of hepatitis and human immunodeficiency virus (HIV) transmission after allogeneic transfusion. These statistics have changed markedly over the last decade with improvements in screening of blood products. Despite the relatively low risk for viral transmission with current screening techniques, a variety of strategies have been developed to reduce the use of allogeneic blood transfusion after orthopedic procedures. This is particularly true in the care of patients undergoing revision total hip arthroplasty. These strategies have included stricter criteria for transfusion of autologous blood, use of autogenous blood products, intraoperative methods for reducing blood loss, intraoperative blood salvage, postoperative reinfusion, and use of recombinant human erythropoietin therapy.

CONSIDERATIONS IN ALLOGENEIC TRANSFUSION

In 1981, a National Institutes of Health–sponsored panel determined that 25% of whole blood transfusions are unnecessary. Although this conclusion reflected opinion rather than specific irrefutable fact, it was based on consensus from a group of experts knowledgeable about the use of blood products. Historically, most unnecessary allogeneic transfusions were likely because the traditional guidelines for transfusion have been too liberal. Reflexive transfusion based on hemoglobin concentration alone is not justified because shock rarely

C. L. Nelson: Department of Orthopaedic Surgery, University of Arkansas for Medical Sciences, Little Rock, Arkansas 72205.

J. H. Lonner: Department of Orthopaedic Surgery, University of Pennsylvania School of Medicine, Philadelphia, Pennsylvania 19104.

occurs from anemia alone. Tissue perfusion and oxygen tension are critical determinants of the need for transfusion. Unfortunately, determination of tissue hypoxia is difficult. Patient symptoms, vital signs, estimation of oxygen delivery, estimation of blood loss, and physician experience all should be considered in the evaluation of need for transfusion.

It is intuitive that the cardiac and pulmonary status of the patient and duration of anemia are important factors that effect oxygen delivery. On the basis of the cardiovascular, pulmonary, and metabolic status, each patient has minimal oxygen requirements that change under stress. At rest, oxygen is delivered to the tissues at four times what is consumed. Under stressful conditions, however, oxygen delivery falls relative to consumption. Factors that may enhance oxygen diffusion include increasing oxygen saturation by means of addition of inhaled oxygen and increasing cardiac output.

Patients with normal cardiopulmonary function often can withstand very low hemoglobin levels. Some Jehovah's Witnesses have been able to survive intraoperative hemoglobin levels as low as 3 to 5 g/dL. However, hemoglobin levels less than 10 g/dL in other patients have been associated with increases in adverse cardiac events. Therefore, among older patients with underlying cardiopulmonary disease, transfusion needs must be individualized.

A study by Carson et al. (3) involving 125 surgical patients who declined blood transfusion for religious reasons demonstrated an association between mortality rate and preoperative hemoglobin as well as surgical blood loss. The authors found that mortality rates rose from 7.1% among patients with preoperative hemoglobin levels in excess of 10 g/dL to 61.5% among those with levels less than 6 g/dL. Mortality rates also rose from 8% for those who lost less than 500 mL intraoperatively to 42.9% for those with intraoperative blood loss in excess of 2 L. The authors reiterated that compromised cardiac reserve and greater metabolic needs should be considered for transfusion in a timely manner.

RISKS OF ALLOGENEIC TRANSFUSION

Allogeneic transfusion risks may be divided into three categories—contamination by infectious agents, transfusion reaction, and transfusion of incorrect blood caused by error.

Contamination of Allogeneic Blood by Infectious Agents

Because of developments in testing and improved criteria for the selection of donors, the safety of blood transfusion has increased progressively, making the present supply of donated blood safer than in any other previous period. Unfortunately, the screening tests currently used are not infallible. All of the screening tests performed for viruses other than hepatitis B surface antigen are indirect tests that reflect the antibody formed by the host to the virus. Consequently, there is a period of time, referred to as the *window period,* between the instant when the host is infected and the time that detectable antibodies are present. This window period has been estimated to be 45 days for HIV and 28 days for the hepatitis C virus (20). During this window period, because the host is infected but antibodies are not detectable, false-negative tests results may occur. It has been calculated that risk for a false-negative test result for HIV and human T-cell lymphotropic virus-I (HTLV-I) during the time from infection to detectable antibody formation is one in 360,000 and that the overall risk of infection is one in 225,000 per unit (20). It is likely that most HIV transmission after allogeneic transfusion occurs from blood that has been collected within the 45-day window period, when antibodies are not yet detected.

Hepatitis is the most common infectious agent transmitted through transfusion, mostly representing hepatitis C virus (HCV), or non-A, non-B hepatitis. Eighty to 90 percent of cases of post-transfusion non-A and non-B hepatitis are caused by HCV. Among donors whose units passed all screening tests, the risks of giving blood during an infectious window period were for HIV, 1 in 493,000 (95% confidence interval [CI], 202,000 to 2,778,000); for HTLV, 1 in 641,000 (95% CI, 256,000 to 2,000,000); for HCV, 1 in 103,000 (95% CI, 28,000 to 288,000); and for hepatitis B virus (HBV), 1 in 63,000 (95% CI, 31,000 to 147,000). HBV and HCV accounted for 88% of the aggregate risk of 1 in 34,000 (17,21). New screening tests that shorten the window periods for the four viruses should reduce the risks by 27% to 72% (23).

New screening tests will reduce the risk even further. Transfusion-associated HCV infection may result in a 20% incidence of chronic active hepatitis, 50% incidence of cirrhosis, and a 5% risk for hepatocelluar carcinoma 4 years after transfusion.

Other less common viral and nonviral diseases may be transmitted by means of transfusion of allogeneic blood products including cytomegalovirus infection, syphilis, malaria, toxoplasmosis, *Yersinia enterocolitica* infection, and *Trypanosoma cruzi* infestation. Fortunately the risk for transmission of these diseases by blood products has been reported to be less than one in 1 million per unit (6).

Transfusion Reactions

Transfusion reactions can be divided into acute intravascular immune reactions, delayed intravascular immune reactions, and febrile reactions. Transfusion reactions occur among 5% of blood transfusion recipients; febrile reactions occur among 1%; nonfatal hemolytic reactions occur among 1 in 25,000, and fatal hemolytic reactions occur among 1 in 100,000 (5). There is also the risk for transfusing the wrong unit of allogeneic blood to a patient, which may be fatal.

In a study of approximately 1.2 million units transfused during a 2-year period in New York state, the risk of a patient's receiving the wrong unit of blood was about 1 in 12,000 units transfused. Human and computer error remain the most common culprits of this egregious error, despite stringent regulations, inspections, policy for documentation, and intrahospital awareness. In this study, there were 54 ABO incompatible transfusions, 3 of which were fatal. Most errors occurred after the blood left the blood bank, incorrect identification accounting for 43% of the errors, and improper labeling accounting for 11%.

A study by the American College of Pathologists reviewing transfusions of more than 126,000 units of autologous blood in 596 hospitals found that no patient had an incorrect transfusion with another patient's preoperatively donated autologous blood. In contrast, 17 patients, or 1 in 42,000 units, had incorrect transfusions with blood from the allogeneic pool. In spite of the reported paucity of errors with autologous blood, instances of erroneous transfusions of autologous blood may occur, and not all adverse events are reported to regulatory agencies (2).

In a review by AuBuchon and Kruskall (2) an avoidable transfusion death attributable to misidentification of the samples, the unit, or the recipient occurred once in every 587,000 transfusions between 1976 and 1978, once in every 630,000 transfusions in the period 1976 to 1985, and once in every 600,000 transfusions from 1990 to 1991. Even these numbers may be an underestimation of the mortality associated with ABO errors. David Kessler, MD, former commissioner of the U.S. Food and Drug Administration (FDA), suggested that only a small fraction of serious adverse events that occur, perhaps as few as 1 in 100, are reported to the FDA and other regulatory agencies (2).

Immunomodulation

Immunomodulatory effects of allogeneic transfusion are concerning. The effects of transfusion on cellular immune function are thought to include down regulation of the effector cells, activation of latent viral infection, and prolonged circulation of donor immunocompetent cells. This is supported by results with several series that have shown higher incidences of infections and recurrence of tumors after transfusions of blood products containing immunosuppressive components than with transfused blood cell concentrates alone (22). Although these issues have been recorded, there is no universal agreement on the interpretation of the data.

PREOPERATIVE AUTOLOGOUS BLOOD DONATION

Deposit of autologous blood before an operation has been successfully incorporated into elective orthopedic surgical procedures and is particularly helpful in total hip and knee arthroplasty and scoliosis operations. Several studies have identified that preoperative deposit of autologous blood may reduce considerably the need for allogeneic transfusion (26,27). Woolson et al. (27) found that in 92% of total hip arthroplasties for which autologous blood had been donated homologous transfusion was not necessary (27). In 1987, Thomson et al. (26) reported that 64% of patients from a series who underwent 139 consecutive total hip arthroplasty procedures needed only autologous blood that had been preoperatively deposited. Techniques of intraoperative salvage of red blood cells were not been performed in that series, in contrast to the series by Woolson et al. (27).

These and other encouraging results have influenced the transfusion practices of many orthopedic surgeons performing total hip arthroplasty in the United States. Preoperative deposit of autologous blood should be encouraged before all elective total hip arthroplasty procedures, provided there are no contraindications, such as a low hematocrit or religious beliefs (9,16,25). Conditions that require patients to receive medical clearance before donation of autologous blood are unstable angina, severe aortic stenosis, and uncontrolled hypertension. In general a hematocrit less than 34 precludes autologous blood donation.

Blood that is deposited before on operation can be stored in a liquid or frozen state. Frozen red blood cells can be stored indefinitely; blood stored in the liquid state contains anticoagulants and therefore can be stored for only 35 days unless additional units of anticoagulant are added. Frozen red blood cells take several hours to thaw and must be used within 24 hours of thawing. Anemia may be induced by donated blood, so adequate time must be allowed after the collection of autologous blood for the hematocrit to equilibrate. It is therefore recommended that 5 to 7 days be allowed between donations, and the last donation should be made at least 3 days before the operation. In our practices, patients are generally given iron supplements during the period of donation. Clearly, excessive preoperative donation of autologous blood may result in waste, which has prompted evaluation of the cost of preoperative deposit of blood. In a retrospective analysis involving 54 patients undergoing primary total hip arthroplasty, Kirk et al. (13) found that of the 62% of patients who deposited blood before the operation, only 58% underwent reinfusion without exposure to allogeneic blood. The authors thus questioned the cost effectiveness of routine preoperative donation of autologous blood for hip arthroplasty. Other authors, however, have suggested that routine transfusion of autologous blood immediately after an operation and before a marked decrease in hemoglobin level may reduce the incidence of nonsurgical complications, including arrhythmia, myocardial infarction, confusion, hypotension, and lethargy (15). Lotke et al. (15) thus have 100% utilization of preoperatively donated blood in total joint arthroplasty.

OTHER PERIOPERATIVE TECHNIQUES TO REDUCE THE USE OF ALLOGENEIC TRANSFUSION

Other methods that have been used to limit blood transfusions have included hemodilution, intraoperative salvage and reinfusion, postoperative salvage and reinfusion, modifying surgical technique, reducing the hematocrit trigger, and withholding transfusion. These techniques have been in use for a considerable period of time, although clinical application to orthopedic practice is a relatively recent phenomenon.

Acute Normovolemic Hemodilution

Acute normovolemic hemodilution is a helpful technique for controlling intraoperative blood loss. In this technique, blood is withdrawn from the patient and replaced simultaneously with colloid or crystalloid, thereby maintaining normovolemia as the hematocrit diminishes. As a result, the patient loses blood at a lower hematocrit, and at the conclusion of the operation the patient may be reinfused with his or her own blood with a normal hematocrit. For instance, if a patient with a preoperative hematocrit of 35% undergoes hemodilution to a hematocrit of 25% and subsequently loses 1 L of blood, the patient has effectively lost 250 mL of red blood cells rather than 350 mL. Oishi et al. (19) evaluated this technique prospectively with a random series of 33 patients undergoing total hip arthroplasty. Only 41% of patients who underwent acute preoperative normo-volemic hemodilution required autologous blood transfusion, compared with 75% of the control group in whom no preoperative hemodilution was performed. The hemodilution group needed a lower mean quantity of autologous blood transfusion (41% of the estimated blood loss) compared with the control group (71%). The procedure was considered safe with few expected side effects.

This technique does raise some concern inasmuch as a decrease in arterial oxygen content may reduce peripheral organ perfusion. However, experimental models have demonstrated that compensatory mechanisms exist to increase cardiac output and coronary perfusion. Because of these concerns, careful patient selection is advisable. It is recommended that patients with underlying coronary artery disease, cardiac dysfunction, or peripheral vascular disease not be considered for this technique.

Adjusting the Transfusion Trigger

Unnecessary use of homologous blood may be reduced by means of changing the trigger that has been historically used to guide transfusion, namely a hemoglobin of 10 g/dL and a hematocrit of 30%. In realty, many patients do not need a transfusion until their hemoglobin falls well below 10 g/dL, provided tissue perfusion is maintained. Some experts even suggest that patients at low risk may not need routine postoperative blood tests. Patients at high risk, on the other hand, may need invasive cardiopulmonary monitoring to assess pulmonary arterial pressure and cardiac output and continuous monitoring of the electrocardiogram and arterial oxygen saturation (18).

For patients at low risk, fluid replacement with crystalloid or colloid may adequately manage hypovolemia. If there is to be an automatic transfusion trigger based on hemoglobin and hematocrit, it might empirically be about 7 g/dL of hemoglobin or a hematocrit of 20%. Patients at high risk may need monitoring with a different set of criteria. Even when central venous pressure, pulmonary capillary wedge pressure, and other objective measurements are within normal limits, tachycardia, tachypnea, and low mixed venous oxygen saturation may be present. In such cases, transfusion with packed red blood cells should be administered.

Although a precise formula for calculating blood volume is available, a crude rule for estimating blood volume is simply to multiply 75 times body weight in kilograms, which gives blood volume in milliliters. This calculation prepares the surgeon by providing a mathematical approach to blood loss and subsequent replacement. For example, a 500-mL blood loss from an 85-kg patient with an estimated blood volume of 6,375 mL (75 × 85 kg) is a blood volume loss of 8% in contrast to a 40-kg patient (blood volume of 3,000 mL) with a similar amount of blood loss, which would represent a 17% blood volume loss. Blood volume and hematocrit are key components of red blood cell volume, one of the essential measurements of oxygen delivery. For example, the red blood cell volume of a patient with a total blood volume of 6,000 mL and hematocrit of 20% is the same as that of a patient with a total blood volume of 4,000 mL and a hematocrit of 30%. Thus the surgeon has a better appreciation of which patient will be most effected by a given blood loss if hematocrit and blood volume are known. It has been suggested that this calculation be made before the operation to determine the amount of preoperatively deposited blood to order. Appropriate calculations also can be made intraoperatively or postoperatively to anticipate the potential physiologic response of the patient to surgical blood loss.

Hypotensive Anesthesia

Hypotensive anesthesia has been shown to reduce intraoperative blood loss during total hip arthroplasty (16,24). Particularly for patients who refuse homologous transfusion because of their religious beliefs, such as Jehovah's Witnesses, this technique has proved effective. Nelson et al. (16) used the technique of hypotensive anesthesia with sodium nitroprusside to treat 100 patients who were Jehovah's Witnesses. Intraoperative blood loss is primary total hip arthroplasty was reduced by 43% compared with the situation for matched controls among whom hypotensive conditions were not induced. Among patients who had undergone operations on the hip before total hip arthroplasty, a 30% reduction in intraoperative blood loss was achieved, compared with results for matched controls who were operated on with normotensive anesthesia. Of the 100 patients studied, none were given an allogeneic transfusion, and there were no instances of myocardial infarction, cerebral vascular accidents, or renal failure attributed to the hypotensive anesthesia. Furthermore, postoperative blood loss was statistically similar, whether the operation was performed in hypotensive or normotensive conditions (16).

Epidural anesthesia has been reported to be an effective method for inducing hypotension during total hip arthroplasty. One potential disadvantage, however, compared with general anesthetic techniques, is that the level of hypotension cannot be titrated on a minute by minute basis. Nonetheless, Sharrock et al. (24) found that induction of hypotension to a systolic mean arterial pressure of 60 mm Hg or less can effectively reduce blood loss and contribute to shorter operative times and improved cementing technique.

Perioperative Red Blood Cell Salvage

Perioperative red blood cell salvage and reinfusion is another technique for reducing the need for homologous blood transfusion. Intraoperative red cell salvage with a cell saver entails collecting blood with a heparin-treated double-lumen suction catheter, washing the filtered blood with normal saline solution, and centrifuging the contents to separate a supernatant layer. This layer contains white blood cells, aggregated red blood cells, platelets, free hemoglobin, fibrinogen, plasma coagulation factors, and other proteins that can be discarded. The final product—packed red blood cells in saline solution—is reinfused. Guerra and Cuckler (10) found that the cell saver salvaged a mean of 450 mL of red blood cells, reducing the percentage of patients exposed to banked blood by 40% and decreasing the mean homologous transfusion requirement from 2.5 to 1.5 units per patient ($p < .05$). The blood salvaged represented 58% of the mean estimated blood loss in the study group.

Law and Wiedel (14) found that an average of 3.9 units of intraoperative blood may be salvaged in revision total hip arthroplasty. They observed that use of intraoperative blood salvage and autologous blood transfusions provided 72% of the replenished blood pool. However, the amount of allogeneic blood transfused to patients without stored autologous blood was nearly three times that of patients with autologous blood available, potentially implicating autologous blood availability as a more important factor in the decision to transfuse blood. This concern was corroborated by Guerra and Cuckler (10), who found that for those who had donated autologous blood, the cell saver did not decrease the number of postoperative homologous transfusions required or the percentage of patients exposed to homologous blood. However, for those without preoperatively donated autologous blood, the cell saver was effective in statistically decreasing the percentage of patients exposed to allogeneic transfusion by 40% and significantly decreasing the mean number of units of homologous blood transfused from 2.5 to 1.5 units per patient.

Intraoperative salvage and washing of red blood cells appears to be safe, because most contaminants within the joint fluids, such as fat and bacteria, are removed, and no adverse reactions to reinfusion of washed cells have been reported. There are, however, disadvantages to using intraoperative cell-saver devices. There must be at least 400 mL of drainage to make the procedure feasible; the cost of the apparatus and the need for trained personnel to supervise the procedure make it relatively expensive; and it can only be performed in the operating or recovery rooms.

Postoperative collection and subsequent reinfusion of wound drainage after total hip arthroplasty is common as well. This blood, although filtered, is usually reinfused without centrifugation or washing. Unwashed red blood cell salvage can begin in the operating room and can continue for up to 6 hours after completion of the operation. Postoperative salvage of unwashed blood yields an average of about 450 mL per total hip arthroplasty with a hematocrit in the rage of 25% to 35% (1,4). Although postoperative reinfusion of salvaged blood, washed or unwashed, may effectively decrease the need for blood transfusion, several authors have seen adverse reactions to unwashed drainage, including febrile reactions, chills, and tachycardia, occur in as many as 10% of cases, particularly when reinfusion is delayed (4,7). Transient episodes of hypotension after the use of unwashed cells have been postulated to be associated with a commonly used anticoagulant, acid citrate dextrose, because hypotension has not occurred in washed or unwashed salvage without anticoagulation (4). Free fat within the salvaged blood also represents a possible concern because of its potential for fat embolism. This risk can be avoided by means of washing the salvaged blood or, if an unwashed salvage system is used, by means of excluding the top layer of the drainage, where most of the fat resides.

Miscellaneous Intraoperative Techniques

Blood loss occurs at an insensible, constant rate once the surgical procedure has started. Therefore insensible blood loss is related in part to the duration of the operation. Peak intraoperative blood loss occurs consistently during three stages of total hip arthroplasty—cutting the femoral neck, reaming the acetabulum and reaming the femur. Controlling bleeding during these peak periods can reduce blood loss and optimize surgical exposure. Packing sponges into prepared spaces may prevent profuse blood loss. Sponges soaked in epinephrine in a concentration of 1 in 1 million parts also may reduce blood loss. Hemostatic agents, such as thrombin-soaked gelatin foam, to cover bleeding bone after it has been cut or reamed also are effective. Finally, expeditious, yet meticulous, surgical technique may limit blood loss. A well-planned surgical procedure that progresses methodically in a controlled and efficient manner can reduce surgical time and thus the amount of blood loss. Nelson and Bowen (16) found that reduction in surgical time can account for a 15% reduction in intraoperative blood loss.

Pharmacologic Agents

The perioperative administration of pharmacologic agents to reduce surgical blood loss is a relatively new concept. Desmopressin, a synthetic analogue of vasopressin, showed early promise in reducing blood loss in cardiac surgery and in spinal surgery. However, a recent double-blind, randomized, prospective clinical trial by Karnezis et al. (12) concluded that desmopressin in fact did not reduce blood loss or transfusion requirements after total hip or knee arthroplasty.

Aprotinin is a protease inhibitor with an unknown mechanism of action that has been used successfully to reduce blood loss during cardiac operations and more recently during total joint replacement in Europe (11). In a prospective, double-blind, randomized study, Janssens et al. (11) found that intraoperative administration of aprotinin reduced total blood loss and the amount of blood transfused perioperatively. No side effects observed among patients who had received aprotinin. Clinical studies evaluating aprotinin in the United States have not been completed, and more work is necessary to document its safety and efficacy.

Erythropoietin is a naturally occurring glycoprotein hormone that regulates the production of erythrocytes in the human body. Its production is naturally regulated and stimulated by hypoxia. This hypoxia is sensed by the kidneys, which leads to increased production and secretion of erythropoietin. Erythropoietin then travels through the blood stream, where it stimulates erythroid progenitor cells to differentiate into red blood cells. Advances have led to the production of recombinant human erythropoietin, which is being applied in a variety of areas and may play an important role in the orthopedic care of patients. The drug has been used successfully both experimentally and to treat patients with anemia or chronic disease. With a series of subcutaneous injections of recombinant human erythropoietin before surgical intervention complex revision hip arthroplasty may be performed safely with a reduced need for allogeneic transfusion (25). Therapy with recombinant human erythropoietin also has been shown to increase the ability of patients to donate autologous blood before elective surgical procedures (8).

SUMMARY

There is no substitute for sound clinical judgment in deciding when patients should undergo transfusion. Perioperative measures for reducing blood loss, enhancing blood salvage, and alternatives for allogeneic blood transfusion should be considered and adopted as routine practice in revision total hip arthroplasty. In 1995, at the Blood Management Practice Guidelines Conference, 11 policies for surgical blood management and interventions were identified. These policies included the following:

1. Assess transfusion requirements on a case by case basis.
2. Transfuse one unit of blood at a time and assess benefit and further need.
3. Limit exposure to allogeneic blood to appropriate need. This involves modifying the transfusion trigger on the basis of hemoglobin and hematocrit levels.
4. Prevent or control perioperative blood loss. Consider stopping aspirin, nonsteroidal antiinflammatory drugs, warfarin, heparin, similar anticoagulant drugs, and thrombolytic agents before the operation; identify and address any existing coagulopathy; restrict perioperative phlebotomy to necessary tests; consider use of regional anesthesia or hypotensive anesthesia.
5. Consider use of autologous blood an alternative to allogeneic transfusion. Consider preoperative autologous blood procurement, intraoperative acute normovolemic hemodilution, and intraoperative and postoperative autologous blood salvage and autotransfusion.
6. Make efforts to maximize oxygen delivery for surgical patients. Manage underlying cardiopulmonary disease and use invasive cardiac monitoring judiciously.
7. Increase or restore red blood cell mass by means other than red blood cell transfusion. Replace iron stores and consider use of erythropoietin.
8. Involve the patient in the transfusion decision.
9. Document the reasons for and the results of transfusion decisions.
10. Develop hospital policies and procedures as a cooperative effort with input from all those involved in the transfusion decision.
11. Assess transfusion practices, both individual and institutional, yearly or more often.

REFERENCES

1. Ayers DC, Murray DG, Duerr DM. Blood salvage after total hip arthroplasty. *J Bone Joint Surg Am* 1995;77:1347–1351.
2. AuBuchon JP, Kruskall MS. Transfusion safety: realigning efforts with risks. *Transfusion* 1997;37:1211–1215.
3. Carson JL, Spence RK, Poses RM, Bonavita G. Severity of anemia and operative mortality and morbidity. *Lancet* 1988;1:727–729.
4. Clements DH, Sculco TP, Burke SW, Mayer K, Levine DB. Salvage and reinfusion of postoperative sanguineous wound drainage. *J Bone Joint Surg Am* 1992;74:646–651.
5. Consensus Conference. Perioperative red blood cell transfusion. *JAMA* 1988;260:2700–2703.
6. Dodd RY. The risk of transfusion transmitted infected. *N Engl J Med* 1992;327:419–420.
7. Faris PM, Ritter MA, Keating EM, Valeri CR. Unwashed filtered shed blood collected after knee and hip arthroplasty: a source of autologous red blood cells. *J Bone Joint Surg Am* 1991;73:1169–1178.
8. Goodnough LT, Rudnick S, Price TH, et al. Increased preoperative collection of autologous blood with recombinant human erythropoietin therapy. *N Engl J Med* 1989;321:1163–1168.
9. Goodnough LT, Wasman J, Corlucci K, Chernosky A. Limitations to donating adequate autologous blood prior to elective surgery. *Arch Surg* 1989;124:494–496.
10. Guerra JJ, Cuckler JM. Cost effectiveness of intraoperative autotransfusion in total hip arthroplasty surgery. *Clin Orthop* 1995;315:212–222.
11. Janssens M, Joris J, David JL, Lemaire R, Lamy M. High dose aprotinin reduces blood loss in patients undergoing total hip replacement surgery. *Anesthesiology* 1994;80:23–29.
12. Karnezis TA, Stulberg SD, Wixson RL, Reilly P. The hemostatic effects of desmospressin on patients who had total joint arthroplasty: a double blind randomized trial. *J Bone Joint Surg Am* 1994;76:1545–1550.
13. Kirk PG, Auffrey C, Rozen A, Robinson M. Cost effectiveness of autologous blood donation in patients undergoing total hip and total knee replacement. In: *Proceedings of the American Association of Hip and Knee Surgeons;* 1997 Nov 61.
14. Law JK, Wiedel JD. Autotransfusion in revision total hip arthroplasties using uncemented prostheses. *Clin Orthop* 1989;245:145–149.
15. Lotke PA, Garino JP, Barth P. Autogenous blood after total knee arthroplasty: reduction in non-surgical complications. In: *Proceedings of the 64th Annual Meeting of the American Academy of Orthopaedic Surgeons;* 1997 Feb 13–17; San Francisco. 1997:153.

16. Nelson CL, Brown WS. Total hip arthroplasty in Jehovah's Witnesses without blood transfusion. *J Bone Joint Surg Am* 1986;68:350–353.
17. Nelson K, Donahue J, Munoz A, et al. Risk of transfusion transmitted HIV-1 and HTLV-1 and 2. [Abstract] *Transfusion* 1991;31[Suppl]47S.
18. Nelson CL, Nelson RL, Cone J. Blood conservation techniques in orthopaedic surgery. *Instr Course Lect* 1990;39:425–529.
19. Oishi CS, D'Lima DD, Morris BA, Hardwick ME, Berkowitz SD, Colwell CW Jr. Hemodilution with other blood reinfusion techniques in total hip arthroplasty. *Clin Orthop* 1997;339:132–139.
20. Peterson LR, Satten GA, Dodd R, et al. Duration of time from onset of human immunodeficiency virus type I infectiousness to development of detectable antibody: the HIV seroconversion study group. *Transfusion* 1994;34:283–289.
21. Public Health Service. Interagency guidelines for screening donors of blood plasma, organs, tissues, and semen for evidence of hepatitis C. *MMWR Morb Mortal Wkly Rep* 1991;40:1–17.
22. Quintiliani L, Buzzonetti A, DiGiorolamo M, et al. Effects of blood transfusion on the immune responsiveness in survival of cancer patients: a prospective study. *Transfusion* 1991;31:713–718.
23. Schreiber GB, Busch MP, Kleinman SH, Korelitz JJ. The risk of transfusion-transmitted viral infections: the Retrovirus Epidemiology Donor Study. *N Engl J Med* 1996;334:1685–1690.
24. Sharrock NE, Mineo R, Urquhart B, Salvati EA. The effect of two levels of hypotension on intraoperative blood loss during total hip arthroplasty performed under lumbar epidural anesthesia. *Anesthes Analg* 1993;76:580–584.
25. Sparling EA, Nelson CL, Lavender R, Smith J. The use of erythropoietin in the management of Jehovah's Witnesses who have revision total hip arthroplasty. *J Bone Joint Surg Am* 1996;78:1548–1552.
26. Thomson JD, Callaghan JJ, Savory CG, Stanton RP, Pierce RN. Prior deposition of autologous blood in elective orthopaedic surgery. *J Bone Joint Surg Am* 1987;69:320–324.
27. Woolson ST, Watt JM. Use of autologous blood in total hip replacement: a comprehensive program. *J Bone Joint Surg Am* 1991;73:76–80.

Subject Index

Figures are indicated in *bold italic type.* Tables are indicated by page number followed by a t.